DISEASES OF THE
ORBIT

DISEASES OF THE
ORBIT

A Multidisciplinary Approach

Jack Rootman,
M.D., F.R.C.S.(C), Diplomate A.A.O.

Professor of Ophthalmology and Pathology
Department of Ophthalmology and Pathology
University of British Columbia
Vancouver General Hospital

Chairman
Ocular and Orbital Pathology Group
Cancer Control Agency of British Columbia
Vancouver, British Columbia

With 18 contributors

J.B. LIPPINCOTT COMPANY *Philadelphia*

London   Mexico City   New York
St. Louis   São Paulo   Sydney

OPTOMETRY

Sponsoring Editor: Sanford Robinson
Manuscript Editor: Virginia Barishek
Indexer: Sandra King
Designer and Coordinator: Susan Hess Blaker
Production Manager: Kathleen Dunn
Production Coordinator: George V. Gordon
Compositor: Progressive Typographers
Printer/Binder: Halliday Lithograph

6 5 4 3 2 1

Library of Congress Cataloging-in-Publication Data

Rootman, Jack.
    Diseases of the orbit.

    Includes bibliographies and index.
    1. Eye-sockets—Diseases.   I. Title.   [DNLM:
1. Orbital Diseases. WW 202 R783d]
RE711.R66   1988   617.7'8   87-21433
ISBN 0-397-50651-1

The authors and publisher have exerted every effort to ensure that drug selection and dosage set forth in this text are in accord with current recommendations and practice at the time of publication. However, in view of ongoing research, changes in government regulations, and the constant flow of information relating to drug therapy and drug reactions, the reader is urged to check the package insert for each drug for any change in indications and dosage and for added warnings and precautions. This is particularly important when the recommended agent is a new or infrequently employed drug.

This book is dedicated to those who sacrificed the most for its achievement: my wife, Jenny; our children, Russell, Katie, and Daniel; and our parents, Sydney and Lillian Rootman, and Leo and Rebeka Puterman.

Contributors

Larry H. Allen, M.B.B.Ch., F.R.C.S. (C)
Lecturer of Ophthalmology
University of Western Ontario
  and Victoria Hospital
London, Ontario

Craig W. Beattie, M.D.
Head, Electrodiagnostic Ophthalmology Unit
Vancouver General Hospital
Vancouver, British Columbia

K.W. Chan, M.B., F.R.C.P. (C)
Associate Professor of Oncology
Division of Hematology
Department of Pediatrics
University of British Columbia
  and British Columbia Children's Hospital
Vancouver, British Columbia

Roy Cline, M.D.
Clinical Instructor
Department of Ophthalmology
University of British Columbia
Vancouver, British Columbia

Peter Dolman, M.D.
Fellow, Department of Pathology
University of British Columbia
Vancouver, British Columbia

Stephen M. Drance, O.C., M.D.
Professor and Head
Department of Ophthalmology
University of British Columbia
Vancouver, British Columbia

D.G. Fitzpatrick, M.D., F.R.C.S. (C)
Clinical Assistant Professor
University of British Columbia
Active Staff, Vancouver General Hospital
  and British Columbia Children's Hospital

Consulting Staff, Cancer Control Agency of British
  Columbia
Vancouver, British Columbia

Douglas A. Graeb, M.D.
Associate Professor of Radiology
University of British Columbia
Vancouver, British Columbia

Ewan G. Kemp, M.B., F.R.C.S., D.O.
Consultant Ophthalmologist
Heathfield Hospital
Ayr, Scotland

Jocelyn S. Lapointe, M.D.
Associate Professor of Radiology
University of British Columbia
Vancouver, British Columbia

Janet M. Neigel, M.D.
Clinical Assistant Professor
Department of Ophthalmology
University of Medicine and Dentistry of New Jersey
Newark, New Jersey

Robert A. Nugent, M.D.
Assistant Professor of Radiology
University of British Columbia
Vancouver, British Columbia

John Pratt-Johnson, M.D.
Head, Department of Ophthalmology
British Columbia Children's Hospital
Professor of Pediatric Ophthalmology
University of British Columbia
Vancouver, British Columbia

Joseph Ragaz, M.D., L.R.C.P., M.R.C.S. (UK), F.R.C.P. (C)
Medical Oncologist
Associate Professor
University of British Columbia
Vancouver, British Columbia

William D. Robertson, M.D.
Professor of Radiology
University of British Columbia
Vancouver, British Columbia

Jack Rootman, M.D., F.R.C.S.(C)
Professor of Ophthalmology and Pathology
Department of Ophthalmology and Pathology
University of British Columbia
Vancouver General Hospital
Chairman, Ocular and Orbital Pathology Group
Cancer Control Agency of British Columbia
Vancouver, British Columbia

Bruce Stewart, B.F.A.
Senior Medical Artist
Coordinator, Art Division
Biomedical Communications
University of British Columbia
Vancouver, British Columbia

Valerie A. White, M.D., F.R.C.S.
Clinical Fellow
Department of Pathology
Vancouver General Hospital
Vancouver, British Columbia

Foreword

The efflorescence of interest in orbital diseases is now almost 20 years old — and it is still redolent. At one time a no-man's-land that few were intrepid enough to enter, the territory of the orbit is now a well-defined subspecialist precinct of ophthalmology, with many individuals who have acquired abundant clinical experience and produced an enormous amount of research data. The reasons for the increased devotion to orbital diseases are manifold, but the most obvious are the following: dramatic improvements in imaging, commencing with ultrasonography, through computed tomography, and most recently magnetic resonance imaging; the development of orbital centers and oncology centers, which have allowed well-trained individuals to acquire extensive experience in a difficult area that few other clinicians and surgeons wish to deal with; and the more accessible nature of orbital lesions to biopsy in comparison with intraocular conditions, which has promoted the application of sophisticated pathologic investigative techniques to elucidate the pathogenesis of orbital diseases.

Diseases of the Orbit is the latest in a series of substantial contributions to a comprehensive understanding of orbital disorders. Is there the need for another book on orbital diseases? The answer is emphatically yes! The field of orbital diseases is evolving so rapidly that every effort at synthesis should be appreciated by the ophthalmic community. This book will also be heavily relied upon by nonophthalmic specialists who occasionally share an interest in orbital disease with the ophthalmic surgeon: head and neck surgeons, otolaryngologists, neurosurgeons, and general oncologists.

Jack Rootman's latest contribution to integrating our understanding of orbital diseases has several distinctive virtues. First, the elegant anatomical prolegomenon is far more detailed than that found in any other textbook on orbital diseases. An enormous expenditure of energy, time, talent, and finances is clearly discernible in this section. Some of the artwork has no rival elsewhere in the literature, and the succinct and highly accurate rendition of orbital anatomy will repay serious attention by the beginning resident as well as by the advanced ophthalmic surgeon. The second distinction is the conceptual organization and breadth of Rootman's effort. This textbook is not a ponderous catalogue or a desiccated list of orbital diseases, but rather is a logical approach to diagnosis and management that combines features of the clinical history along with the results of advanced diagnostic tests. Finally and most importantly, this work is the synthesis of firsthand observations of a well-trained and alert ophthalmic orbital surgeon with training in ophthalmic pathology, who has closely analyzed his unique collection of cases. While this textbook clearly updates the pertinent literature on a spectrum of orbital diseases, its cornerstone is the author's reflections on his own surgical and pathologic experience.

Those who will enjoy the clean prose, delight in the beautiful illustrations and artwork, and profit from the codified experiences incorporated into this book should know something about Jack Rootman. In the early 1970s, Jack completed his residency in ophthalmology in Canada, and thereafter did sequential fellowships with Professor Norman Ashton in ophthalmic pathology at the Institute of Ophthalmology in London, with Dr. Robert Ellsworth in clinical oncology at the Harkness Eye Institute of the Columbia-Presbyterian Medical Center in New York City, and with Mr. John Wright in orbital surgery in London. I met Jack when he was doing his fellowship at the Harkness Eye Institute, and when we were both toiling away on our early scientific articles. We met in the library many times, and discussed orbital diseases and other more encompassing and mutually resonating topics about life, the arts, and science. It was clear to me that Jack possessed a first-class mind and a highly developed personal and professional ethical system; moreover, he exhibited the requisite industry to become an undisputed leader in any field of ophthalmology that he chose to enter.

I believe that the single event of Jack's professional

career that cemented all of these ingredients into a highly productive clinical and research effort was his recruitment by Professor Stephen Drance to be in charge of a new oncology and orbital section of the Department of Ophthalmology at the University of British Columbia in Vancouver. Jack's diagnostic and surgical skills quickly became known to a region that had not seen his likes before, and seemingly out of the woodwork came a backlog of cases. He has continued to enlarge his referral practice, which testifies to his mastery of his field. One of my observations about orbital diseases is that different centers and different individuals somehow seem to attract different groups of patients with disparate clinical and pathologic profiles. Jack has applied his expertise to an in-depth analysis of orbital anatomy, orbital inflammations (Graves' orbitopathy and idiopathic orbital inflammation), lymphoproliferative lesions, and vascular tumors. Chapters on these topics in this textbook represent in my opinion the acme of clinical experience and contemplative analysis for the entire field of ophthalmology.

I admire Jack Rootman greatly, and marvel at his energy and resourcefulness. Only someone who has written

a book can appreciate the dimensions of his undertaking, dedication, and success. I believe that his comparative youth, his neuronal plasticity, and his superb preparation upon entering the field of orbital diseases have enabled him to be consistently creative and original. Even while writing this book, and continuing to cultivate an enormous diagnostic and surgical referral practice, Jack did not neglect the aesthetic and spiritual side of his nature. A gifted artist, he has enrolled himself in art school, and has won several prizes for his canvas work.

His charming wife, Jenny, has been an inestimable support to Jack, and has sustained him through this scientific enterprise with patience and love. It is with great excitement that one contemplates the professional growth and rewards that await Jack Rootman at future stages of his career. It is furthermore with enlightened self-interest that I look forward to the elegant fruits of his ongoing research efforts, so that I and my colleagues can continue to learn from this man's hard-earned and enviable experience.

Frederick A. Jakobiec, M.D.

Foreword

It was with pleasure that I accepted Dr. Jack Rootman's invitation to herald this major medical treatise. I am especially honored to be associated with a scholarly work of this magnitude to which so much time and care have been devoted in the consummation of its final publication. I recall with pride that Dr. Rootman, early in his career, was an exceptionally able research worker in my Department of Pathology at the Institute of Ophthalmology in London, where I like to think his enthusiasm for ocular pathology was first aroused. It is good to see—so many years later—this authoritative work presenting up-to-date knowledge of the anatomic, clinical, and pathologic aspects of diseases of the orbit, in the light of his own extensive clinical experience and that of his co-authors.

This work, although describing in meticulous detail the pathologic features of orbital disease, preceded by a beautifully illustrated account of the anatomy of the orbit, is essentially directed towards diagnosis, management, and prognosis. I have no doubt that the extensive material so clearly marshalled and eruditely presented, with the considerable technological and therapeutic advances of today, will prove a valuable textbook and a reference work for those having a special interest in orbital disease.

Norman Ashton, C.B.E., D.Sc., F.R.C.P., F.R.C.S., F.R.C.Path., F.R.S.

Foreword

Considerable advances have been made in recent years in the diagnostic accuracy and management of orbital disease. The orbit as a subspecialty area has attracted teams of ophthalmologists and neurosurgeons with special talents who tackle lesions that were previously considered inoperable and usually led to blindness.

Dr. Rootman, who is a specialist in diseases of the orbit, has the advantage of also being a trained and practicing ocular pathologist. He created the Orbital Referral Center at the Vancouver General Hospital and the University of British Columbia, which has attracted large numbers of patients with orbital disease from far away.

He is in an excellent position to synthesize the diagnostic, pathologic, and therapeutic know-how that has resulted in the publication of this book, which I am sure will serve as a classic in this area of our specialty.

The Department of Ophthalmology has benefited from the advice that he has given as a consultant, and I am sure that the specialties of ophthalmology, neurosurgery, and radiology will benefit from the care and comprehensiveness of the present text. The department is proud to have been associated with this endeavor.

Stephen M. Drance, o.c., m.d.

Preface

The great 12th century physician and philosopher, Maimonides, invoked physicians to love their art, serve their fellow man, take counsel from learned physicians, and have an insatiable desire to acquire knowledge, correct errors, and reexamine their knowledge. The development of this book has allowed me to address many of these duties of a physician. Certainly this has afforded an opportunity to analyze patient care and scientific knowledge in the field of orbital disease, and to formalize my thinking and teaching processes. When Paul Henkind asked me some four years ago to write a "manual" on orbital disease, I immediately grasped the task with enthusiasm because of these opportunities. Little did I know when I began how daunting it would be to assemble the local experience, place it in the context of general knowledge, and rationalize it for a broader community.

Working in a medical system with a good, up-to-date clinical community and an environment of excellence in many areas including radiology, pathology, surgery, ophthalmology, medical biophysics, oncology, and the many subspecialties available in our center has afforded a unique opportunity to integrate the many disciplines for the study and management of orbital disease. This task would have been impossible without three major factors: a good scientific and medical background for which I am grateful to my many mentors and teachers; an equitable medical system in which to practice for which I am grateful to the people of Canada, in particular, British Columbia; and a good scientific community for which I am grateful to the University of British Columbia, the Vancouver General Hospital, and the Departments of Ophthalmology and Pathology.

Not all of what is written in black and white is truly (that) well-defined. In fact, we all discover that knowledge is open to interpretation. Examining our experience and that of others gave me the opportunity to explore the "gray" areas and develop an approach to the diagnosis and management of orbital disease. This task has re-quired a concurrence of epidemiologic, pathologic, clinical, and technical knowledge. The fact that this occurred within an environment where there are many students helped to organize my knowledge and provided a framework to the body of information so that it may be understood by the student.

There has been an attempt in this text to divide the material into two major areas. The first part of the book deals with the development of anatomic and physiologic information necessary for understanding the broad conceptual basis of orbital disease. Following this, I have attempted to fit the information within the context of patient investigations and epidemiology of orbital disease. This whole section, therefore, would provide a framework for the examination and logical interpretation of the patients encountered in clinical practice. The remainder of the book consists of a more detailed coverage of specific orbital disorders and their management. I have attempted to consolidate all information in the book by illustrating both concepts and disease processes with specific case material carried from the clinical level to the laboratory and therapeutic setting.

I recognize that it is unusual for a single author to embark on such an undertaking, and at its completion I realize why. The advantage, of course, is that the text presents a relatively uniform outlook governed by a particular approach with a melding of the various disciplines.

If I have a single message to emphasize, it is that our surest knowledge comes from a rational, organized, and compassionate approach to patient care. The demands of this particular environment force the physician to explore and manage disease carefully. When all is said and done, a good analytical approach is the best tool for patient care regardless of the degree of sophistication of one's environment.

Jack Rootman, M.D.

Acknowledgments

This book could never have been put together without the dedicated care of many people in our institution, and a few words of thanks simply do not go far enough to express my gratitude. In particular, the members of our department of neuroradiology, William Robertson, Robert Nugent, Jocelyn Lapointe, Douglas Graeb, and their technical staff have dedicated a great deal of time to the review and organization of the enormous amount of visual material that contributed to this text. The expert advice of many of my colleagues in the pathology department allowed for critical analysis of my own interpretations and has been fundamental to my understanding of the pathogenesis of orbital disease; in particular, the chairman of the department, Dr. David Hardwick, and the chairman of the division of anatomic pathology, Dr. Noel Quenville, have given me both the latitude of time and the depth of their expertise. Dr. James Dimmick, chairman of the pediatric pathology group, has provided expert guidance as has Dr. Anne Worth, an oncologic pathologist par excellence with a vast knowledge and experience. Dr. Clarisse Dolman, neuropathologist, kindly reviewed the discussion of neurogenic lesions and Dr. Barad Benny reviewed the chapter on lymphoproliferative diseases. Many of my students spent hours reviewing the text and offering advice from a student's point of view, in particular, Dr. Peter Dolman and Dr. Janet Neigel. Many physicians have contributed to portions of the text and they are acknowledged specifically throughout the book. I would be remiss in not mentioning Dr. Stephen Drance, the chairman of the Department of Ophthalmology, who provided the environment that allowed this task to come to fruition. Gedy Gudauskas (Pharm. D.) and Doug Hoffart gave time and advice in the development of a computer retrieval system that formed the basis for analysis of my patients. Finally, I had an enormous amount of secretarial help from Pat Ring, Pam Cusick, and Liz Wong. In particular, Liz served as a stable, unflappable influence throughout the maelstrom of the development of this book. In addition, she always seemed to be able to remember the case that neither I nor the computer could find. Finally, my sincere gratitude to those teachers who affected my life the most: Professor T.A.S. Boyd, Professor Norman Ashton (C.B.E.), Mr. John Wright, Dr. Robert Ellsworth, and Dr. Felix Durity for his neurosurgical expertise and kindness. A number of professional friends have given me advice and encouragement during the development of this book, in particular, William Stewart and Frederick Jakobiec.

Many of the technical and intellectual aspects of this book have been contributed by the people involved in the meticulous preparation of histologic and photographic material. I am grateful to Gloria McLeod and Eva Chang for the many hours of preparation and retrieval of histologic and electron-microscopic material. The members of our Biomedical Communications Department, Jean-Marc Thomas, Ron Thorpe, and Michael Robertson, devoted an enormous amount of time and care to the photographic material in this text, as will be obvious from the quality of reproduction. Marguerite Drummond did some of the fine illustrations in the chapter on surgery. My thanks to Irvie Hollenberg and Jack Abramson, who contributed financially towards the development of the orbital illustrations. I wish to make special mention of Bruce Stewart, who did the superb illustrative work for this book. His commitment to accurate and informative illustration has made a major impression on this work. Finally, I would like to acknowledge the support of the J.B. Lippincott Company staff, especially Virginia Barishek and Sanford Robinson for their editorial expertise and Susan Blaker and George Gordon for their design and production contributions.

Contents

DISEASES OF THE
ORBIT

PART I

Anatomy of the Orbit

Jack Rootman, Bruce Stewart,
Robert Nugent, and William Robertson

CHAPTER 1

Basic Anatomic Considerations

Jack Rootman

The complex of neurosensory, vascular, motor, and secretory structures within the orbit are confined to 30 cm³ bounded anteriorly by the lids and surrounded by bone, nasal sinuses, intracranial contents, and deep facial structures. Disease may originate from, or affect, any of these spaces independently or conjointly and lead to deterioration of visual and/or ocular function. Knowledge of orbital and periorbital anatomy is fundamental to understanding the effect of disease and planning surgical intervention. The important features of orbital anatomy are the relationship to surrounding tissues, its structural integrity, anatomic uniformity, and essential symmetry. Although anatomic variations exist, in clinical and surgical situations we can rely on the fundamental structural uniformity of this organ complex.

Bony Anatomy

The orbit is pyramidal in shape with an overall volume of 30 cm³ of which the eye constitutes 7 cm³ (Fig. 1-1). The base of the pyramid is a quadrangular anterior opening that measures 4 cm horizontally and 3.5 cm vertically. The widest dimension is 1 cm to 1.5 cm from the anterior orbital margin. The apex is formed by the optic canal and the superior orbital fissure.

The medial walls of the orbit are 2.5 cm apart, roughly parallel, and 4.4 cm to 5 cm long. The lateral walls are 4.5 cm to 5 cm long and lie at right angles to each other. The distance from the inferior orbital rim anteriorly to the infraorbital groove posteriorly is 2.5 cm to 3 cm. The depth of the temporalis fossa laterally is 2 cm.

Orbital growth is completed between 7 years of age and puberty. It is believed that enucleation in childhood retards bony growth.

The orbital roof (Fig. 1-2) is triangular. It is composed of the lesser wing of the sphenoid and the frontal bones, which may have within it a posterior extension of the frontal sinus. Apically, the lesser wing contains the optic canal, which is 5 mm to 6 mm in diameter, 10 mm to 12 mm in length, and has an axis of 36 degrees to the coronal plane. Thus, the optic canals are separated anteriorly by 3 cm and posteriorly by 2.5 cm. The orbital roof is 3 mm thick posteriorly, and is thinnest just behind the superior rim. Anterolaterally is the lacrimal fossa, located just above the frontozygomatic suture line.

The lateral wall (see Fig. 1-2) is composed of the greater wing of the sphenoid, frontal, and zygomatic bones, and is at an angle of 45 degrees to the medial wall. It is 4.5 cm to 5.0 cm long, and is the strongest orbital wall. Posteriorly, it is separated from the roof by the superior orbital fissure (which is 2.2 cm long) and from the floor by the inferior orbital fissure (which is 2 mm long). Laterally, it forms a portion of the temporalis fossa, which is thinnest at the suture line between the greater wing of the sphenoid and the zygomatic bone (where it can be fractured easily at surgery). Posteriorly, the inferior orbital fissure communicates with the pterygopalatine and infratemporal fossae.

The oblong medial wall is the thinnest (0.2 mm to 0.4 mm) and is made up of the maxillary, lacrimal, ethmoid and lesser wing of sphenoid. About 20 mm behind the anterior medial orbital margin is the anterior ethmoid foramen, and 12 mm behind this, the posterior ethmoid foramen, which is 5 mm to 8 mm from the optic canal. These foramina mark the horizontal level of the cribriform plate at the fronto-ethmoid suture line. The ethmoid and frequently the sphenoid and maxillary sinuses form part of the medial wall.

The floor (see Fig. 1-2; Fig. 1-3) is shorter, triangular, and is made up of the maxillary, zygomatic, and palatine bones. The infraorbital sulcus originates about 2.5 cm to 3 cm from the inferior orbital rim and forms a canal halfway along its course. The canal opens on the maxilla at the infraorbital foramen. The maxillary and often some of the ethmoid sinuses are immediately adjacent to the floor. The floor is 0.5 mm to 1 mm thick. The thinnest point is medial to the infraorbital sulcus and canal,

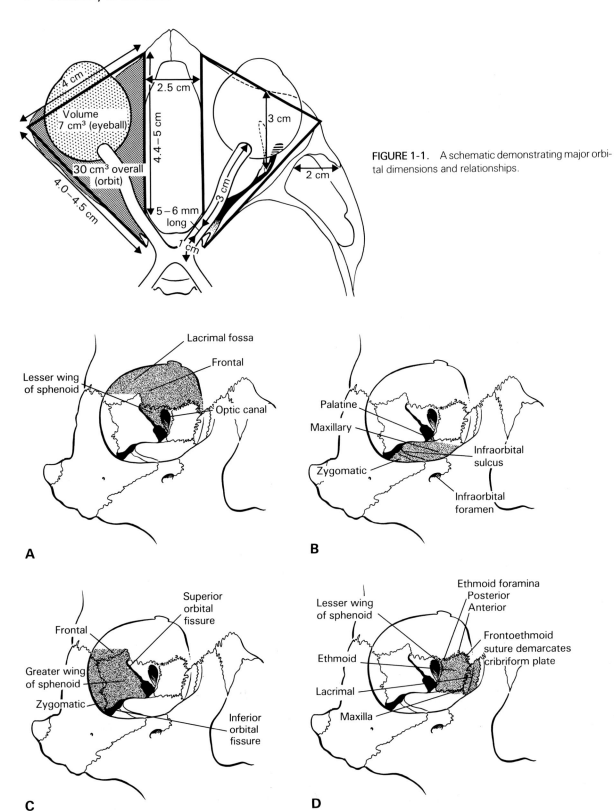

FIGURE 1-1.   A schematic demonstrating major orbital dimensions and relationships.

A

B

C

D

FIGURE 1-2.   Schematic of bony anatomy of the orbital walls showing constituents of the roof *(A)*, floor *(B)*, lateral wall *(C)*, and medial wall *(D)*.

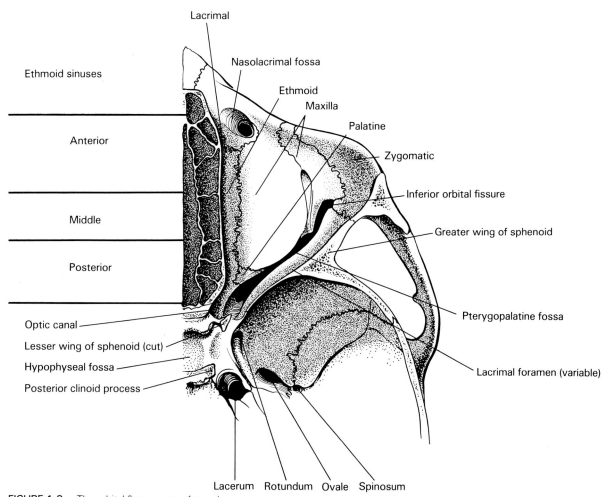

Lacrimal

Ethmoid sinuses

Nasolacrimal fossa

Ethmoid

Maxilla

Palatine

Zygomatic

Anterior

Inferior orbital fissure

Greater wing of sphenoid

Middle

Posterior

Pterygopalatine fossa

Optic canal

Lesser wing of sphenoid (cut)

Hypophyseal fossa

Posterior clinoid process

Lacrimal foramen (variable)

Lacerum   Rotundum   Ovale   Spinosum

FIGURE 1-3.   The orbital floor as seen from above.

where it can be fractured easily at the time of decompression surgery. Anteromedially is the nasolacrimal fossa (5 mm by 17 mm) and duct formed by the lacrimal and maxillary bones. It contains the lacrimal sac, which drains into the duct. Immediately posterior to the nasolacrimal fossa is the origin of the inferior oblique muscle. The duct is 17 mm to 20 mm long and runs inferolaterally and 15 degrees posteriorly, where it opens under the inferior turbinate at the junction of the anterior one third and posterior two thirds. Table 1-1 summarizes the sites and contents of the orbital fissures and canals.

Periorbita and Septa

The periosteum or periorbita (Fig. 1-4) is generally loosely adherent to the surrounding bones except at the anterior orbital margin, lacrimal crests, and the margins of the fissures and canals. Posteriorly, it is continuous

with the dura of the optic nerve and that surrounding the superior orbital fissure, and anteriorly with the periosteum of the orbital margins. Thus, surgery or trauma posteriorly may result in cerebrospinal fluid leaks.

In descriptive terms, the orbit has been divided into the extraperiosteal, extraconal, and intraconal spaces. The latter two are separated by the rectus muscles and intermuscular septa, which are denser in the anterior orbit. Disease processes may be roughly contained within these spaces, and the concept serves some practical value. However, work by Koornneef has shown that the intraconal and extraconal spaces are highly complex and are divided by radial fibrovascular connective tissue septa, which also bridge between the muscles and the periorbita. Further, these septa connect to and provide support to all of the intraorbital structures, thereby forming complex surgical spaces. They invest the orbital fat that surrounds all the structures as lobules. In general, the septa

(Text continues on p. 8.)

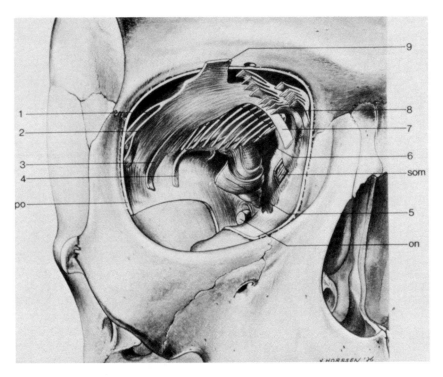

FIGURE 1-4. Demonstrates the connective tissue apparatus of the superior, lateral, inferior, and medial orbit. *(A)* Connective tissue of the superior levator palpebrae/superior rectus muscle complex and of the superior oblique muscle. *1*, superior part of the lateral aponeurosis; *2*, middle part of the aponeurosis; *3*, inferior part of the aponeurosis; *4*, connections with the lateral rectus muscle connective tissue; *po*, periorbit; *on*, optic nerve; *5*, contributions to the superior ophthalmic vein hammock; *som*, superior oblique muscle; *6*, connections of the superior oblique muscle tendon connective tissue to the medial upper part and hind surface of the eye; *7*, medial aponeurosis; *8*, area of the superior oblique muscle trochlea; *9*, attachment to the superior tarsal plate.

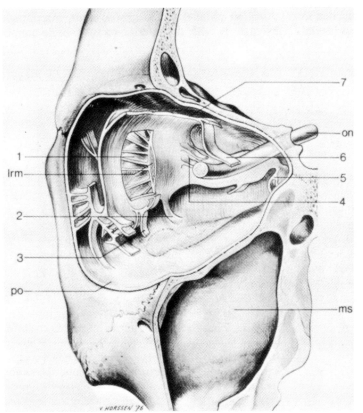

(B) Lateral rectus muscle connective tissue apparatus. *1*, area of attachment to the lateral orbital wall; *lrm*, lateral rectus muscle; *2*, connections with the connective tissue of the inferior oblique muscle connective tissue septa; *po*, periorbit; *ms*, maxillary sinus; *4*, relationships with the optic nerve; *5*, connections with Müller's muscle in the inferior orbital fissure; *6*, contribution to the superior ophthalmic vein hammock; *on*, optic nerve; *7*, connection to the lateral aponeurosis of the superior levator palpebrae/superior rectus muscle complex.

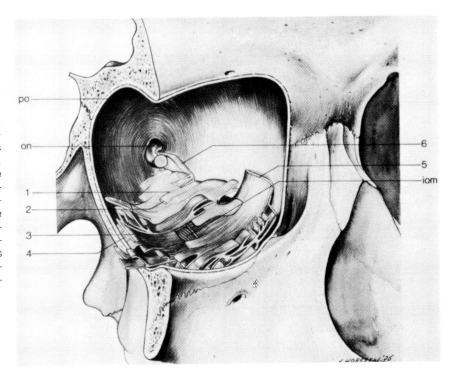

(C) Connective tissue of the inferior rectus and inferior oblique muscles. *po*, periorbit; *on*, optic nerve; *1*, inferior rectus muscle connective tissue; *2*, septal connections with the lateral rectus muscle; *3*, connections of the inferior oblique muscle connective tissue to the lateral rectus muscle connective tissue; *4*, fingerlike offshoots to the inferolateral orbital wall; *iom*, inferior oblique muscle; *5*, septal connections with the medial rectus muscle connective tissue; *6*, contributions to the superior ophthalmic vein hammock.

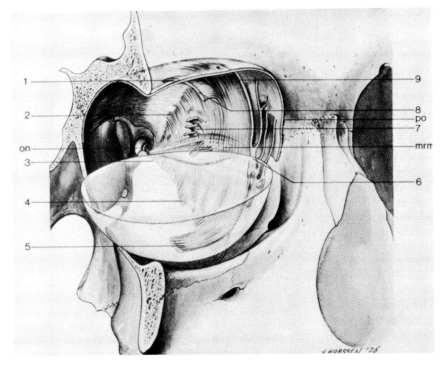

(D) Connective tissue system of the medial rectus muscle. *1*, superior ophthalmic vein hammock; *2*, area of attachment to the orbital roof; *on*, optic nerve; *3*, connective tissue septa to Müller's muscle; *4*, area of attachment to the orbital floor; *5*, connections with the connective tissue systems of the inferior oblique and inferior rectus muscles; *6*, medial conglomeration area; *mrm*, medial rectus muscle; *7*, relationships with the optic nerve and hind surface of the eyeball; *po*, periorbit; *8*, connection to the medial aponeurosis of the superior levator palpebrae muscle; *9*, connections to the orbital roof. (Reproduced with permission from Koornneef L: Orbital connective tissue. In Duane TD, Jaeger EA (eds): Biomedical Foundations of Ophthalmology, Vol 1, Chap 32. Philadelphia, Harper & Row, 1982)

TABLE 1-1.
CONTENTS OF ORBITAL FISSURES AND CANALS

	Location	Contents
Optic canal	Lesser wing of sphenoid	Optic nerve Meninges Ophthalmic artery Sympathetic fibers

Superior orbital fissure	Lesser and greater wing of sphenoid	Nerves
		  Motor
		    III Superior and inferior divisions
		    IV Trochlear
		    VI Abducens
		  Sensory
		    V1 Frontal lacrimal, nasociliary
		  Sympathetic fibers
		Vessels
		  Superior ophthalmic vein
		  Anastomosis of recurrent lacrimal and middle meningeal artery

Inferior orbital fissure	Greater wing of sphenoid, palatine, zygomatic, and maxillary bones	Nerves
		  Sensory
		    V2 infraorbital and zygomatic
		  Parasympathetic
		  Branches from pterygopalatine ganglion
		Vessels
		  Inferior ophthalmic vein and branches to pterygoid plexus

Anterior ethmoid canal	Frontal and ethmoid	Nerve: Anterior ethmoid becomes dorsal nasal Vessel: Anterior ethmoid artery
Posterior ethmoid canal	Frontal and ethmoid	Nerve: Posterior ethmoid Vessel: Posterior ethmoid artery
Nasolacrimal fossa	Lacrimal and maxillary bones	Nasolacrimal sac and duct

are more complex and dense anteriorly, where surgical dissection is therefore more difficult. The connective tissue system also supports intraorbital structures and accounts for the anatomic uniformity of the tissue relationships. Roughly, the system is best understood in relationship to the extraocular muscles, as demonstrated schematically (see Fig. 1-4). Disruption of the orbit with alterations in the connective tissue architecture accounts for many of the clinical results of fractures and trauma.

Orbital Contents

EXTRAOCULAR MUSCLES

The six striated extraocular muscles, including the four recti and two oblique muscles, control eye movement. (See Chapter 2, Atlas of Orbital Anatomy.) The rectus muscles arise from the annulus of Zinn at the apex, where

it is continuous with the dural sheath of the optic nerve and periorbita and apical component of the connective tissue system. The annulus has an upper tendon (of Lockwood) and lower tendon (of Zinn). Because of this intimate relationship apical disease frequently affects all of these structures simultaneously. In addition, surgical removal of the optic nerve must be done within the annulus, which is most safely entered superomedially after removing the orbital roof. Anteriorly, the recti insert on the globe 5 mm to 7 mm posterior to the limbus. The superior oblique originates just superior to the annulus, and passes forward through the trochlea (4 mm posterior to the orbital margin just medial to the supraorbital notch) from whence it extends in a slight posterolateral plane to insert on the superior aspect of the globe. The inferior oblique arises from the bone just posterolateral to the nasolacrimal fossa, then it extends in a slight posterolateral direction coursing beneath the inferior rectus, and inserts on the inferolateral aspect of the eye. The superior oblique is innervated by the trochlear nerve, the lateral rectus by the abducens nerve, and the remaining muscles by the branches of the oculomotor nerve. The levator palpebrae (oculomotor innervation) originates from the annulus and inserts on the upper lid. Müllers' muscle, a sympathetically innervated smooth muscle, is attached anteriorly to the levator muscle and aponeurosis. Disease, such as thyroid orbitopathy, affecting either of these muscles may alter lid position or function. The approximate anteroposterior length of the recti and the superior oblique muscles is 4 cm. Their nerve supply enters at the junction of the posterior and middle third of the muscle belly. The inferior oblique is 3.5 cm in length, and its motor supply from the inferior division of the oculomotor nerve enters its belly posteriorly after coursing just lateral to the inferior rectus, just behind the equator of the globe.

OPTIC NERVE

The optic nerve (see Fig. 1-1 and Chapter 2) is a nerve fiber tract, 4.5 cm to 5 cm long and about 4 mm in diameter, that extends from the globe to the chiasm. It is divided into four portions: intraocular (1 mm), intraorbital (3 cm), intracanalicular (5 mm to 6 mm), and intracra-

nial (1 cm). Because the distance from the globe to the orbital apex is 20 mm, the intraorbital portion of the nerve tends to form an S-shaped configuration. The subarachnoid space and meningeal linings sheathe the nerve and extend from the canal forward to the globe. The ophthalmic artery is encased by dura in the optic canal where it lies inferolateral to the nerve. At the orbital end of the canal, it loses the dural coat and crosses medially in the intraconal space. The central retinal artery, a branch of the ophthalmic artery, enters inferomedially about 1 cm behind the globe. The remaining arterial supply of the optic nerve is from collateral branches via the pia-arachnoid. The optic nerve is related intracranially to the frontal lobe, anterior cerebral, anterior communicating, middle cerebral, and internal carotid arteries as well as the cavernous sinus.

PERIPHERAL NERVES

The major sensory innervation of the orbit is by means of the ophthalmic division of the trigeminal, with the maxillary (by means of the infraorbital and zygomatic branches) supplying the inferior orbital, cheek, and temporal regions (Fig. 1-5). (See Chapter 2.) The frontal and

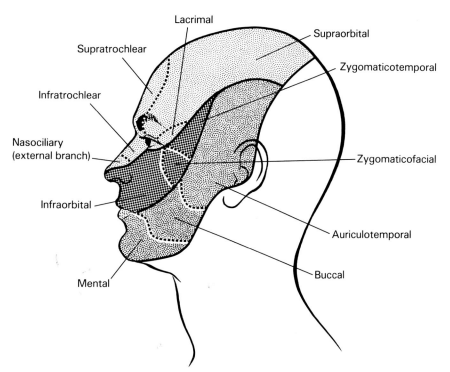

FIGURE 1-5. Schematic demonstrates the sensory dermatomes of the fifth nerve: V$_1$ ophthalmic division *(fine stippling)*, V$_2$ maxillary division *(dark stippling)*, V$_3$ mandibular division *(intermediate stippling)*.

lacrimal branches of the ophthalmic nerve enter the orbit outside the annulus of Zinn and run forward between the periorbita and the levator complex to supply the forehead and lacrimal gland. The nasociliary branch is intraconal, crosses medially over the optic nerve, and terminates as the ethmoidal and infratrochlear nerves. The trochlear nerve extends forward in the same space as the frontal and lacrimal.

The oculomotor nerve enters the muscle cone within the annulus of Zinn as a superior division (supplying the levator and superior rectus) and an inferior division (supplying the medial and inferior rectus and inferior oblique). Just temporal to the optic nerve (1.5 cm to 2 cm from the globe) in the apex is the ciliary ganglion. It is chiefly a ganglion where the parasympathetic fibers from the inferior division of the oculomotor nerve form a synapse. In addition, sensory fibers from the nasociliary nerve and sympathetic fibers from the plexus around the internal carotid artery (via the superior orbital fissure) pass through the ganglion. The sensory root subserves the cornea, iris, and ciliary body; the parasympathetic supplies the iris sphincter, ciliary body, and lacrimal gland; and the sympathetic supplies ocular vessels, the iris dilator (by means of ciliary nerves), the lacrimal gland, and sympathetic muscles of the upper and lower lids. The secretory fibers to the lacrimal gland (postganglionic from the sphenopalatine) arrive by the zygomatic and lacrimal nerves.

The seventh nerve (Fig. 1-6) is the motor supply for the orbicularis, and by the nervus intermedius gives the parasympathetic supply to the lacrimal gland. The facial nerve enters the parotid gland and divides into temporal facial (upper) and cervical facial (lower) branches. It innervates the orbicularis by the upper division, which forms temporofrontal and zygomatic branches. Numerous anatomic variations exist (see Fig. 1-6). Surgically, when operating laterally it is important to avoid this nerve by entering anteriorly over the frontozygomatic process and staying in a plane just superficial to the temporalis fascia.

VASCULAR ANATOMY

Arterial Supply

The major arterial supply of the orbit is from branches of the ophthalmic artery, which generally arises from the internal carotid artery just inferomedial to the optic nerve. (See Chapter 2.) Rarely, the ophthalmic artery may arise from the middle meningeal and enter the orbit through the superior orbital fissure. In the optic canal it courses forward and laterally within the dural sheath, and at the orbital apex penetrates laterally through the dura and then crosses in 82.6% of subjects to the medial orbit over the nerve. In the remaining 17.4% of subjects the artery courses under the nerve. The branches of the ophthalmic artery with some variations in origin are as follows: central retinal, lateral posterior ciliary, lacrimal, medial posterior ciliary, muscular, supraorbital, posterior and anterior ethmoidal, nasofrontal, supratrochlear, and dorsonasal arteries. (See Chapter 2.) The ophthalmic artery frequently has anastomotic branches to the external carotid system by means of the middle meningeal and lacrimal arteries, which pass through the superior orbital fissure, and by means of the anterior deep temporal, superficial temporal, and lacrimal arteries (Fig. 1-7). The major distribution and anatomic variations of the ophthalmic artery have been described by Hayreh (Table 1-2).

The posterior ciliary arteries supply the globe by 15 to 20 short (to choroid and optic nerve head) and two long (to ciliary muscle, iris, and anterior choroid) branches. There are two main muscular branches: the lateral (supplying levator, superior rectus, and superior oblique) and the medial (supplying medial and inferior recti and inferior oblique muscles). Anteriorly, the arteries in the recti divide into two anterior ciliary arteries, which supply the anterior globe. The lacrimal artery branches into recurrent meningeal, zygomatic, glandular, and lateral palpebral arteries (which form the arcades of the lid). The zygomatic branches anastomose with the anterior deep temporal (by the zygomaticotemporal) and the transverse facial (by the zygomaticofacial) arteries. The supraorbital artery supplies the eyebrow and forehead and has small branches contributing to the superior rectus, superior oblique, and levator muscles.

The posterior ethmoid artery supplies the posterior ethmoid air cells, and the anterior ethmoid artery supplies the remaining ethmoid cells, frontal sinus, dura in the anterior cranial fossa, and the lateral wall of nose and septum. The marginal arcades of the lid are formed from the medial and lateral palpebral arteries and lie 4 mm from the upper lid margin and 2 mm from the lower. The remaining terminal arteries are the dorsal nasal and supratrochlear branches.

The major external carotid branches supplying the orbit are the facial (medially), superficial temporal (laterally), and maxillary (deep) arteries. The facial forms the angular branch, which anastomoses with the dorsal nasal artery. The superficial temporal artery forms the transverse facial, which anastomoses with infraorbital; the zygomatic, which anastomoses with lacrimal and palpebral branches of the ophthalmic; and the frontal, which anastomoses with supraorbital and frontal arteries of the ophthalmic. The maxillary artery forms the infraorbital branch (supplying the lacrimal gland, inferior rectus, inferior oblique, lacrimal sac, and lower eyelid) and anastomoses with branches of the facial artery.

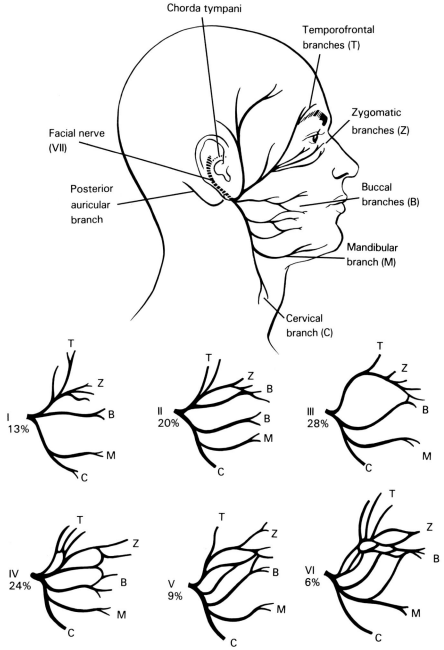

FIGURE 1-6. A schematic demonstrating the peripheral course of the seventh nerve, with six varying patterns that have been described (Davis, 1956). (Adapted from Miehlke A: Surgery of the Facial Nerve. Philadelphia, WB Saunders, 1973)

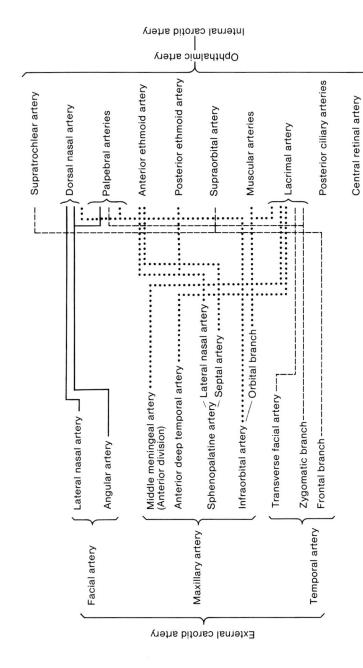

FIGURE 1-7. The major anastomoses of the ophthalmic artery to branches of the external carotid artery (Hayreh SS: Arteries of the orbit in the human being. Br J Surg 50:938, 1963).

TABLE 1-2.
ORDER OF ORIGIN OF BRANCHES OF OPHTHALMIC ARTERY

Order of Origin	Ophthalmic Artery Crossed	
	Over Optic Nerve	Under Optic Nerve
1	Central retinal and medial posterior ciliary	Lateral posterior ciliary
2	Lateral posterior ciliary	Central retinal
3	Lacrimal	Medial muscular
4	Muscular to superior rectus or levator	Medial posterior ciliary
5	Posterior ethmoid and supraorbital, jointly or separately	Lacrimal
6	Medial posterior ciliary	Muscular to superior rectus and levator
7	Medial muscular	Posterior ethmoid and supraorbital, jointly or separately
8	Muscular to superior oblique and medial rectus, jointly/separately/to either	Muscular to superior oblique and medial rectus, jointly/separately/to either
9	To areolar tissue	Anterior ethmoid
10	Anterior ethmoid	To areolar tissue
11	Medial palpebral or inferior medial palpebral	Medial palpebral or inferior medial palpebral
12	Superior medial palpebral	Superior medial palpebral
Terminal	1. Dorsal nasal 2. Supratrochlear	1. Dorsal nasal 2. Supratrochlear

(Hayreh SS: The ophthalmic artery. III: Branches. Br J Ophthalmol 46:212, 1962)

Venous System

The orbital veins are valveless, the superior ophthalmic draining into the cavernous sinus by the superior orbital fissure, and the inferior into the superior ophthalmic vein and the pterygoid plexus. (See Chapter 2.) The venous system has a different course than that of the arteries, and lies within the connective tissue septa of the orbit. In contrast, the arteries pass through the septa. The superior is the larger, and is formed by the confluence of the angular, nasofrontal, and supraorbital veins. It has three sections, the first extending posterolaterally to the medial border of the superior rectus in the anterior third of the orbit. The second section of the superior ophthalmic vein enters the muscle cone, passing to the lateral orbit beneath the superior rectus muscle. The third section extends posteromedially along the lateral border of the superior rectus into the superior orbital fissure, where it drains into the cavernous sinus. The more variable inferior ophthalmic vein forms inferolaterally as a plexus, and

passes posteriorly adjacent to the inferior rectus muscle. It anastomoses with the superior ophthalmic vein, and has a similar branch that connects with the pterygoid plexus through the inferior orbital fissure. The tributaries are muscular, medial collateral, vortex, and lateral collateral.

Anterior venous drainage may be through the facial by means of the angular vein medially, and a plexus from the inferior ophthalmic to the facial vein laterally.

Cavernous Sinus

The cavernous sinus (Fig. 1-8) lies in the middle cranial fossa adjacent to the sphenoid sinus and pituitary fossa, just below the anterior and posterior clinoid processes and inferomedial to the temporal lobe. It is a dural venous sinus that communicates with the ophthalmic, central retinal, inferior cerebral, superficial middle cerebral, and middle meningeal veins. In addition, it communicates with the inferior and superior petrosal sinuses and the pterygoid plexus. Structurally, the cavernous sinus consists of a complex of venous channels. Within the sinus are the carotid siphon and sympathetic plexus.

The lateral wall contains within its inner loose fibrillar or deep layer the oculomotor, trochlear, abducens, and ophthalmic and maxillary divisions of the fifth nerve. The relationship of these nerves within the sinus changes from posterior to anterior (see Fig. 1-8). The oculomotor nerve moves from a superior to an inferior position in relationship to the trochlear nerve, and the abducens shifts down in relationship to the ophthalmic division of the trigeminal nerve. Anterior to the sinus the lacrimal, frontal, and trochlear nerves enter the orbit outside the annulus of Zinn and the oculomotor, abducens, and nasociliary enter the orbit within the annulus. Because of the complex and intimate relationships involved in the cavernous sinus, lesions in this area frequently involve multiple functional abnormalities of the sensory and motor nerves of the orbit.

LACRIMAL SYSTEM

The lacrimal gland, situated in a shallow fossa in the superolateral orbit, weighs 78 g and measures 20 mm by 12 mm by 5 mm. It is divided into palpebral and orbital (larger) lobes by the lateral horn of the levator aponeurosis. (See Chapter 2.) The orbital lobe is superior to the palpebral, and the isthmus between the two extends through a gap in the lateral extension of the levator aponeurosis, which can be best visualized at lacrimal surgery by identifying the levator superiorly and following the fibers of the aponeurosis inferolaterally. The ducts (10 to 12) pass through the palpebral lobe, where they can be seen in the superolateral conjunctival fornix 4 mm to 5

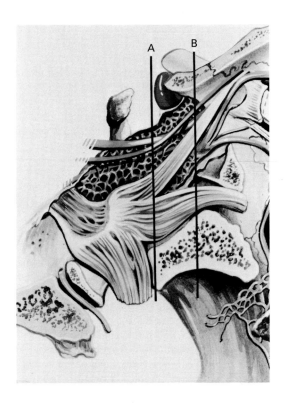

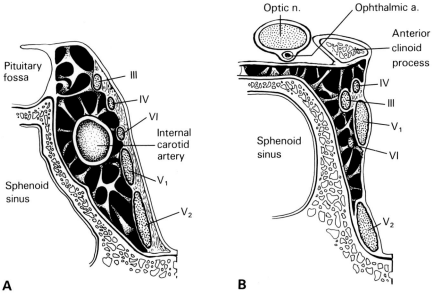

FIGURE 1-8.   Lateral view *(top)* and coronal sections *(bottom)* of the cavernous sinus demonstrating the relationships of the third, fourth, fifth, and sixth nerves, carotid artery, and optic nerve at the level of the pituitary fossa *(A)* and anterior clinoid *(B)*.

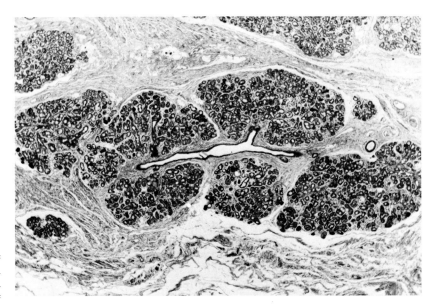

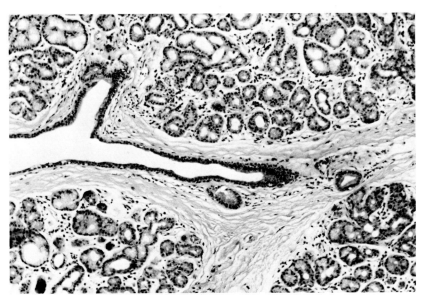

FIGURE 1-9. Photomicrograph of lobules of the lacrimal gland and interlobular duct (*top,* H&E, original magnification ×2.5). The acini consist of columnar cells surrounded by an incomplete layer of myoepithelial cells (*bottom,* H&E, original magnification ×10).

mm from the tarsal border. Thus, resection of the palpebral lobe functionally destroys the gland. The borders of the gland are related anteriorly to the orbital septum, posteriorly to the orbital fat, and medially to the superior rectus, globe, and lateral rectus. The inferior surface rests on the lateral rectus. The lacrimal gland is a serous gland, and the acini have a tubuloracemose arrangement. The acini consist of columnar cells surrounded by an incomplete layer of myoepithelial cells. Acinar secretions drain into intralobular, then interlobular, and thence into the main ducts (Fig. 1-9). Grossly the lacrimal gland has a

nodular surface with a fine connective tissue pseudocapsule. It is pinkish-gray, in contrast to orbital fat, which is yellow-gray. The gland is supported by Whitnall's ligament and the lateral horn of the levator aponeurosis as well as by septal attachments to the superior periorbita. The lacrimal artery penetrates it posteriorly, and the vein from it drains into the superior ophthalmic. Lymphatic drainage is by means of the lid and conjunctiva to the preauricular nodes. The lacrimal nerve and sometimes branches of the zygomatic carry the sensory afferents, the parasympathetic efferents (by the nervus intermedius, facial, greater superficial petrosal, vidian, sphenopalatine ganglion, infraorbital, and lacrimal nerves), and the sympathetic efferents (from the carotid plexus through the sphenopalatine ganglion). This pathway is believed to account for reflex tearing. In addition to the lacrimal gland, there are accessory glands (of Krause and Wolfring) in the lids and conjunctiva. There are 20 to 40 glands of Krause in the upper fornix, and six to eight in the lower fornix. The glands of Wolfring are fewer, consisting of three at the upper border of the superior tarsus and one at the lower border of the inferior tarsus.

Tears flow across the eye and are drained into the lacrimal sac through the canaliculi of the upper and lower lid by a pump system initiated by blinking. The tear film consists of a superficial lipid, central aqueous, and deep mucus layer. The upper and lower canaliculi originate at the puncta, and have a 2.0-mm vertical portion and an 8.0-mm horizontal portion, which fuse into a common canaliculus. The common canaliculus enters the lateral wall of the lacrimal sac by means of the valve of Rosenmüller, which prevents reflux. The canaliculi are lined by squamous epithelium, whereas the sac and duct are lined by columnar epithelium, goblet cells, and ciliated cells. The lacrimal sac is 13 mm to 15 mm in vertical length, and has a fundal portion (3 mm to 5 mm) behind and above the medial canthal ligament and a body (10 mm) below it. It fills the lacrimal fossa and is enveloped by the periorbita and the medial canthal ligament, superficial and deep heads of the pretarsal, and deep head of the preseptal muscles. This complex constitutes the lacrimal pump system. The tears drain through the nasolacrimal duct just beneath the inferior turbinate through a fold in the duct (called the valve of Hausner) in the lateral wall of the nose.

Lids

The orbit forms a complex interdigitation with the lid and brow region that accounts for the structural barrier of the orbit anteriorly. (See Chapter 2.)

The brow is a thick multilaminar structure at the upper orbital margin in men. It is located slightly higher in women. It consists of four layers including a thick skin, muscle, fat, and aponeurotic layer. The muscle layer is made up of the frontalis superiorly, which fuses medially with the vertically oriented procerus muscle and obliquely orientated corrugator superciliaris. The corrugator, procerus, and frontalis are in turn attached to fibers of the orbicularis. Deep to the muscles is a layer of fat, which extends over the brow to lie on the orbital septum. The muscle and adipose tissue are attached to an aponeurotic layer arising from the deep galea insertion, particularly in the medial portion. Laterally, the muscular

layers are less firmly attached, which accounts for the development of lateral brow ptosis in this region.

The lids and orbital septum are integral to and form the anterior boundary of the orbit. The anatomy of the upper lid is similar to that of the lower lid, except for differences in the upper and lower lid retractors. Very thin keratinizing epithelium covers the lids and is loosely attached to the underlying orbicularis muscle. This muscle is divided into orbital, preseptal, and pretarsal portions. Laterally, the orbital fibers extend continuously around to the lower lid and attach medially to the orbital margin, frontal bone, and frontal process of maxillary bone. Medially, the preseptal and pretarsal muscles form a complex relationship to the lacrimal sac and medial canthal ligament by dividing into interdigitating deep and superficial heads. The superficial preseptal head inserts into the medial canthal ligament and the deep head into the fascia of the lacrimal sac. Pretarsal orbicularis divides into an anterior head that attaches to the medial canthal tendon in front of the canaliculus, and a deep head that attaches to the lacrimal fascia and posterior crest. The medial canthal ligament also has a deep head (thin; attached to posterior lacrimal crest), a superficial head (thick; attached to frontal process of maxillary bone), and a fine superior branch. Laterally, the preseptal muscles form an indistinct raphe and the pretarsal muscles form the lateral canthal ligament, which inserts on the lateral orbital tubercle.

Deep to the orbicularis, the orbital septum fuses with the periosteum of the orbital rim peripherally, except medially, where it splits to attach to the anterior and posterior lacrimal crests. The septum is confluent with the levator aponeurosis in the upper lid and the capsulopalpebral fascia in the lower lid. Preaponeurotic orbital fat is retained by the septum and divided into several pads in the upper and lower lids.

Both the upper and lower lid retractors attach to anterior orbital condensations, which act as suspensory ligaments. The superior transverse ligament of Whitnall is 15 mm to 20 mm above the tarsus. It attaches medially near the trochlea and laterally through the lacrimal gland to the orbital wall. The aponeurotic portion of the levator begins just below the ligament, as does Müller's muscle. These two lamellae can be separated surgically, Müller's attaching to the upper tarsal border and the aponeurosis to the anterior border of tarsus, orbicularis, and subcuticular tissue. Laterally, the horn of the levator aponeurosis divides the orbital and palpebral lobes of the lacrimal gland and inserts on the lateral orbital tubercle, retinaculum, and tendon. The medial horn attaches posteriorly to the canthal ligament.

In the lower lid the retractors are the capsulopalpebral fascia. This is a fibrous layer that extends from the inferior rectus, surrounds the inferior oblique, and fuses to the suspensory ligament of Lockwood. Thence, it incorporates the inferior tarsal muscle (in the fornix) and inserts as a fascial aponeurosis into the lower lid. Additional attachments are to the septum and Tenon's capsule. The inferior tarsal muscle does not attach to the tarsus, but is incorporated in the fascia 2 mm to 3 mm below it. Lockwood's ligament forms complex attachments to the anterior orbital fascia and the lower lid retractors.

The tarsus is composed of dense regular connective tissue and contains the meibomian glands (25 in the upper and 20 in the lower). They are sebaceous glands that produce lipid secretions. The follicles of the lids also contain sebaceous glands of Zeis and apocrine glands of Moll. Additionally, the skin of the lids contains eccrine sweat glands. The arterial supply of the pretarsal lid is from the external carotid system by means of the superficial temporal and facial arteries. Venous drainage is through the anterior facial and superior temporal veins. The post-tarsal lid is supplied by the terminal branches of the ophthalmic artery, and is drained by the ophthalmic veins. The lids have lymphatic drainage laterally to the preauricular and intraparotid lymph nodes, and medially to the submental and submandibular nodes. There are no lymphatics in the deep orbit.

Surface Anatomy

The supraorbital notch (present in 75% of persons) or foramen (present in 25%) is palpable at the junction of the medial one third and lateral two thirds of the superior margin. A vertical line from this point intersects the inferior margin 3 mm to 4 mm in front of the origin of the inferior oblique muscle (which is adjacent to the opening of the nasolacrimal duct). Four millimeters directly below is a palpable indentation created by the infraorbital foramen. Medial to the supraorbital notch, the trochlea may be palpated 4 mm posterior to the margin. Below this, the medial canthal ligament can be felt at the level of the upper margin of the lacrimal sac. (Thus, cystic masses felt above it are generally ethmoidal in origin, and below it lacrimal sac in origin.) The frontozygomatic suture can be felt 6 mm above the marginal tubercle of the zygomatic bone and is the surface marking for the inferior border of the lacrimal gland.

The eyelids extend superiorly to the eyebrow and lateral orbital rim and inferiorly to the nasojugal (medial) and malar (lateral) folds. Generally, the upper lid crease is 8 mm to 11 mm above the margin, and is due to the firm attachment of the levator aponeurotic fibers below this point. This fold separates the loosely adherent (upper) preseptal portion from the more firmly attached tarsal portion. The inferior lid crease, which is more evident in

the young, is 2 mm to 3 mm below the lower lid margin medially and 5 mm to 6 mm laterally. The lids are divided horizontally by the puncta into an inner (one-sixth) lacrimal portion and outer ciliary or bulbar portion. The ciliary portion of the lid margin contains the lashes and adnexa and is separated by the gray line from the tarsal (posterior) portion, which contains the meibomian orifices. The lateral commissure is at the level of the superior attachment of the helix of the ear.

Bibliography

GENERAL

Beard C, Quickert M: Anatomy of the Orbit. Birmingham. Aesculapius, 1977

Doxanas MT, Anderson RL: Clinical Orbital Anatomy. Baltimore, Williams & Wilkins, 1984

Duke-Elder S: Anatomy of the visual system. In Duke-Elder S: System of Ophthalmology, Vol 2. London, Kimpton, 1961

Henderson JW: Orbital Tumours. New York, BC Decker, 1980

Hogan MJ, Alvarado JA, Weddell JE: Histology of the Human Eye. Philadelphia, WB Saunders, 1971

Jakobiec FA: In Duane TD, Jaeger EA (eds): Biomedical Foundations of Ophthalmology, Vol 1. Philadelphia, Harper & Row, 1982

Jones IS, Jakobiec FA: Diseases of the Orbit. Philadelphia, Harper & Row, 1979

Jones LT, Wobig JL: Surgery of the Eyelids and Lacrimal System. Birmingham, Aesculapius, 1976

Last RJ: Eugene Wolff's Anatomy of the Eye and Orbit. Philadelphia, WB Saunders, 1968

Lockhart RD, Hamilton GF, Fyfe FW: Anatomy of the Human Body. London, Faber & Faber, 1959

Miller NR: Walsh and Hoyt's Clinical Neuro-Ophthalmology, 4th ed. Baltimore, Williams & Wilkins, 1982

Whitnall SE: The Anatomy of the Human Orbit and Accessory Organs of Vision, 2nd ed. London, Oxford University Press, 1932

PERIORBITA AND SEPTA

Koornneef L: Spatial Aspects of Orbital Musculo-fibrous Tissue in Man. Amsterdam, Swets & Zeitlinger, 1977

Koornneef L: New insights in the human orbital connective tissue: Results of a new anatomic approach. Arch Ophthalmol 95:1269, 1977

Koornneef L: Details of the orbital connective tissue system in the adult. Acta Morphol Neerl Scand 15:1, 1977

Koornneef L: Orbital septa: Anatomy and function. Ophthalmology 86:876, 1979

Koornneef L: Orbital connective tissue. In Duane TD, Jaeger EA (eds): Biomedical Foundations of Ophthalmology, Vol 1, Chap 32. Philadelphia, Harper & Row, 1982

EXTRAOCULAR MUSCLES

Apt L: An anatomical reevaluation of rectus muscle insertions. Trans Am Ophthalmol Soc 78:365, 1980

Helveston EM, Merriam WW, Ellis FD et al: The trochlea: A study of the anatomy and physiology. Ophthalmology 89:124, 1982

NERVES

Davis RA, Anson BJ, Budinger JM et al: Surgical anatomy of the facial nerve and parotid gland based upon a study of 350 cervicofacial halves. Surg Gynecol Obstet 102:385, 1956

Gudmundsson K, Rhoton AL, Jr, Rushton JG: Detailed anatomy of the intracranial portion of the trigeminal nerve. J Neurosurg 35:592, 1971

Henderson WR: A note on the relationship of the human maxillary nerve to the cavernous sinus passing through the foramen ovale. J Anat 100:109, 1966

VASCULAR

Bergen MP: Spatial aspects of the orbital vascular system. In Duane TD, Jaeger EA (eds): Biomedical Foundations of Ophthalmology, Vol 1, Chap 32. Philadelphia, Harper & Row, 1982

Brismar J: Orbital phlebography. II: Anatomy of the superior ophthalmic vein and its tributaries. Acta Radiol [Diagn] (Stockh) 15:481, 1974

Brismar J: Orbital phlebography. III: Topography of orbital veins. Acta Radiol [Diagn] (Stockh) 15:577, 1974

Harris FS, Rhoton AL, Jr: Anatomy of the cavernous sinus: A microsurgical study. J Neurosurg 45:169, 1976

Hayreh SS: The ophthalmic artery. III: Branches. Br J Ophthalmol 46:212, 1962

Hayreh SS: Arteries of the orbit in the human being. Br J Surg 50:938, 1963

Hayreh SS, Dass R: The ophthalmic artery. I: Origin and intracranial and intra-canalicular course. Br J Ophthalmol 46:65, 1962a

Hayreh SS, Dass R: The ophthalmic artery. II: Intra-orbital course. Br J Ophthalmol 46:165, 1962b

Henderson WR: A note on the relationship of the human maxillary nerve to the cavernous sinus and to an emissary sinus passing through the foramen ovale. J Anat 100:905, 1966

Kaplan HA, Browder J, Krieger AJ: Intercavernous connections of the cavernous sinus: The superior and inferior circular sinuses. J Neurosurg 45:166, 1976

Renn WH, Rhoton AL, Jr: Microsurgical anatomy of the sellar region. J Neurosurg 43:288, 1975

Umansky F, Hilel N: The lateral wall of the cavernous sinus: With special reference to the nerves related to it. J Neurosurg 56:228, 1982

LACRIMAL SYSTEM

Doane MG: Interactions of eyelids and tears in corneal wetting and the dynamics of the normal human eyeblink. Am J Ophthalmol 89:507, 1980

Doane MG: Blinking and the mechanics of the lacrimal drainage system. Ophthalmology 88:844, 1981

Egeberg J, Jensen OA: The ultrastructure of the acini of the human lacrimal gland. Acta Ophthalmol 47:400, 1969

Hurwitz JJ, Welham RAN, Lloyd GAS: The role of intubation macro-dacryocystography in the management of problems of the lacrimal system. Can J Ophthalmol 10:361, 1975

Jones LT: The lacrimal secretory system and its treatment. Am J Ophthalmol 62:47, 1966

Jones LT, Wobig JL: Surgery of the Eyelids and Lacrimal System, p. 58. Birmingham, Aesculapius, 1976

Rosenstock T, Hurwitz JJ: Functional obstruction of the lacrimal drainage passages. Can J Ophthalmol 17, No. 6:249, 1982

Smith B, Petrelli R: Surgical repair of the prolapsed lacrimal gland. Arch Ophthalmol 96:113, 1978

LIDS

Anderson RL: Medial canthal tendon branches out. Arch Ophthalmol 95:2051, 1977

Anderson RL, Beard C: The levator aponeurosis: Attachments and their clinical significance. Arch Ophthalmol 95:1437, 1977

Anderson RL, Dixon RS: The role of Whitnall's ligament in ptosis surgery. Arch Ophthalmol 97:705, 1979

Collin JRO, Beard C, Wood I: Experimental and clinical data on the insertion of the levator palpebrae superioris muscle. Am J Ophthalmol 85:792, 1978

Hawes MJ, Dortzbach RK: The microscopic anatomy of the lower eyelid retractors. Arch Ophthalmol 100:1313, 1982

Jones LT: The anatomy of the lower eyelid and its relation to the cause and cure of entropion. Am J Ophthalmol 49:29, 1960

Jones LT: A new concept of the orbital fascia and rectus muscle sheaths and its surgical implications. Trans Am Acad Ophthalmol 72:755, 1968

Kuwabara T, Cogan DG, Johnson CC: Structure of the muscles of the upper eyelid. Arch Ophthalmol 93:1189, 1975

Lemke BN, Stasior OG: The anatomy of eyebrow ptosis. Arch Ophthalmol 100:981, 1982

CHAPTER 2
Atlas of Orbital Anatomy

Jack Rootman and Bruce Stewart

Orbital anatomy is best understood in the clinical and surgical context by developing a three-dimensional image of the complex relationships within and surrounding it. In this atlas, we have attempted to present the anatomy from three traditional surgical points of view, superolateral, anterior, and lateral. Emphasis has been placed on developing three-dimensional images of the bony anatomy, muscular structures, motor and sensory nerves, and vascular supply from each of these points of view. Colors are used to represent structures as follows: red, arteries; blue, veins; yellow, sensory nerves; and orange, motor nerves. Finally, the complex relationships and structures of the lid and anterior orbit have been rendered. A minimum of labelling and a maximum of imagery will provide the framework for developing an orbital engram from a surgeon's viewpoint.

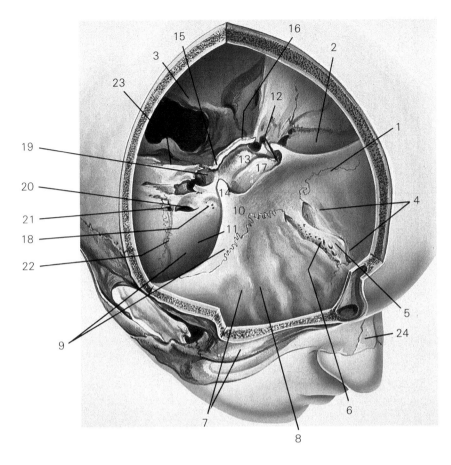

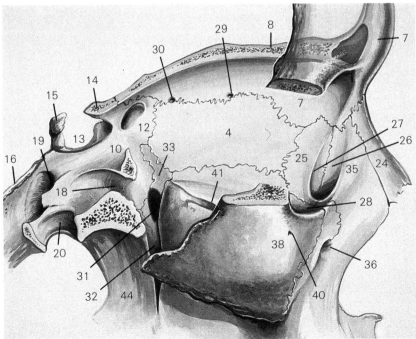

Bony structures

1 Anterior cranial fossa
2 Middle cranial fossa
3 Posterior cranial fossa
4 Ethmoid bone
5 Crista galli
6 Cribriform plate
7 Frontal bone
8 Orbital plate
9 Sphenoid bone
10 Lesser wing of sphenoid
11 Greater wing of sphenoid
12 Optic canal
13 Hypophyseal fossa
14 Anterior clinoid process
15 Posterior clinoid process
16 Dorsum sellae
17 Tuberculum sellae
18 Foramen rotundum
19 Foramen lacerum
20 Foramen ovale
21 Foramen spinosum
22 Groove for middle meningeal
   artery
23 Groove for superior petrosal sinus
24 Nasal bone
25 Lacrimal bone
26 Lacrimal fossa
27 Lacrimal crest
28 Fossa for inferior oblique
   muscle
29 Anterior ethmoid foramen
30 Posterior ethmoid foramen
31 Pterygopalatine foramen
32 Pterygopalatine fossa
33 Palatine bone
34 Maxillary bone
35 Frontal process of maxilla
36 Infraorbital foramen
37 Supraorbital notch
38 Zygomatic bone
39 Frontal process of zygomatic
   bone
40 Zygomaticofacial foramen
41 Infraorbital groove
42 Superior orbital fissure
43 Inferior orbital fissure
44 Lateral pterygoid lamina

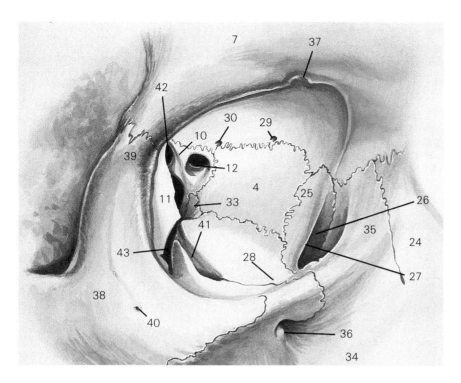

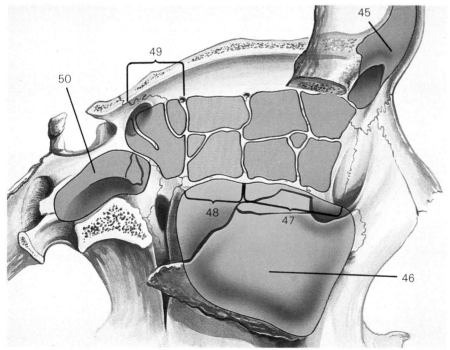

Sinuses

45 Frontal
46 Maxillary
47 Ethmoid: anterior
48 Ethmoid: middle
49 Ethmoid: posterior
50 Sphenoid

21

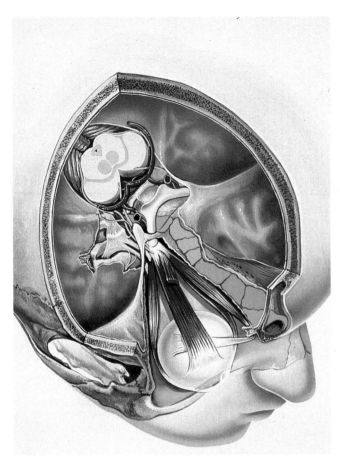

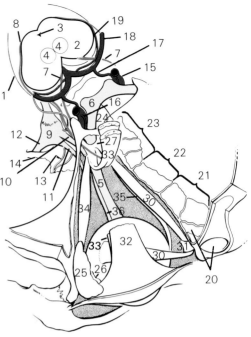

Intracranial structures

1 Tentorium cerebelli
2 Midbrain
3 Cerebral aqueduct
4 Red nucleus
5 Optic nerve (II)
6 Optic chiasm
7 Oculomotor nerve (III)
8 Trochlear nerve (IV)
9 Trigeminal nerve (V), Gasserian ganglion
10 Ophthalmic nerve (V^1)
11 Maxillary nerve (V^2)
12 Mandibular nerve (V^3)
13 Meningeal branches
14 Dura (cut edge)
15 Internal carotid artery
16 Ophthalmic artery
17 Posterior communicating artery
18 Posterior cerebral artery
19 Superior cerebellar artery
20 Frontal sinus
21 Ethmoid sinus: anterior
22 Ethmoid sinus: middle
23 Ethmoid sinus: posterior
24 Sphenoid sinus
25 Lacrimal gland (orbital part)
26 Lacrimal gland (palpebral part)

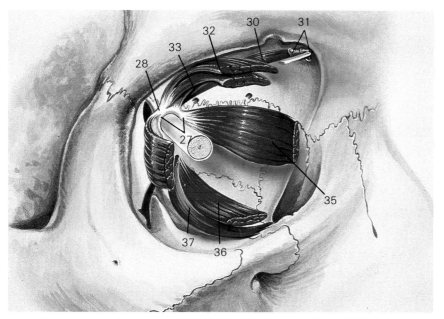

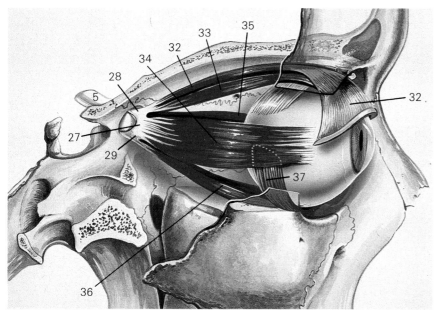

Extraocular muscles

27 Annulus of Zinn
28 Upper tendon (of Lockwood)
29 Lower tendon (of Zinn)
30 Superior oblique
31 Trochlea
32 Levator palpebrae
33 Superior rectus
34 Lateral rectus
35 Medial rectus
36 Inferior rectus
37 Inferior oblique

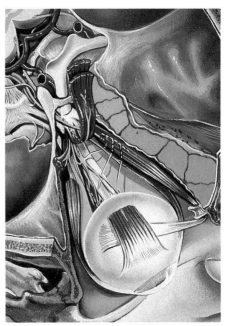

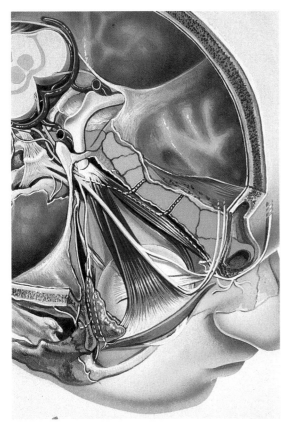

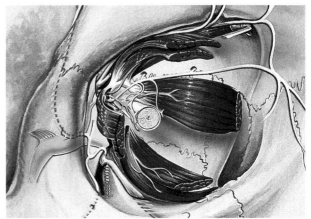

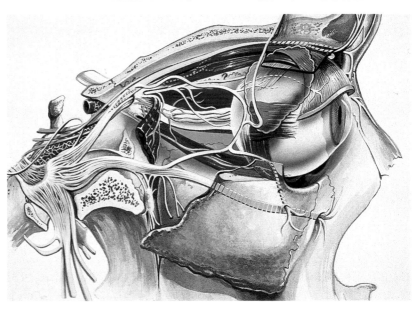

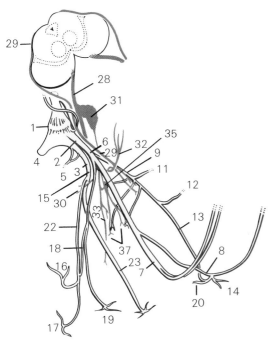

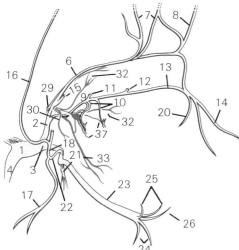

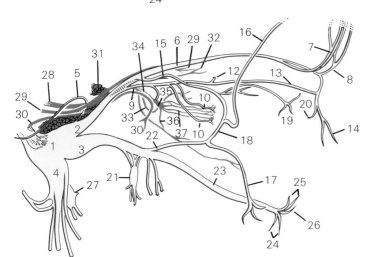

Sensory nerves

1 Trigeminal (Gasserian) ganglion
2 Ophthalmic (first) division
3 Maxillary (second) division
4 Mandibular (third) division
5 Meningeal branch
6 Frontal
7 Supraorbital
8 Supratrochlear
9 Nasociliary
10 Sensory (long) posterior ciliary
11 Posterior ethmoidal
12 Anterior ethmoidal
13 Infratrochlear
14 External nasal
15 Lacrimal
16 Zygomaticotemporal
17 Zygomaticofacial
18 Anastomosis with lacrimal
19 Lateral palpebral
20 Medial palpebral
21 Pterygopalatine ganglion
22 Zygomatic
23 Infraorbital
24 Superior labial branches
25 Inferior palpebral branches
26 Lateral nasal branch
27 Otic ganglion

Motor nerves

28 Oculomotor (III)
29 Trochlear (IV)
30 Abducent (VI)
31 Carotid plexus (sympathetic)
32 Oculomotor, upper division
33 Oculomotor, lower division

Ciliary ganglion

34 Sympathetic root from carotid plexus
35 Ciliary ganglion
36 Parasympathetic root to inferior division of oculomotor nerve
37 Short posterior ciliary

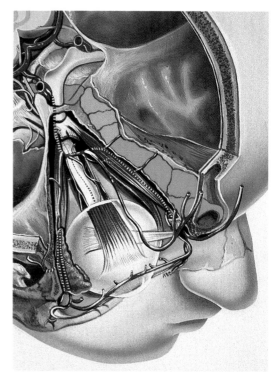

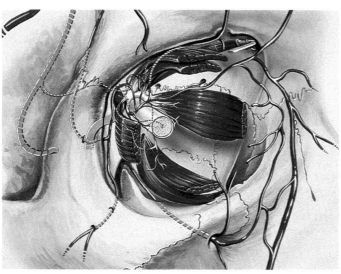

Arteries

1. Middle meningeal
2. Carotid
3. Ophthalmic
4. Central artery of retina
5. Lateral posterior ciliary
6. Medial posterior ciliary
7. Short ciliary
8. Long ciliary
9. Lateral muscular: branches to levator palpebrae, superior rectus, and superior oblique
10. Medial muscular: branches to inferior rectus, inferior oblique, and lateral rectus

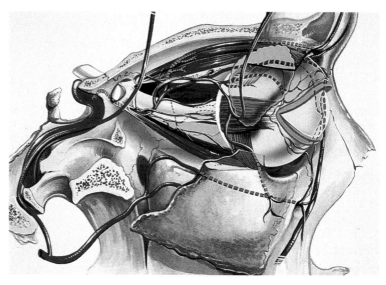

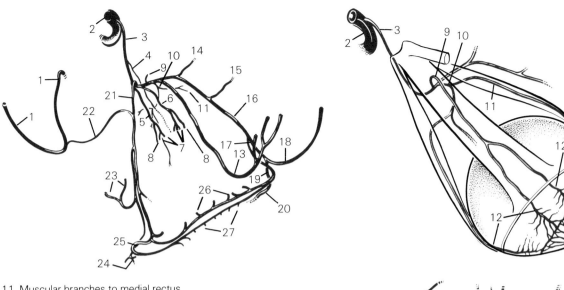

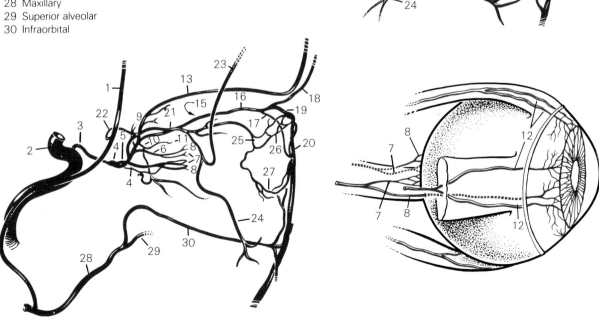

11 Muscular branches to medial rectus
12 Anterior ciliary
13 Supraorbital
14 Posterior ethmoid
15 Anterior ethmoid
16 Nasofrontal
17 Medial palpebral
18 Supratrochlear
19 Dorsal nasal
20 Angular
21 Lacrimal
22 Recurrent meningeal artery communicating through foramen
   lacrimale or superior orbital fissure
23 Zygomaticotemporal
24 Zygomaticofacial
25 Lateral palpebral
26 Superior marginal palpebral arcade
27 Inferior marginal palpebral arcade
28 Maxillary
29 Superior alveolar
30 Infraorbital

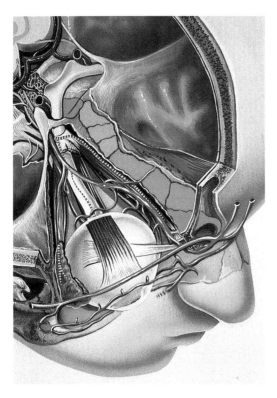

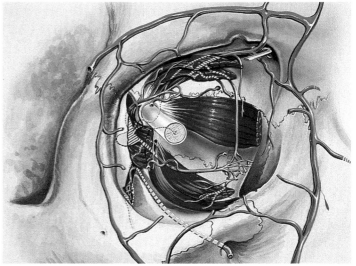

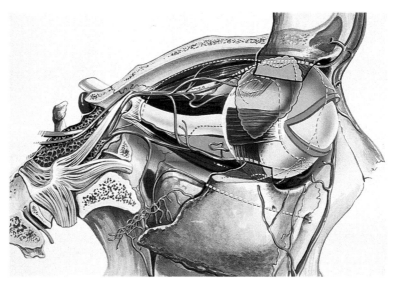

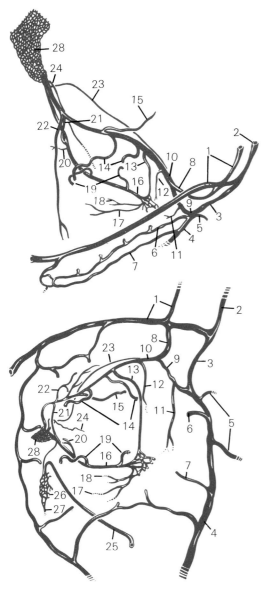

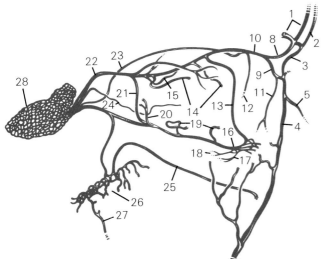

Veins

1 Supraorbital
2 Supratrochlear
3 Angular
4 Anterior facial
5 Nasal branches
6 Superior palpebral
7 Inferior palpebral
8 Superior root of superior ophthalmic
9 Inferior root of superior ophthalmic
10 Superior ophthalmic
11 Anterior collateral
12 Muscular branch from medial rectus
13 Medial collateral
14 Vena vorticosa (superior medial, superior lateral)
15 Anterior ethmoid
16 Inferior ophthalmic
17 Muscular branches from inferior oblique
18 Muscular branches from inferior rectus
19 Vena vorticosa (inferior medial, inferior lateral)
20 Muscular branches from lateral rectus
21 Lateral collateral
22 Lacrimal
23 Medial ophthalmic
24 Central vein of retina
25 Infraorbital
26 Pterygoid plexus
27 Posterior superior alveolar
28 Cavernous sinus

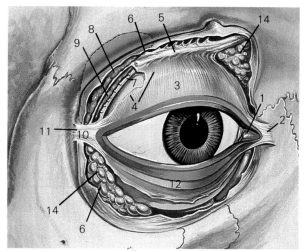

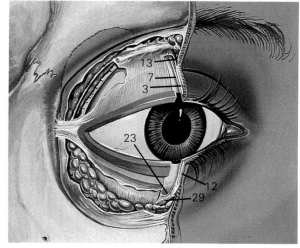

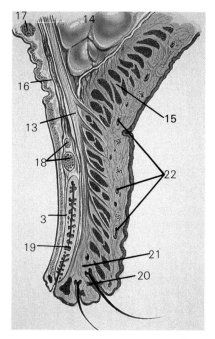

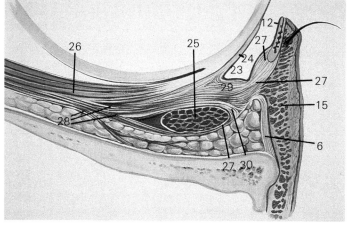

Lids

1 Caruncle
2 Medial canthal ligament
3 Superior tarsus
4 Levator aponeurosis
5 Whitnall's ligament
6 Orbital septum
7 Conjunctiva
8 Lacrimal gland (orbital part)
9 Lacrimal gland (palpebral part)
10 Lateral canthal ligament
11 Lateral orbital tubercle
12 Inferior tarsus
13 Levator palpebrae muscle
14 Orbital fat

15 Orbicularis oculi muscle
16 Müller's muscle
17 Gland of Krause
18 Glands of Wolfring
19 Meibomian gland
20 Gland of Zeis
21 Gland of Moll
22 Marginal arcade
23 Fornix of conjunctiva
24 Tenon's capsule
25 Inferior oblique muscle
26 Inferior rectus muscle
27 Capsulopalpebral fascia
28 Capsulopalpebral head
29 Inferior tarsal muscle
30 Lockwood's ligament

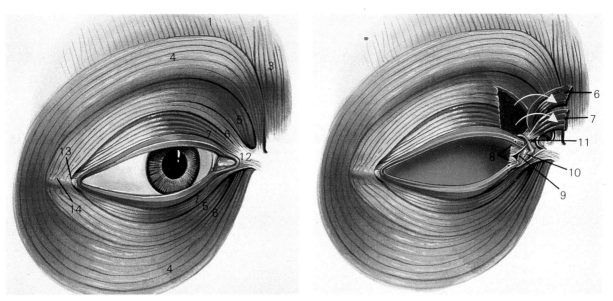

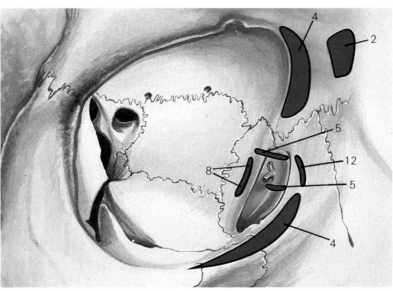

1 Frontalis muscle
2 Corrugator supercilii muscle
3 Procerus muscle
 Orbicularis oculi muscle:
4   Orbital portion
5   Preseptal portion: deep head
6   Preseptal portion: superficial head
7   Pretarsal portion: superficial head
8   Pretarsal portion: deep head (Horner's muscle)
9 Lacrimal sac
10 Inferior lacrimal canaliculus
11 Superior lacrimal canaliculus
12 Medial canthal ligament
13 Lateral canthal ligament
14 Lateral palpebral raphé

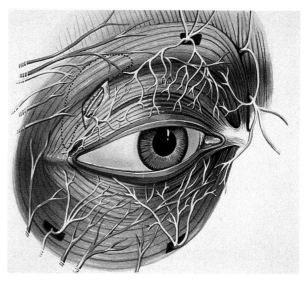

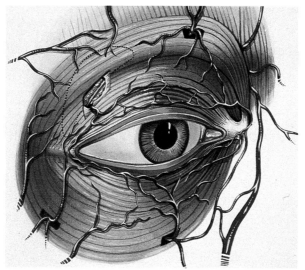

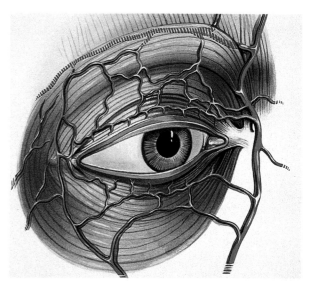

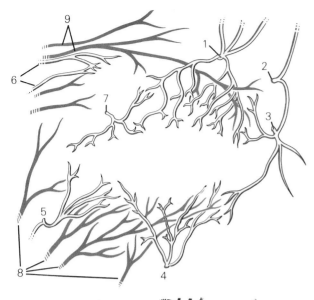

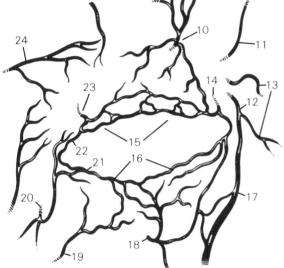

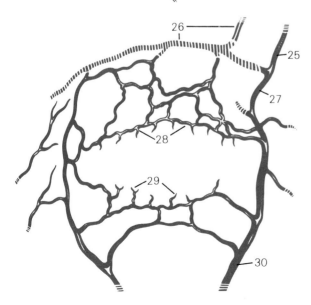

Lids

Sensory nerves

1 Supraorbital
2 Supratrochlear
3 Infratrochlear
4 Infraorbital
5 Zygomaticofacial
6 Zygomaticotemporal
7 Lacrimal

Motor nerve

8 Facial nerve (VII), zygomatic branches
9 Facial nerve (VII), temporofrontal branches

Arteries

10 Supraorbital
11 Supratrochlear
12 Dorsal nasal
13 Nasal branches
14 Superior medial palpebral
15 Superior marginal palpebral arcade
16 Inferior medial palpebral arcade
17 Angular
18 Infraorbital
19 Transverse facial
20 Zygomaticofrontal
21 Inferior lateral palpebral
22 Superior lateral palpebral
23 Lacrimal
24 Frontal branch of superficial temporal

Veins

25 Supratrochlear
26 Supraorbital
27 Angular
28 Superior palpebral
29 Inferior palpebral
30 Anterior facial

CHAPTER 3

Applied Investigative Anatomy

*Robert Nugent, Jack Rootman,
and William Robertson*

Advances in radiographic imaging of the orbit in the past decade have provided exquisite detail, particularly with modern CT scanners. Magnetic resonance imaging (MRI) has yet to reach its full potential, but promises to provide exciting new details of orbital disease. Traditional techniques, such as plain film radiography, may be helpful but have a diminished role. This chapter describes normal radiographic orbital anatomy available with each of these imaging techniques and discusses the role of each in assessing orbital disease.

Plain Films of the Orbits

Plain film assessment of the orbits includes a 23-degree PA (Caldwell), a 37-degree PA (Waters), and a true lateral view. Other projections may be obtained, including a basal and an oblique view to show the optic canal (Fig. 3-1D). These provide a relatively inexpensive assessment of the bony orbit and paranasal sinuses without giving direct information about orbital soft tissues. They are useful in assessing bony defects and injuries or developmental abnormalities. In addition, many foreign bodies can be detected, although this technique is less sensitive than CT and not as useful for localization.

Several important bony landmarks are easily identified on plain films. The Caldwell view (Fig. 3-1A) is particularly useful for demonstrating the anterior orbital rim, with the exception of the inferior portion, which is best seen on the Waters' view. In addition, the Caldwell view shows portions of the medial, superior, and posterior walls well, with the superior orbital fissure visualized between the lesser and greater sphenoid wings posteriorly. Frequently, the palpebral fissure will produce a transverse radiolucent line across the orbit that may mimic a fracture line.

The Waters' view (Fig. 3-1B) gives the best demonstration of the orbital floor, lateral rim, and infraorbital canal. It is particularly useful with suspected blowout fractures of the floor.

The lateral view (Fig. 3-1C) demonstrates the orbital roof and is also useful for the floor and posterolateral wall, formed by the greater wing of sphenoid.

The basal view may sometimes give added information about the optic canal. It is particularly useful for assessment of the lateral orbital wall.

Complex Motion Tomography

Tomography is helpful in defining bony anatomy. It may be performed in different planes, including the Caldwell, basal, lateral, or oblique view. However, this technique is more expensive and time consuming and requires more technician skill than routine plain films. Moreover, it involves a considerable increase in the radiation dose to the eye, estimated at 5 rad to 10 rad per imaging plane. Because of this and the lack of information regarding orbital soft tissues, this technique has been largely replaced by computed tomography.

Computed Tomography

Because of its high-contrast resolution and ability to define different soft tissues, computed tomography (CT) has become the method of choice for imaging the orbit. Radiation dose to the lens is slightly less than that of complex motion tomography, averaging 5 rad per imaging plane. Moström and co-workers have emphasized the higher doses obtained with scan protocols designed for orbital study with a mean of 86 mGy per study.

TECHNIQUE

Routine assessment of the orbits includes contiguous axial and coronal views. Each image or "slice" is 3 mm in thickness. Thin slices have the advantage of less volume

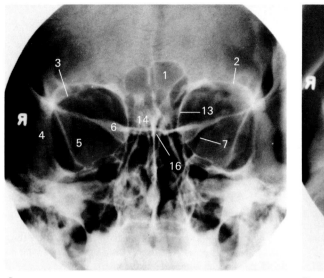

A

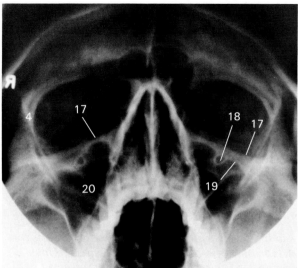

B

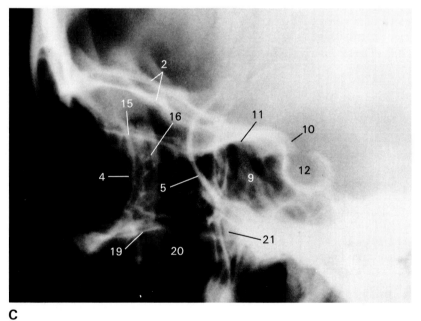

C

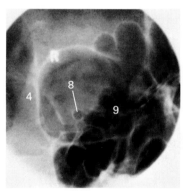

D

1	Frontal sinus	8	Optic canal	15	Roof of ethmoid sinus
2	Orbital roof	9	Sphenoid sinus	16	Cribriform plate
3	Superior orbital rim	10	Anterior clinoid	17	Inferior orbital rim
4	Lateral orbital rim	11	Planum sphenoidale	18	Infraorbital canal
5	Greater wing of sphenoid	12	Sella turcica	19	Floor of orbit
6	Lesser wing of sphenoid	13	Medial orbital rim	20	Maxillary sinus
7	Superior orbital fissure	14	Ethmoid sinus	21	Pterygopalatine fossa

FIGURE 3-1.   Plain film views of the orbits: *(A)* Caldwell view, *(B)* Waters' view, *(C)* lateral view, and *(D)* optic canal view of right orbit.

averaging with adjacent structures, thus providing finer spatial resolution. Some institutions prefer to do 1.5-mm-thick images in the axial plane and use computer reformatting ability to produce images in other planes. These reformatted images help reduce the overall radiation dose as well as avoid dental filling artifacts or patient discomfort related to the coronal position. However, reformatted images do not match the resolution capability of the direct images.

The axial slices are normally obtained at an angle parallel to Reid's baseline (inferior orbital rim to the external auditory canal) (Fig. 3-2I). However, the best view of the optic canal is obtained at an angle of −30 degrees because the canal passes inferiorly and obliquely from posterior to anterior.

ROLE OF INTRAVENOUS OR INTRATHECAL CONTRAST

The high radiographic density of iodine in the contrast medium provides increased density or "enhancement" because the contrast agent will be more abundant in vascular structures following intravenous infusion. Normally, extraocular muscles demonstrate moderate enhancement, as does the lacrimal gland. The optic nerve has minimal central enhancement with more prominent enhancement of the dural sheath. Arteries and veins within the orbit demonstrate prominent enhancement, as does the scleral uveal rim.

Orbital masses tend to be readily identified even without contrast enhancement, because of surrounding low-density fat. However, contrast is essential in identifying extraorbital extension, particularly with tumors extending intracranially where there is no low-density fat to highlight the lesion. In addition, intravenous contrast enhancement frequently aids in the differential diagnosis of the lesion because tumors may have variable vascularity and different degrees of enhancement. Contrast use may help define venous thrombosis, cystic masses, and optic nerve lesions, particularly meningioma and glioma.

The subarachnoid space extends into the optic nerve sheath from the intracranial compartment. In approximately 30% of patients who have had a cisternogram performed with water-soluble agents, contrast material can be seen in the optic nerve sheath on CT. This technique is seldom indicated.

NORMAL CT ANATOMY

Axial and coronal views of the orbit are complementary for showing bony and soft tissue anatomy. The axial view is superior for demonstrating the lateral and medial bony margins, the superior orbital fissure, and the optic canal.

(See Fig. 3-2.) Coronal views are best for assessing the floor and roof (Fig. 3-3). The lacrimal sac and nasolacrimal duct as well as the inferior orbital fissure and infraorbital canal are equally well seen on axial or coronal images.

The optic nerve has a slightly serpiginous course with minimal inferior and lateral bowing in its midportion. Because of this, thin slices may not show the entire course of the nerve on any one axial slice. The nerve can be well defined through its entire course, except within the optic canal. The postcanalicular portion as well as the optic chiasm can be identified. The dural sheath along the optic nerve is particularly well defined with intravenous contrast. On coronal views immediately posterior to the globe, a small central density within the nerve represents the central retinal artery and vein.

The extraocular muscles generally have a course parallel to the adjacent orbital wall. Consequently, only the medial and lateral rectus muscles may be seen in their entirety on an axial view. The tapering of these muscles in their tendinous portions as well as their origins at the annulus of Zinn are well seen. On a coronal view, they are vertically oriented. The superior and inferior rectus muscles are only partially visualized on any one axial slice and on coronal views are seen cross sectionally to lie in a slightly oblique horizontal plane. This is related to the superior slope of the floor and the inferior slope of the roof from lateral to medial. The levator palpebrae superioris merges with the superior rectus and is only identified separately on anterior coronal images where it diverges and separates from the superior rectus. The superior oblique muscle is best seen on coronal views, lying superior and slightly medial to the medial rectus muscle. The trochlea is well seen on axial views, and is occasionally calcified. The least well-defined muscle is the inferior oblique, with only its insertion well seen on axial views and the muscle belly somewhat poorly defined on anterior coronal views.

The lacrimal gland is readily identified in the lacrimal fossa on both coronal and axial views. The anterior soft tissue densities merging with the globe medially and laterally are the orbital septum, eyelids, and conjunctiva. The lacrimal sac can be identified by noting the position of the anterior and posterior lacrimal crest on axial views. The superior portion of the nasolacrimal duct, where it extends inferiorly from the lacrimal sac, can be readily identified on axial and coronal CT.

Vascular structures in the orbit can be seen without intravenous contrast, but are highlighted with contrast. The ophthalmic artery is seen in the apex of the orbit as it swings laterally before looping over the optic nerve. Several of its branches, including the anterior and posterior ethmoidal and posterior ciliary branches, can usually be identified.

(Text continues on p. 42.)

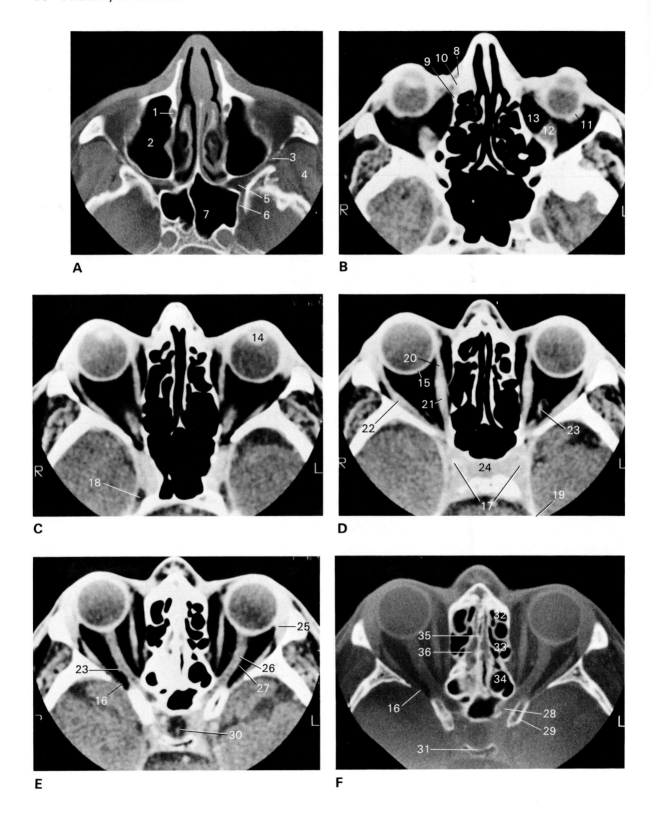

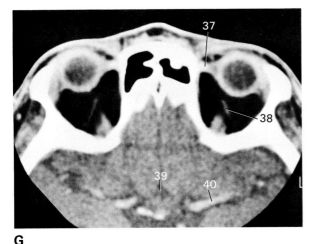

G

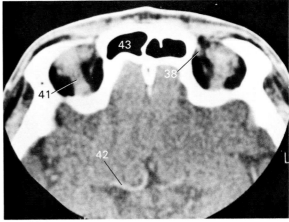

H

I

FIGURE 3-2. Axial CT scans. Selected axial scans, performed with intravenous contrast enhancement, demonstrate anatomy progressing from an inferior level to a superior position in the orbit. *A* through *F* highlight bone anatomy, whereas the others have been done on standard settings to demonstrate soft tissue anatomy. *(I)* Lateral scout view demonstrates the usual plane chosen for axial slices.

1	Nasolacrimal duct	16	Superior orbital fissure	31	Dorsum sellae
2	Maxillary sinus	17	Cavernous sinus		Ethmoid sinuses
3	Inferior orbital fissure	18	Gasserian ganglion	32	Anterior
4	Temporal fossa	19	Tentorium	33	Middle
5	Pterygopalatine fossa	20	Medial rectus muscle tendon	34	Posterior
6	Foramen rotundum	21	Medial rectus muscle belly	35	Crista galli
7	Sphenoid sinus	22	Lateral rectus muscle	36	Olfactory groove
8	Anterior lacrimal crest	23	Ophthalmic artery	37	Trochlea (calcified)
9	Posterior lacrimal crest	24	Pituitary gland	38	Superior ophthalmic vein
10	Lacrimal fossa	25	Lacrimal gland	39	Optic chiasm
11	Inferior oblique insertion	26	Optic nerve	40	Middle cerebral artery
12	Inferior rectus muscle	27	Optic nerve sheath	41	Superior rectus/
13	Orbital fat	28	Optic canal		levator palpebrae superioris
14	Lens	29	Anterior clinoid	42	Anterior cerebral artery
15	Scleral uveal rim	30	Pituitary stalk	43	Frontal sinus

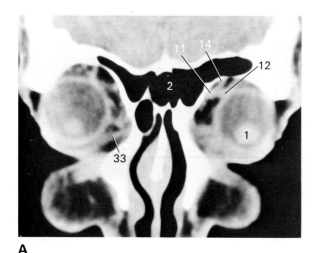

A

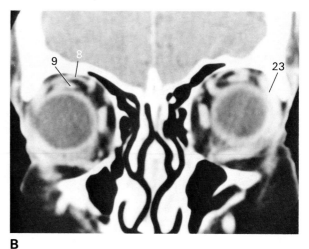

B

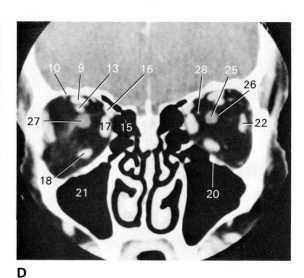

C

D

1	Lens	12	Superior oblique tendon	23	Lacrimal gland
2	Frontal sinus	13	Superior ophthalmic vein	24	Inferior orbital fissure
3	Lesser wing of sphenoid	14	Supratrochlear vein	25	Optic nerve
4	Superior orbital fissure	15	Ethmoid sinus	26	Optic nerve sheath
5	Greater wing of sphenoid	16	Superior oblique muscle	27	Central retinal artery/vein
6	Annulus of Zinn	17	Medial rectus muscle	28	Ophthalmic artery
7	Sphenoid sinus	18	Inferior rectus muscle	29	Crista galli
8	Levator palpebrae superioris	19	Zygomatic branch of infraorbital nerve	30	Cribriform plate
9	Superior rectus muscle	20	Infraorbital canal	31	Nasolacrimal duct
10	Frontal nerve (of V_1)	21	Maxillary sinus	32	Inferior turbinate
11	Trochlea	22	Lateral rectus muscle	33	Inferior oblique

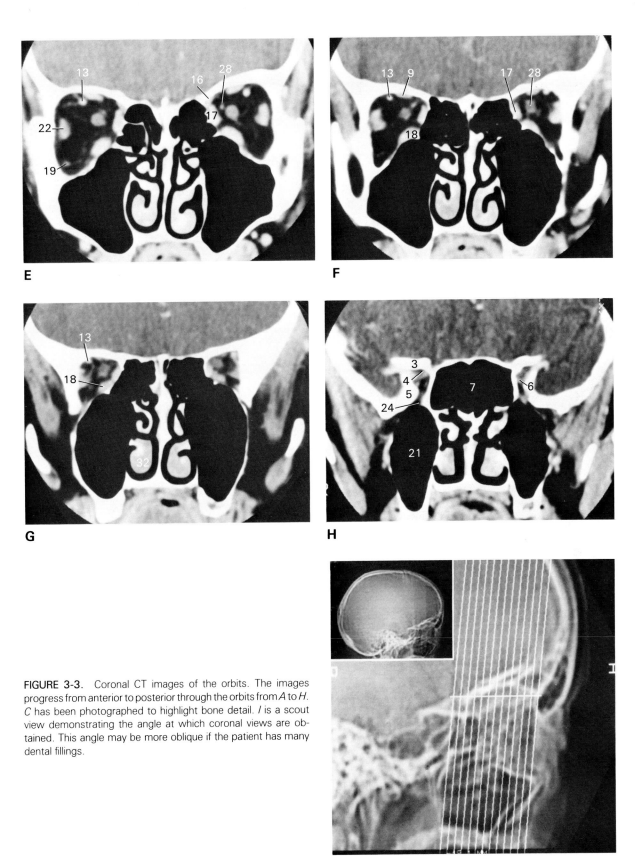

FIGURE 3-3. Coronal CT images of the orbits. The images progress from anterior to posterior through the orbits from A to H. C has been photographed to highlight bone detail. I is a scout view demonstrating the angle at which coronal views are obtained. This angle may be more oblique if the patient has many dental fillings.

41

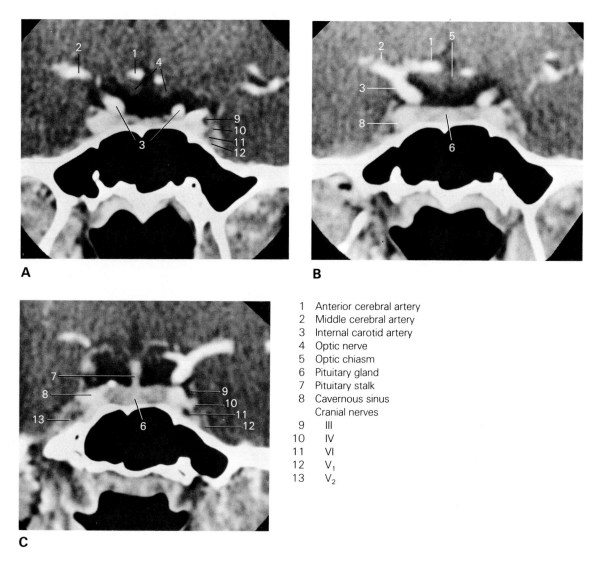

A

B

C

1	Anterior cerebral artery
2	Middle cerebral artery
3	Internal carotid artery
4	Optic nerve
5	Optic chiasm
6	Pituitary gland
7	Pituitary stalk
8	Cavernous sinus
	Cranial nerves
9	III
10	IV
11	VI
12	V_1
13	V_2

FIGURE 3-4. Coronal images with intravenous contrast enhancement of the cavernous sinus region. *A* is most anterior and *C* is most posterior.

The superior ophthalmic vein is routinely identified in axial and coronal views as it courses near the trochlea to pass through the muscle cone inferior to the superior rectus and superior to the optic nerve, to exit the orbit through the superior orbital fissure. The inferior ophthalmic and connecting veins are seen inconsistently.

A line joining the lateral orbital margins in the axial plane will normally intersect the globe near its midportion, with at least one third of the globe posterior to this line. The sclera, choroid, and retina form a well-defined band that enhances with intravenous contrast. The lens is normally high density on CT.

Nerves can occasionally be identified within the orbit, although position may be variable. In particular, the frontal, supraorbital, and inferior divisions of the third nerve may be seen. However, they may be difficult to differentiate from vascular structures, particularly when the study is done without intravenous contrast.

The cavernous sinus (Fig. 3-4) is particularly well seen with intravenous contrast. The third, fourth, and first divisions of the fifth nerve and the sixth intracranial nerve appear as round, low-density structures on coronal views through the uniformly enhancing cavernous sinus.

The optic chiasm is more readily identified than the

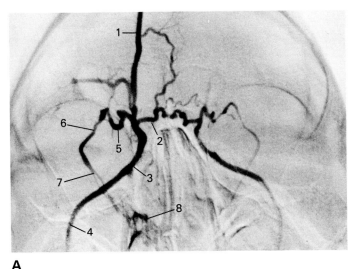

A

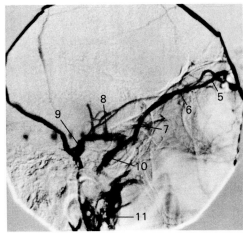

B

1	Frontal vein	8	Cavernous sinus
2	Prenasal vein		Petrosal sinus
3	Angular vein	9	Superior
4	Facial vein	10	Inferior
	Superior ophthalmic vein	11	Deep cervical plexus
5	First segment		
6	Second segment		
7	Third segment		

FIGURE 3-5.   Orbital venograms: *(A)* Waters' view, *(B)* lateral view.

postcanalicular portion of the optic nerves, because the former is surrounded by CSF in the suprasellar cistern.

Orbital Venography

Orbital venography is used to assess intraorbital venous abnormalities and the cavernous sinus. Since the advent of CT scanning, this technique is no longer required for assessment of mass lesions within the orbit.

The technique consists of injecting contrast by means of a midline vein in the forehead, while the patient applies finger compression over the area of the angular vein to encourage flow of contrast through the superior ophthalmic vein. Films are obtained in the Caldwell, Waters, and lateral projections (Fig. 3-5). Generally, the superior ophthalmic vein can be identified bilaterally with variable filling of the inferior ophthalmic and connecting channels.

The first segment of the superior ophthalmic vein starts near the trochlea and extends posteriorly in the anterior one third of the orbit, before entering the muscle cone along the medial border of the levator palpebrae

superioris. The second part of the superior ophthalmic vein passes posteriorly, superior to the optic nerve and inferior to the superior rectus muscle. The third segment extends between the origins of the lateral and superior rectus muscles, through the superior orbital fissure, and into the anteroinferior part of the cavernous sinus. This vein can be well seen through its entire intraorbital course on both axial and coronal views.

Orbital Angiography

The role of angiography in assessment of avascular intraorbital mass lesions has been eliminated with the advent of CT scanning. However, angiography remains essential in the assessment of vascular lesions, particularly arteriovenous malformations and fistulas (Fig. 3-6). In addition, it may aid in the differential diagnosis of lesions shown on CT scan, particularly optic nerve meningiomas and gliomas. Preoperative assessment of the arterial anatomy may occasionally be desirable.

This technique is invasive, requiring femoral artery puncture and selective catheterization of the internal and

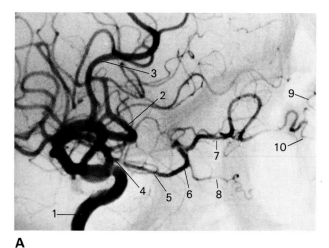

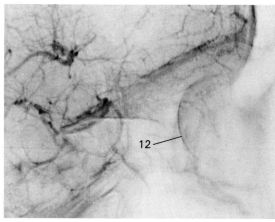

1   Internal carotid artery
2   Middle cerebral artery
3   Anterior cerebral artery
    Ophthalmic artery
4   Intracranial
        Intraorbital
5   First portion
6   Second portion
7   Third portion
8   Inferior muscular artery
9   Frontal
10 Angular
11 Lacrimal
12 Choroidal crescent

FIGURE 3-6. Normal orbital angiograms: *(A)* lateral view obtained during the arterial phase; *(B)* lateral view obtained during the venous phase; *(C)* Caldwell view obtained during the arterial phase.

external carotid artery. Super-selective catheterization of branches of the external carotid is frequently done as well. The high cost and moderate to high radiation doses are other drawbacks of angiography.

The ophthalmic artery has intracranial, intracanalicular, and intraorbital portions. In more than 80% of patients it originates from the subdural extracavernous portion of the carotid artery prior to entering the optic canal. In approximately 10% of the population it originates from the cavernous portion of the carotid artery and enters the orbit via the superior orbital fissure. Rarely, the ophthalmic artery originates from the middle meningeal artery.

The intracranial portion is relatively short. On a lateral film, it is seen bending superiorly as it passes medial and inferior to the anterior clinoid. In the optic canal, it lies inferior to the optic nerve, and is relatively straight as it passes anteroinferiorly. This is well seen on lateral and AP films.

The intraorbital portion of the ophthalmic artery consists of three parts. The most posterior portion extends from the optic canal to the point where it starts to bend laterally around the optic nerve. The second portion crosses superior to the optic nerve from lateral to medial in more than 80% of patients. In approximately 15% to 20%, the artery passes inferior to the optic nerve.

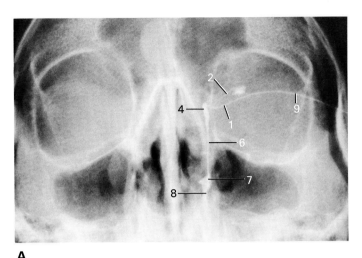

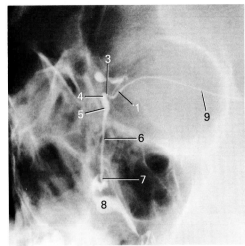

A

B

1	Inferior canaliculus	6	Nasolacrimal duct
2	Superior canaliculus	7	Valve of Hasner
3	Common canaliculus	8	Contrast in nose
4	Lacrimal sac	9	Cannula
5	Valve of Krause		

FIGURE 3-7. Demonstrates normal dacryocystography: *(A)* Waters' view, *(B)* oblique view.

The third part of the orbital portion extends from the superomedial aspect of the optic nerve to pass forward under the superior oblique and above the medial rectus muscles. It passes below the trochlea before dividing into the frontal and angular branches.

The lacrimal artery originates from the second portion of the ophthalmic artery within the orbit, but the proximal portion is not well seen. In the lateral view, this vessel usually projects above the ophthalmic artery and extends anterior to the choroidal crescent, unlike the ciliary arteries. In the AP view, it can be seen passing towards the superolateral angle of the orbit.

The supraorbital artery is the most superior vessel on the lateral view, closely related to the orbital roof. In the AP view, it courses upward and medially towards the supraorbital foramen. The posterior and anterior ethmoidal arteries are relatively small branches noted in the midorbit and posterior orbit. The inferior muscular artery is the most inferior of the branches on the lateral film.

The choroidal crescent is a characteristic vascular blush outlining the posterior two thirds of the globe. It is best seen in the early venous phase, and may be indented by intraconal lesions. The superior and inferior vorticose veins can be seen in the venous phase passing posteriorly from the upper and lower margins of the globe. They outline the boundaries of the muscle cone.

Several anastomoses exist between the ophthalmic artery branches and those of the external carotid. In particular, anastomoses are present with the supraorbital, ethmoidal, lacrimal, infraorbital, and zygomaticofacial branches. Therefore, complete vascular assessment of the orbit should also include an external carotid arteriogram.

Dacryocystography

Dacryocystography is useful in patients presenting with epiphora, in which there may be a mechanical obstruction, inflammatory disease, tumor, fistula, diverticulum, lacrimal concretion, or postoperative failure (Fig. 3-7). CT scan shows the lacrimal sac and nasolacrimal duct but does not demonstrate the canaliculi or the site of stenosis or occlusion.

When radiographic contrast material, usually a water-soluble agent, is injected via a cannula into the inferior canaliculus, good opacification of the superior, inferior, and common canaliculi will be seen at the medial

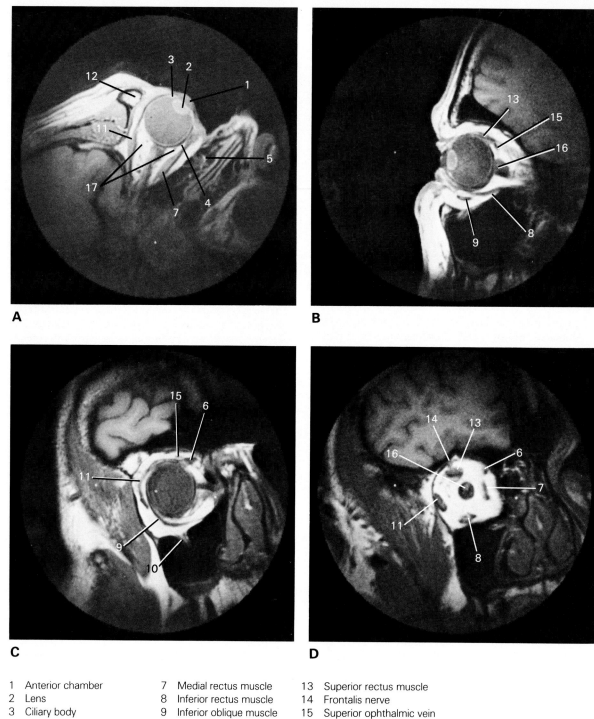

1	Anterior chamber	7	Medial rectus muscle	13	Superior rectus muscle
2	Lens	8	Inferior rectus muscle	14	Frontalis nerve
3	Ciliary body	9	Inferior oblique muscle	15	Superior ophthalmic vein
4	Sclera	10	Infraorbital nerve	16	Optic nerve
5	Ethmoid air cells	11	Lateral rectus muscle	17	Long posterior ciliary artery
6	Superior oblique muscle	12	Zygomatic bone		

FIGURE 3-8. MRI orbital images: *(A)* axial view of the mid-left orbit; *(B)* sagittal view through the mid-orbit; *(C)* coronal view through the anterior portion of the right orbit; and *(D)* coronal view through the mid-portion of the right orbit. (Reproduced with permission from the General Electric Company, 1985)

aspect of the orbit on the AP view. The Caldwell view is useful for showing these structures as well as the lacrimal sac and nasolacrimal duct. A narrowing at the inferior margin of the lacrimal sac, relating to the valve of Krause, is normally seen, as is a similar narrowing in the midportion of the nasolacrimal duct at Taillefer's valve. Narrowing at the distal end of the nasolacrimal duct is related to Hasner's valve. Contrast can normally be demonstrated extending into the inferior meatus where the duct empties.

This technique has the advantage of being relatively simple and inexpensive, and it provides exquisite anatomical detail of the nasolacrimal system.

Magnetic Resonance Imaging

Magnetic resonance imaging (MRI) is a recently developed imaging modality that already has proven superior to CT scanning for many intracranial applications (Fig. 3-8). In addition, the recent development of surface coil techniques has further improved spatial resolution of the orbit and subsequent application to certain orbital diseases. It is conceivable that in the future this technique will surpass CT for assessment of orbital disease.

MRI has remarkable sensitivity in demonstrating different tissue "intensities" as opposed to CT, which has good contrast resolution based on differences in tissue "densities." MRI signal intensity depends upon several parameters: hydrogen proton density as well as T1 and T2 relaxation times, which are specific for different tissues. CT densities depend primarily on differences in tissue electron density.

MRI has several advantages compared to CT scanning. MRI is noninvasive and does not involve any radiation. Images may be obtained in a variety of planes without repositioning the patient. Therefore, sagittal, coronal, axial, or oblique views are easily obtained. It is not as susceptible to image degradation from artifact, such as that caused by dental fillings. The remarkable sensitivity of MRI may permit it to be competitive with ultrasonography for assessing intraocular lesions.

The disadvantages of MRI relative to CT include greater sensitivity to patient motion, slightly less spatial resolution, and higher cost. MRI can adversely affect pacemaker function, and it can be hazardous in patients with intraorbital magnetic foreign bodies or intracranial aneurysm clips. Therefore, these patients should be excluded.

Soft tissue anatomy with MRI is very similar to that shown with CT. Orbital fat is very high intensity and serves to highlight other intraorbital structures, as it does

with CT scanning. The structure of the globe is better defined on MRI. Because of the lack of signal from cortical bone, the intracanalicular portion of the optic nerve can be better imaged with MRI than with CT. The optic chiasm is also more readily identified because of high signal intensity. MRI appears to provide superior definition of the optic nerve when mass lesions surround the nerve and obscure its boundary on CT scan. However, calcification gives no signal, and is therefore not readily identified on MRI. Thus, a subtle optic sheath meningioma is better identified with CT. This text emphasizes CT because of its common usage at the present time.

Summary

The imaging modalities described in this section are complementary in evaluating orbital disease. Angiography, venography, and dacryocystography have very specific indications. Plain films and complex motion tomography are primarily limited to bony assessment. CT scan provides excellent anatomical definition of bony and soft tissue anatomy and remains the primary imaging modality for orbital disease. MRI is still developing, and has proven complementary to CT in the study of certain orbital diseases.

Bibliography

Bilaniuk LT, Schenck JF, Zimmerman RA et al: Ocular and orbital lesions: Surface coil MR imaging. Radiology 156:669, 1985

Chambers EF, Manelfe C, Cellerier P: Metrizamide CT cisternography and perioptic subarachnoid space imaging. J Comput Assist Tomogr 5, No. 6:875, 1981

Daniels DL, Herfkins R, Gager WE et al: Magnetic resonance imaging of the optic neves and chiasm. Radiology 152:79, 1984

Dojon DL, Aron-Rosa DS, Ramee A: Orbital veins and cavernous sinus. In Newton TH, Potts DG (eds): Radiology of the Skull and Brain. Vol 2, Book 3, Angiography, p 2220. St Louis, CV Mosby, 1974

Forbes GS, Earnest IVF, Waller RR: Computed tomography of orbital tumors including late-generation scanning techniques. Radiology 142:387, 1982

Hammerschlag SB, O'Reilly GVA, Naheedy MH: Computed tomography of the optic canals. AJNR 2:593, 1981

Kline LB, Acker JD, Donovan Post MJ, Vitak JJ: The cavernous sinus: A computed tomographic study. AJNR 2:229, 1981

Lloyd GAS: Radiology of the Orbit. Philadelphia, WB Saunders, 1975

Moret J, Vignaud J: Topographic arteriography applied to the analysis of orbital masses and carotid cavernous fistulae. In Bergeron RT, Osborn AG, Som PM (eds): Head and Neck Imaging—Excluding the Brain, p 618. St Louis, CV Mosby, 1984

Moström U, Ytterberg C, Bergström K: Eye lens dose in cranial computed tomography with reference to the technical development of CT scanners. Acta Radiol [Diagn] (Stockh) 5:599, 1986

Peyster RG, Hoover ED, Hershey BL et al: High-resolution CT of lesions of the optic nerve. AJNR 4:169, 1983

Sargent EN, Ebersole C: Dacryocystography: The use of sinografin for visualization of the nasolacrimal passages. AJR 102:4:831, 1968

Tate E, Cupples H: Detection of orbital foreign bodies with computed tomography: Current limits. AJNR 2:363, 1981

Weinstein MA, Modic MR, Risius B et al: Visualization of the arteries, veins, and nerves of the orbit by sector computed tomography. Radiology 138:83, 1981

Pathophysiologic and Anatomic Principles of Classification, Diagnosis, and Investigation of Orbital Disease

CHAPTER 4
Pathophysiologic Patterns of Orbital Disease

Jack Rootman

Five processes can occur, either independently or together, within and around the orbit: inflammation; neoplasia; structural abnormality (acquired and congenital); vascular lesions; and degeneration and depositions. The processes are not mutually exclusive and may occur in concert, but for the most part in our experience one process is the dominant underlying pathophysiology of presentation. Based on over 1400 cases seen at the Orbital Clinic of the University of British Columbia, their incidence is as follows:

- Inflammation (overall): 57.3%
    Thyroid orbitopathy: 47.1%
    Other inflammations: 10.2%
- Neoplasia: 22.3%
- Structural abnormality: 15.8%
    Congenital: 7.1%
    Acquired: 8.7%
- Vascular lesions: 2.8%
- Degeneration and depositions: 1.7%

Inflammation

Overall, we found that inflammation accounts for close to 60% of primary orbital disease processes. The underlying pathophysiologic substrate determines the nature of the clinical presentation and development. The substrate ranges in character from acute inflammatory cells and their chemical intermediates, to delayed infiltrates in the case of some misdirected immune responses. Specifically in acute inflammation, polymorphonuclear leucocytes are usually the dominant cells inciting a rapid, frequently destructive process. In contrast, slower, more progressive disorders may have a substrate of lymphocytes, plasma cells, histiocytes, and fibroblasts (idiopathic sclerosing inflammations and Graves' disease), or a granulomatous infiltrate (lipogranulomatous inflammation and Wegeners' granulomatosis). As we learn more about the lymphocyte, it has become evident these cells can react with varying patterns ranging from a rapid to slow influx of cells, with corresponding clinical patterns.

The character and location of the infiltrate affects the clinical presentation, which may vary from acute (dominated by pain, injection, systemic malaise, and loss of function) to chronic, which may be characterized by an infiltrative picture dominated by entrapment or may simply produce a mass effect. This scheme reflects the fundamental and established pathophysiologic patterns of inflammatory disease, which may be acute, subacute, or chronic.

ACUTE INFLAMMATION

Acute inflammation is characterized by rapid development (days) and flagrant features of inflammation (warmth, injection, swelling, malaise, and loss of function). Infective cellulitis is the model for acute inflammation. It is inferred by rapid onset (days to weeks) of proptosis, pain, injection, and ultimately damage to the orbital and ocular structures. The majority of inflammatory disorders in this category are of sinus origin, especially in children, but they may be ocular, pyemic, or due to secondary infection of a wound. The location of the process determines the effect on the orbital structures. For instance, a preseptal infection rarely affects function of orbital structures initially, but may lead to damage of the lid structures (Fig. 4-1). On the other hand, sinusitis with orbital spread may have a profound and sudden effect on optic nerve and orbital function early in the course of the disease (Fig. 4-2).

Pathologically, acute bacterial infections draw polymorphonuclear leucocytes and their pharmacologic intermediates, which lead to necrosis and rapid destruction of tissue planes. Thus, the early manifestations are edema, injection, pain, loss of function, and systemic malaise with subsequent abscess formation and localization or spread if unchecked. On investigation, the progressive features reflect tissue swelling, infiltration, and

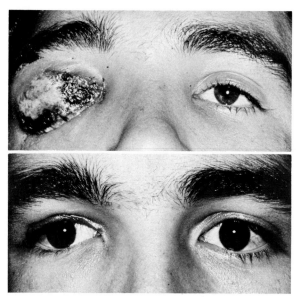

FIGURE 4-1. An acute necrotizing infective lesion of the preseptal lid is shown before *(above)* and after *(below)* treatment with systemic antibiotics and local measures. Note minor damage to lid structures only.

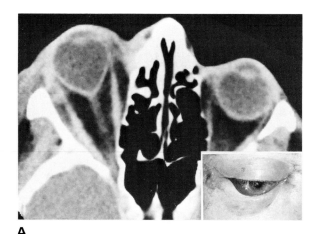

A

B

FIGURE 4-2. Acute sinus infection caused sudden and profound effects on ocular and orbital structures. *(A)* Note the marked tense proptosis with tenting of the globe and stretching of the optic nerve. *(B)* Proptosis and orbital tension were due to the sudden extension of purulent material into the superior subperiosteal space from a frontal sinus abscess. (*A:* Rootman J: The clinical evaluation and pathology of tumors of the eye, orbit and lacrimal apparatus. In Thawley SE (ed): Comprehensive Management of Head and Neck Tumors, Vol 2, Chap 68. Philadelphia, WB Saunders, 1987)

destruction with irregular margins, leading to abscess formation, loss of normal planes, separation of structures, and contrast enhancement.

The limited and practical differential diagnosis of acute inflammation might include about six disorders: infective cellulitis; acute (nonspecific) idiopathic inflammation of the orbit; acute ocular inflammation (uveitis, keratitis, scleritis); acute myositis (infective and noninfective); a sudden event in a pre-existing lesion (*e.g.,* a hemorrhage in a lymphangioma); and more rarely a fulminant neoplasm (such as chloroma, rhabdomyosarcoma, or metastasis). Fulminant neoplasia more commonly presents with patterns suggestive of subacute inflammation.

SUBACUTE INFLAMMATION

Subacute inflammation generally has two patterns, which take weeks to months to develop and tend to be associated with more subtle signs of inflammation. The first is a slow onset of displacement, injection, pain, and loss of function (*i.e.,* mass and functional effects), and the second is a remitting pattern with progressive signs and symptoms.

Many cases of infiltrative thyroid orbitopathy are good examples of progressive slower onset of inflammatory disease. The underlying immunopathogenic mechanism consists of lymphocytic, mast cell, and plasmacytic infiltration with increased mucopolysaccharides, connective tissue, and water content, affecting primarily the extraocular muscles and fat. Thus, the clinical pattern consists of swelling of the lids and conjunctiva, proptosis, injection, and diplopia. If the infiltration is significant, problems secondary to proptosis and motor involvement dominate the pattern. On the other hand, apical disease affects the optic nerve and extraocular movements at an early stage regardless of the degree of proptosis (Fig. 4-3).

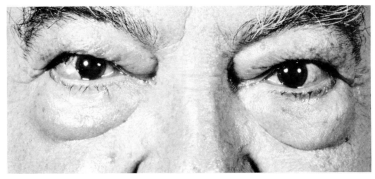

A

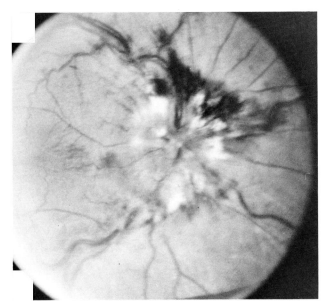

B

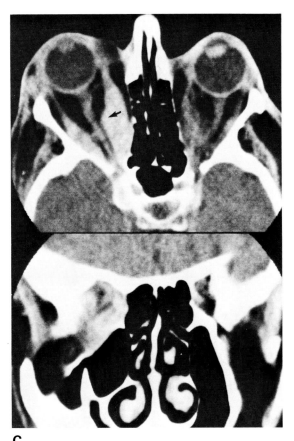

C

FIGURE 4-3.   Subacute inflammatory disease in a patient with infiltrative thyroid orbitopathy. *(A, B)* He showed lid swelling, chemosis, symmetrical limitation of movement, and papilledema. *(C)* These features were due to profound apical muscle swelling, leading to compressive optic neuropathy as shown on CT scan. Note posterior angulation of the muscle due to compression of the optic nerve *(arrow)*. (A, C: Rootman J: The clinical evaluation and pathology of tumors of the eye, orbit and lacrimal apparatus. In Thawley SE (ed): Comprehensive Management of Head and Neck Tumors, Vol 2, Chap 68. Philadelphia, WB Saunders, 1987)

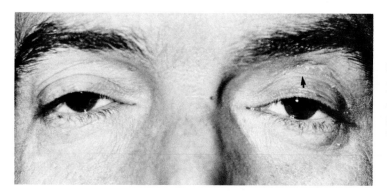

FIGURE 4-4.   The patient demonstrates a fistula *(arrow)* in the left upper lid, which was due to tracking of pus from the frontal sinus. He suffered from intermittent subacute inflammation as the result of recurrent closing and opening of the fistula.

The second subacute pattern is remitting. It is characterized by abeyance and exacerbations. A good example of this is an orbital inflammation that may occur secondary to sinus disease, especially in the adult. The remitting course is brought about by two factors. The first is the development of natural defense mechanisms such as fistula formation or drainage (Fig. 4-4). The second and more frequent cause is iatrogenic due to incomplete or inappropriate treatment for sinusitis with orbital cellulitis. To summarize, the subacute pattern is either slow and progressive or remitting in character. The basic differential diagnosis includes thyroid orbitopathy, infective cellulitis (especially fungal), idiopathic (nonspecific) orbital inflammations (especially granulomatous or persistent lymphocytic infiltrates), primary ocular inflammation (such as scleritis or uveitis), collagen vascular disease, and rapidly developing (fulminant) malignancies. Rarely, the vascular dilatation and tissue exudation associated with arteriovenous fistulas may produce a picture that can be confused with inflammation.

CHRONIC INFLAMMATION

Chronic orbital inflammation is dominated by silent or extremely low-grade signs of inflammation with a progressive pattern of displacement with or without evidence of entrapment and interference with orbital function. Thus, chronic inflammation may produce infiltrative disease (entrapment) or simply act to produce a mass effect. A classic chronic infiltrative pattern can be seen in the idiopathic sclerosing inflammations and some granulomatous orbital inflammations (Fig. 4-5). The inflammation stimulates a desmoplastic response that infiltrates the orbit, leading to fixation of structures. Investigations generally demonstrate loss of tissue planes with an irregular infiltrative mass. In the case of some destructive lesions, especially those arising from or adjacent to bone, infiltration and irregularity of bone may be noted. The differential diagnosis for chronic infiltrative inflammation includes lymphoproliferative disorders, thyroid ophthalmopathy, primary and secondary neoplasia, col-

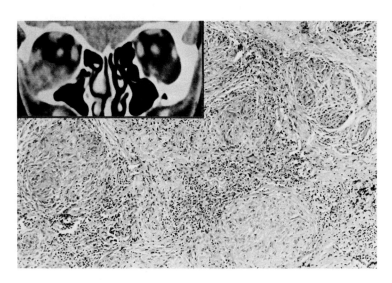

FIGURE 4-5.   Chronic infiltrative granulomatous inflammation of the orbit. Note the irregular infiltration of the inferior and lateral portion of the right orbit. Upgaze and abduction were limited due to entrapment of the inferior and lateral rectus muscles.

lagen vascular disease, idiopathic sclerosing infiltrations, and rare disorders such as amyloidosis.

On the other hand, chronic inflammatory lesions may simply produce a mass effect without evidence of infiltration or entrapment of orbital structures. The location of the mass will affect the clinical presentation. For example, a case of cholesterol granuloma in the roof of the orbit eroded bone and caused simple downward displacement without features of orbital entrapment (Fig. 4-6). The simple differential diagnosis of chronic inflammatory disease with mass effect includes any primary or secondary mass within the orbit.

Neoplasia

Neoplasia accounts for 22% of the orbital disease cases we have seen. The specific list of new growths is as long as the number of soft tissue tumors seen anywhere in the body, and is getting longer all the time. However, from a practical clinical and decision making point of view, they can be defined pathophysiologically on the basis of general biologic behavior. That is, they are either benign or malignant and may display infiltrative or noninfiltrative behavior. Clinically, the benign noninfiltrative masses are usually associated solely with mass effect without destruction or entrapment. In contrast, an infiltrative mass is usually associated with evidence of functional damage or entrapment. On investigation, both types are characterized by mass effect with displacement; however, malignant and infiltrative lesions may have irregular margins, entrap structures, and destroy bone, as opposed to smooth, regular, noninfiltrative masses.

The schwannoma is a good example of a benign, slow-growing, and progressive neoplasm that is associated with displacement of orbital structures. An example is a 60-year-old man who had right proptosis for 24 years before presenting with blurred vision and intermittent diplopia (Fig. 4-7, *A* and *B*). On CT scan, he had a well-defined intraconal mass with focal calcification, and on ultrasonography a solid mass. Angiography showed downward displacement of the ophthalmic artery without tumor blush or puddling; schwannoma was histologically confirmed (Fig. 4-7, *C* and *D*). Other tumors in this category include an array of soft tissue lesions such as cavernous hemangioma.

Benign infiltrative tumors include many types of locally invasive lesions. For example, we saw a case of granular cell tumor that was infiltrating and entrapped the anterior orbital structures, leading to restricted extraocular movements, proptosis, indentation of the posterior pole, and reduced vision (Fig. 4-8). Other benign neoplasias that may be infiltrative include fibrous histiocytoma and hemangiopericytoma.

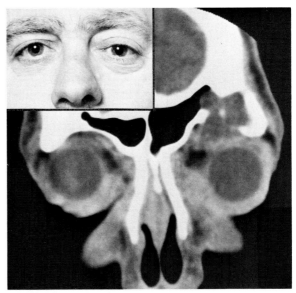

FIGURE 4-6.   This patient demonstrates the mass effect of a cholesterol granuloma that destroyed the superolateral bone of the orbit and displaced the orbital structures downward without infiltrating them. (Rootman J: The clinical evaluation and pathology of tumors of the eye, orbit and lacrimal apparatus. In Thawley SE (ed): Comprehensive Management of Head and Neck Tumors, Vol 2, Chap 68. Philadelphia, WB Saunders, 1987)

Histologically, malignant lesions can also have these two patterns of behavior. This is well demonstrated by two cases of the same tumor in the lacrimal gland that showed infiltrative and non-infiltrative behavior. A 70-year-old man presented with a 10-year history of slowly progressing proptosis and downward displacement of his left eye, with a sudden increase in signs and symptoms over the previous 6-months. He had marked proptosis, edema, ptosis, limitation of movement, and chemosis with a sensory deficit affecting the distribution of the lacrimal division of the fifth nerve. Investigations confirmed an infiltrative mass lesion arising from the lacrimal gland and destroying bone (Fig. 4-9). Histologically, it was a poorly differentiated mucoepidermoid carcinoma.

As demonstrated above, malignant lesions usually have infiltrative and destructive effects leading to displacement (mass effect) and functional deficits (motor, sensory, or visual). On the other hand, histologically malignant lesions can be less aggressive, as shown by another patient with a history of downward displacement of the eye and no evidence of interference with sensory or motor function. She had a lacrimal gland lesion without bone destruction but with excavation of the lacrimal fossa shown on plain films and CT scans, suggesting a long-standing noninfiltrative mass (Fig. 4-10). At surgery, it was well encapsulated. It proved to be a well-differentiated mucoepidermoid carcinoma of the lacrimal gland.

(Text continues on p. 62.)

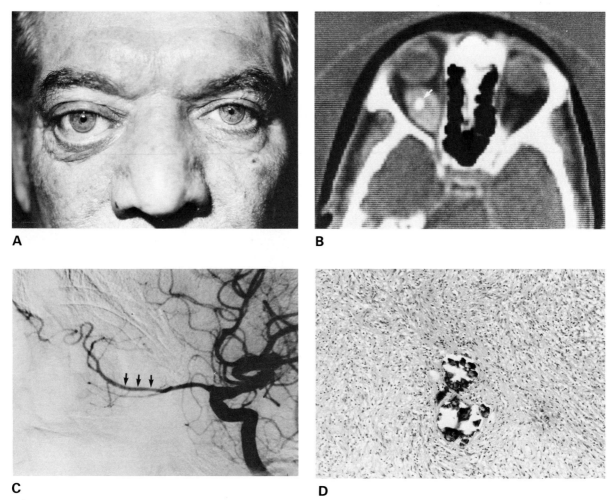

FIGURE 4-7.   This 60-year-old patient illustrates the features of a benign progressive noninfiltrative neoplasm. *(A)* He had long-standing proptosis of the right eye with recent slight blurring of vision and diplopia. *(B)* CT scan showed a well-defined intraconal mass with focal calcification. *(C)* Angiography showed downward displacement and slight narrowing of the ophthalmic artery *(arrows)* without tumor blush (ruling out meningioma) or pooling of contrast (weighing against cavernous hemangioma). *(D)* Histologically, it was a typical schwannoma with an area of calcification. (*C*: Rootman J: The clinical evaluation and pathology of tumors of the eye, orbit and lacrimal apparatus. In Thawley SE (ed): Comprehensive Management of Head and Neck Tumors, Vol 2, Chap 68. Philadelphia, WB Saunders, 1987)

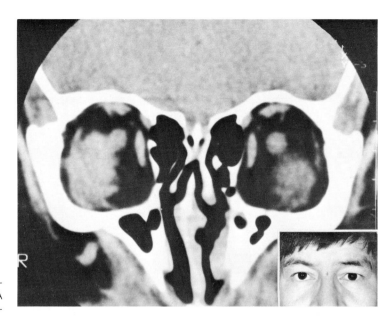

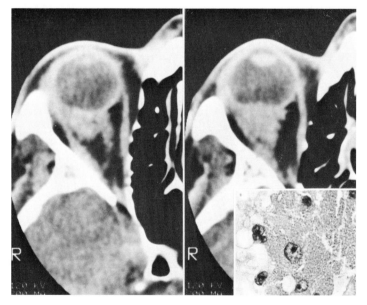

FIGURE 4-8.   *(Top)* This patient has a locally infiltrative benign neoplastic process. *(Bottom)* A granular cell tumor *(inset,* H&E, original magnification ×100) infiltrated the anterior portion of the orbit, restricting ocular movements, indenting the posterior pole, and reducing vision.

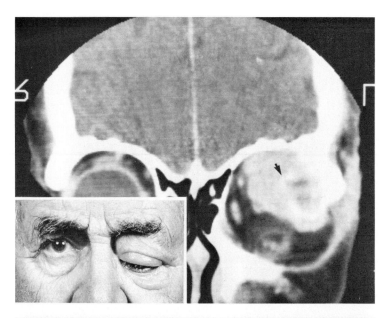

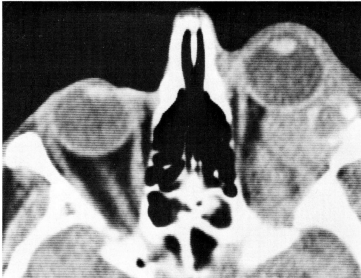

FIGURE 4-9.   The features of an infiltrative malignant epithelial tumor of the lacrimal gland. *(Top)* Clinically, the patient had a long-standing lesion with sudden growth over a 6-month period leading to ptosis, chemosis, and edema with limitation of ocular movements. *(Bottom)* Note irregular bony invasion and destruction, calcification, and apical infiltration of the orbit. Histologically, it was a poorly differentiated mucoepidermoid carcinoma.

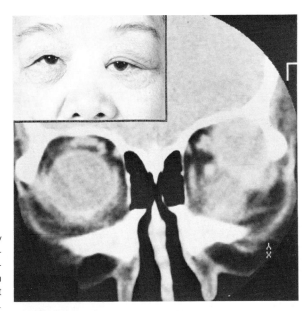

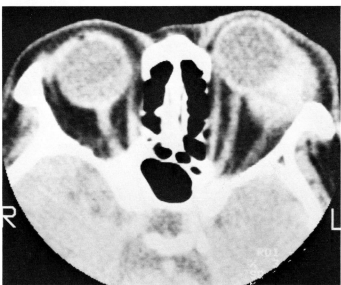

FIGURE 4-10.   *(Top)* This patient had a histologically diagnosed low grade malignant mucoepidermoid carcinoma of the lacrimal gland with features of long-standing growth. *(Bottom)* Note bony expansion in contrast to the irregular invasion seen in the malignant mucoepidermoid carcinoma shown in Figure 4-9. (Rootman J: The clinical evaluation and pathology of tumors of the eye, orbit and lacrimal apparatus. In Thawley SE (ed): Comprehensive Management of Head and Neck Tumors, Vol 2, Chap 68. Philadelphia, WB Saunders, 1987)

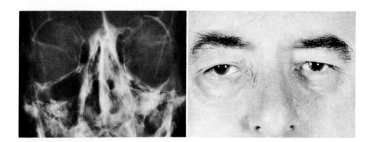

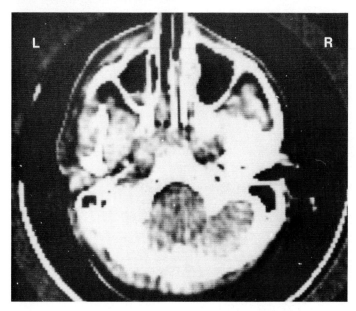

FIGURE 4-11. *(Top)* A patient with a congenital structural abnormality presented with apparent right proptosis; in fact, he has left enophthalmos. It was due to left maxillary hypoplasia resulting in enlargement of the left orbit shown on radiographs *(top)* and CT scan *(bottom)*. (Rootman J: The clinical evaluation and pathology of tumors of the eye, orbit and lacrimal apparatus. In Thawley SE (ed): Comprehensive Management of Head and Neck Tumors, Vol 2, Chap 68. Philadelphia, WB Saunders, 1987)

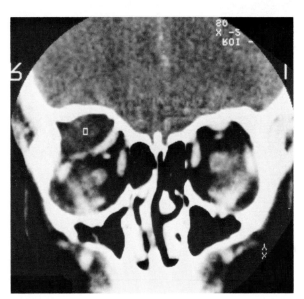

FIGURE 4-12. CT scan features of an irregular dermoid cyst that is a congenital ectopia. Note the low-density (fat-containing) lesion with irregular margins arising in bone above the level of the frontozygomatic suture.

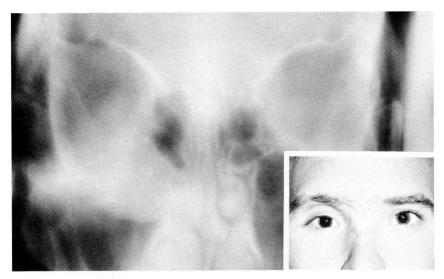

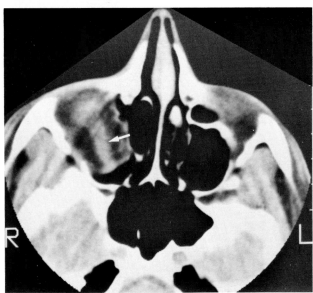

FIGURE 4-13. An acquired traumatic structural abnormality. *(Top)* The patient had right enophthalmos and globe ptosis due to a blow-out fracture shown on hypocycloidal polytomography. *(Bottom)* Axial CT scan shows the inferior rectus muscle and surrounding fat herniating through the defect *(arrow)*. (Rootman J: The clinical evaluation and pathology of tumors of the eye, orbit and lacrimal apparatus. In Thawley SE (ed): Comprehensive Management of Head and Neck Tumors, Vol 2, Chap 68. Philadelphia, WB Saunders, 1987)

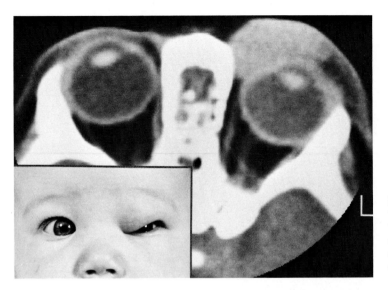

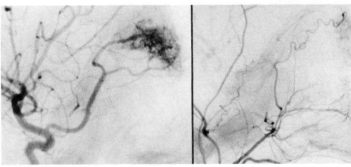

FIGURE 4-14.   This patient demonstrates an infantile capillary hemangioma with high arterial flow. *(Top)* Note the left-sided enhancing mass on CT scan. *(Bottom)* Rapid arterial filling is shown on both external and internal carotid angiography.

Structural Abnormalities: Congenital and Acquired

Structural lesions include congenital bony abnormalities such as Crouzon's disease or craniofacial dysostosis, maxillary hypoplasia, and facial asymmetry (Fig. 4-11). Structural abnormalities of a congenital nature include ectopias, such as dermoid cysts (Fig. 4-12). Acquired structural abnormalities are really posttraumatic lesions of the orbit, following all types of physical damage. The most common injury is a direct physical blow (Fig. 4-13), but other injuries result from thermal, chemical, and radiation-induced orbital damage. Included in this category are some of the cysts (dermoids, implantations, lacrimal cysts, mucoceles), and ectopias.

Vascular Lesions

Vascular lesions of the orbit constitute an important component of disease. In our experience, they were the fourth most common orbital process. Pathologically, a large number of diseases are included in this category; pathophysiologically, a few fundamental patterns can be seen based on the character of flow or the lack thereof (hemodynamics). The nonobstructive vascular lesions on the arterial side may be either high or low flow (including tumors, malformations, and fistulas). Venous lesions are either large or small venous anomalies (distensible and nondistensible varix). Hemodynamically, lymphangiomas are relatively isolated vascular anomalies. The obstructive lesions may be on the arterial or venous side.

A classic example of a high-flow tumor on the arterial side is seen in some infantile capillary hemangiomas (Fig. 4-14). These include the facial strawberry hemangiomas, which may have a spectrum of involvement from local superficial infantile hemangioma to massive facial lesions (combined infantile hemangiomas) with and without multiple external and internal hemangiomatosis. Histologically, they have many vascular channels and typically undergo spontaneous regression with time. However, these high-flow tumors may be intraorbital (deep infantile hemangiomas) and manifest pulsating exophthalmos due to their rich blood supply.

(Text continues on p. 67.)

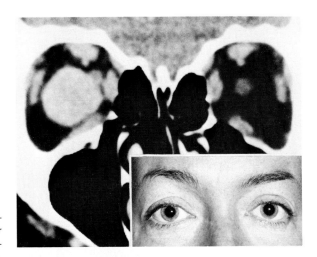

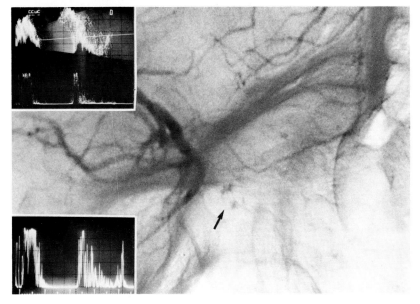

FIGURE 4-15.   This cavernous hemangioma is an example of a vascular tumor with low arterial flow. *(Top)* Note contrast enhancement on CT scan. *(Bottom)* There is late minimal pooling of contrast *(arrow)* on angiography. *Insets* demonstrate ultrasound features of this well-circumscribed echogenic mass on B scan with high and medium internal reflectivity and well-defined highly reflective borders on A scan.

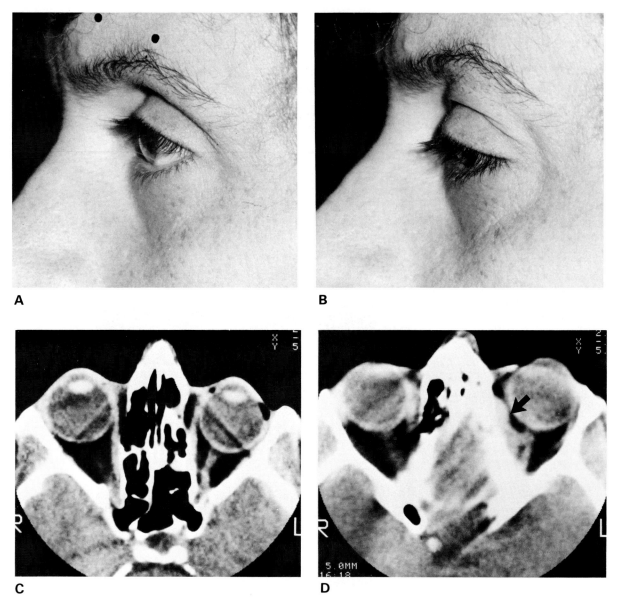

FIGURE 4-16.   This patient has the clinical and CT features of a distensible venous anomaly. *(A,C)* Note enophthalmos at rest, and *(B,D)* proptosis on Valsalva maneuver due to filling of the medial varix *(arrow)*. *(A – C*: Rootman J: The clinical evaluation and pathology of tumors of the eye, orbit and lacrimal apparatus. In Thawley SE (ed): Comprehensive Management of Head and Neck Tumors, Vol 2, Chap 68. Philadelphia, WB Saunders, 1987)

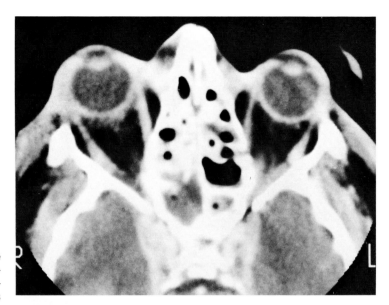

FIGURE 4-17. CT features of an obstructive vascular lesion. Sphenoid sinusitus led to cavernous sinus thrombosis. The cavernous sinus is enlarged and contains irregular low-density areas representing thrombus. *(Top)* Both orbits are engorged. *(Bottom)* An area of infarction is seen in the right frontal lobe as a result of cortical venous thrombosis. (Rootman J: The clinical evaluation and pathology of tumors of the eye, orbit and lacrimal apparatus. In Thawley SE (ed): Comprehensive Management of Head and Neck Tumors, Vol 2, Chap 68. Philadelphia, WB Saunders, 1987)

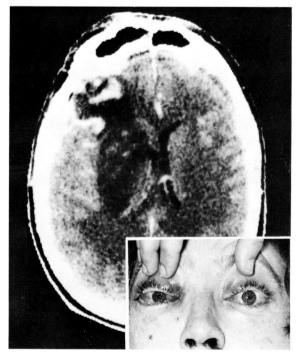

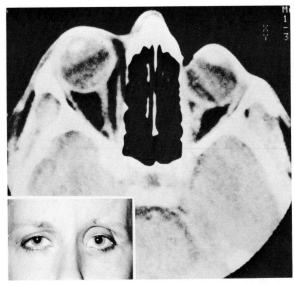

FIGURE 4-18.   This patient has a degenerative disease process. Linear scleroderma was associated with focal frontal dermal and orbital fat atrophy, with scarring of the lid and medial rectus muscle.

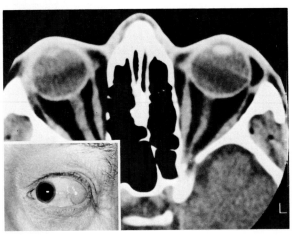

FIGURE 4-19.   A degenerative lesion of the orbit. Note the superior lateral fat prolapse due to a defect in Tenon's capsule.

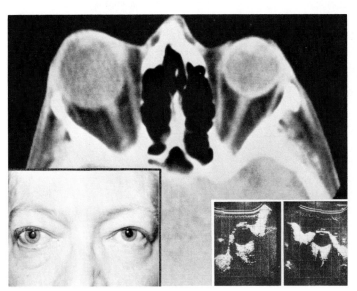

FIGURE 4-20.   Another degenerative process leading to pseudoproptosis is progressive myopia. Note enlarged right myopic globe on CT scan and ultrasound. (Rootman J: The clinical evaluation and pathology of tumors of the eye, orbit and lacrimal apparatus. In Thawley SE (ed): Comprehensive Management of Head and Neck Tumors, Vol 2, Chap 68. Philadelphia, WB Saunders, 1987)

The cavernous hemangioma is a vascular tumor with low arterial flow. It grows slowly in the orbit of the adult. It is a well-defined lesion on ultrasonography, enhances on contrast CT scanning, and shows minimal late pooling on angiography (Fig. 4-15).

With congenital or acquired arteriovenous fistulas and malformations, the site of arteriovenous communication (shunt) may also be either large or small, resulting in high-flow or low-flow lesions. The larger the shunt, the more profound the orbital findings. A high-flow shunt demonstrates pulsating exophthalmos, bruit, and marked orbital swelling clinically, which may be substantiated on CT scan and on arteriography. In contrast, a low-flow carotid–cavernous fistula may manifest milder elevations of venous pressure leading to dilated episcleral, orbital, and intraocular veins and features of milder proptosis, raised intraocular pressure, and an absent or minimal bruit.

On the venous side of the circulation, there are a number of lesions that may have either large venous connections (distensible) or small venous connections (nondistensible). For example, the clinically nondistensible varix has minimal flow, and thus tends to present as a spontaneous thrombosis or hemorrhagic episode. However, these may also present as slowly progressive asymptomatic tumors resulting from microscopic thrombosis and hemorrhage. In contrast, the large venous shunts frequently present with enophthalmos and have intermittent proptosis on raising the jugular venous pressure (Fig. 4-16). Some of the foregoing lesions have either arterial or venous obstructive elements. However, arterial and venous obstruction can be part of other systemic and local processes. An example is a patient with sudden chemosis, edema, and retinal venous dilatation due to orbital vein thrombosis secondary to sphenoid sinusitis (Fig. 4-17).

Degenerations and Depositions

Degenerations include orbital diseases characterized by atrophy, deposition, and cicatrization. Progressive myopathy and amyloid deposition are examples of degenerative processes and depositions. Another example we have encountered was noted in a patient with linear scleroderma with facial and orbital atrophy associated with cicatrization of the lid and medial extraocular muscles (Fig. 4-18). On the other hand, orbital fat prolapse through Tenon's capsule may present with the patient having noted a tumor, especially when pressure was applied to the eye. This results from weakening of the orbital connective tissue with age (Fig. 4-19). Progressive myopia is another degenerative process that may present as pseudoproptosis (Fig. 4-20). Finally, localized amyloidosis is an example of a deposition that may occur in the orbit, and lead to functional and structural changes that may reflect an underlying inflammatory pathogenesis.

The foregoing is meant to serve as a logical, clinically based formulation for thinking about orbital disease. As in all simplifications, it has exceptions. However, for the most part it provides an accurate method of viewing orbital disease in the clinical setting.

CHAPTER 5

Anatomic Patterns of Orbital Disease

Jack Rootman

The effect of any disease process in the orbit is governed not only by the primary nature of the process (pathophysiology) but also by the anatomic pattern of involvement. Location profoundly affects clinical presentation; for instance, a small tumor in the orbital apex may produce an early disturbance of the second, third, fourth, fifth, or sixth nerves. An example is a case of a hemangiopericytoma that presented with the rapid loss of vision (Fig. 5-1A). In contrast, a more laterally placed apical meningioma affected the structures of the superior orbital fissure before the optic nerve (Fig. 5-1B). In simple terms, disease can be viewed as having either functional or mass effect. It is the character of these effects that helps to discern location of disease. Functional effect interferes with the motor, sensory, or secretory physiology of orbital structures. Mass effect shifts or displaces orbital structures by occupying space (positive effect), by increasing space (bone expansion, a negative effect), or by cicatrization (negative effect). For instance, an ethmoidal mass causes lateral displacement (positive effect), whereas destruction of the orbital floor leads to enophthalmos and downward displacement (negative effect). A desmoplastic process such as a metastatic carcinoma may tether and trap structures and lead to traction of structures toward it as well as entrapment (negative effect) (Fig. 5-2).

The patterns of anatomic involvement can be divided into anterior, diffuse, apical, lacrimal, myopathic, ocular, intraconal, optic nerve, periorbital, and lacrimal drainage system. Disease in any of these areas tends to produce signs and symptoms that reflect their location. For instance, using inflammatory disease as examples, the effect of location on presentation can be demonstrated. We have classified acute idiopathic (nonspecific) orbital inflammatory disease using an anatomic model. This includes five locations of anterior, diffuse, apical, lacrimal, and myopathic idiopathic inflammations. All of the acute and subacute idiopathic inflammations are characterized by the rapid onset of clinical features of inflammation in the orbit and differ in presentation on the basis of primary site of involvement.

Anterior

The anterior or periocular idiopathic inflammations may be characterized by pain, diplopia, chemosis, lid swelling, injection, uveitis, papillitis, optic neuropathy, and even exudative inflammatory retinal detachment (Fig. 5-3). All of these features relate to the location and severity of the process anteriorly within the orbit adjacent to and affecting the globe. A typical patient presents with proptosis, chemosis, lid injection, retinal venous dilatation, and possible uveitis. Characteristically, on CT investigation a contrast-enhancing anterior orbital infiltration intimately related to the globe produces scleral and choroidal thickening, obscuring the junction of the globe and optic nerve extending variably along the sheath. Ultrasonography localizes the anterior inflammatory process and demonstrates a sclerotenonitis.

Diffuse

Diffuse idiopathic inflammation is similar in clinical presentation to anterior, but is more severe with profound features of inflammation consisting of uveitis and papillitis (Fig. 5-4). It is frequently associated with optic neuropathy and motor and sensory orbital deficits. CT scan shows the entire orbit to be involved by a diffuse, poorly defined contrast-enhancing infiltrate.

Apical

Perineural or apical acute idiopathic inflammation produces less proptosis, pain, or visible inflammation, but is associated with the early development of optic neuropa-

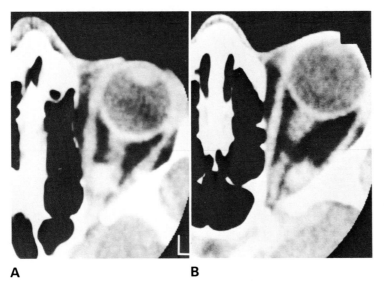

A   B

FIGURE 5-1. Two apical lesions in which slightly different locations affected presentation. The hemangiopericytoma *(A)* presented with the sole feature of visual deterioration due to compressive optic neuropathy. In contrast, the meningioma *(B)* presented with proptosis, venous congestion, and mild optic neuropathy reflecting compression of structures passing through the superior orbital fissure. (Rootman J: The clinical evaluation and pathology of tumors of the eye, orbit and lacrimal apparatus. In Thawley SE (ed): Comprehensive Management of Head and Neck Tumors, Vol 2, Chap 68. Philadelphia, WB Saunders, 1987)

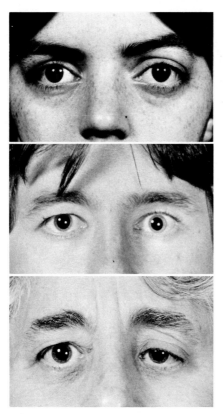

FIGURE 5-2. Three different mass effects. *(Top)* A positive mass effect led to lateral displacement of the left eye from an ethmoidal fibrous dysplasia. *(Middle)* A negative effect of enophthalmos and downward displacement of the left eye was due to a blow-out fracture with depression of the orbital floor. *(Bottom)* A cicatrizing metastatic carcinoma caused a negative effect of left enophthalmos.

thy or motor and sensory symptoms (Fig. 5-5). In addition, when a process affects the superior orbital fissure at the apex, vascular congestion due to obstruction of the superior or inferior ophthalmic veins may be a clinical feature. Thus, the patient characteristically reports pain, limitation of movement, or visual deficit typical of the so-called orbital apex syndromes. CT scans confirm apical and perineural inflammation consistent with the clinical syndrome.

Lacrimal

Acute idiopathic lacrimal inflammation typically presents with localized pain, tenderness, injection of the temporal lid and fornix with a palpable lacrimal gland, an S-shaped deformity of the lid, and often pouting of the lacrimal ducts (Fig. 5-6). The anatomic localization on CT scan and ultrasonography reveals an irregular, poorly defined infiltrate confined to the superolateral aspect of the orbit, adjacent to and obscuring the lateral part of the globe, which is displaced down and in.

Myopathic

Acute idiopathic inflammations of muscle are characterized by pain with eye movement, localized injection of the globe over the insertion of the affected muscle, and reduced ocular motility (Fig. 5-7). On CT scan and ultrasonography, the contrast-enhancing irregular infiltrate involves one or more extraocular muscles with relatively diffuse enlargement extending up to the globe and usually including the tendon.

(Text continues on p. 75.)

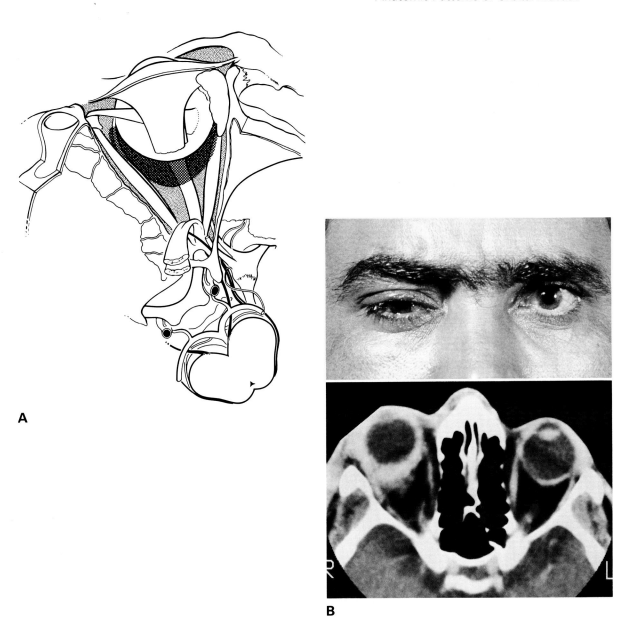

A

B

FIGURE 5-3.   *(A)* Schematic of anterior (periocular) pattern of involvement in a case of acute anterior idiopathic inflammation. *(B, top)* Clinically, it was characterized by pain, right ptosis, chemosis, injection, proptosis (3 mm), and mild exudative retinal detachment with decreased vision (20/60). *(B, bottom)* CT scan with contrast shows an irregular enhancing lesion of the anterior orbit associated with a thickened sclerochoroidal rim. These features may be indistinguishable from scleritis. The patient responded promptly to oral corticosteroids.

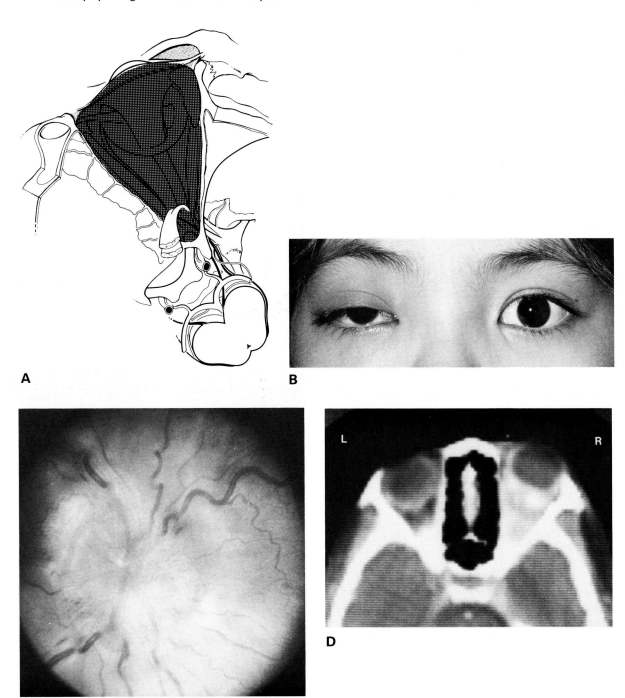

FIGURE 5-4. *(A)* Schematic of diffuse orbital disease in a case of acute idiopathic inflammation. *(B)* The adolescent patient presented with ptosis, chemosis, injection, uveitis, *(C)* papillitis, and limited painful extraocular movements. *(D)* Contrast-enhanced CT scan demonstrates an irregular contrast-enhancing lesion affecting the whole orbit and posterior portion of the globe. The patient responded promptly to oral corticosteroids.

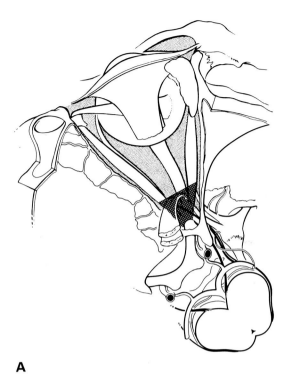

A

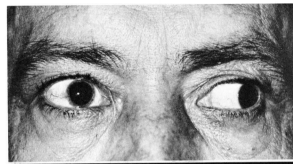

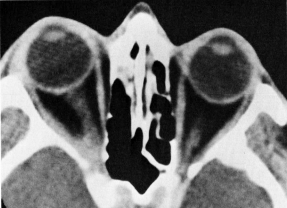

B

FIGURE 5-5.   *(A)* Schematic demonstrates the major orbital structures affected by the apical pattern of disease. *(B, top)* Clinical features of an acute idiopathic apical inflammatory disease are shown in a middle-aged patient who presented with sudden onset of a painful ophthalmoplegia with limitation of right ocular movement, profound optic neuropathy (hand movements), mild proptosis, and minimal signs of ocular or lid inflammation. *(B, bottom)* CT scan demonstrates an irregular infiltration of the orbital apical structures with mild swelling of the optic nerve. The patient responded rapidly to oral corticosteroids.

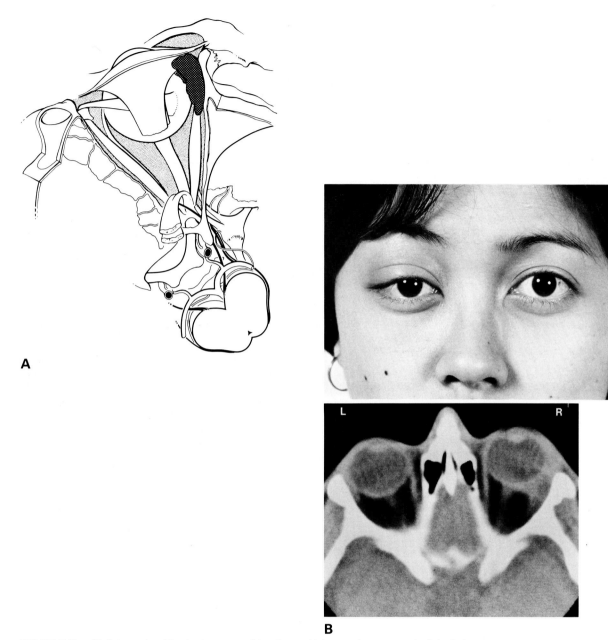

FIGURE 5-6. *(A)* Schematic of lacrimal pattern of location, which was demonstrated clinically in a 25-year-old woman who presented with an idiopathic inflammatory lesion of the right lacrimal gland. *(B, top)* Note superolateral lid swelling, S-shaped deformity of the lid, mild local chemosis, lid swelling, and injection. *(B, bottom)* CT scan shows an irregular lacrimal mass that proved inflammatory on biopsy, and responded to oral corticosteroids.

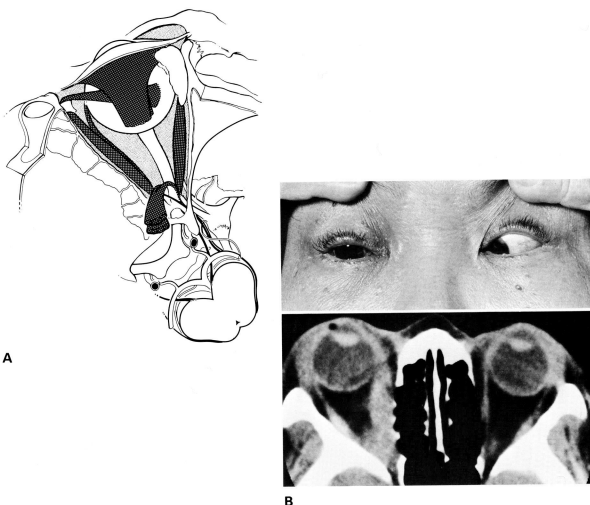

A

B

FIGURE 5-7.   *(A)* Schematic demonstrates myopathic pattern of orbital disease. A 60-year-old woman presented with painful subacute idiopathic myositis. *(B, top)* Note limitation of ocular movement on the right, medial chemosis and injection, swollen lid, and mild ptosis and proptosis. *(B, bottom)* Diffuse swelling and contrast enhancement of the entire medial rectus muscle and tendon confirmed the diagnosis. The patient responded promptly to systemic corticosteroids.

The remaining anatomic patterns of disease can be demonstrated using an inflammatory model. They include ocular, periorbital, intraconal, optic nerve, and lacrimal drainage locations.

Ocular

Ocular inflammation obviously can extend to involve surrounding orbital structures as demonstrated by a patient presenting with keratitis, uveitis, conjunctivitis, and scleritis due to Cogan's syndrome (Fig. 5-8). In addition, there was clinical evidence of anterior orbital inflamma-

tion leading to ptosis and lid swelling. Investigations show thickening of the globe and anterior orbital infiltration on CT scan with evidence of sclerotenonitis on ultrasonography. A conjunctival biopsy confirmed perivasculitis.

Periorbital

Diseases originating from the sinuses, face, and intracranial cavity may extend into and affect the orbit by contiguity or as the result of damage to neurosensory or vascu-

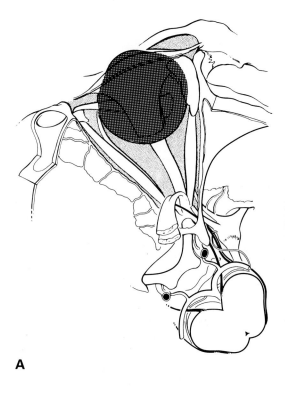

A

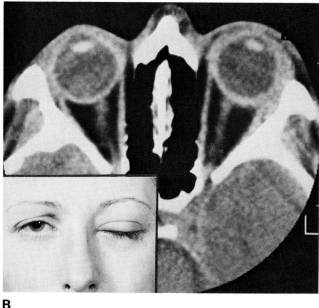

B

FIGURE 5-8. *(A)* Schematic of ocular pattern of orbital disease. *(B, inset)* Clinically, the patient had acute left lid swelling, ptosis, and mild proptosis. This was associated with hearing loss. On slit lamp examination, she had superficial corneal infiltrates. Conjunctival biopsy showed perivasculitis. These features were all consistent with a diagnosis of Cogan's syndrome. *(B)* The CT scan shows mild thickening of the globe, lid, and lacrimal gland. (*B*: Rootman J: The clinical evaluation and pathology of tumors of the eye, orbit and lacrimal apparatus. In Thawley SE (ed): Comprehensive Management of Head and Neck Tumors, Vol 2, Chap 68. Philadelphia, WB Saunders, 1987)

lar structures shared with the orbit. This is well demonstrated in sinus inflammation where the clinical presentation varies depending on the location of primary sinus disease and the stage of the process. These may include diffuse cellulitis, fistulization, recurrent inflammation, or acute proptosis secondary to subperiosteal abscess formation (Fig. 5-9C). Intracranial lesions may also secondarily affect structures supplying the orbit or may indeed extend into the orbit (Fig. 5-9B).

Intraconal

Lesions within the muscle cone produce axial displacement and functional deficit of the eye, optic nerve, muscles, and ciliary ganglion. Figure 5-10 shows bilateral in-

traconal sclerosing inflammation that led to axial proptosis and limitation of extraocular movements.

Optic Nerve

Included in this category of anatomic involvement are diseases primarily affecting the optic nerve (Fig. 5-11). Here the effect of disease is also governed by whether or not the process is intrinsic to the nerve or affects the nerve from the sheath outside its axis. The difference is demonstrated by intrinsic optic neuritis versus optic sheath inflammations. However, the pathophysiology of the difference is better defined by tumors, where the onset, character, progression, and clinical signs and

(Text continues on p. 80.)

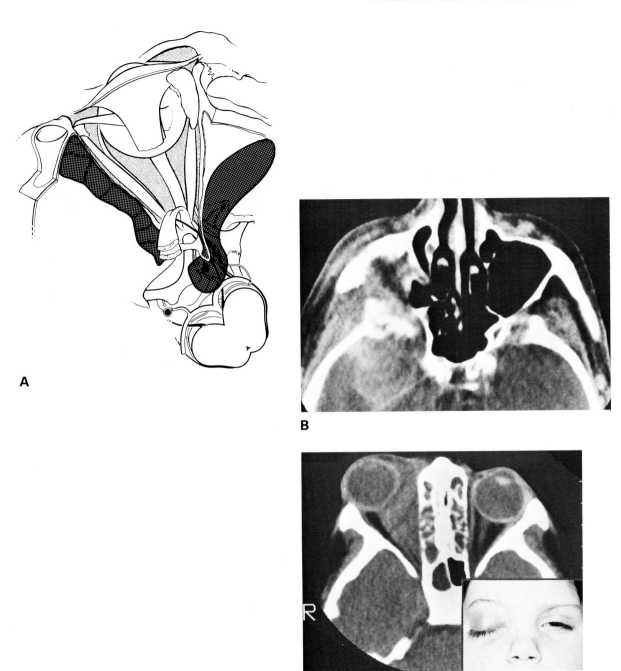

FIGURE 5-9. *(A)* Schematic demonstrates periorbital sources of disease, which may arise from the sinuses, bone, or intracranial structures. *(B)* CT scan shows a metastatic carcinoma of the prostate, which caused bony destruction (bilateral) of the sphenoid wing with soft tissue involvement of the right middle cranial fossa, floor of the orbit, and maxillary sinus. *(C)* Ethmoid sinus infection and a subperiosteal abscess caused sudden tense proptosis, lateral displacement, ptosis, and optic neuropathy. (*C*: Rootman J: The clinical evaluation and pathology of tumors of the eye, orbit and lacrimal apparatus. In Thawley SE (ed): Comprehensive Management of Head and Neck Tumors, Vol 2, Chap 68. Philadelphia, WB Saunders, 1987)

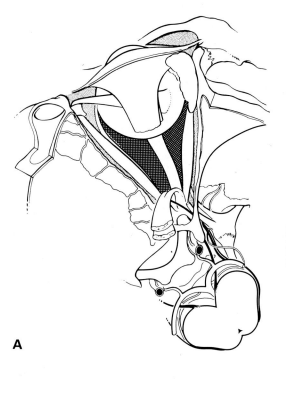

A

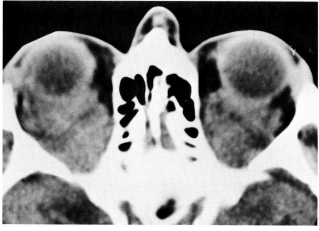

B

FIGURE 5-10. *(A)* Schematic of intraconal location. *(B)* Clinically, bilateral intraconal infiltrative disease was found, which proved on biopsy to be idiopathic sclerosing inflammation of the orbit.

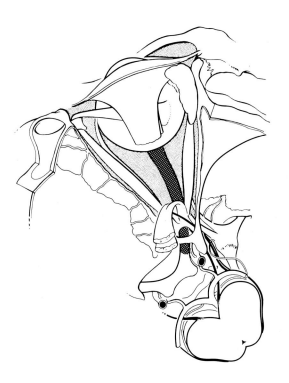

FIGURE 5-11. Schematic of optic nerve location of disease. Clinically, it is primarily associated with psychophysical abnormalities.

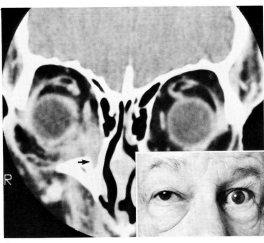

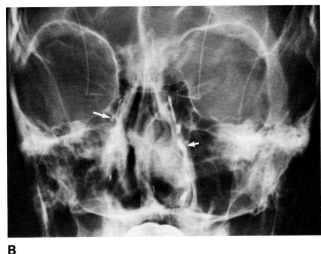

A   **B**

FIGURE 5-12.   *(A)* Lacrimal drainage system location is demonstrated in a patient who presented with swelling of the right lower lid, upward displacement of the globe, limitation of elevation, and tearing. CT scan shows an irregular infiltrative mass *(arrow)* involving the anterior inferior orbit with entrapment of the inferior oblique muscle and lacrimal drainage system. *(B)* A dacryocystogram of the same patient shows obstruction on the right *(long arrow)* in contrast to the open system on the left *(short arrow)*. Biopsy showed an idiopathic sclerosing inflammatory process. *(A, B*: Rootman J: The clinical evaluation and pathology of tumors of the eye, orbit and lacrimal apparatus. In Thawley SE (ed): Comprehensive Management of Head and Neck Tumors, Vol 2, Chap 68. Philadelphia, WB Saunders, 1987)

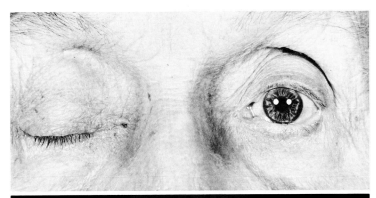

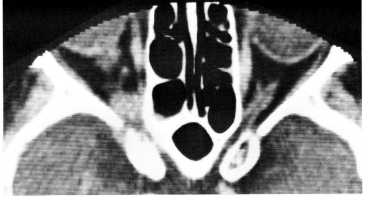

FIGURE 5-13.   Clinical photograph demonstrates right ptosis *(top)*, which was associated with compressive optic and motor neuropathy due to an apical metastatic carcinoma *(bottom)*.

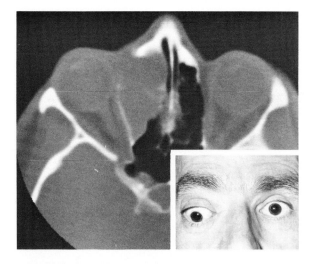

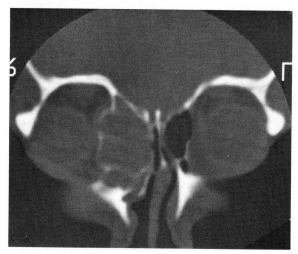

FIGURE 5-14.   A mass (mucocele) arising in the right frontoethmoid complex caused downward and outward displacement of the globe *(top)*, demonstrating the effect of the periorbital location of disease *(bottom)*. (Rootman J: The clinical evaluation and pathology of tumors of the eye, orbit and lacrimal apparatus. In Thawley SE (ed): Comprehensive Management of Head and Neck Tumors, Vol 2, Chap 68. Philadelphia, WB Saunders, 1987)

symptoms may be different for intrinsic tumors (gliomas) versus optic sheath tumors (meningiomas).

Lacrimal Drainage System

Inflammation in the lacrimal drainage system can lead to tearing, anterior orbital and lid swelling, upward or lateral displacement, and fistulization (Fig. 5-12). The effect depends on the severity and nature of the primary process.

Summary

Inflammatory disease has for the most part been used to demonstrate the anatomic pattern of disease, but all other diseases can be viewed in a similar manner. The effects of these disease processes are governed by the pathophysiologic disturbance they cause in that location. For instance, neoplasia may be lacrimal, periorbital, neural, or apical in the case of benign mixed tumor of the lacrimal gland, carcinoma of the sinus, optic nerve glioma, and sphenoid wing meningioma, respectively. The major difference is that neoplasms are usually dominated by noninflammatory mass effects or infiltration (entrapment). Anterior lesions cause greater direct ocular effects due to the immediate relationship to the globe, whereas diffuse diseases involve motor and sensory structures of the entire orbit and may lead to fixation of the globe and sensory deficits (pain, paresthesia, or loss of visual function). Apical disease tends to affect the optic, motor, and sensory nerves earlier as in a case of minimal apical infiltration by a metastatic carcinoma with profound early motor loss (ptosis and limitation of movement), sensory deficit (paresthesia), and visual loss without much evidence of mass effect (proptosis) (Fig. 5-13). Lacrimal pathology is dominated by functional (tearing or drying) and structural alterations of the gland, lacrimal fossa, and the outer third of the upper lid. A tumor here may cause displacement of the globe down and in, sensory defects of the frontotemporal and frontozygomatic nerves, and a S-shaped deformity of the lid. Myopathic disease such as thyroid ophthalmopathy leads to restriction of ocular movement due to a combination of mass effect, scarring, or neuromuscular dysfunction. Ocular diseases have symptomatic functional changes (*e.g.,* visual loss, floaters, photopsia, pain, photophobia) affecting primarily vision, and are usually readily accessible to clinical examination of the globe. Processes within the tight periorbital space can cause profound and even sudden effects (*e.g.,* an abscess), with the displacement governed by the site of involvement. A mass arising from the ethmoids causes lateral; the roof, downward (Fig. 5-14); and the floor upward displacement. Disease of the lacrimal drainage system is usually characterized functionally by obstruction leading to tearing with or without recurrent infection. Mass effect here leads to lateral and upward displacement with anterior tumefaction.

Because of the complicated nature of the orbit as an organ system, location of disease can usually be defined from the signs and symptoms produced. Awareness of the effect of site on the signs and symptoms of orbital disease makes clinical analysis more pertinent and accurate.

CHAPTER 6

Pathophysiologic Approach to Clinical Analysis of Orbital Disease

Jack Rootman

When confronted with a patient suspected of having orbital disease, the clinician may feel confused. Yet, there are basic clinical patterns that provide a framework for analyzing each case. The clinical analysis sets the stage for other investigations and is still our most reliable tool. I like to analyze a case by trying to locate and characterize the process induced by the disease. Essentially, history-taking and physical examination should be directed to answering two questions:

- Where is the disease located?
- How has the disease affected the orbital structures, that is, what dynamic alteration has it caused?

With the answers to these two questions synthesized, the clinician is ready to formulate a plan for further investigation.

Principles

LOCATION OF DISEASE

The "where" question is usually the easiest to answer. Clues to location can be obtained by analysis of mechanical displacement of orbital structures. When a disease process shifts orbital structures, the direction of shift is a clue to the location of the disease. The effect can be viewed as positive if the disease occupies space and pushes structures away (Fig. 6-1) and negative if it draws structures towards it through cicatrization (Fig. 6-2), excavation (Fig. 6-3), or both. An excavating effect may be due to atrophy of contents or enlargement of the orbit secondary to hypoplasia of adjacent structures, expansion, trauma, or lytic disturbances of bone.

The physical examination should provide information on the degree and direction of displacement of the affected orbital structures. Displacement of the eye should be measured in the following manner:

1. Measure horizontal displacement by recording the distance at the level of the canthi from the center of the nose to the medial edge of the limbus with the patient looking in the axial direction (Fig. 6-4A).
2. Measure vertical displacement by recording the position of the globe above or below the level of the canthi (Fig. 6-4B).
3. Measure proptosis with an exophthalmometer, one eye at a time, with the patient regarding an object (preferably your eye) along his central axis (Fig. 6-4C).

In addition to mechanical clues to location, functional deficits may help in defining the "where" of disease. For instance, apically located disease may have disproportionate visual, sensory, and motor deficit when compared to the degree of displacement of structures. Or a disease primarily affecting motor function may direct attention to the neuromuscular structures of the orbit.

DYNAMIC ALTERATION

Dynamic alteration is more difficult to assess and requires the analysis of two basic clinical features of disease: temporal change and the abnormal process.

Temporal Change

Evidence of temporal change in the disease, such as diurnal variation or an intermittent nature, should be extracted from the patient's history, with special emphasis

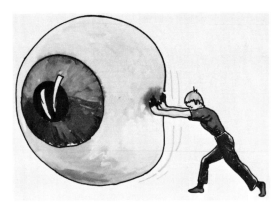

FIGURE 6-1. Positive effect of orbital disease: the lesion pushes orbital structures (in this case, the globe) away from it. (Rootman J: An approach to diagnosis of orbital disease. Can J Ophthalmol 18:102, 1983)

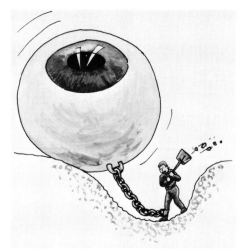

FIGURE 6-3. Ocular displacement may be due either to cicatrization of orbital contents, or to traumatic or lytic dehiscence of bone with or without surrounding atrophy. (Rootman J: An approach to diagnosis of orbital disease. Can J Ophthalmol 18:103, 1983)

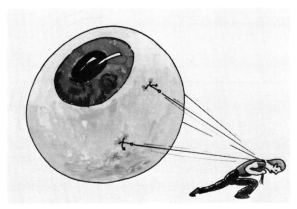

FIGURE 6-2. Negative effect of orbital disease: the disease process draws structures towards it. (Rootman J: An approach to diagnosis of orbital disease. Can J Ophthalmol 18:103, 1983)

on time of onset and rapidity of development. For example, many patients with thyroid ophthalmopathy have more proptosis, lid edema, and diplopia in the morning as a result of accentuation of orbital swelling due to lying prone all night.

Both the time and the rapidity of onset of the change may provide a clue to the nature of the underlying disease. A catastrophic change occurring over several hours suggests either hemorrhage in a pre-existing lesion or fulminant inflammation with or without a pre-existing lesion. A change that is somewhat less rapid but progressive suggests either an inflammatory process or fulminant neoplasia. On the other hand, an insidious change may be due to low-grade inflammation or neoplasia, either benign or malignant. Finally, an intermittent change, such as pulsation or alteration with a Valsalva maneuver, sug-

gests either a bony defect in the wall of the orbit or a relation between the lesion and the vascular system.

The Abnormal Process

Abnormal changes can be divided into four basic clinical categories. They are not necessarily independent, but provide a working framework for characterization of a particular orbital problem. One tends to associate certain clinical signs with each of these processes.

- *Inflammatory signs.* Inflammation is characterized by and can be inferred from signs and symptoms of pain, warmth, loss of function, and a mass effect. The degree to which one categorizes the process as either acute or chronic is related to the severity of the signs and symptoms and the rapidity of their onset.
- *Mass effect.* A mass effect consists of displacement with or without signs of involvement of sensory or neuromuscular structures. Displacement points to the location of the disease and may help to characterize its nature.
- *Infiltrative change.* Infiltrative diseases are usually associated with evidence of destruction, entrapment, or both. This includes effects on ocular movement or neurosensory function (*e.g.,* diplopia, muscle restriction or fibrosis, optic neuropathy, pain, or paresthesia).
- *Vascular change.* Alteration in the character, size, and structural integrity of vessels may imply an underlying vascular process. The major features implying vascu-

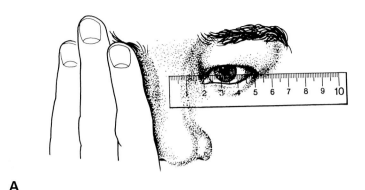

A

FIGURE 6-4. *(A)* Measurement of horizontal displacement of eye by recording distance (in millimeters) at level of canthi from center of nose to medial edge of limbus. *(B)* Measurement of vertical displacement of eye by recording position of globe above or below level of canthi. *(C)* Measurement of proptosis with exophthalmometer: with other eye occluded, patient looks along central axis. (*C:* Rootman J: An approach to diagnosis of orbital disease. Can J Ophthalmol 18:103, 1983)

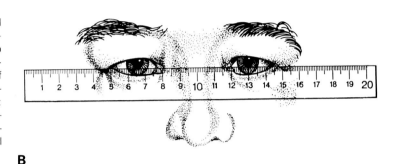

B

C

lar disease consist of venous dilatation, tissue exudation, hemorrhage, infarction, and structural alterations of vascular components.

Examination of the Orbital Patient

Examination of the orbit should seek to glean information that provides for a pathophysiologic analysis of the patient. Although I personally disparage a mechanical approach to patients, it is useful to have a conceptual framework for obtaining the necessary information. This information can then be synthesized and an appropriate plan of investigation established.

HISTORY OF PRESENT ILLNESS

The history of the present illness should place emphasis on elucidating temporal dynamics and major physiologic symptoms. The temporal dynamics include questions concerning the onset, duration, intermittency, and chronicity of disease. It is frequently useful to ask patients for old photographs or observations of family members. Symptoms suggesting various physiologic disturbances can be thought of as sensory, motor, psychophysical, structural, and functional.

Sensory symptoms include pain, which should be characterized in terms of severity, location, radiation, and associations with ocular movements or exposure to light. Loss of or modifications in sensation should be elucidated by seeking symptoms of numbness, tingling, and cold.

Symptoms suggestive of motor abnormalities include diplopia, which should be characterized in terms of variation with direction of gaze, pain, and any sensations of tightness on movement that may reflect a cicatricial or restrictive component.

Psychophysical symptoms primarily relate to variations in visual acuity, color vision, and awareness of either positive or negative scotomata. With development of early and often subtle defects of the optic nerve, patients can often be aware of slight graying of their vision or color desaturation, which may be intermittent or gaze related. It is useful to elicit this information specifically.

Structural changes symptomatically are associated with an awareness of displacement of the globe. Patients may have become aware of proptosis, enophthalmos, or horizontal or vertical displacements. In addition they may be conscious of fullness of the lids, intermittent swelling, or masses, which may or may not be tender.

Other functional abnormalities related to orbital disease include increased lacrimation or dry eyes. Symptoms reflecting vascular disease include swelling, redness, hyperemia, and epibulbar vascular dilatation.

GENERAL INQUIRY

Orbital disease is often associated with systemic abnormalities. Inquiry concerning the present state of health, current and past drug treatment, allergies, and significant dermatologic abnormalities should be elicited. Past illnesses should also be elicited, particularly endocrine disorder, immunologic disease, cancer, infections, surgery, and major medical disease. Some emphasis should be placed on symptoms of central nervous system disease including headache, sensory, and motor symptoms. Sometimes a family history of disease can aid in uncovering a diagnosis, particularly as relates to immunologic, neoplastic, endocrine, and infectious diseases.

PHYSICAL EXAMINATION OF THE ORBIT

Physical examination of the orbit can be divided into categories of general, psychophysical, orbital, ocular movement, and ocular assessment.

General assessment of the patient should include observations concerning the facial contours, and lateral and vertical symmetry of facial, lid, orbital, and ocular structures. Particular attention should be paid not only to alterations in contour but changes in color and pigmentation. The orbital and periorbital structures should be pal-

pated as should the preauricular and cervical nodes. The lids and conjunctiva should be assessed for position and alterations in structure. I usually measure the interpalpebral fissure bilaterally and document both upper and lower lid retraction, lid lag, and degree of scleral show. Measurement of maximum levator function should be included. Injection of both the conjunctiva and lids should be documented and graded (usually I use a four-point system). The degree of preseptal, pretarsal, and conjunctival edema should also be documented (using a subjective or four-point system).

Psychophysical examination includes a study of the best corrected visual acuity, confrontation visual fields, a central visual acuity using an Amsler grid, and color vision assessment. In addition, the sensory functions of the fifth nerve should be assessed both for light touch and pain. Pupillary examination should assess size, symmetry, light, and near reaction as well as check for afferent pupillary defects.

Orbital examination should document the degree of horizontal and vertical displacement of the globe, the ease of ballotment (which can be either measured subjectively in a four-point system or by millimeter measurement). Exophthalmometry should be documented and the width of the exophthalmometer recorded. Normal exophthalmometry measurements will vary according to age, sex, and race. The mean normal protrusion values are 16.5 mm in white men, 18.5 mm in black men, 15.4 mm in white women, and 17.8 mm in black women. Values above 21 mm are usually considered abnormal; however, Migliori and Gladstone have noted that the upper limits of normal were 21.7 mm for white men, 24.7 for black men, 20.1 mm for white women, and 23 mm for black women.

Ocular movements can be documented by recording ductions in the four cardinal positions by degrees. Cover and cross cover tests with prism measurements should assess manifest deviations. I also do Maddox rod testing using a Risley prism in the primary position, upgaze, downgaze, right, and left gaze. Any evidence of abnormalities of movements will require a forced duction examination, which can be recorded subjectively as one through four.

Ocular examination should include measurement of the intraocular pressure in the primary position and upgaze. Frequently, in the presence of a duction abnormality there is a pressure rise in the position of gaze opposite to a cicatrized muscle. Biomicroscopy of the cornea, conjunctiva, and fornices should be carefully done. Finally the fundus, optic nerve head, retinal blood vessels, and choroid should be carefully examined with direct and indirect ophthalmoscopy. In particular, evidence of choroidal folds, disc edema, and optociliary vessels should be ruled out. Indentation of the globe may be noted, and if it is due to a mass the indentation may shift as you observe the fundus with an indirect ophthalmoscope and the patient alters his ocular position.

Following history taking and physical examination, it is useful to develop an analysis profile of the patient in which location and dynamics, both temporal and physiologic, can be summarized. This then should lead to the development of a differential diagnosis and an investigative plan.

Prospective follow up should include a record of management, outcome, or progression of disease with and without therapy. A chart profile for documentation is provided in Table 6-1.

Examples

The foregoing principles can best be appreciated through specific clinical examples that emphasize aspects of this approach to the diagnosis of orbital disease.

LOCATION OF DISEASE

Mechanical Features

A mass lesion arising in the area of the lacrimal fossa and producing a positive effect leads to downward and in-

TABLE 6-1.
PATIENT PROFILE

I. **History of Illness**
  Symptoms
  Temporal
  Dynamics
    Sensory
    Motor
    Structural
    Psychovisual
    Functional

II. **General Status**
  Allergy
  Drugs
  Past illness
  Systemic disorders
  Family history
  Functional inquiry

III. **Physical Examination**   OD   OS
  A. Psychophysical
    VA
      Refraction
      Distance
      Near
    Color vision
    Visual field
    Amsler grid
    Sensory function
      V1
      V2
      V3
    Pupil
  B. General
    Facial contours
    Palpation
    Lacrimal gland
    Lids
      Interpalpebral fissure
      Lid fold
      Retraction
      Maximum levator function
    Edema (1 – 4)
      Preseptal
      Pretarsal
      Chemosis
    Injection (1 – 4)
      Conjunctival
      Lid

          Lid lag   OD   OS
          Lagophthalmos
          Auscultation
          Nodes
  C. Orbital
      Displacement
      Vertical (mm)
      Horizontal (mm)
      Ballotment (1 – 4 or mm)
      Exophthalmometry
  D. Ocular movement
      Ductions
      Cover test

      Maddox rod

          Forced ductions
  E. Ocular examination
      Biomicroscopy
        Conjunctiva
        Fornix
        Cornea
        Anterior chamber
        Iris
        Lens
      Schirmer test
      Intraocular pressure
        Primary position
        Up
        Other
      Vitreous
      Fundus

IV. **Analysis Profile**
      Location
      Dynamics
        Temporal
        Physiologic

V. **Plan**
      Differential diagnosis
      Investigations

VI. **Management**

VII. **Outcome**

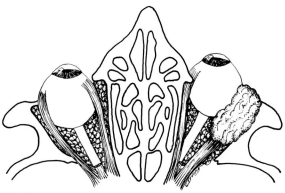

FIGURE 6-5.   Positive mass effect of lacrimal tumor: downward and inward displacement of globe. (Rootman J: An approach to diagnosis of orbital disease. Can J Ophthalmol 18:104, 1983)

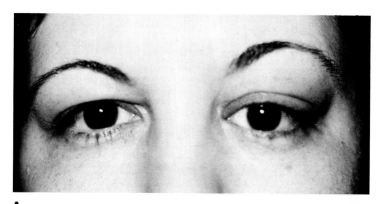

A

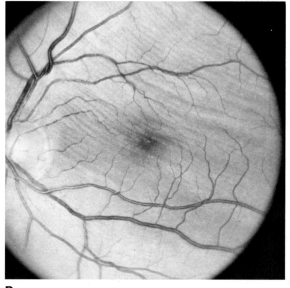

B

FIGURE 6-6.   (A) Downward and inward displacement of the left globe, with fullness and S-shaped deformity of lid, in a patient with a benign mixed tumor of the lacrimal gland. (B) Superotemporal choroidal folds in the same patient. (Rootman J: An approach to diagnosis of orbital disease. Can J Ophthalmol 18:104, 1983)

ward displacement with or without indentation of the globe (see Fig. 6-1; Fig. 6-5). This picture, associated with superotemporal choroidal folds, was evident in a patient who proved to have a benign mixed tumor of the lacrimal gland (Fig. 6-6). On the other hand, a negative process due to cicatrization in the same area may result in enophthalmos and upward and outward displacement of the globe, as in the patient shown in Figure 6-7, who had a sclerosing carcinoma.

Within the muscle cone a positive or a negative process produces axial displacement of the globe (Fig. 6-8). For example, an intraconal schwannoma leads to positive displacement and axial proptosis (Fig. 6-9), and an orbital metastasis of sclerosing breast carcinomas leads to axial enophthalmos (Fig. 6-10). In rare instances both a positive and a negative effect may occur under different circumstances. The patient in Figure 6-11 was normally enophthalmic (Fig. 6-11A), but owing to an orbital venous anomaly, showed increasing axial proptosis and fullness of the lid during a Valsalva maneuver or when bending over (Fig. 6-11B).

Functional Features

The patient with myositis shown in Figure 6-12 demonstrates a functional deficit that helps point to location. She had pain on ocular movement, swelling of the lid, and local injection over the affected medial rectus muscle suggesting a process located in the muscle.

DYNAMIC ALTERATION

A catastrophic temporal change suggests either hemorrhage in a pre-existing lesion or fulminant inflammation with or without a pre-existing lesion. The patient in Figure 6-13 presented with sudden proptosis and sixth nerve palsy after a normal night's sleep (Fig. 6-13A). He proved to have a large orbital hemorrhage within a pre-existing vascular lesion. The diagnosis was supported by the orbital asymmetry seen in a photograph taken 5 years earlier (Fig. 6-13B), an elicited history of spontaneous proptosis followed by subconjunctival hemorrhage at age 5 years, and the fact that the lesion resolved over the next month while the patient was under observation (Fig. 6-13C). His case history demonstrates how eliciting a history of temporal change can aid in precise diagnosis.

Temporal change may be continuous and rapid or insidious, implying different processes. On the other hand, intermittent change, such as pulsation or alteration with a Valsalva maneuver, suggests either a bony defect or a relation between the lesion and the vascular system. The child in Figure 6-14 had pulsating exophthalmos due to the rich vascular supply of an infantile orbital hemangioma.

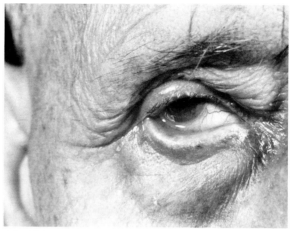

FIGURE 6-7. Upward and outward displacement of eye and lid in a patient with sclerosing carcinoma in the superolateral orbit. (Rootman J: An approach to diagnosis of orbital disease. Can J Ophthalmol 18:104, 1983)

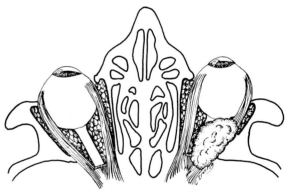

FIGURE 6-8. Schematic of axial proptosis due to intraconal mass. (Rootman J: An approach to diagnosis of orbital disease. Can J Ophthalmol 18:105, 1983)

The Abnormal Process

Clinically inflammation is categorized on the basis of the severity of the signs and the rapidity of their onset. For instance, in acute infective cellulitis there is a sudden development of features of orbital inflammation, with marked limitation of movement, proptosis, injection, and pain (Fig. 6-15). In contrast, a more insidious process, such as some cases of idiopathic inflammatory disease or thyroid ophthalmopathy, may have all or most of the features of inflammation, but they will be much more subtle (Fig. 6-16).

A mass effect consists of displacement of orbital structures with or without compromise of function. For instance, with a well-encapsulated lesion there tends to

(Text continues on p. 93.)

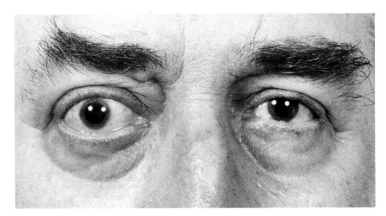

FIGURE 6-9. The clinical appearance of axial proptosis in a patient with a right-sided intraconal schwannoma. (Rootman J: An approach to diagnosis of orbital disease. Can J Ophthalmol 18:105, 1983)

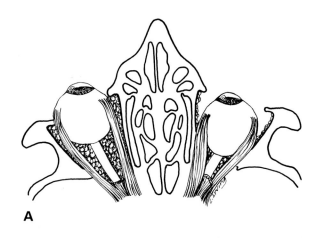

A

FIGURE 6-10. (A) Schematic demonstrating axial enophthalmos due to intraconal cicatrization or atrophy. (B) Left-sided enophthalmos and ptosis due to orbital metastasis of a sclerosing breast carcinoma. (Rootman J: An approach to diagnosis of orbital disease. Can J Ophthalmol 18:105, 1983)

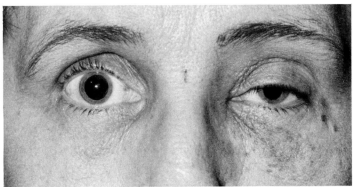

B

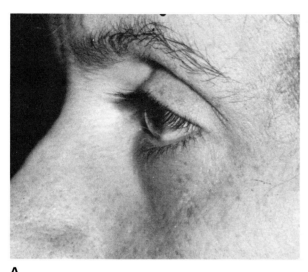

A

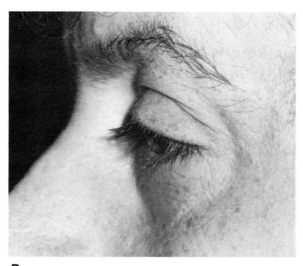

B

FIGURE 6-11.   *(A)* Enophthalmos due to fat atrophy and enlargement of the orbit in a patient with distensible orbital venous anomaly. *(B)* Exophthalmos, increased fullness of lids, and loss of deep upper sulcus in the same patient during Valsalva maneuver. (Rootman J: An approach to diagnosis of orbital disease. Can J Ophthalmol 18:106, 1983)

FIGURE 6-12.   *(A)* Clinical photograph of a patient with myositis demonstrates lid swelling and local injection over the muscle insertion. *(B)* CT scan demonstrates enlarged medial rectus muscle and tendon.

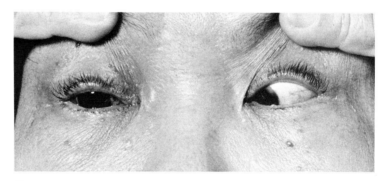

A

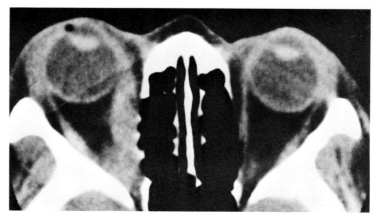

B

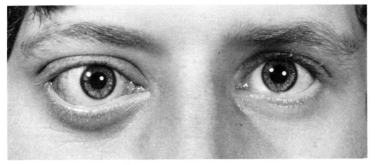

A

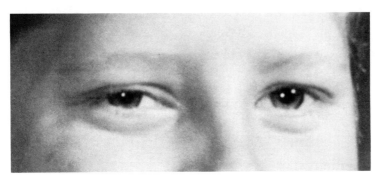

B

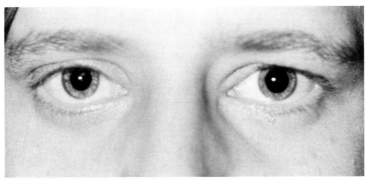

C

FIGURE 6-13. *(A)* Right-sided proptosis and sixth nerve palsy that developed overnight in a 16-year-old boy with an orbital vascular anomaly. *(B)* Orbital asymmetry in the same boy 5 years earlier. *(C)* Photograph taken 1 month later demonstrates resorption of blood and minimal residual proptosis. (Rootman J: An approach to diagnosis of orbital disease. Can J Ophthalmol 18:106, 1983)

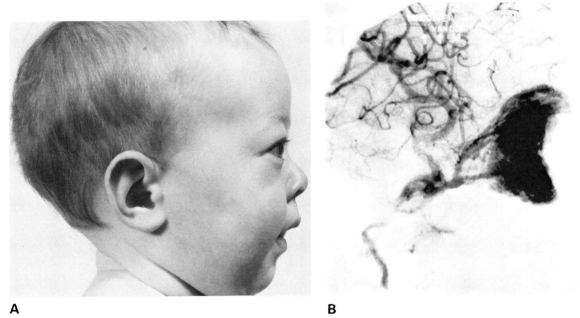

A   **B**

FIGURE 6-14.   *(A)* Axial proptosis that pulsated. *(B)* Vascular capillary hemangioma of orbit, demonstrated by arteriography, in the same infant. (Rootman J: An approach to diagnosis of orbital disease. Can J Ophthalmol 18:106, 1983)

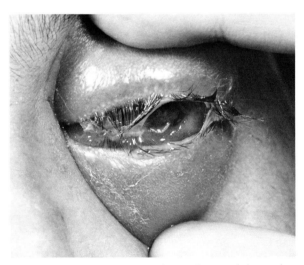

FIGURE 6-15.   Lid edema, injection, and proptosis in a patient with acute orbital cellulitis secondary to pyemic endophthalmitis. The patient also had marked limitation of ocular movement and pain. (Rootman J: An approach to diagnosis of orbital disease. Can J Ophthalmol 18:107, 1983)

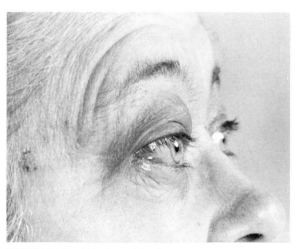

FIGURE 6-16.   Lid edema, injection, and chemosis in a patient with insidious orbital inflammation due to thyroid orbitopathy. The patient also had limitation of ocular movement, but little pain. (Rootman J: An approach to diagnosis of orbital disease. Can J Ophthalmol 18:107, 1983)

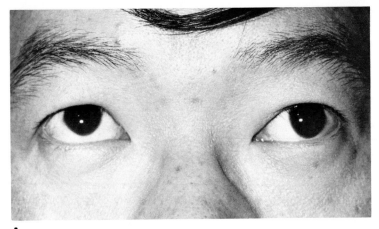

A

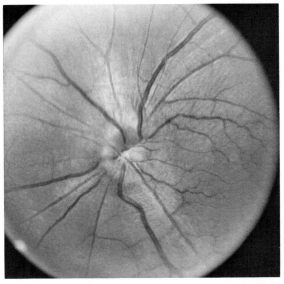

B

FIGURE 6-17. *(A)* Left-sided proptosis and limitation of upward gaze (he is looking up) in a patient with rapidly progressive signs of infiltration. *(B)* Sight papilledema (note superior disc injection and engorged retinal veins) due to orbital metastasis of colonic adenocarcinoma in the patient shown in *A*. (Rootman J: An approach to diagnosis of orbital disease. Can J Ophthalmol 18:107, 1983)

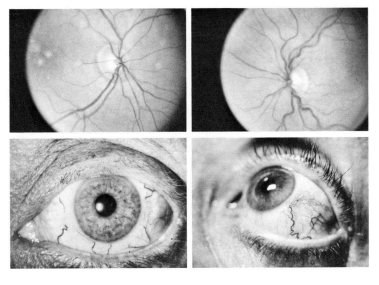

FIGURE 6-18. Clinical manifestations of low-flow arteriovenous shunts. *Upper right* photo shows vascular dilatation and tortuousness in the right posterior pole, compared with a normal right posterior pole *(upper left)*. This was associated clinically with epibulbar vascular dilatation *(lower left)* and 3 mm of proptosis that occurred spontaneously in a 72-year-old woman. Epibulbar vascular dilatation and tortuousness in a 74-year-old woman *(lower right)* who presented with a mild sixth nerve palsy, raised intraocular pressure (34 mm Hg) and 2 mm of proptosis due to a low-flow dural arteriovenous shunt.

be displacement without much effect, other than mechanical indentation, on any of the orbital structures (see Figs. 6-6 and 6-9).

The process of infiltration leads to entrapment and damage of orbital structures, as seen in the enophthalmos, ptosis, and limitation of ocular movement of the patient with an orbital metastasis of sclerosing breast carcinoma (see Fig. 6-10). On the other hand, the patient in Figure 6-17 presented with progressive proptosis, limitation of ocular movement, and papilledema of relatively rapid onset but no clinical evidence of inflammation; these signs pointed to a malignant or a destructive inflammatory process. The patient proved to have an orbital metastasis.

Vascular change is well demonstrated in patients showing episcleral venous dilatation, slightly increased intraocular pressure, retinal venous dilatation, and modest tissue engorgement due to arteriovenous shunts (Fig. 6-18).

Trying to answer the two questions about disease location and resultant dynamic alteration in all cases makes orbital examination more fun, more productive, and more accurate. To make a clinical diagnosis of orbital disease one should bring together information from the history and physical examination that identifies displacement, characterizes temporal development, and defines the disease process. Diseases of the orbit present virtually every combination of location and dynamic alteration. Defining these by clinical means does not necessarily provide absolute proof of the disease, but it does give a reasonable framework for investigation. It remains the most powerful tool for studying the patient.

Bibliography

Migliori ME, Gladstone GJ: Determination of the normal range of exophthalmometric values for black and white adults. Am J Ophthalmol 98:438, 1984

Rootman J: An approach to diagnosis of orbital disease. Can J Ophthalmol 18:102, 1983

CHAPTER 7

Investigation of Orbital Disease and Its Effect on Function

Jack Rootman

Investigative procedures based on a framework of clinical analysis as outlined in the preceding chapters should elucidate a diagnosis by defining the structural and dynamic (both temporal and process related) characteristics as well as location of orbital lesions. The categories of investigation are clinical examination, ocular and visual function assessment, orbital imaging, systemic survey, and pathologic study. Ocular and psychophysical investigations provide evidence of the functional effect of disease on the visual apparatus. Imaging methods help to pinpoint location and suggest features of inflammatory, mass, infiltrative, vascular, and structural change. Systemic investigation is particularly important in the assessment of the patient because endocrine, vascular, infectious, immunologic, and neoplastic disease may have orbital manifestations. Histopathologic analysis, the final arbiter, has become increasingly sophisticated. Its proper use requires an awareness of technical change to maximize use of biopsy material for diagnosis, prognosis, and research. Therapeutic decisions are then made on the basis of the clinical findings and subsequent investigations.

■ OCULAR AND VISUAL FUNCTION EXAMINATION IN ORBITAL DISEASE

Craig Beattie, Stephen Drance, and Jack Rootman

To assess the effect of disease on ocular and orbital function, there are an array of methods to study psychophysical function, ocular motility, blood supply, and lacrimal dynamics. Optic nerve function may be delineated by study of color vision, electroretinography, visually evoked responses, and visual fields. Dysfunction of the muscles or neuromuscular apparatus may be detected early, documented, and studied on a temporal basis for similar reasons. Tear production, content, and drainage can be studied with simple or sophisticated technology.

Psychophysical Study

Although physical examination will always be the cornerstone for diagnosis of disease processes in the orbit, psychophysical and electrophysiological investigations frequently contribute to the understanding of the overall clinical picture.

The role played by psychophysical (color vision, visual field, and contrast sensitivity testing) and electrophysiological investigations can best be illustrated by cases in which these techniques have been employed usefully. Psychophysics plays a role mainly in two specific clinical settings: the identification of early visual function pathology where clinical evidence is scanty or "soft," and for the follow up of patients in whom it is imperative that progression of disease be identified or postoperative improvement monitored.

APICAL HEMANGIOMA, LEFT ORBIT

The patient, a 36-year-old man, had a history of long-standing left proptosis with a recent onset of central visual problems. He had a visual acuity reduced to 20/80 (OD 20/20), a slightly swollen optic nerve head, and a small superotemporal focal elevation of the peripapillary retina due to a presumed subretinal hemorrhage. Normal pattern VEP results were obtained from the right eye with a very prolonged delay and reduction of VEP voltage from the left eye (Fig. 7-1). Color vision assessment showed virtually no pathology on testing with Ishihara and Dvorine plates or the Farnsworth Pane D15, but hue discrimination testing on the Farnsworth-Munsell 100 Hue test revealed a marked abnormality of color performance (patient's score 368 left eye, 95th percentile limit for this age group 120). Visual field studies show that there was a small central scotoma and expansion of the blind spot (Fig. 7-2A). On CT investigation, he had a large intraconal enhancing mass crowding the apex of the orbit (Fig. 7-3). Clinically, it appeared to be a hemangioma. It was removed by lateral orbitotomy.

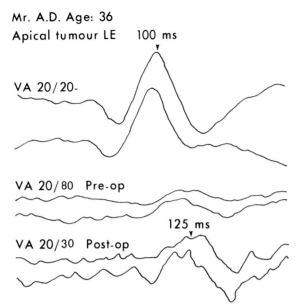

Mr. A.D. Age: 36
Apical tumour LE   100 ms

VA 20/20-

VA 20/80 Pre-op

125 ms

VA 20/30 Post-op

FIGURE 7-1. VEP of normal right eye and abnormal left eye preoperatively and postoperatively in a patient with an apical compressive hemangioma of the orbit. VEP implicit time improved, but not to normal levels.

The patient was assessed again 6 months postoperatively. Visual acuity had improved to 20/30. This was confirmed also by VEP and color vision testing. For the left eye, VEP implicit time had shortened and voltage had increased, though still not to normal values (see Fig. 7-1). He had a small persistent visual field defect (see Fig. 7-2B) and a persistent focal superotemporal peripapillary scar. The Farnsworth-Munsell 100 Hue score had decreased to 200 left eye, a significant improvement, though still abnormal.

Comment: The VEP changes in this patient are typical of compressive lesions in the orbit affecting optic nerve function. VEP voltage drops more or less in parallel with the changes in visual acuity, whereas the changes in VEP implicit time indicate better the extent of optic nerve dysfunction. Improvement in visual function was also documented by increased visual acuity and color vision even with a persistent visual field defect.

THYROID ORBITOPATHY

Preoperatively, the patient, a women with compressive thyroid orbitopathy and marked soft tissue and oculomotor signs, exhibited visual field defects (greater on the left) and visual acuity of 20/40+ right eye, 20/70— left eye. VEP and color vision assessments were performed also. VEP studies showed normal recordings from the right eye, but with reduced and delayed major peaks from studies of the left eye (Fig. 7-4). Color vision studies confirmed the severe optic nerve dysfunction in the left eye, showing major color confusion errors on Ishihara and Dvorine testing, and predominantly red/green losses on both Farnsworth D15 and Farnsworth-Munsell 100 Hue testing. Scores for the right eye were within normal limits on all tests.

Testing was conducted 3 months after orbital decompression. Central visual acuity had worsened somewhat (20/60 right eye, 20/80 left eye), but both VEP and color vision performance had improved significantly (see Fig. 7-4). VEP implicit time was nearly normal, although the amplitude of the major positive peak remained in the subnormal range. The acquired red/green defect remained present on color vision assessment, but had decreased in severity.

This case illustrates the fact that VEP and color vision testing can sometimes provide documentation of a visual function change not evident on visual acuity testing alone. The improvement in conduction and decrease in vision pointed to additional retinal pathology rather than compressive optic neuropathy.

Visual Field Assessment

The function of the optic nerve is frequently impaired by disease of the orbit, optic canal, and intracranial lesions anterior to the chiasm. Although the visual field defects are not pathognomonic of the type of disturbance, be it compression, infiltration, or inflammation, they are more likely to indicate location of disease at these sites. The defect may suggest direction of compression in the case of mass lesions or whether the entire nerve is involved in some infiltrative process. A single examination of the field may not be characteristic, but the type of progression, nature of onset, and possible regression will help in the clinical evaluation of the dynamics of orbital disease.

INVOLVEMENT OF THE OPTIC NERVE IN THE ORBIT

Tumors in the anterior part of the orbit are less likely to involve the optic nerve than tumors at the apex, where there is less space for expansion and the optic nerve is more fixed. Field defects due to apical orbital disease are predominantly centrocecal scotomas, which may be dense when the patient first presents or may start as small paracentral nuclei between the blind spot and fixation, and gradually progress to become centrocecal defects (Fig. 7-5). Such scotomas may break through to the periphery, a feature that we have noted particularly in the optic neuropathy of thyroid orbitopathy where the

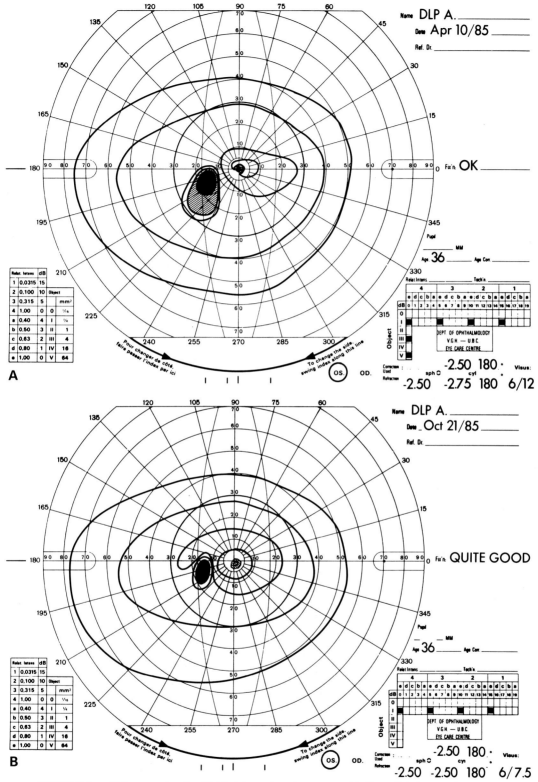

FIGURE 7-2. *(A)* Preoperative visual field of the patient demonstrated in Figure 7-1 shows enlargement of the blind spot and a small paracentral relative scotoma. The enlargement of the blind spot corresponded to a focal area of subretinal neovascularization above the disc. Central vision at this point was 20/80. *(B)* Visual field of the same patient 6 months after removal of an apical cavernous hemangioma. There was an improvement in central visual acuity (20/30), with an increase in the size of the central isopters but a persistence of the scotoma.

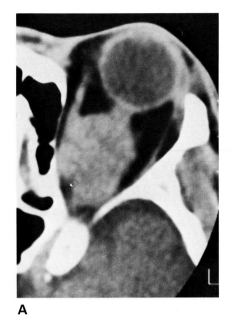

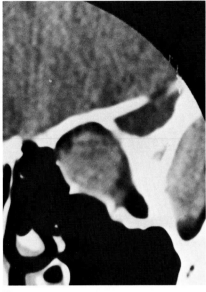

A   **B**

FIGURE 7-3. Axial and coronal CT scans of the patient in Figures 7-1 and 7-2 show a well-defined lobular mass surrounding and obscuring the optic nerve and extending to the orbital apex.

breakthrough is more often inferior than superior (Fig. 7-6).

Generalized contraction of the isopters may also occur, but is a nonspecific finding and always difficult to interpret. When the patient's visual acuity remains good and there is no disturbance of the clarity of the media (so that no other cause for a contraction of the isopters exists), contraction should raise the suspicion of optic nerve involvement.

The visual field may also show abnormalities of localized sectors. Those most commonly involved are the temporal visual field, from medial compression, and the inferior sectors, presumably from superior pressure or compression of the nerve against superior structures. The

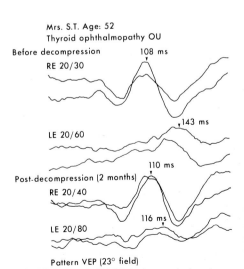

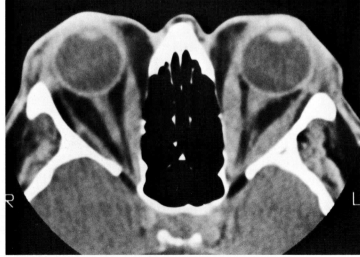

FIGURE 7-4. *(Left)* VEP before and after decompression in a patient with compressive thyroid optic neuropathy. Note improvement in the implicit time with slight deterioration of vision, which was due to concurrent retinal pathology. *(Right)* Axial CT scan of the same patient shows apical compression on the left. Note distention of the left retrobulbar nerve sheath.

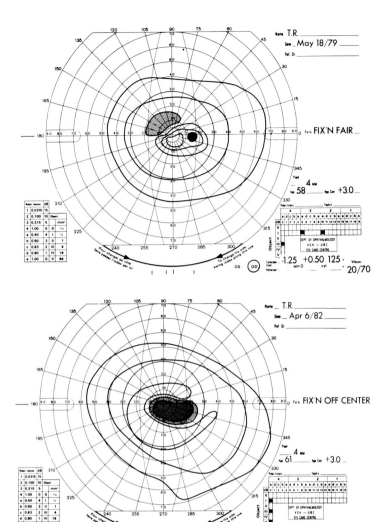

FIGURE 7-5. Visual fields of a patient with compressive thyroid orbitopathy who showed progression of a central *(top)* to a centrocecal *(middle)* defect. *(Bottom)* Axial CT scan of the same patient shows apical compression and massive medial rectus muscles. Note bilateral bowing of the lamina papyracea (Coca Cola sign).

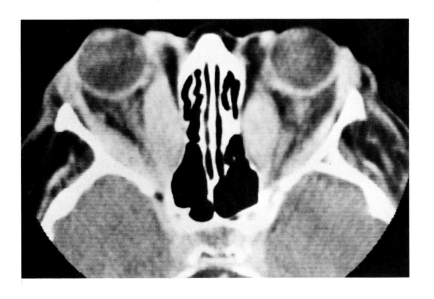

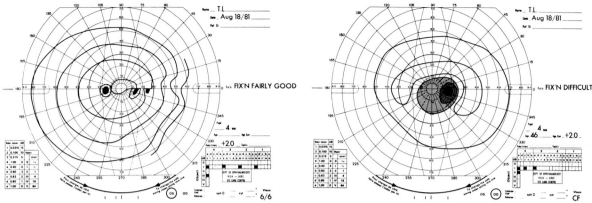

FIGURE 7-6. Visual fields of a patient with a bilateral longstanding compressive optic neuropathy that is worse on the right than on the left. The right visual field shows a dense centrocecal scotoma whereas the left shows an inferior nerve fiber bundle defect with some nasal peripheral isopter indentation. The early field defect on the left was a frequent type seen in a series of thyroid orbitopathy with optic neuropathy.

visual field defects of thyroid orbitopathy as well as those from compressive tumors at the orbital apex suggest that the temporal and nasal fibers are already well segregated into those that will cross in the chiasm and those that will remain uncrossed on their way to the lateral geniculate body. Therefore, it is not unusual to find evidence of a vertical step in optic nerve compression at the apex of the orbit. In bilateral orbital disease, particularly thyroid orbitopathy, if both visual fields have a temporal defect with a vertical step, chiasmal disease may be suspected. In our series of thyroid orbitopathy with optic neuropathy, there were a number of such cases wherein chiasmal disease was excluded by CT studies and the orbital pathologic process could not possibly have involved the junction of the optic nerves. Thus, bitemporal field defects could be misleading in terms of the location of the lesion. In addition, we have had several unusual experiences with patients having thyroid orbitopathy and temporal field defects, which emphasize the necessity for a broad approach to field defects. In one instance the patient had, in addition to thyroid orbitopathy, a parasellar dermoid; and in another patient, a basilar aneurysm accounted for the field defect. Both patients clinically had thyroid orbitopathy but did not have the usual constellation of features associated with thyroid orbitopathy and optic neuropathy, leading to a suspicion of another cause for the field defect.

Nerve fiber bundle defects of the arcuate or inferior altitudinal types may also occur with compression of the optic nerve. However, they are more unusual.

INTRACRANIAL COMPRESSION OF THE OPTIC NERVE

Intracranial compression is most likely to occur from meningiomas of the optic nerve or surrounding structures, aneurysms of the anterior part of the circle of Willis, craniopharyngiomas, and pituitary tumors. Visual field defects in these circumstances are not unlike those occurring due to lesions at the apex of the orbit. Centrocecal scotomas, frequently with breakthrough to the superior periphery, are the most common defects. Classic nerve fiber and altitudinal defects are also common. The closer the lesion is to the chiasm, the more likely is a defect of the opposite visual field due to involvement of the anterior knee of von Willebrand. This produces the classic junctional scotoma, a temporal defect with a vertical step, which may go on to involve the entire upper temporal quadrant of the opposite field. The visual field study is useful in assessing the extent of optic nerve tumors and ruling out chiasmal involvement. Although such a combination is suggestive of involvement of the optic nerve intracranially, we have already drawn attention to the fact that in bilateral apical compression due to thyroid orbitopathy, vertical steps and temporal field defects may occur and be misleading.

Progression of disease may be monitored with ongoing visual field examinations, particularly in the case of meningiomas. The rate of progression of visual field defects due to meningiomas is variable, but tends to be slow. Improvement can be noted following surgical decompression of the lesion (Fig. 7-7).

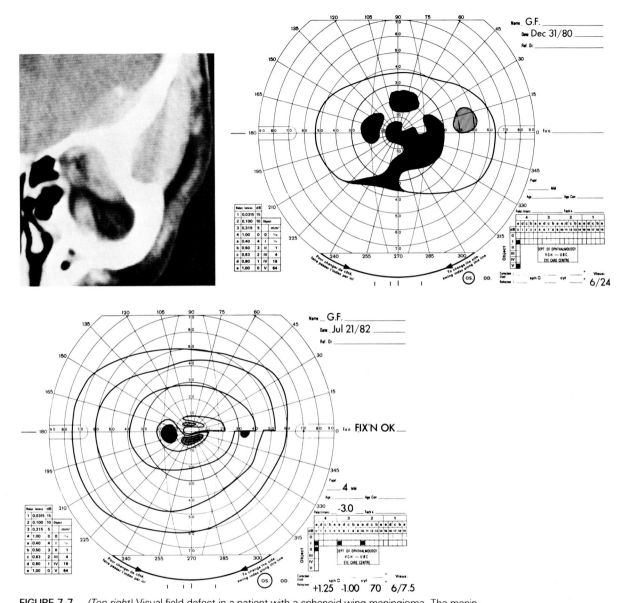

FIGURE 7-7. *(Top right)* Visual field defect in a patient with a sphenoid wing meningioma. The meningioma had encroached on the apical orbit and the optic nerve intracranially. There is a dense central scotoma breaking through inferiorly. Two other dense paracentral scotomas are present. The CT scan shows a meningioma involving the apex of the orbit, temporalis fossa, and anterior cranial fossa. *(Bottom right)* Visual field of the same patient after surgical resection of the meningioma, which led to improvement of vision from 6/24 to 6/7.5. The central scotoma disappeared with good visual recovery. An upper and lower nerve fiber bundle defect remained.

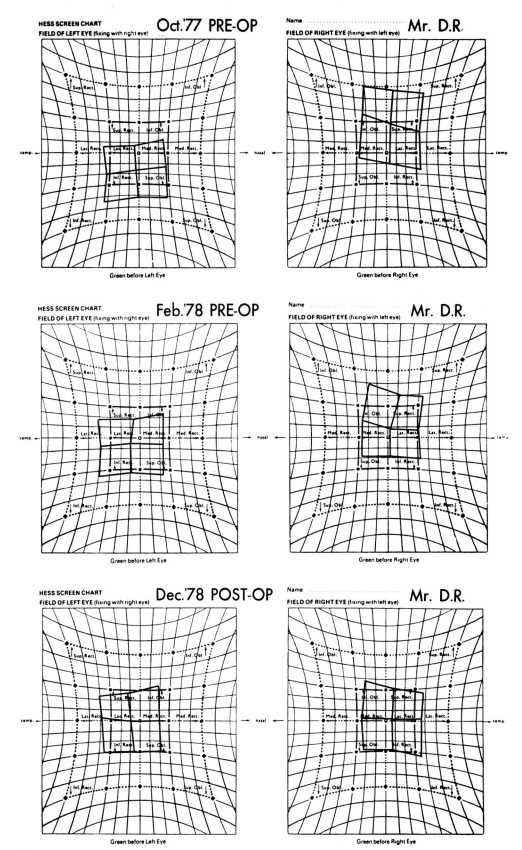

A

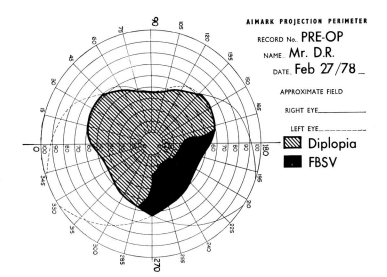

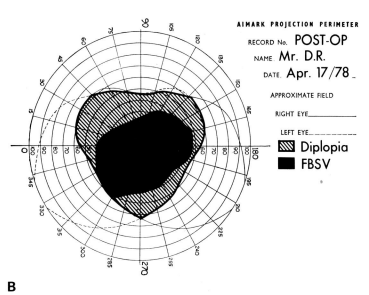

B

FIGURE 7-8. *(A, top and middle)* Preoperative Hess screen tests of a 50-year-old patient with thyroid orbitopathy and myopathy done in October 1977 and February 1978. There was evidence of stabilization and reduction in the cyclovertical element with flattening of the top and bottom. He had a 25-D hypertropia and a 6-D exophoria. *(Bottom)* Postoperative Hess screen of the same patient following a left inferior rectus adjustable recession. Note marked improvement in vertical element. *(B, top)* Preoperative binocular field of vision of the same patient. *(Bottom)* Postoperative binocular field of vision showing restoration of the central field.

Oculomotor Examination

Accurate oculomotor examination is useful in differentiating between infiltrative and noninfiltrative (mass effect or paresis) restrictions caused by orbital disease. Forced ductions help to distinguish between infiltrative and noninfiltrative myopathies. In addition, prospective documentation with objective measurements, including the use of Hess screens, allows documentation of primary features and progression of disease. For example, preoperative evaluation of patients with progressive myopathies, particularly when thyroid related, helps to define the need for and timing of intervention (Fig. 7-8A). Documentation of the binocular field of vision is also a useful adjunctive test in following treatment of thyroid orbitopathy (Fig. 7-8B).

■ ORBITAL IMAGING

Recent advances allow for increasing specificity in definition of the position, nature, and progress of lesions. Imaging procedures can provide information on location, relationship to adjacent structures, evidence of infiltration, capsular definition, tissue characteristics, and relationship to the vascular system. In addition, change in a lesion with time can aid in diagnosis or assessment of treatment.

For example, in the differential diagnosis of the patient with axial proptosis, computed tomography (CT) localized the disease to the intraconal space in the case of a hemangioma and to the orbital apex and medial wall in a case of chondrosarcoma of the sinus (Fig. 7-9). CT scanning can help to define the difference between an

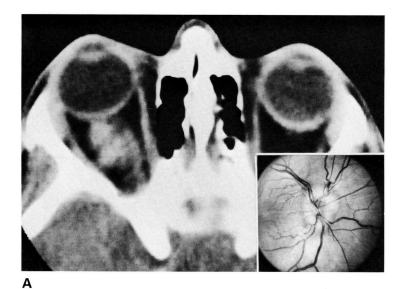

A

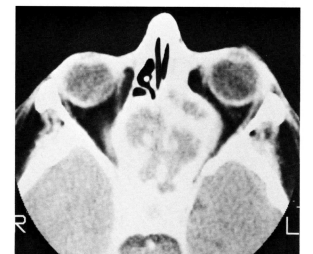

B

FIGURE 7-9. *(A,B)* Both of these patients had presented with axial proptosis in one instance due to an intraconal hemangioma with some displacement of the optic nerve *(A)* and in the other a chondrosarcoma arising from the ethmoid sinus complex *(B)*.

infiltrative and noninfiltrative orbital mass, as illustrated by cases of mucocele and carcinoma invading the orbital roof (Fig. 7-10). Localization of tumors preoperatively or for ancillary diagnostic procedures such as aspiration needle biopsy can be done accurately (Fig. 7-11). Finally, disease progress or the effect of treatment can be monitored, as shown in a patient with Ewing's sarcoma of the orbit and nasopharynx before and after treatment with radiotherapy and systemic chemotherapy (Fig. 7-12).

Routine Radiographic Methods

Routine radiographic and conventional tomographic studies may contribute to the study of orbital disease, particularly in terms of the effect of the disease process on bony structures. Dense tumors such as osteomas may be clearly defined and separated from soft tissue components of disease (Fig. 7-13). Generalized expansion of the orbit in childhood masses and localized expansion in

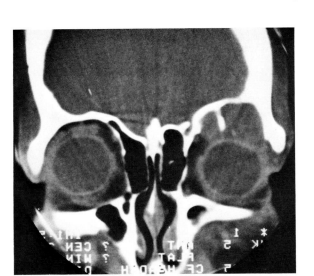

A

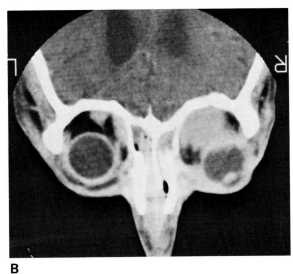

B

FIGURE 7-10. *(A,B)* The CT scan helps to differentiate a cystic noninfiltrative mass in the roof of the orbit *(A)* from a solid infiltrative lesion in the same location *(B)*.

FIGURE 7-11. This demonstrates the value of orbital imaging for localization during a needle aspiration biopsy of a patient with progressive proptosis, ptosis, third nerve palsy, and an infiltrative mass extending from the apex of the maxillary sinus into the orbit. Ultrasound can be used in the same manner.

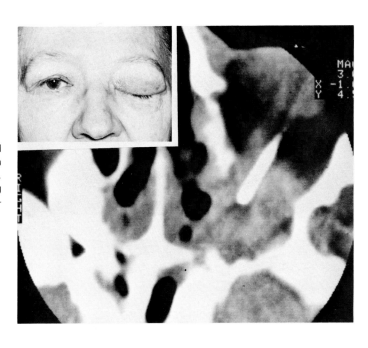

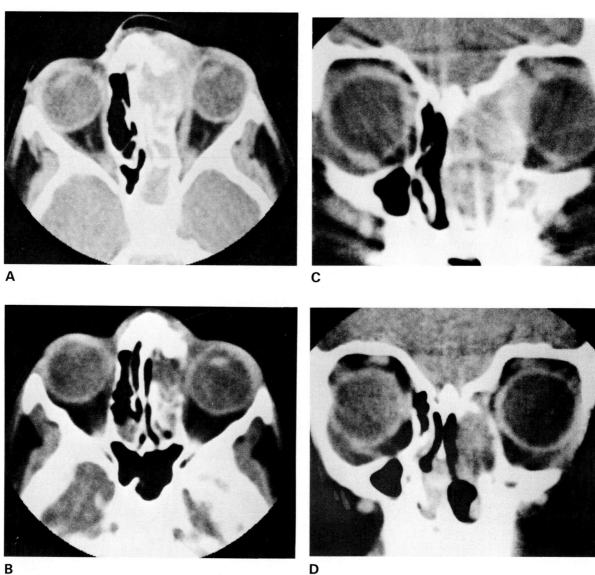

FIGURE 7-12. Regression of a Ewing's sarcoma can be demonstrated by comparison of axial and coronal scans prior to *(A, C)* and after *(B, D)* radiotherapy and chemotherapy.

long-standing lesions of the adult may be studied. Bony erosion in the case of destructive lesions and the site, extent, and degree of fractures can be identified.

COMPUTED TOMOGRAPHY

In the study of disease processes, a CT scan can define the lesion margin as smooth, nodular, or infiltrative. A post-contrast study may show rim enhancement in the case of a deep orbital lymphangioma, tumor blush in a heman-

gioma, or nonenhancement of a mucocele or some solid sinus tumors. Density differentiation can be made between fat, calcium, and soft tissues (Fig. 7-14). Site of origin and degree of extension can be defined in combined orbito-nasopharyngeal-intracranial lesions (Fig. 7-15). Bony erosion in destructive masses and expansion in chronic progressive masses can be differentiated. Erosion of bone adjacent to a lesion suggests an aggressive disease process (malignancy), whereas expansion implies a long-standing noninfiltrative disease. However, there is one instance in which orbital expansion may occur with a

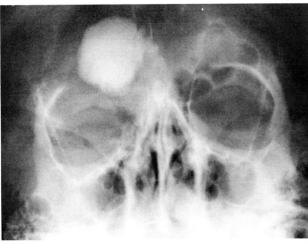
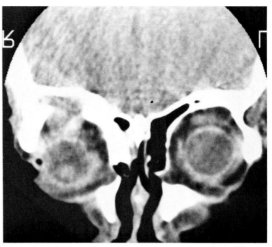

A   **B**

FIGURE 7-13.   *(A)* A routine radiograph of a patient who presented with downward and axial displacement of the right eye. Note the solid, bony osteoma. *(B)* CT scan of the same patient shows a mucocele due to frontal sinus obstruction caused by the osteoma. The mucocele accounted for the clinical features of a superior orbital mass.

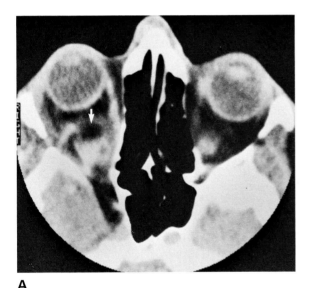
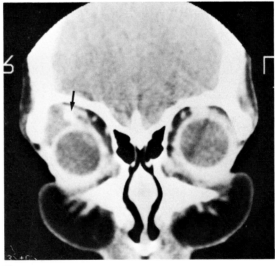

A   **B**

FIGURE 7-14.   *(A)* An axial CT scan of an intraconal apical orbital mass showing an anterior area of decreased density due to the presence of fat *(arrow)* in an orbital dermoid cyst. *(B)* A coronal CT scan of a patient who presented with a relatively long-standing history of downward displacement of the right globe. Note a focal area of calcification in this noncontrast scan *(arrow)* as well as evidence of local excavation or expansion of the adjacent bone, which was due to an epithelial cyst.

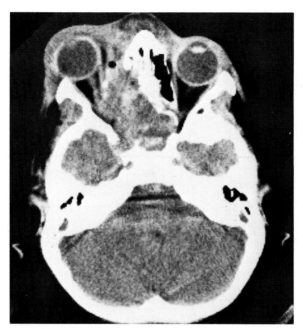

FIGURE 7-15. Axial CT scan of a patient who presented with a rapid, regular onset of proptosis on the right side. It was due to the presence of a solid aneurysmal bone cyst that had led to destruction of the sinuses, nasopharynx, and adjacent wall of the middle cranial fossa.

relatively aggressive lesion, and that is in childhood where the bones are more pliable and expansion rather than erosion may occur with an aggressive infiltrative disease process. In some instances, features of both erosion and expansion may be noted. In trauma, the site, extent, and degree of fracture as well as the presence or absence of a foreign body may be documented (Fig. 7-16). In addition, the structural effects of trauma on soft tissues can be delineated. Contrast enhancement combined with dependent positioning or Valsalva maneuver may demonstrate orbital varices, allowing preoperative localization of an essentially intermittent lesion.

VASCULAR STUDIES AND PROCEDURES

Vascular studies, including both arterial and venous phases, are useful in assessing selected aspects of orbital tumors and vascular lesions. Magnified and subtracted views of the arterial supply can aid in defining the location and the character of the blood supply of tumors preoperatively (Fig. 7-17). Indeed, therapy of highly vascular tumors and fistulas can be performed with selected arterial embolization and occlusion. Phlebography is rarely indicated in the study of orbital disease, except for varices where specific localization and definition may be possible (Fig. 7-18). Orbital venograms are routinely done by the angular tributaries, but the venous system may also be studied by means of the retrograde jugular venous supply in selected circumstances. In some instances, the

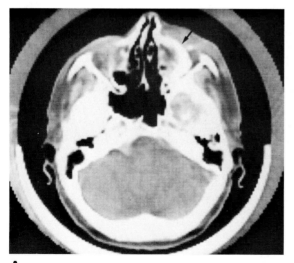

A

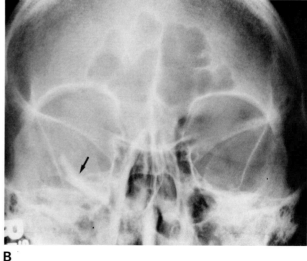

B

FIGURE 7-16. (A) Axial CT scan of a patient who presented with a right infraorbital laceration due to a large fragment of glass that lodged within the maxillary sinus and the floor of the right orbit (arrow). (B) Routine radiograph of the same patient shows two large shards of glass in the sinus and orbit (arrow).

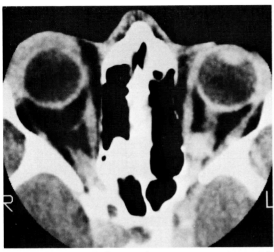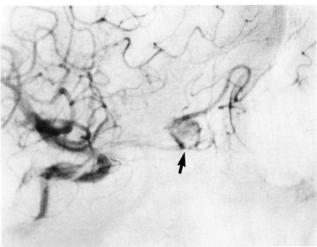

FIGURE 7-17. *(Left)* CT scan demonstrates a contrast-enhancing apical orbit mass that displaced the optic nerve and led to optic neuropathy. *(Right)* The angiogram demonstrates an early uniform fine mesh of enhancing vessels suggestive of either an angiomeningioma or a vascular tumor.

introduction of digital subtraction methods may circumvent the need for direct and complicated intra-arterial injection studies.

ECHOGRAPHY

Jack Rootman and Allan Maberly

Orbital echography, which is a noninvasive ultrasonographic technique, provides useful information regarding the location, size, shape, tissue characteristics, and vascular features of orbital disease. The technique of standardized echography combines information obtained from A-mode, B-mode, and Doppler echography. The reflections of sound waves of an A-scan are emitted from a small probe, and can be displayed on an oscilloscope. These can differentiate the reflectivity, structure, sound attenuation, location, shape, size, borders, mobility, and compressibility of lesions. With the added two-dimensional modality of B-scan, location and size can be graphically demonstrated. Doppler echography provides information concerning vascularity.

Depending on the type of lesion being studied, the overall technique should involve a combination of these methods. We utilize echography primarily as an adjunctive imaging modality. It is particularly useful in showing lesions that involve the globe and adjacent orbit, such as scleritis (Fig. 7-19). In addition, ultrasonography is good for the study of cystic lesions of the orbit (Fig. 7-20). In the case of tumors, location, tissue density, and margins can be defined and differences between smooth, nodular,

and infiltrative lesions documented (Figs. 7-21, 7-22). Finally, inflammatory lesions, such as myositis or abscesses, may be distinguished with ultrasonography.

METHODS OF STUDY OF THE LACRIMAL DRAINAGE SYSTEM

The lacrimal drainage system can be assessed by tomographic and CT studies. In the case of obstruction, contrast injection of the drainage system can help to outline intraluminal masses or sites of the obstruction secondary to extraluminal pressure. This may be particularly useful in the study of combined nasopharyngeal and orbital lesions or lesions of the lacrimal sac. Biochemical analysis of tear lysozyme and angiotensin-converting factor may help to differentiate between sarcoidosis and Sjögren's disease affecting the lacrimal gland. (Both angiotensin-converting enzyme and tear lysozyme levels increase in sarcoidosis.)

NEW IMAGING MODALITIES

Magnetic resonance imaging and positron emission tomography may provide added structural and physiologic information about the effect of disease. The nature of magnetic resonance imaging has been previously outlined in Chapter 3, Investigative Anatomy. Research and development in these areas will define their value in study of orbital disease.

(Text continues on p. 112.)

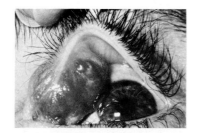
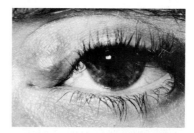

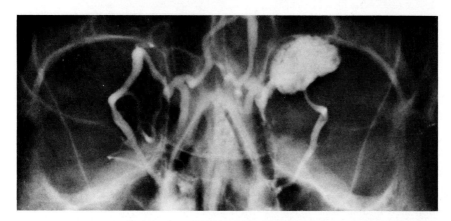

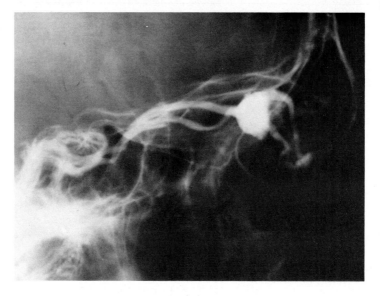

FIGURE 7-18. The clinical photograph shows the anterior component of a varix without *(right)* and with *(left)* distention. The venograms demonstrate the posterior component of the varix on AP and lateral views.

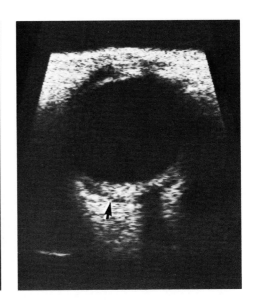

FIGURE 7-19. These B-mode ultrasound images demonstrate features of posterior scleritis. In both instances there is evidence of thickening of the scleral envelope posteriorly, and fluid accumulation in Tenon's space *(arrow)*.

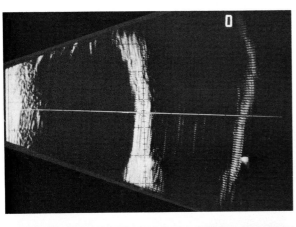

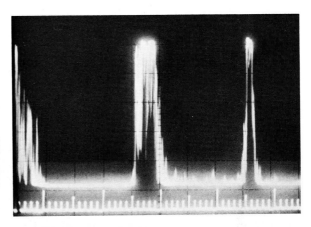

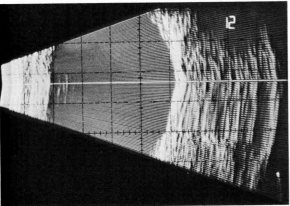

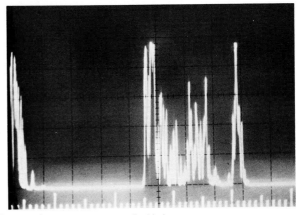

FIGURE 7-20. *(Top)* These ultrasound images demonstrate the differences between two types of orbital cysts. The images are B-mode and A-mode scans of a mucocele invading the orbit. They show high reflectivity of both the anterior and posterior walls of the cyst, with low internal echoes (A mode) suggesting a fluid-filled cavity. *(Bottom)* Scans of a dermoid cyst of the orbit. The cyst appears to have a high echo at its anterior and posterior surfaces with many echoes within the lesion. The posterior portion of the lesion evidences some echo-free areas, suggesting that the content of the cyst was less homogeneous than the above mucocele.

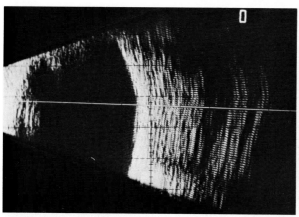
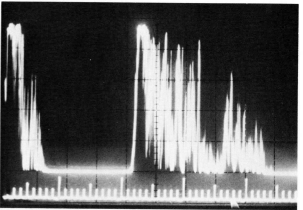

FIGURE 7-21.   *(Left)* B-mode and *(right)* A-mode scan ultrasound images of a recurrent fibrous histiocy-toma of the orbit. There is an irregular mass directly behind the right globe. In addition, there is marked sound wave attenuation throughout the lesion and the posterior aspect of the tumor was somewhat difficult to delineate. The tumor appeared to be irregular and infiltrating.

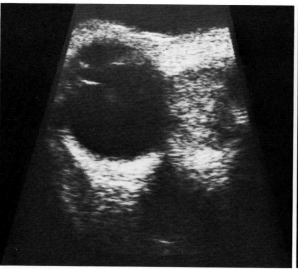
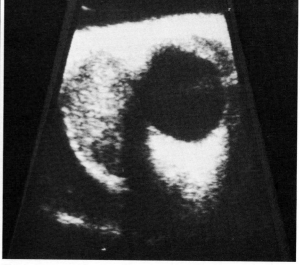

A   **B**

FIGURE 7-22.   Both of these B-mode scans demonstrate large, well-defined masses in the superotem-poral orbit. These are consistent with solid tumors with no cystic or anechoic areas within the lesions. Both were tumors of the lacrimal gland; *A* was a pleomorphic adenoma and *B* an adenoid cystic carcinoma.

■ PATHOLOGIC ASSESSMENT

Frequently, orbital lesions are not easily accessible and considerable technical expertise is required to obtain material both for biopsy or for total removal. Once material is obtained, it is important to have a clear plan for the disposition of tissue based on a presumptive diagnosis. Four major areas of diagnostic tissue pathology are cytology, histochemistry, immunohistochemistry, and elec-

tron microscopy. The value of these methods can best be demonstrated by a few practical case examples.

Routine cytologic methods and ancillary technology including histochemistry and electron microscopy applied to these specimens are readily available in most treatment centers. In the orbit, this has facilitated fine needle aspiration, which is particularly useful in the diagnosis of secondary invasions where this procedure might avoid open biopsy. For instance, aspiration of a progres-

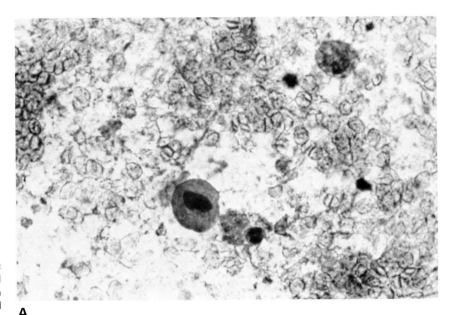

FIGURE 7-23. *(A)* Histopathologic photograph of cytology obtained from aspirate of tumor shown in Figure 7-11. Note large squamoid cells (H&E, original magnification × 100). *(B)* An electron micrograph of the aspirate obtained from the same tumor shows desmosomes *(arrows)* and subcellular organelles consistent with squamous cell origin. (Rootman J, Quenville N, Owen D: Recent advances in pathology as applied to orbital biopsy. Ophthalmology 91:708, 1984)

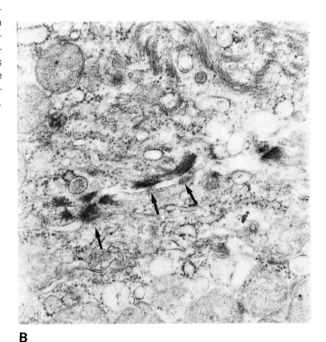

B

sive infiltrative lesion of the orbit arising from the maxillary antrum (see Fig. 7-11) yielded a specimen that proved to be a squamous cell carcinoma on histology and electron microscopy (Fig. 7-23).

Routine histochemical methods offer a broad range of standard techniques for identifying myofilaments, amyloid, fibrin, reticulin, neuroglial tissues, and so forth. Further, the introduction of immunohistochemical techniques, particularly the immunoperoxidase method with monoclonal antibodies, has allowed for an ever-increasing range of specificity in tissue diagnosis. Immunohistochemistry is most successful with fresh frozen tissue or tissue briefly fixed in acetone, Bouin's solution, or Carnoy's solution. Proper management of the tissues is important to obtain accurate results. Methods for identifying component antigens are routinely available for immunoprotein, muscle, keratin, glial protein, prostatic

(Text continues on p. 117.)

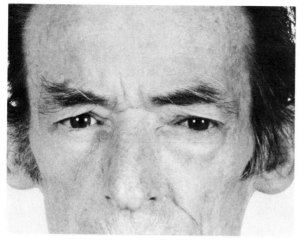

A

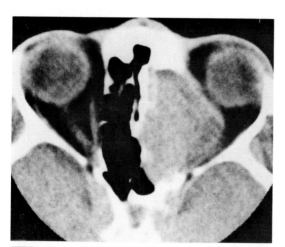

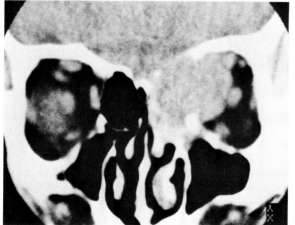

B

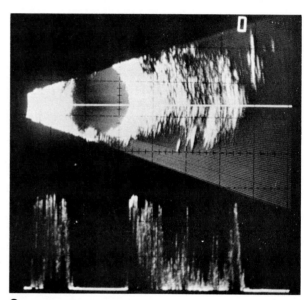

C

FIGURE 7-24. *(A)* This patient presented with lateral and axial displacement of the left globe due to a mass within the sinus and nasopharynx, which is shown on axial *(B, top)* and coronal *(B, bottom)* CT scan. Note bone destruction and infiltration. *(C)* Ultrasound image of the same patient (A and B modes) shows multiple interfaces characteristic of a solid infiltrating orbital mass.

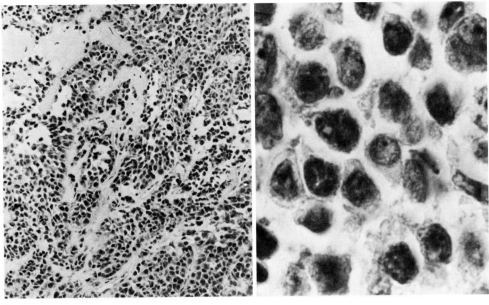

D

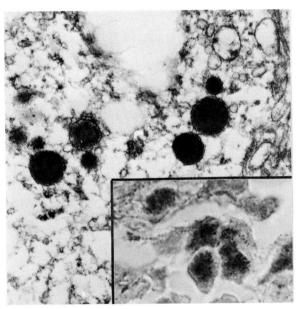

E

FIGURE 7-24. *(Continued)* *(D)* Low- and high-power photomicrograph of a biopsy of this lesion. It is a poorly differentiated round cell tumor of the nasopharynx (H&E, original magnification *left* × 10, *right* × 100). *(E, inset)* A grimelius stain was positive for argyrophil granules (grimelius, original magnification × 100). The electron micrograph of the same lesion shows membrane-bound neuroendocrine granules, confirming a diagnosis of neuroendocrine carcinoma. (Rootman J, Quenville N, Owen D: Recent advances in pathology as applied to orbital biopsy. Ophthalmology 91:708, 1984)

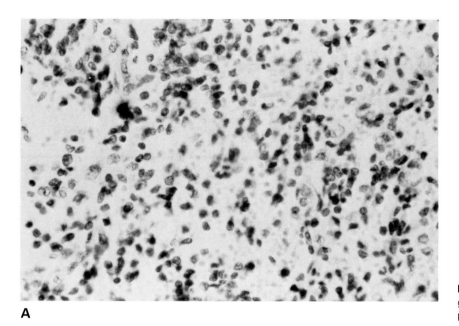

A

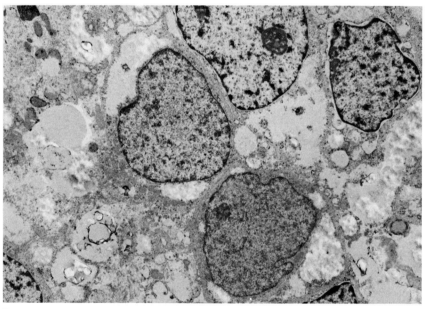

B

FIGURE 7-25. *(A)* Photomicrograph of a biopsy obtained from the patient shown in Figure 7-12. It demonstrates a poorly differentiated round cell tumor of childhood (H&E, original magnification × 25). *(B)* Electron micrograph demonstrates pools of glycogen with few subcellular organelles, suggestive of the diagnosis of Ewing's sarcoma.

antigen, endocrine granules, and many others. Immuno-histochemical methods can even be applied to aspiration biopsy material.

An example demonstrating the gamut of technology is shown in a case of a nasopharyngeal carcinoma. On routine histology, it appeared to be a poorly differentiated malignancy with a wide-ranging differential diagnosis (Fig. 7-24A – D). Immunoperoxidase stain ruled out immunoglobulin, myoglobulin, and glial fiber protein. Routine histochemistry stained for argyrophil granules was strongly positive, suggesting a carcinoma with neuroendocrine features (Fig. 7-24E).

Ultrastructural methods are particularly useful in distinguishing tissue types, as demonstrated in this same case, which showed membrane-bound neuroendocrine granules (Fig. 7-24E). In another case of a poorly differentiated round cell tumor of the nasopharynx seen in a child, electron microscopy showed pools of glycogen and cell membrane junctions with the absence of other subcellular components, leading to a diagnosis of Ewing's sarcoma (see Fig. 7-12; Fig. 7-25). Electron microscopy is valuable in the study of round cell tumors of childhood, where we are attempting to differentiate between rhabdomyosarcoma, lymphoma, neuroblastoma, and rarer tumors such as granulocytic sarcoma, Ewing's sarcoma, and histiocytosis X. In the case of rhabdomyosarcoma, the electron microscope allows identification of the banding typical of myoblastic origin. The pools of glycogen and the presence of cell membrane junctions with the absence of other subcellular components help to identify Ewing's sarcoma. Granulocytic sarcomas contain granules and lysosomes, and in the case of histiocytosis X there are typical Birbeck's granules (X bodies or Langerhans granules). Similarly, electron microscopy of poorly differentiated tumors of the adult can help to distinguish between lymphoma (convoluted nuclei, cytoplasmic indentations, nuclear vacuoles, and nuclear bridges), carcinomas (villi, neuroendocrine granules, intracellular bridges, microgland formation, and so on), and melanomas (melanosomes). It is important following surgical biopsy to get appropriate fixation (glutaraldehyde) and rapid transportation to the lab for maximal electron microscopy results.

We do not wish to review comprehensively the myriad of details applied to the technology demonstrated, but rather to emphasize the value of an informed multidisciplinary approach to biopsy. It is not necessary for all of us to be experts in the area of pathology, but to be aware of increasing and changing sophistication and specificity. Practically, the message is that the clinician should have a clear plan for the disposition of the specimen prior to the biopsy. The best way of handling material is to alert the pathologist in advance, discuss the differential diagnosis, and ask for guidance in the handling of the tissue. This will assure maximum diagnostic information.

Conclusion

This chapter is meant to provide the basis for a rational approach to the clinical evaluation and investigation of disease processes in the orbit. In particular, it is intended to give the framework for establishing the presence, location, effect, and specific identity of disease. In the final analysis it is the multidisciplinary integration of a broad background of knowledge of anatomy, clinical presentation, pathophysiology, and investigative technology that leads to the rational management of disease in the orbit.

Bibliography

Amemiya T, Yoshida H: Electron microscope study of the orbital lesion of Hand-Schüller-Christian disease. J Pediatr Ophthalmol 14:242, 1977

Basset F, Escaig J, LeCrom M: A cytoplasmic membranous complex in histiocytosis X. Cancer 29:1380, 1972

Byrne SF, Glaser JS: Orbital tissue differentiation with standard echography. Ophthalmology 90, No. 9:1071, 1983

Carriere VM, Karcioglu ZA, Apple DJ et al: A case of prostate carcinoma with bilateral orbital metastases and the review of the literature. Ophthalmology 89:402, 1982

Char DH, Sobel D, Kelly WM et al: Magnetic resonance scanning in orbital tumor diagnosis. Ophthalmology 92, No. 10:1305, 1985

Churg A, Ringus J: Ultrastructural observations on the histogenesis of alveolar rhabdomyosarcoma. Cancer 41:1355, 1978

Crist WM, Edwards RH, Pereira F: Rhabdomyosarcoma diagnosed by electron microscopy in a child with acute lymphocytic leukemia. J Pediatr 93:893, 1978

deLuise VP, Tabbara KF: Quantitation of tear lysozyme levels in dry-eye disorders. Arch Ophthalmol 101:634, 1983

Dresner SC, Kennerdell JS, Dekker A: Fine needle aspiration biopsy of metastatic orbital tumors. Surv Ophthalmol 27:397, 1983

Dubois PJ, Kennerdell JS, Rosenbaum AE et al: Computed tomographic localization of fine needle aspiration biopsy of orbital tumors. Radiology 131:149, 1979

Duke-Elder S: System of Ophthalmology, Vol 13. London, Henry Kimpton, 1984

Falini B, Taylor CR: New developments in immunoperoxidase techniques and their application. Arch Pathol Lab Med 107:103, 1983

Frable WJ: Fine-needle aspiration biopsy: A review. Hum Pathol 14:9, 1983

Freeman AI, Johnson WW: A comparative study of childhood rhabdomyosarcoma and virus-induced rhabdomyosarcoma in mice. Cancer Res 28:1490, 1968

Friedman B, Gold H: Ultrastructure of Ewing's sarcoma of bone. Cancer 22:307, 1968

Friedman B, Hanaoka H: Round-cell sarcomas of bone. J Bone Joint Surg [Am] 53:1118, 1971

Ghadially FN: Diagnostic electron microscopy of tumours. London, Butterworth, 1980

Giorno R, Goetz G. Immunohistologic analysis of lymphocyte surface markers. Lab Med 13:554, 1982

Henderson DW, Raven JL, Pollard JA et al: Bone marrow metastases in disseminated alveolar rhabdomyosarcoma: A case report with ultrastructural study and review. Pathology 8:329, 1976

Henderson JW: Orbital Tumors, 2nd ed. New York, Thieme-Stratton, 1980

Horvat BL, Caines M, Fisher ER: The ultrastructure of rhabdomyosarcoma. Am J Clin Pathol 53:555, 1970

Hou-Jensen K, Priori E, Dmochowski L: Studies on ultrastructure of Ewing's sarcoma of bone. Cancer 29:280, 1972

Hurwitz JJ, Welham RAN, Lloyd GAS: The role of intubation macrodacryocystography in the management of problems of the lacrimal system. Can J Ophthalmol 10:361, 1975

Jakobiec FA (ed): Ocular and Adnexal Tumors. Birmingham, Aesculapius, 1978

Jones IS, Jakobiec FA: Diseases of the Orbit. New York, Harper & Row, 1979

Kadin ME, Bensch KG: On the origin of Ewing's tumor. Cancer 27:257, 1971

Kameya T, Shimosato Y, Adacho I et al: Neuroendocrine carcinoma of the paranasal sinus: A morphological and endocrinological study. Cancer 45:330, 1980

Kaminsky DB: Aspiration biopsy for the community hospital. Masson Monographs in Diagnostic Cytopathology, Vol 2. New York, Masson, 1981

Kennerdell JS, Dekker A, Johnson BL et al: Fine-needle aspiration biopsy: Its use in orbital tumors. Arch Ophthalmol 97:1315, 1979

Khalil MK, Huang S, Viloria J et al: Extramedullary plasmacytoma of the orbit: Case report with results of immunocytochemical studies. Can J Ophthalmol 16:39, 1981

Kline TS: Handbook of fine needle aspiration biopsy cytology. St. Louis, CV Mosby, 1981

Knowles DM II, Jakobiec FA: Ocular adnexal lymphoid neoplasms: Clinical, histopathologic, electron microscopic, and immunologic characteristics. Hum Pathol 13:148, 1982

Kroll AJ, Kuwabara T, Howard GM: Electron microscopy of rhabdomyosarcoma of the orbit: A study of two cases. Invest Ophthalmol 2:523, 1963

Kroll AJ: Fine-structural classification of orbital rhabdomyosarcoma. Invest Ophthalmol 6:531, 1967

Mahoney JP, Alexander RW: Ewing's sarcoma: A light and electron microscopic study of 21 cases. Am J Surg Pathol 2:283, 1978

Mesa-Tejada R, Pascal RR, Fenoglio CM: Immunoperoxidase: A sensitive immunohistochemical technique as a "special stain" in the diagnostic pathology laboratory. Hum Pathol 8:313, 1977

Mierau GE, Favara BE: Rhabdomyosarcoma in children: Ultrastructural study of 31 cases. Cancer 46:2035, 1980

Morales AR, Fine G, Horn RC, Jr: Rhabdomyosarcoma: An ultrastructural appraisal. Pathol Annu 7:81, 1972

Morales AR: Electron microscopy of human tumors. Prog Surg Pathol 1:51, 1980

Mukai K, Rosai J: Applications of immunoperoxidase techniques in surgical pathology. Prog Surg Pathol 1:15, 1980

Nakayama I, Tsuda N, Muta H et al: Fine structural comparison of Ewing's sarcoma with neuroblastoma. Acta Pathol Jpn 25:251, 1975

Ossoinig KC: Standardized echography: Basic principles, clinical application and results. Int Ophthalmol Clin 19:127, 1979

Ossoinig KC, Blodi FC: Preoperative differential diagnosis of tumors with echography. Part 4: Diagnosis of orbital tumors In Blodi FC (ed): Current Concepts of Ophthalmology, p 313. St. Louis, CV Mosby, 1974

Rice RW, Cabot A, Johnston AD: The application of electron microscopy to the diagnostic differentiation of Ewing's sarcoma and reticulum cell sarcoma of bone. Clin Orthop 91:174, 1973

Rootman J, Quenville N, Owen D: Recent advances in pathology as applied to orbital biopsy: Practical considerations. Ophthalmology 91, No. 6:708, 1984

Rosenstock T, Hurwitz JJ: Functional obstruction of the lacrimal drainage passages. Can J Ophthalmol 17:249, 1982

Sarkar K, Tolnai G, McKay DE: Embryonal rhabdomyosarcoma of the prostate: An ultrastructural study. Cancer 31:442, 1973

Schyberg E: Fine needle biopsy of orbital tumours. Acta Ophthalmol [Suppl] 125:11, 1975

Sharma OP, Vita JB: Determination of angiotensin-converting enzyme activity in tears: A noninvasive test for evaluation of ocular sarcoidosis. Arch Ophthalmol 101:559, 1983

Sheehan DC, Hrapchak BB: Theory and Practice of Histotechnology, 2nd ed. St. Louis, CV Mosby, 1980

Spoor TC, Kennerdell JS, Dekker A et al. Orbital fine needle aspiration biopsy with B-scan guidance. Am J Ophthalmol 89:274, 1980

Taylor CR: Immunoperoxidase techniques: Practical and theoretical aspects. Arch Pathol Lab Med 102:113, 1978

Triche TJ: Round cell tumors in childhood: The application of newer techniques to the differential diagnosis. Perspect Pediatr Pathol 7:279, 1982

Van Lith GHM, Vijfvinkel-Bruinenga S, Graniewski-Wijnands S: Pattern evoked cortical potentials and compressive lesions along the visual pathways. Documenta Ophthalmologica 52:347, 1982

Westman-Naeser S, Naeser P: Tumours of the orbit diagnosed by fine needle biopsy. Acta Ophthalmol 56:969, 1978

Winkler CF, Goodman GK, Eiferman RA et al: Orbital metastasis from prostatic carcinoma: Identification by an immunoperoxidase technique. Arch Ophthalmol 99:1406, 1981

Zimmerman LE, Font RL, Tso MOM et al: Application of electron microscopy to histopathologic diagnosis. Trans Am Acad Ophthalmol Otolaryngol 76:101, 1972

CHAPTER 8

Frequency and Differential Diagnosis of Orbital Disease

Jack Rootman

The aim of the preceding chapters has been to establish an intelligent, analytical approach to the examination, investigation, and diagnosis of orbital disease within the context of pathophysiology and location. This approach should provide a reasoned differential diagnosis *appropriate* to the specific patient being examined. Personally, I eschew the philosophy of "listing" diseases, but it is useful to have some broad concept of overall incidence for different age groups and for specific clinical presentations. This chapter will provide an overview of our personal experience and some differential diagnoses for age groups and specific presentations. All of this should be viewed in the context that any series is prejudiced by factors of regional epidemiology, choice of nosology and classification, and special areas of expertise that may lead to referral. Thus, only a broad picture can be obtained from such a review, but it should provide a framework for the analysis of orbital disease. There are a number of excellent series that review incidence of orbital diseases. The reader is referred to these for comparison with our experience, in particular, the texts by Jones and Jakobiec, Duke-Elder, Henderson, Krohel and co-workers, as well as articles by Shields, Kennedy, and Iliff and Green.

Age Distribution of Orbital Disease

DISTRIBUTION PROCESS

Figure 8-1 demonstrates our experience with the broad categories of disease processes seen in the University of British Columbia Orbital Clinic, and Table 8-1 outlines the specific diagnosis in each category. The major trends that can be noted are the bimodal distribution of neoplasia, the dominance of thyroid orbitopathy in middle life, the gradual decrease in structural disease throughout life, and a relatively uniform occurrence of inflammatory, vas-

cular, and degenerative lesions. The specific changing profiles in each diagnostic category can be seen in Table 8-1 and will be outlined in the next section.

DISTRIBUTION BY DIAGNOSIS

All of the specific diseases will be discussed in detail later in this book; however, it is useful to look at their overall occurrence within the broad age groups of childhood and adolescence (0 to 20 years), middle adult life (20 to 60 years), and the elderly (over 60 years).

The incidence and order of occurrence of orbital lesions in childhood and adolescence provides a framework for the differential diagnosis in this age group (Table 8-2). The inflammatory lesions were most common and were roughly divided 3:2 between infection and acute/subacute idiopathic orbital inflammations, both of which are dominated clinically by obvious inflammatory signs and symptoms. Dermoids, epidermoids, and implantation cysts were next most frequent. Third was thyroid orbitopathy, which was usually seen in the adolescent age group and was relatively mild in nature. Vascular lesions collectively are the most frequent orbital lesion, but the different subtypes are easily distinguished clinically. Of these, capillary hemangiomas occur mostly in infants and children as rapidly progressive, obviously vascular, frequently high-flow lesions dominated by mass effect. These were the fourth most common orbital lesion of childhood. In contrast, lymphangiomas and low-flow varices are characterized by episodic changes precipitated by intralesional hemorrhage and thrombosis, and placed seventh and ninth in frequency. Trauma constituted the fifth most frequent orbital disorder in the first two decades; sixth most common were rapidly growing neoplasms, usually malignant primary or secondary tumors. The majority of these tended to be

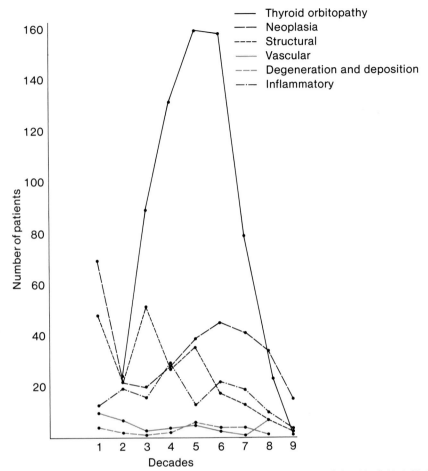

FIGURE 8-1. Age distribution of orbital lesions, University of British Columbia Orbital Clinic, 1976–1986.

associated with rapidly developing mass effect. The adenoid cystic carcinomas of the lacrimal gland were slower to develop but manifest clinically as abrupt lesions. Optic nerve gliomas presented because of visual complaints with mild proptosis and optic nerve head changes. A substantial number of other lesions occurred less frequently, including neurofibromas (largely orbital) and paraorbital plexiform or diffuse lesions (involving the globe and orbit). Orbital asymmetry with pseudoproptosis was not infrequent in this age group, and should be considered in the differential diagnosis of orbital disease in childhood and adolescence.

In middle adult life (20 to 60 years), seven disorders constitute the most common cause of orbital disease (Table 8-3). In order of occurrence they were thyroid orbitopathy, primary and secondary neoplasia, inflammatory diseases, orbital asymmetry, cystic lesions, and lymphoproliferative and vascular disorders. The most common primary neoplasms (occurring in roughly equal numbers) were cavernous hemangiomas, lacrimal gland

tumors, and schwannomas. The secondary neoplasms or tumors invading by contiguity were dominated by meningioma and nasopharyngeal tumors. There were roughly twice as many meningiomas as there were either nasopharyngeal tumors or metastatic lesions. It should also be noted that in middle life we had about a 4:3 occurrence of primary versus secondary and metastatic neoplasms. Of the inflammatory lesions, the acute and subacute idiopathic inflammations occurred most commonly, followed in order by infective and specific inflammatory disorders. Patients in this period of life may also present with orbital asymmetry as a cause of pseudoproptosis. The order of occurrence of cystic lesions was mucoceles, dermoids, and lacrimal cysts; mucoceles occurred roughly twice as many times as dermoids or lacrimal cysts. Lymphoproliferative and vascular lesions, in particular arteriovenous shunts, begin to appear in this age group.

The profile for orbital disease in late life (ages 60 to 90

(Text continues on p. 124.)

TABLE 8-1.
AGE DISTRIBUTION OF ORBITAL DISEASE, UNIVERSITY OF BRITISH COLUMBIA ORBITAL CLINIC, 1976–1986

Type of Lesion	1	2	3	4	5	6	7	8	9	Total	Percentage
Thyroid Orbitopathy		24	89	131	159	158	79	23	1	664	47.1
Neoplasia											
Neurogenic											
Optic nerve glioma	11	2	1			1				15	
Meningioma											
Optic nerve			2		3		1	1		7	
Sphenoid wing		1	1	3	5	7	3	2		22	
Other	1					1				2	
Other optic nerve tumors											
Dural melanoma					1					1	
Leukemia		1								1	
Medulloblastoma	1									1	
Carcinoma				1						1	
Peripheral nerve sheath											
Neurofibroma											
Plexiform	8	1	3	1						13	
Solitary							1			1	
Schwannoma											
Benign			2	3		2				7	
Malignant			1		1					2	
Rare neurogenic											
Granular cell					1					1	
Total neurogenic	21	5	10	8	11	11	5	3		74	
Lymphoproliferative											
Lymphocytic											
Reactive lymphoid hyperplasia					2	1				3	
Atypical lymphoid hyperplasia					1	3		2		6	
Lymphomas				1	5	8	6	13	4	37	
Plasma cell tumors											
Reactive								1		1	
Myeloma						1	2	2		5	
Other											
T-cell lymphoma						1				1	
Hodgkin's			1							1	
Histiocytoses											
Histiocytosis X	3									3	
Malignant histocytosis					1					1	
Total lymphoproliferative	3		1	1	9	14	8	18	4	58	
Vascular Neoplasia											
Capillary hemangioma	22	1								23	
Cavernous hemangioma				5	1	4	2			12	
Lymphangioma	11	3	3	1	1					19	
Hemangiopericytoma			1		1					2	
Total vascular neoplasia	33	4	4	6	3	4	2			56	
Secondary Tumors											
Nasopharynx											
Squamous		1			2	1	2	2	1	9	
Transitional cell					2	1				3	
Adenoid cystic						1	2			3	
Mucoepidermoid					1					1	
Neuroendocrine					1					1	
Melanoma							1			1	
Basal cell							1			1	

(continued)

TABLE 8-1. *(Continued)*

Type of Lesion	____ Decade ____									Total	Percentage
	1	2	3	4	5	6	7	8	9		
Lid											
Basal cell					1		1		1	3	
Squamous							1		1	2	
Sebaceous				1						1	
Melanoma						1		1		2	
Conjunctiva											
Melanoma				1		2	1			4	
Squamous							3		2	5	
Ocular											
Melanoma						2		2		4	
Lacrimal sac											
Transitional							1	1		2	
Squamous							1			1	
Fibrous histiocytoma				1						1	
Total secondary tumors		1		3	7	10	12	6	5	44	
Mesenchymal											
Striated muscle											
Rhabdomyosarcoma	5									5	
Fibrous tissue											
Fibrosarcoma	1									1	
Histiocytic											
Fibrous histiocytoma	1			1	1		1			4	
Bone tumors											
Fibrous dysplasia	2	5	2							9	
Reactive											
Reparative granuloma		1								1	
Aneurysmal bone cyst	1	1								2	
Brown tumor								1		1	
Xanthoma				1	1					2	
Neoplasia											
Ewing's sarcoma	1	1								2	
Osteoma		2	1	1			1			5	
Chondrosarcoma					2					2	
Osteogenic sarcoma				1						1	
Total mesenchymal	11	10	3	4	4		2	1		35	
Metastatic											
Carcinoma											
Breast					1	4	5	1	1	12	
Prostate							1		2	3	
Gastrointestinal				1			1	2		4	
Lung								1		1	
Thyroid							2			2	
Unknown							1		2	3	
Sarcoma											
Liposarcoma							1			1	
Neuroblastoma	1									1	
Melanoma				1						1	
Fibrosarcoma	1									1	
Total metastatic	2			2	1	4	11	4	5	29	
Lacrimal											
Pleomorphic adenoma			1	2	3					6	
Adenoid cystic		2		1		2				5	
Mucoepidermoid							1	1		2	
Spindle cell					1					1	
Total lacrimal		2	1	3	4	2	1	1		14	

(continued)

TABLE 8-1. *(Continued)*

Type of Lesion	Decade 1	2	3	4	5	6	7	8	9	Total	Percentage
Unknown			1	1				1	1	4	
Total Neoplasia	70	22	20	28	39	45	41	34	15	314	22.3
Structural Lesions											
Congenital											
Cystic											
Dermoids and epidermoids	23	4	5	2	1		1			36	
Microphthalmos with cyst	3									3	
Sweat gland cyst	1		1							2	
Rathke pouch		1								1	
Muscle cyst					1					1	
Bony anomalies											
Asymmetry	6	1	9	7	9	9	4	1	1	47	
Von Recklinghausen	1			1						2	
Ectopia											
Dermolipoma	7		1							8	
Acquired											
Cystic											
Mucocele		2	4	4	6	1	3	5	1	26	
Implantation	1	1	1	1						4	
Lacrimal			1	1	4	2				8	
Polyposis					1				1	2	
Trauma											
Fractures	5	11	21	8	9	3	4			61	
Soft tissue			6	1	1	1	1			10	
Foreign bodies		2	1	1	1					5	
Pseudoproptosis	1		1	1	3	1				7	
Total structural lesions	48	22	51	27	36	17	13	7	2	223	15.8
Inflammatory											
Infectious											
Microbial											
Sinusitis	7	7	4	5	1	2	1	1	1	29	
Other	3		3	4	2	4	1	3	1	21	
Nonmicrobial	1			1						2	
Nonspecific Inflammation											
Acute and subacute idiopathic inflammation											
Anterior	1	3	3	2	2	5	1	1		18	
Diffuse	1	1								2	
Myositic		3	2	6	1	3	4			19	
Apical		1			1	2	1			5	
Lacrimal		2	2	2	1	1	2		1	11	
Sclerosing		1		1	1	2	1			6	
Nonspecific granulomatous				2			1	2		5	
Other Orbital Inflammations											
Sarcoidosis			1		1					2	
Sjögren's syndrome						1		1		2	
Vasculitis											
Systemic lupus			1							1	
Wegener's granulomatosis				1			3			4	
Orbital vasculitis							4	1		5	
Ocular with orbital signs											
Scleritis		1		2	2	1		1		7	
Cogan's syndrome				1						1	
Tolosa-Hunt syndrome				2	1	1				4	
Total inflammatory	13	19	16	29	13	22	19	10	3	144	10.2

(continued)

TABLE 8-1. *(Continued)*

Type of Lesion	Decade									Total	Percentage
	1	2	3	4	5	6	7	8	9		
Vascular											
AV Shunts											
Malformations	3	1	1							5	
Acquired		1	1	3	3	2	1	2		13	
Venous											
Nondistensible varix	5	3	1		1					10	
Distensible varix	2	2			1					5	
Thrombosis								2		2	
Lymphedema				1		1		2		4	
Spontaneous hemorrhage								1		1	
Total vascular	10	7	3	4	5	3	1	7		40	2.8
Degenerative											
Atrophy											
Postirradiation	4	1	1		1					7	
Post-trauma					1	2				3	
Idiopathic senile (lipodystrophy)					1					1	
Other											
Myopia				1	1		1			3	
Scleroderma				1						1	
Fat prolapse		1			2	1	2	1		7	
Amyloid								1		1	
Progressive external ophthalmoplegia							1			1	
Total degenerative	4	2	1	2	6	4	4	1		24	1.7
Overall Total	241			908			260			1409	

TABLE 8-2.
ORBITAL DISEASE IN CHILDHOOD AND ADOLESCENCE (AGES 0–20 YEARS)

Type of Lesion	Number of Lesions	Percentage
Inflammatory lesions	31	12.9
Infections 18		
Idiopathic 13		
Dermoids and epidermoids	27	11.2
Thyroid orbitopathy	24	10.0
Capillary hemangioma	23	9.5
Trauma	18	7.5
Rapidly growing neoplasia	17	7.1
Rhabdomyosarcoma 5		
Metastatic and secondary 5		
Histiocytosis X 3		
Ewing's sarcoma 2		
Adenoidcystic carcinoma 2		
Lymphangioma	14	5.8
Optic nerve glioma	13	5.4
Varix	12	5.0
Other	62	25.7
Total, all types	241	

years) changes from that of middle adult life (Table 8-4). Although thyroid orbitopathy remains the leader, it more nearly equals other major causes. The second most common disease in this age group was neoplasia, with secondary and metastatic tumors roughly outnumbering primary tumors in a 4 : 1 ratio. Among the secondary lesions, the dominant neoplasms are contiguous malignancies, which roughly outnumber metastases 3 : 2. Inflammatory disease also demonstrates a change in profile with the emergence of the vasculitides and granulomatous inflammations, which, together with the acute and subacute idiopathic inflammations, dominate inflammatory disease in this age group. The fourth most common orbital disease in the elderly was lymphoproliferative disorders, primarily lymphoma. Mucoceles remained a common disorder in this age group. The least frequent lesions were vascular diseases, primarily arteriovenous shunts.

The profile of orbital disease experienced in the various age groups allows for some useful generalizations. For example, nonthyroid orbital inflammatory disease is dominated by infections in childhood, by nonspecific inflammations in adulthood, and by vasculitides and granulomas in the elderly. Neoplastic disease shows a similar change in patterns: childhood and adolescence is dominated by rapidly growing primary tumors, middle life by equal occurrence of primary and secondary tumors, and late life by secondary, generally malignant neoplasms. As would be expected, children and adolescents suffer traumatic and congenital structural lesions, whereas middle-aged and elderly patients develop acquired structural lesions (primarily mucoceles and trauma). The orbital lymphoproliferative processes appear in middle adult life and include the gamut of reactive and atypical lymphoproliferative lesions as well as lymphomas. In contrast, lymphomas predominate in late adult life.

DISTRIBUTION BY CLINICAL PRESENTATION

Where possible, we have attempted to analyze our orbital cases in terms of the pathophysiology of onset with regard to both temporal change and the abnormal process. It was not possible in all instances to establish with assurance the nature of onset or dynamics. However, this was ascertainable in the majority of instances.

TABLE 8-3.
ORBITAL DISEASE IN ADULT MIDDLE LIFE (AGES 20–60 YEARS)

Type of Lesion	Number of Lesions	Percentage
Thyroid orbitopathy	537	59.1
Neoplasia	105	11.6
Primary		
Cavernous hemangioma 10		
Lacrimal gland tumors 10		
Schwannoma 9		
Others 31		
Secondary and metastatic		
Sphenoid wing meningioma 16		
Nasopharyngeal tumors 9		
Metastatic tumors 7		
Others 13		
Inflammatory	74	8.1
Acute and subacute idiopathic inflammation 33		
Infective 26		
Specific inflammation 15		
Asymmetry	34	3.7
Cystic lesions	31	3.4
Mucocele 15		
Dermoid 8		
Lacrimal cysts 8		
Lymphoproliferative	25	2.8
Vascular lesions	17	1.9
Other	85	9.36
Total, all types	908	

TABLE 8-4.
ORBITAL DISEASE IN LATE ADULT LIFE (AGES 60–90 YEARS)

Type of Lesion	Number of Lesions	Percentage
Thyroid orbitopathy	103	39.6
Neoplasia	60	23.1
Secondary		
Contiguous 28		
Metastatic 20		
Primary		
Cavernous hemangioma 2		
Lacrimal gland tumors 2		
Optic nerve tumors 2		
Other 6		
Inflammatory	32	12.3
Vasculitis and granulomatous inflammation 11		
Acute and subacute idiopathic inflammation 9		
Microbial infection 8		
Other 4		
Lymphoproliferative	30	11.5
Mucoceles	9	3.5
Vascular lesions (shunts and thrombosis)	8	3.1
Other	18	6.9
Total, all types	260	

Temporal Onset

Temporal onset has been divided into five categories: catastrophic (hours), acute (days), subacute (days to weeks), chronic (months), and chronic (years). Each type of onset has been divided into childhood and adolescence (0 to 20 years), middle life (20 to 60 years), and late life (over 60 years) to assess changes in profile. Further, temporal onset has been divided into patients with and without thyroid orbitopathy. It can be seen from Table 8-5 that thyroid orbitopathy dominated the acute and subacute inflammations in a 4:3 ratio when compared to other causes. The patients with thyroid orbitopathy tended to present with a chronic disorder in about 60 percent of instances, and it can be seen that as patients get older, there is a greater tendency for acute and subacute onset of the orbitopathy. This is discussed more fully in Chapter 11 on Graves' orbitopathy. Finally, the major diseases in each category of onset have been summarized (see Table 8-5).

The least frequent temporal onset of nonthyroid orbital disease was catastrophic, wherein the majority were related to trauma or hemorrhage in a preexisting lesion. The rarer causes included infections that presented in a fulminant manner, one instance of metastasis and one of an arteriovenous shunt developing over a very short period of time.

TABLE 8-5.
TEMPORAL ONSET OF ORBITAL DISEASE, UNIVERSITY OF BRITISH COLUMBIA ORBITAL CLINIC, 1976–1986

Onset	0–20 yr		20–60 yr		60–90 yr		Summary	
Catastrophic (hours to day)	Trauma	15	Trauma	33	Trauma	3	Trauma	51
	Infection	2	Hemorrhage in preexisting lesion	3	Infection	1	Hemorrhage	6
	Hemorrhage in preexisting lesion	2	Infection	1	Spontaneous hemorrhage	1	Infection	4
			Shunt	1	Metastasis	1	Shunt	1
							Metastasis	1
Total		19		38		6		63
Acute (days)	Inflammatory Infection 13 Nonspecific 5	18	Inflammatory Infection 10 Nonspecific 16	26	Inflammatory Infection 6 Nonspecific 8	14	Inflammatory Infection 29 Nonspecific 29	58
	Hemorrhage in preexisting lesion	5	Trauma	5	Neoplasia, metastatic and secondary	2	Trauma	9
	Trauma	4	Hemorrhage in preexisting lesion	2	Superior ophthalmic vein thrombosis	1	Hemorrhage in preexisting lesion	7
	Neoplasia, primary	1	Shunt	2	Shunt	1	Neoplasia Primary 1 Secondary or metastatic 4	5
	Cyst	1	Neoplasia, secondary	2			Vascular	4
							Cyst	1
Total		29		37		18		84
Subacute (days to weeks)	Neoplasia Primary 6 Secondary or metastatic 3	9	Inflammatory Infection 5 Nonspecific 21	26	Inflammatory: nonspecific	11	Inflammatory Infection 7 Nonspecific 38	45
	Inflammatory Infection 2 Nonspecific 6	8	Neoplasia Primary 2 Secondary or metastatic 3	5	Lymphoma and leukemia	6	Neoplasia Primary 9 Secondary or metastatic 9	18
	Structural Cyst 3 Trauma 2	5	Structural Cyst 5 Trauma 4	9	Neoplasia Primary 1 Secondary or metastatic 3	4	Structural Cyst 10 Trauma 7	17
	Vascular: varix	2	Lymphoma or leukemia	4	Structural Cyst 2 Trauma 1	3	Lymphoma and leukemia	11
	Leukemia	1			Vascular: vein thrombosis	1	Vascular	3
					Degenerative fat prolapse	1	Degenerative fat prolapse	1
Total		25		44		26		95
Thyroid orbitopathy, acute and subacute onset*		3		203		55		261
Chronic (months)	Neoplasia Primary 21 Secondary and metastatic 4	25	Neoplasia Primary 14 Secondary and metastatic 12	26	Neoplasia, secondary and metastatic	25	Neoplasia Primary 35 Secondary 41	76
	Structural Cyst 14 Ectopic 4 Asymmetry 3	21	Structural Cyst 13 Asymmetry 5 Trauma 4 Pseudoproptosis 1 Polyposis 1	24	Lymphoproliferative	14	Structural	50
	Vascular anomaly	1	Vascular Shunt 4 Lymphedema 1 Varix 1	6	Structural Old fracture 2 Cyst:mucocele 2 Asymmetry 1	5	Lymphoproliferative	14
	Degenerative fat prolapse	1	Degenerative atrophy	2	Vascular Shunt 2 Lymphedema 1	3	Vascular	10
			Inflammatory Nonspecific 4 Sarcoid 1 Sclerosing 2 Sjögren 1	8			Inflammatory	8
							Degenerative	3
Total		48		66		47		161

* Thyroid orbitopathy patients were grouped into a broader combined category of acute and subacute onset.

TABLE 8-5. *(Continued)*

Onset	0–20 yr		20–60 yr		60–90 yr		Summary	
Chronic (years)	Neoplasia	16	Neoplasia	43	Neoplasia	20	Neoplasia	79
	Primary 14		Primary 23		Primary 7		Primary 44	
	Secondary and		Secondary and		Secondary and		Secondary and	
	metastatic 2		metastatic 20		metastatic 13		metastatic 35	
	Structural	17	Structural	41	Structural	11	Structural	69
	Dermoids 6		Dermoids 6		Asymmetry 5		Degenerative	15
	Asymmetry 5		Asymmetry 22		Mucosal 2		Lymphoprolifera-	
	Implantation		Mucocele 5		Dermoid 1		tive	14
	cyst 1		Pseudoprop-		Polyposis 1		Vascular	12
	Absent sphe-		tosis 5		Pseudoproptosis 2		Inflammatory	8
	noid wing 2		Cyst 3		Lymphoproliferative	6		
	Microphthal-		Lymphoprolifer-		Degenerative	7		
	mous 2		ative	7	Atrophy 2			
	Dermolipoma 1		Degenerative	6	Fat prolapse 3			
	Vascular	5	Scleroderma 1		Amyloid 1			
	Degenerative		Post-trauma 4		Progressive			
	atrophy	2	Postirradia-		ophthalmoplegia	1		
	Inflammatory		tion 1		Inflammatory	3		
	sclerosing	1	Vascular	5	Wegener's 1			
	Lymphoma	1	A-V 2		Sclerosing 1			
			Varix 3		Recurrent			
			Inflammatory	4	cellulitis 1			
			Granuloma-		Vascular	2		
			tous	1	Varix 1			
			Fistula 1		Edema 1			
			Nonspecific 2					
Total		42		106		49		197
Thyroid orbitopathy, chronic		21		333		49		403
Total with onset history		187		827		250		1264

In general, acute diseases developing over days were, in order of occurrence, inflammatory processes, trauma, hemorrhage in preexisting lesions, and occasional neoplastic and vascular disorders (including shunts and thrombosis). The incidence of inflammatory disease was equally divided between infectious and nonspecific inflammations, except in childhood where infections dominated.

When presentation was from days to weeks (subacute), the nonspecific inflammations tended to dominate the inflammatory syndromes in contrast to the more acute presentation of infectious disease. The next most frequent subacute disorder was neoplasia, which was roughly divided equally between primary and secondary or metastatic lesions. The structural lesions included a number of cystic diseases as well as trauma with orbital changes noted days to weeks after the primary episode. Lymphomas and leukemias were next most frequent in order of occurrence. Vascular diseases included a single case of vein thrombosis and two varices that presented with subacute onset. In the single case of fat prolapse with this onset, the patient had a history suggesting a subacute onset.

Overall, acute and subacute onset occurred in about 40% of our patients. These categories were dominated by inflammatory disease. The major additional processes included hemorrhage in preexisting lesions, trauma, and some neoplasia.

In contrast, about 60% of patients had chronic onset of disease that occurred either over months or years in about equal instances. In terms of chronic diseases occurring over months, the two major categories were neoplastic and structural lesions, both categories of which also were noted as chronic processes occurring over years. The neoplasms were about equally divided between primary and secondary or metastatic disease. The structural lesions included dermoids, orbital asymmetry, mucoceles, polyposis, pseudoproptosis, and cysts. Degenerative lesions largely occur in this category, as do the vascular diseases wherein arteriovenous anomalies tend to dominate. Lymphoproliferative disorders usually have a chronic onset and may even develop over years, as noted. The inflammatory diseases with chronic onset include low-grade nonspecific inflammations, sclerosing lesions, sarcoidosis, Sjögren's syndrome, occasional granulomatous disorders, fistulas, and some of the vasculitides.

In summary, catastrophic onset is largely due to trauma and hemorrhage; acute and subacute disorders are dominated by inflammation, with a relatively small number of neoplasms; and chronic disorders are dominated by neoplasms, structural lesions, and lymphoproliferations. This review may provide a simple framework for the differential diagnosis of disease according to temporal onset.

Clinical Onset

The four clinical processes alluded to in Chapter 6 on pathophysiologic analysis include inflammatory, mass effect, vascular, and infiltrative presentations (Table 8-6). Patients who had clinically obvious inflammatory disease were, of course, largely those whose final diagnosis included infection and nonspecific and specific inflammations. A small minority of patients with neoplastic, structural, and vascular disorders (generally in middle or later life) presented with pseudoinflammatory syndromes. The neoplasms that we encountered in this group include occasional lymphomas, meibomian carcinoma, and metastatic disease. The structural lesions that had inflammatory features included two dermoid cysts, a mucocele with fistulas, and a case of polyposis with recurrent inflammation. In addition, we saw several patients with pyomucoceles that had some features suggestive clinically of inflammation. The two vascular diseases that had the appearance of inflammation included lymphedema secondary to nodal irradiation and superior ophthalmic vein thrombosis. The major category of clinical presentation was mass effect; close to 70% of patients presented with some sort of displacement. The two categories of disease presenting primarily as displacement were structural and neoplastic lesions with a rare occurrence of either inflammatory or vascular disease. The inflammatory diseases that appeared primarily as masses were largely low-grade chronic disorders such as granulomas, sarcoid, and sclerosing inflammations. Many of the varices presented as either slowly or intermittently developing orbital masses or in patients with variable degrees of proptosis. Arteriovenous shunts, particularly when low grade, may masquerade as a proptosis without features suggestive of vascular disease.

Patients who presented with an onset that suggested vascular disease included those with varices and obvious surface lesions or a variable proptosis related to jugular venous distention. The majority of arteriovenous shunts were clinically detectable as vascular disorders. The patients with lymphangiomas often had a mass effect, but could be suspected in the superficial and the combined category if surface lesions suggested a vascular abnormality. Two patients with a superior ophthalmic vein thrombosis had vascular features, and a single case of lymphedema was noted in this group.

Patients who presented with infiltrative disease with limitation of ocular movement, functional damage, or cicatricial effect had for the most part secondary or metastatic tumors. The inflammatory diseases in this group included sclerosing inflammations. A few of the lymphoproliferative disorders had an infiltrative clinical presentation; the majority, of course, were dominated by mass effect alone. Amyloid and scleroderma were rare diseases that had clinical features of infiltration.

The outline of our experience is not meant to replace a careful clinical analysis of the patient population, but does provide a contextual framework for understanding the clinical onset of disease and categorizing patients following clinical examination prior to investigation.

Orbital Differential Diagnosis

BILATERAL PROPTOSIS

The lesions that can cause bilateral proptosis are listed below. From a practical point of view the most common causes include thyroid orbitopathy, acute and subacute idiopathic inflammations, congenital craniofacial disorders, myopia, lymphomas and leukemias, metastatic lesions, and arteriovenous shunts. The potential causes of bilateral proptosis are as follows:

Inflammatory
  Thyroid orbitopathy
  Acute and subacute idiopathic inflammations
  Vasculitis and Wegener's granulomatosis
  Idiopathic sclerosing inflammation
  Trichinosis
Neoplastic
  Lymphoma and leukemia
  Metastatic carcinoma
  Metastatic neuroblastoma
  Histiocytosis X
  Diffuse optic nerve glioma in neurofibromatosis
  Chordoma and chondrosarcoma
  Midline fibrous dysplasia
  Sinus carcinomas
  Meningiomas
Structural
  Congenital craniofacial dysostosis
  Mucocele
Degenerative
  Myopia
Vascular
  Arteriovenous shunt
  Bilateral varix
  Cavernous sinus thrombosis
Bilateral lacrimal lesions
  Lymphoma
  Sarcoid
  Sjögren's syndrome
  Acute and subacute idiopathic inflammation
  Lacrimal cysts

TABLE 8-6.
**THE NATURE OF CLINICAL ONSET OF NONTHYROID ORBITAL DISEASE (THE ABNORMAL PROCESS),
UNIVERSITY OF BRITISH COLUMBIA ORBITAL CLINIC, 1976–1986**

Onset	Process	0–20 yr	20–60 yr	60–90 yr	Total
Inflammatory onset	Infection	19	17	7	43
	Nonspecific inflammation	10	29	12	51
	Specific inflammation	2	19	10	31
	Neoplastic		4	2	6
	Structural		4	3	7
	Vascular		2		2
Total inflammatory		31	75	32	138
Mass effect	Neoplasia				
	Primary	57	46	9	112
	Secondary or metastatic	16	32	15	63
	Lymphoproliferative	3	11	22	36
	Inflammatory		5	4	9
	Vascular				
	Varix	8	4	1	13
	AV shunt	2		1	3
	Structural				
	Cyst	32	29	11	72
	Asymmetry	9	29	6	44
	Trauma	20	53	4	77
	Other	7	9		16
	Degenerative	3	3	6	12
Total mass effect		157	221	79	457
Vascular	Varix	3	2		5
	AV shunt	3	10	2	15
	Lymphangioma	12			12
	Superior ophthalmic vein thrombosis			2	2
	Lymphedema			1	1
Total vascular		18	12	5	35
Infiltrative	Neoplastic	Leukemia 1, Nasopharyngeal cancer 1	Secondary 9, Metastatic 5, Adenoid cystic 1	Secondary 8, Metastatic 10	35
	Lymphoproliferative		3	3	6
	Inflammatory	Sclerosing 1	Sclerosing 3	Sclerosing 1	5
	Degeneration and deposition		Scleroderma 1	Amyloid 1	2
Total infiltrative		3	22	23	48
Total, all types		209	330	141	680

PSEUDOPROPTOSIS

It is important to be aware of a number of disorders that may give the appearance of proptosis, yet not be associated with axial displacement of the globe. These include asymmetries of the bony orbit, globe, and lid fissures. The causes for pseudoproptosis are listed below.

Globe
   Myopia
   Buphthalmos
   Refractive: anisometropia
Altered lid position
   Ptosis
   Lid retraction
   Surgical recession of muscles
   Third nerve palsy
Structural
   Facial asymmetry
   Contralateral enophthalmos

NONAXIAL DISPLACEMENT

The differential diagnosis of nonaxial displacement has been covered in general in Chapter 5 on anatomic principles of classification of orbital disease. The specific disorders we have encountered that have been associated with nonaxial displacement are listed in rough order of occurrence below.

Upward displacement
   Neoplasia of the maxillary sinus (malignant more frequent than benign)
   Lymphomas, inferior
   Orbital asymmetry and contralateral globe ptosis
   Lacrimal sac tumors
   Capillary hemangiomas, inferiorly located
   Childhood neoplasia of sinuses
      Rhabdomyosarcoma
      Ewing's sarcoma
      Carcinoma
   Rare lesions
      Sclerosing inflammation in the inferior orbit
      Carcinomas and melanomas of conjunctiva
      Maxillary cysts: Rathke pouch cyst
      Superior cicatricial lesions
Inward displacement
   Intrinsic and extrinsic tumors of the lacrimal fossa (see Chapter 12, section on lacrimal tumors)
   Sphenoid wing meningioma
Outward displacement
   Mucocele
   Secondary sinus and nasopharyngeal tumors
   Reactive and dysplastic midline lesions of bone

Large intraconal masses
   Metastatic tumors
   Lymphoma
   Lacrimal sac tumors
Downward displacement
   Thyroid orbitopathy
   Neurofibroma
   Mucocele
   Reactive and dysplastic lesions of bone
   Rhabdomyosarcoma
   Medial dermoid cysts
   Neuroblastoma

ENOPHTHALMOS

Enophthalmos is an important and frequently subtle clinical sign that is often overlooked. Three mechanisms alone or in combination can lead to enophthalmos: structural abnormality, fat atrophy, and traction (Table 8-7). The structural abnormalities in order of likeliest causes include trauma with expansion of the orbit, orbital asymmetry, destruction of the orbital floor due to maxillary sinusitis or mucocele, and absence of the sphenoid wing in neurofibromatosis. An additional cause is sympathetic paresis, which may be more apparent than real. Causes of orbital atrophy include: posttraumatic, postinflammatory, and postirradiation fat atrophy; distensible orbital varices; and lipodystrophy. The final mechanism for enophthalmos is traction due to cicatrization. The causes include metastatic carcinoma (particularly from breast, stomach, lung, and prostate), postinflammatory cicatrization of muscle, surgical shortening of extraocular muscles, linear scleroderma, and nystagmus retractorius as well as posttraumatic scarring of orbital soft tissue. In our experience, in 50% of patients with enophthalmos, the presenting symptom was apparent exophthalmos, ptosis, or diplopia, which suggests the sign is often missed both by the patient and the physician. Adequate history, photographic review, family study, and orbital imaging should reveal the diagnosis in all cases.

It is of particular note that patients presenting with enophthalmos due to metastases can be missed for significant periods of time. Enophthalmos secondary to maxillary sinusitis is due to erosion of the orbital floor; surgical correction will obviate the enophthalmos, facial pain, and visual symptoms. Cosmetically disfiguring enophthalmos is also treatable whether due to trauma, microphthalmos, or orbital asymmetry, and may be an important contribution to the patient's needs. In the case of asymmetry, a specific diagnosis will allay the patient's concern. Orbital varices that cause significant pain may require surgical intervention. In summary, enophthalmos is a subtle, frequently missed, but important physical sign that can and should be accurately diagnosed. The range of causes underscores the need for careful and thorough diagnosis.

DYNAMIC LESIONS OF THE ORBIT

The dynamic lesions of the orbit include all those entities that either pulsate, vary with positional change, or alter on Valsalva maneuver (Table 8-8). The basic pathophysiologic mechanism consists either of bony absence with communication of intracranial pulsation or a rich communication between the arterial and venous systems. In addition, venous anomalies that have significant communication with the jugular venous system (distensible varices) may cause intermittent proptosis. (The specific disorders involved in this differential diagnosis are listed later in Table 8-9.) One unusual dynamic lesion that we saw, but have not documented here, was a case of absence of the lateral wall of the orbit associated with neurofibromatosis, which led to bobbing of the eye with chewing as a result of transmission of movement from the temporalis fossa induced by mastication.

ORBITAL IMAGING: DIFFERENTIAL DIAGNOSIS

A number of broad categories of orbital lesions form the basis of differential diagnosis based on their appearances with imaging devices. Again, these lists are not meant to substitute for a rational diagnosis within the context of the entire clinical picture, but may help to form a basis for grasping broad groupings.

TABLE 8-7.
ENOPHTHALMOS

Structural Abnormality
Trauma
Asymmetry
Destruction of the orbital floor
Absence of sphenoid wing
Sympathetic paresis
Atrophy
Post-trauma
Postirradiation
Lipodystrophy
Varix
Cicatrization
Post-trauma
Postinflammation
Metastatic carcinoma
Post-surgical shortening
Nystagmus retractorius
Linear scleroderma

TABLE 8-8.
DYNAMIC LESIONS OF THE ORBIT

Bone Defect
Congenital absence of the sphenoid wing (neurofibromatosis)
Meningoencephalocele
Potentially destructive lesions of bone
  Massive frontal mucocele
  Aneurysmal bone cyst
  Reparative granuloma
  Xanthomatous lesion of bone
  Post-traumatic or postsurgical bone dehiscence
  Dermoid cyst
  Metastatic lytic tumors of bone
  Histiocytosis X
AV Shunts
Capillary hemangioma
High-flow congenital and acquired shunts
Vascular tumors
  Thyroid carcinoma
  Nephroblastoma
  Prostatic carcinoma
Venous Anomalies
Distensible varices

Isolated Circumscribed Lesions

Isolated circumscribed lesions may be benign or malignant, as follows:

Benign
  Cavernous hemangioma
  Benign peripheral nerve sheath tumors
  Fibrous histiocytoma
  Hemangiopericytoma
  Low-grade orbital and lacrimal inflammations (rare)
  Capillary hemangioma (rare)
Malignant
  Lymphomas, frequently nodular
  Carcinoid
  Rhabdomyosarcoma
  Metastatic tumors (occasional)

The major isolated noninfiltrative orbital lesions are cavernous hemangiomas, peripheral nerve sheath tumors including schwannoma and neurofibroma, fibrous histiocytoma, and hemangiopericytoma. The other lesions that can appear to be noninfiltrative are essentially very rare aside from lymphomas. Lymphomas may have well-defined margins, but they are usually nodular; the overall tumor frequently conforms to the adjacent structures in contrast to the other lesions described, which tend to displace and deform the other structures. Some rhabdomyosarcomas and metastatic tumors may appear as relatively circumscribed lesions on CT scan and ultrasonographic study.

Cystic Lesions

Types of cystic lesions and degenerations with cystic change are as follows:

Dermoid cysts
Cysts of conjunctiva
Sweat gland cysts
Microphthalmos with cyst
Lacrimal cysts
Cystic degeneration in rapidly growing neoplasms
   Rhabdomyosarcoma
   Melanoma
   Metastases
Cystic or mucinous degeneration in other neoplasms
   Lymphangioma
   Benign mixed tumor of the lacrimal gland
   Schwannoma
   Isolated neurofibroma
Abscesses
   Microbial
   Parasitic

The major isolated cystic lesions of the orbit are dermoid and various adnexal cysts. A number of the rapidly growing tumors may undergo cystic degeneration, in particular, rhabdomyosarcomas, melanomas, and metastatic lesions. Some of the benign tumors may undergo mucinous degeneration, including benign mixed tumor, schwannoma, and isolated neurofibroma. Lymphangiomas frequently have multiple low-density cystic areas that may be surrounded by an enhancing rim on contrast CT study. Abscesses, whether they are microbial or parasitic, may also appear as cystic lesions with low-density centers and a contrast-enhancing rim.

Isolated Infiltrative Orbital Lesions

The major categories of infiltrative orbital lesions include both benign and malignant neoplastic disease, inflammations, and depositions as listed below.

Benign neoplasms
   Plexiform neurofibromas
   Lymphangiomas
   Capillary hemangiomas
Malignant neoplasms
   Metastatic tumors
   Malignant fibrous histiocytomas
   Some lymphomas
   Leukemias
Inflammations
   Nonspecific orbital inflammations
   Specific orbital inflammations
Depositions: amyloid

The benign lesions, which may have an infiltrative appearance, are plexiform neurofibromas, lymphangiomas, and capillary hemangiomas. All are easily recognized within the context of age of occurrence and the clinical appearance. The malignant lesions and the chronic orbital inflammations may be difficult to differentiate because the clinical syndrome occurs in a similar age group and is characterized by a desmoplastic or cicatricial (infiltrative) response in the orbit. In particular, metastatic and chronic inflammatory disease fall in this category. The nonspecific inflammatory processes and some fulminant neoplasms such as leukemias may present a similar more rapidly developing clinical picture, and may resemble one another on imaging studies. Finally, amyloid deposition may be characterized by infiltration of the orbit with a silent, clinically restrictive disease process.

Lesions of Muscle

Lesions of muscle include the following types:

Inflammatory
   Thyroid orbitopathy
   Myositis
Neoplastic
   Metastatic carcinoma (breast)
   Melanoma (metastatic)
   Lymphomas
Vascular: AV shunts
Deposition: amyloid

The most common lesions of muscle are inflammatory disorders that may be differentiated on clinical as well as radiologic grounds. The specific differential diagnosis between thyroid orbitopathy and myositis is discussed in Chapter 9 in the section on acute and subacute idiopathic inflammations of the orbit. Some of the arteriovenous shunts may present a picture that can be confused with inflammatory disease, and on orbital imaging show relatively uniform enlargement of the extraocular muscles. The neoplastic lesions include metastatic carcinoma, particularly from breast, melanoma, and some lymphomas. Metastatic carcinomas are usually associated with a nodular enlargement of the extraocular muscle and reticular infiltration of the adjacent orbit. In contrast, melanomas tend to produce uniform enlargements of the extraocular muscles. Lymphomas, when they occur in extraocular muscles, can cause marked enlargement of the muscle and tend to involve preferentially the levator, superior rectus, and medial rectus complexes. Amyloid may also deposit in extraocular muscles as a nodular, relatively smooth enlargement.

Destructive Lesions of Bone

Solid Lesions

Primary
   Reparative granuloma

Aneurysmal bone cyst
Ewing's sarcoma
Wegener's granulomatosis
Osteogenic sarcoma
Fibrosarcoma
Secondary
Histiocytosis X
Plasmacytoma
Sinusitis
Bony metastasis
Epithelial malignancies of the sinus and nasopharynx
Lytic meningiomas

A large number of lesions can potentially cause bone destruction with or without a solid soft tissue component. In particular, the inflammatory lesions include chronic sinusitis, osteomyelitis, and Wegener's granulomatosis. Reparative granulomas and aneurysmal bone cysts may also lead to destruction of bone and may have areas of low density within them. Some of the malignancies that have a propensity to involve bone include histiocytosis X, plasmacytoma, and Ewing's sarcoma as well as a number of metastatic tumors, especially neuroblastoma and prostatic carcinoma. Epithelial malignancies of the sinus may and frequently do invade and destroy bone. Some rare lytic meningiomas may also destroy bone.

Cystic Lesions

Dermoid cyst
Mucocele
Reparative granuloma
Xanthomatous lesions

The category of cystic bone lesions includes dermoid cysts, which often have a low-density area due to the presence of fat; they affect a focal area of bone at the site of the suture line, often with a distinct margin. Mucoceles involve the adjacent sinus and the orbital structures with lysis of the intervening bone. Frequently there is an area of dystrophic calcification within the wall of mucoceles. Reparative granulomas and reactive xanthomatous lesions may also lead to bone destruction, and may have low-density cystic areas. The lesions of bone are discussed in greater detail in Chapter 12 in the section on mesenchymal tumors of the orbit.

Hyperostotic Lesions

Prostatic carcinoma (metastatic)
Meningioma
Osteomyelitis
Primary bone tumors
Fibrous dysplasia
Osteomas: ossifying fibromas
Osteosarcoma
Chondrosarcoma

Prostatic carcinoma has a propensity to cause increased

density of bone, as do some meningiomas and chronic osteomyelitis. Several of the primary bone tumors are characterized by a high degree of bone and osteoid formation within them, leading to densely calcified hyperostotic lesions. This includes fibrous dysplasia, osteomas, ossifying fibromas, chondrosarcomas, and osteogenic sarcomas.

Optic Nerve Lesions

Optic nerve lesions include neoplastic and non-neoplastic types, as follows:

Neoplastic
Optic nerve glioma
Optic nerve meningioma
Plexiform neurofibroma
Angiomeningioma
Metastases
Leukemia
Meningeal spread of tumors
Non-neoplastic
Sheath expansion
Apical orbital crowding in thyroid orbitopathy
Pseudotumor cerebri
Chronic papilloedema
Subarachnoid bleeding
Nerve expansion
Optic neuritis
Toxoplasmosis
Tuberculosis
Sarcoidosis
Infarction of the optic nerve

The differential diagnosis of optic nerve meningioma and glioma is discussed in detail in Chapter 12 in the section on neurogenic tumors. A number of non-neoplastic lesions of the optic nerve may lead to expansion (usually uniform) of the nerve or its sheath. Those lesions associated with sheath expansion include apical compression due to thyroid orbitopathy and raised intracranial pressure, in particular pseudotumor cerebri. Bleeding into the subarachnoid space either due to direct orbital or intracranial trauma also leads to expansion of the optic nerve sheath. Expansion of the nerve itself may be associated with a number of inflammatory conditions including optic neuritis, toxoplasmosis, tuberculosis, and sarcoidosis, all of which lead to a uniform density expansion. In contrast, when the nerve is infarcted either by direct vascular obstruction or due to adjacent inflammatory or vasculitic disease, the central portion of the nerve tends to appear as a low-density area.

Orbital Lesions with Calcification

Orbital lesions that show calcification without bone destruction are as follows:

Dystrophic calcification
  Phlebolith
  Varix
  Lymphangioma
  Old thrombosis in AV shunt or malformation
  At a site of old hemorrhage
  Chronic inflammation
Neoplastic
  Malignant and less commonly benign epithelial tumors
    of the lacrimal gland
  Extraosseous mesenchymal chondrosarcoma
  Meningioma
  Occasional lymphomas
  Occasional neuroblastoma
Osseous and cartilaginous soft tissue tumors
Cystic lesions
  Dermoid cyst

Epithelial cyst
  Mucocele
Calcification in the globe
Displaced orbital bone following a fracture
Calcified trochlea

Orbital lesions exhibiting calcification with bone destruction are the following:

Fibro-osseous tumors
Dermoid with bone destruction
Epidermoid
Mucocele

Many lesions in the orbit may be calcified, particularly with dystrophic calcification. Typically, lesions that have undergone thrombosis may form phleboliths including

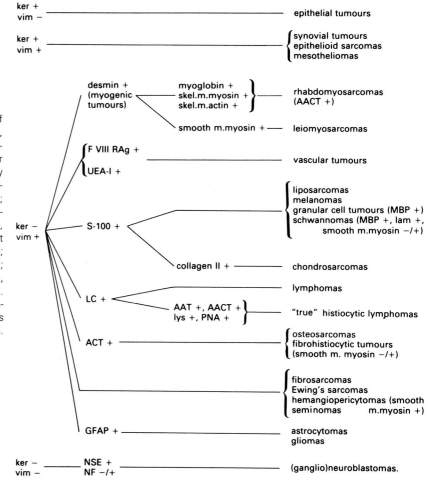

FIGURE 8-2. Flow diagram for use of markers in soft tissue tumors. AAT, alpha-1-antitrypsin; AACT, alpha-1-antichymotrypsin; F VIII RAg, Factor VIII related antigen; GFAP, glial fibrillary acidic protein; ker, cytokeratin; lam, laminin; LC, leukocyte common antigen; lys, lysozyme; MBP, myelin basic protein; NF, neurofilament proteins; NSE, neuron specific enolase; PNA, peanut agglutinin; SBA, soy bean agglutinin; UEA -I, *Ulex europaeus* agglutinin I; vim, vimentin; +, positive staining; −, negative staining; −/+, variable result. (Roholl PJM, De Jong ASH, Ramaekers RCS: Application of markers in the diagnosis of soft tissue tumours. Histopathology 9:1019, 1985)

varices, lymphangiomas, and AV shunts or malformations. Other causes of dystrophic calcification include chronic inflammation. A number of neoplasms are associated with calcification, in particular epithelial tumors of the lacrimal gland. In this category the malignant epithelial tumors are more commonly calcified than the benign ones. The osseous and cartilaginous soft tissue tumors are frequently calcified. Meningiomas, in particular the psammomatous variant, tend to be calcified. Schwannomas, especially ancient ones, may develop dystrophic calcification usually as a focal site. We have seen two lymphomas with focal dystrophic calcification presumably due to areas of necrosis. The cystic lesions of the orbit, including dermoids, epithelial cysts, and mucoceles, are characterized by a tendency to focal calcification, usually in the wall of the cyst.

The numerous causes of calcification within the globe include phthisis bulbi, osteomas, optic nerve drusen, hyalin plaques, and cartilage within dysgenetic and malformed globes.

The lesions that cause bone destruction and may be calcified include the primary fibro-osseous tumors, dermoids, and mucoceles. Both the mucocele and dermoid tend to cause excavation rather than erosion of bone, but we have encountered the rare instance of a ruptured dermoid with granulomatous reaction causing a more irregular infiltration and destruction of bone. The distinguishing feature, however, is the abrupt delimitation to the suture line. The full differential diagnosis of fibro-osseous tumors is discussed in Chapter 12 in the section on mesenchymal tumors.

PATHOLOGIC DIFFERENTIAL DIAGNOSIS

Among the soft tissue tumors of the orbit are two broad categories that may be difficult to diagnose histologically: poorly differentiated round cell tumors and spindle cell neoplasms of the orbit. In most instances, these tumors are distinguishable on the basis of clinical presentation and investigations, but in some circumstances this may not be possible with routine histologic study. Thus, more sophisticated technology is required to identify these tumors. Specific diagnosis is becoming increasingly important, particularly in the instances of childhood tumors where treatment protocols are related to tumor type. Chapter 12 discusses the common clinical and pathologic features of the individual tumor types. This section will deal with the histopathologic differential diagnosis of these tumors when they are not easily diagnosed with routine methods.

Both the round cell and spindle cell tumors can be divided into major subgroups on the basis of presumed cells of origin, which include epithelial, mesenchymal, neural or presumed neural crest, and lymphoreticular (Table 8-9). In broad terms, the need to define the cell of origin determines the histologic, electron-microscopic, and histochemical studies necessary to differentiate tumors in any of these subcategories (Fig. 8-2). It is the purpose of this section to extract from these groups those tumors commonly seen in the orbit that pose a problem of differential diagnosis. For these purposes, they will be divided into the common, poorly differentiated round cell tumors (Table 8-10) and the spindle cell tumors.

TABLE 8-9.
PATHOLOGIC DIFFERENTIAL DIAGNOSIS OF ROUND CELL AND SPINDLE CELL TUMORS

Tissue of Origin	Poorly Differentiated Small or Round Cell	Spindle Cell
Epithelial or presumed epithelial	Undifferentiated carcinoma Oat cell carcinoma Rhabdoid tumor	Spindle cell carcinoma
Mesenchymal	Embryonal rhabdomyosarcoma Ewing's sarcoma Small cell osteosarcoma Mesenchymal chondrosarcoma Thoracopulmonary small cell tumor Undifferentiated sarcoma Synovial sarcomas Epithelial sarcomas Mesotheliomas	Fibrous histiocytoma Fibrosarcoma Leiomyosarcoma Rhabdomyosarcoma Hemangiopericytoma Angiosarcoma Nodular fasciitis Fibromatosis Liposarcoma Osteosarcoma
Neural or presumed neural crest	Neuroblastoma Retinoblastoma Glioblastoma Medulloblastoma Melanoma Alveolar soft part sarcoma	Neurofibroma Schwannoma Meningioma Spindle cell melanoma Granular cell tumor Optic nerve glioma
Lymphoreticular	Lymphoma Leukemia: granulocytic sarcoma Plasmacytoma	

TABLE 8-10.
COMMON ROUND CELL TUMORS OF THE ORBIT

Childhood	Adult
Rhabdomyosarcoma	Anaplastic carcinoma
Granulocytic sarcoma	Oat cell carcinoma
Ewing's sarcoma	Poorly differentiated
Neuroblastoma	lymphoma
Poorly differentiated	Plasmacytoma
lymphoma	Melanoma

Round Cell Tumors of the Orbit

The poorly differentiated round cell tumors are neoplasms characterized by sheets of small cells with round or oval nuclei that usually have minimal cytoplasm. Inclusion in this group implies uncertainty about the tumor's cellular origin, and includes the broad differential diagnosis given above (see Table 8-9). It is worth reiterating that these neoplasms are usually sufficiently differentiated to allow identification by conventional histologic methods; however, the diagnosis of their primitive round cell counterparts, particularly when first identified as an isolated focus in the orbit, may be exceedingly difficult. Fortunately, the list of common round cell tumors found on orbital biopsy without an obvious primary is considerably smaller and can be divided into the broad clinical groups of childhood and adult occurrence (see Table 8-10).

Round Cell Tumors in the Child

Rhabdomyosarcoma. Identification of the poorly differentiated rhabdomyosarcoma implies the need to discern rhabodmyoblastic origin. Routine histochemical stains (phosphotungstic acid–hematoxylin [PTAH], Masson trichrome) rarely may allow recognition of cross striations. The muscle-specific immunoperoxidase stains may be very helpful in differentiating rhabdomyoblastic origin. These include desmin, the M (muscle) subunit of creatine kinase, myoglobin, actin, and skeletal muscle myosin. Skeletal muscle myosin and actin are thought to be more specific for striated muscle than is myoglobin; therefore, they are the most useful for differentiating rhabdomyosarcoma, particularly from desmin-positive myogenic tumors, that is, leiomyosarcoma (see Fig. 8-2).

Electron microscopy may show several features that taken together suggest skeletal muscle origin. These include cytoplasmic actin and myosin filaments, remnants of Z-bands, cytoplasmic glycogen, incomplete basement membrane around the cells, and primitive intercellular junctions. Phagocytosed collagen fibers are frequently seen in rhabdomyosarcoma and never in Ewing's sarcoma cells.

Granulocytic Sarcoma. A not uncommon soft tissue tumor of the orbit in childhood, granulocytic sarcoma is in essence a visceral focus of myelogenous leukemia. The undifferentiated round cells tend to have an indistinct cytoplasm, but may occasionally contain eosinophilic granules. An esterase stain and the immunohistochemical stains for lysosomes may help to distinguish this tumor. Electron microscopy may also aid in differentiating the lysosomal inclusions. Fresh tumor for cytogenetic analysis may demonstrate chromosomal abnormalities in a number of the poorly differentiated tumors of childhood, including Ewing's sarcoma, neuroblastoma, and granulocytic sarcoma. The chromosomal analysis may help in the differential diagnosis of these tumors.

Ewing's Sarcoma. The undifferentiated Ewing's sarcoma usually contains cells that are PAS-positive for cytoplasmic glycogen. Trichrome and reticulin stains show minimal collagenous stroma compared with the abundant reticulin matrix in lymphomas, rhabdomyoblastomas, and neuroblastomas. The immunohistochemical stains demonstrate no reaction to myoglobulins, immunoglobulins, or neuron-specific enolase. Ewing's sarcoma cells are keratin-negative and vimentin-positive, and tissue cultures may demonstrate synthesis of types I, II, and IV collagen compared with lymphoma (which does not make collagen) and neuroblastoma (which makes only type IV). The ultrastructural features consist of medium-sized cells with oval nuclei, a smooth nuclear envelope, scant membranous organelles (in contrast to rhabdomyosarcoma and neuroblastoma), abundant perinuclear glycogen deposits, and primitive intercellular junctions.

Neuroblastoma. Only the better-differentiated neuroblastomas show neurite and rosette formation with central neural processes. All neuroblastomas tend to undergo necrosis and calcification. Unfortunately, in metastatic neuroblastoma, features of neural differentiation may be absent and ancillary techniques become important in differentiating them. Immunohistochemically, the neuroblastomas are keratin-negative and vimentin-negative. Neuron-specific enolase (NSE) is useful as a marker for neuroblastoma, but has been noted in a number of other tumors including amine precursor uptake and decarboxylation (APUD) cell-derived neoplasms and melanomas as well as a number of central nervous system tumors, some carcinomas, schwannomas, and rhabdomyosarcomas.

Electron microscopically, the better-differentiated tumors may demonstrate synaptic junctions. The cytoplasm may contain ribosomes, well-developed Golgi apparatus, neurotubules, and pathognomonic dense core granules.

Cellular products such as catecholamine and its metabolites (vanillylmandelic acid [VMA] or homovanillic acid [HVA] may be found in the urine and blood of 75% of patients with neuroblastoma. However, less than 30% of patients with poorly differentiated tumors have detectable levels. Rapid catecholamine fluorescent techniques such as formaldehyde and glyoxylic acid fluorescence induce autofluorescence in neoplasms containing primary amines (catecholamines), and can identify 80% of undifferentiated neuroblastomas. Tissue cultures of neuroblastomas may allow for differentiation of the cells, wherein they form small aggregations with characteristic neurite outgrowths of slender, branching processes with beadlike varicosites.

So far, no specific markers have been described for neuroblastomas, but a panel of monoclonal antibodies with a high degree of specificity and several neuroblastoma antisera are being evaluated. Chromosomal analysis of tumor may be helpful in differentiating neuroblastoma.

Poorly Differentiated Lymphoma. The majority of lymphomas *when poorly differentiated* are associated with a known systemic syndrome, particularly in the adult. However, the child may have more frequent instances of primary presentation in the orbit, including the Burkitt's, pleomorphic, and lymphoblastic lymphomas. The poorly differentiated lymphoma is keratin-negative and vimentin-positive, but can be distinguished as a rule on the basis of the presence of common leucocyte antigen both in frozen and paraffin section. The traditional surface marker studies that are most useful in differentiating them include sheep red blood cell rosettes with T cells; rosetting of erythrocytes coated with antibody and complement (EAC) indicates complement receptors found on B and T cells and histiocytes; lastly, rosetting of erythrocytes coated with cytophilic antibody (IgGEA) indicates Fc receptors, found on B cells and histiocytes. Immune peroxidase or fluorescence stains can be used to detect cytoplasmic immunoglobulins in formalin or Bouin's-fixed specimens and surface immunoglobulins (IgM, IgD, lambda, kappa) in frozen sections. A large number of specific monoclonal B and T cell markers are available for identification of lymphomas. Ultrastructurally, the lymphomas as a group consist of small round cells with few organelles, minimal glycogen, and no intercellular junctions.

Round Cell Tumors in the Adult

The poorly differentiated lymphomas have already been discussed, leaving the major differential diagnosis of metastatic tumors of the orbit, chiefly anaplastic carcinomas, oat cell carcinoma, and melanoma.

Anaplastic Carcinomas. Metastatic carcinomas of lung, breast, gastrointestinal tract, and prostate may be sufficiently undifferentiated to be difficult to diagnose. In distinguishing them from other round cell tumors, the immunohistochemical stains for keratin are positive and vimentin stains negative in the case of epithelial tumors, in contrast to synovial tumors, epithelioid sarcomas, and mesotheliomas, which are keratin-positive and vimentin-

positive. The mucicarmine and cytokeratin stains may help distinguish squamous carcinomas from adenocarcinomas. The specific monoclonals for various carcinomas are discussed in Chapter 12 in the section on metastatic tumors. Of course, in this age group a careful systemic evaluation for a primary lesion is warranted in undifferentiated tumors.

Melanoma. The poorly differentiated melanomas rarely metastasize to the orbit, and usually are identifiable clinically because of their propensity to involve the extraocular muscle. They are keratin-negative and vimentin-positive, and will usually show a positive reaction to S-100 protein. Ultrastructurally, melanosomes and premelanosomes may be identifiable in these tumors. Histochemically, the Fontana or Warthin-Starry preparation for melanin may identify this tumor.

Oat Cell Carcinomas. An aggressive carcinoma of lung, oat cell carcinoma tends to metastasize early and the orbit is a not infrequent site. Because it belongs to the APUD neuroendocrine class of tumors, ultrastructurally there may be dense core neurosecretory granules and a positive rapid amine fluorescence reflecting the same origin. A primary is usually identifiable on chest x-ray and lung biopsy.

Spindle Cell Tumors of the Orbit

The common spindle cell tumors of the orbit are fibrous histiocytoma, neurofibroma, schwannoma, meningioma, hemangiopericytoma, and optic nerve glioma. The more rare occurrences noted in Table 8-9 are discussed in Chapter 12 in the sections on mesenchymal and neurogenic tumors; the differential diagnoses of meningioma and optic nerve glioma are also dealt with in Chapter 12 in the section on neurogenic tumors. The broad categories of tumor origin can be identified immunohistochemically by separating them into tumors of epithelial, mesenchymal, and neural origin (see Fig. 8-2). The epithelial tumors are keratin-positive and vimentin-negative, whereas the mesenchymal and neural tumors are keratin-negative and vimentin-positive. The subgroups of these tumors may be distinguished with special immunohistochemical stains. True histiocytic lesions are alpha-1-antitrypsin (AAT)-positive and alpha-1-antichymotrypsin (AACT)-positive. These are not absolutely specific to these tumors, because they can be detected in osteosarcomas and some rhabdomyosarcomas, and frequently may be found in spindle cell tumors that have a large cell component. However, it helps to distinguish this group of tumors. Tumors of vascular origin can be distinguished on the basis of their derivation from endothelium. Endothelially derived cells demonstrate factor VIII antigen and several monoclonal antibodies for blood vessel endothelium. The tumors that are of neurogenic origin may be S-100 protein–positive.

Fibrous Histiocytoma

Histologically, fibrous histiocytomas usually have either a storiform or a myxoid pattern. Frequently, there is an admixture of macrophages, which may be lipid or hemosiderin laden. Ultrastructurally, these tumors have interdigitating cell processes with a moderate amount of rough surface endoplasmic reticulum and no basement membrane. The remaining ultrastructural features include the presence of lipid, lysosomes, phagosomes, poorly developed desmosemes, and nonspecific cytoplasmic filaments. Immunohistochemically, they are keratin-negative, vimentin-positive, and reactive to AAT and AACT, as outlined above.

Hemangiopericytoma

With routine histologic analysis, hemangiopericytoma is usually uniformly cellular and has a vascular pattern with a dense reticulin meshwork that surrounds individual cells and distinguishes it from other tumors. It may be difficult to differentiate from fibrous histiocytoma and mesenchymal chondrosarcoma in the orbit. In addition, a number of other tumors may be difficult to differentiate, including hemangioendotheliomas, leiomyosarcomas, malignant schwannomas, angiomeningiomas, mesotheliomas, and liposarcomas. Immunohistochemically, hemangiopericytomas may be vimentin-positive and demonstrate smooth muscle myosin. The electron-microscopic features accentuate perivascular distribution, the presence of few subcellular organelles, and evidence of primitive smooth muscle and fibroblastic differentiation. The nuclei tend to be oval, and there is incomplete basement membrane and poorly developed desmosomes with uncommon pseudolumens surrounding extravasated erythrocytes.

Neurofibroma and Schwannoma

The complete discussion of neurofibroma and schwannoma is in the section on neurogenic tumors in Chapter 12. Only the more poorly differentiated variants cause significant difficulty in differential diagnosis. Both tumors are keratin-negative, vimentin-positive, and S-100 protein–positive. On electron microscopy both contain Schwann cells with a clear cytoplasm; minimal to moderate rough-surfaced endoplasmic reticulum; long, frequently interdigitating cellular processes; basement membranes; occasionally long-spaced collagen in the banded basement membrane; and endoneural fibroblasts. Generally, neurofibromas contain more collagen and perineural fibroblasts, are less distinctively encapsulated, and have demonstrable neurites throughout the tumor, helping to distinguish them from schwannomas. The myxoid variants may contain pools of acid mucopolysaccharide. The electron-microscopic features most readily distinguish these tumors on the basis of the almost exclusive composition by Schwann cells in the case of neurilemmoma.

This chapter has attempted to summarize our experience in the area of orbital disease to provide a framework for the differential diagnosis of orbital lesions. It is by no means comprehensive, but does highlight the major aspects of differential diagnosis in orbital disease.

Bibliography

Adam YG, Farr HW: Primary orbital tumors. Am J Surg 122:726, 1971

Cline RA, Rootman J: Enophthalmos: A clinical review. Ophthalmology 91:229, 1984

Duke-Elder S: System of Ophthalmology, Vol 13, The Ocular Adnexa. London, Henry Kimpton, 1976

Eldrup-Jorgensen P: Primary, histologically confirmed orbital tumours in Denmark 1943–1962: Histopathological and prognostic studies. Acta Ophthalmol 48:657, 1970

Henderson JW, Farrow GM: Orbital Tumors, 2nd ed. New York, Brian C Decker, 1980

Iliff WD, Green WR: Orbital tumors in children. In Jakobiec FA (ed): Ocular and Adnexal Tumors, p 669. Birmingham, Aesculapius, 1978

Jakobiec FA, Font RL: Orbit. In Spencer WH (ed): Ophthalmic Pathology: An Atlas and Textbook, Vol 3, p 2459. Philadelphia, WB Saunders, 1986

Jakobiec FA, Jones IS: Mesenchymal and fibro-osseous tumors. In Duane TD (ed): Clinical Ophthalmology, Vol 2, Chap 44. Philadelphia, Harper & Row, 1985

Jones IS, Jakobiec FA: Diseases of the Orbit. Philadelphia, Harper & Row, 1979

Kandel R, Bedard Y et al: Lymphoma presenting as an intramuscular small cell malignant tumour. Cancer 53:1586, 1984

Kemshead J, Coakham H: The use of monoclonal antibodies for the diagnosis of intracranial malignancies and the small round cell tumours of childhood. J Pathol 141:249, 1983

Kennedy RE: An evaluation of 820 orbital cases. Trans Am Ophthalmol Soc 82:134, 1984

Krohel GB, Stewart WB, Chavis RM: Orbital Disease: A Practical Approach. New York, Grune & Stratton, 1981

Llombart-Bosch A, Blacke R, Peydro-Olaya A: Round cell sarcomas of bone and their differential diagnosis. Pathol Annu 2:113, 1982

McKendrick T, Edwards R: The excretion of a 4-hydroxy-3-methoxy-mandelic acid by children. Arch Dis Child 40:418, 1965

Moss HM: Expanding lesions of the orbit: A clinical study of 230 consecutive cases. Am J Ophthalmol 54:761, 1962

Murray M, Stout A: Distinctive characteristics of the sympathicoblastoma cultivated in vitro: A method for prompt diagnosis. Am J Pathol 23:429, 1947

Reese AB: Expanding lesions of the orbit. Bowman lecture. Trans Ophthalmol Soc UK 91:85, 1971

Reynolds C, German D et al: Catecholamine fluorescence and tissue culture morphology: Techniques in the diagnosis of neuroblastoma. Am J Clin Pathol 75:275, 1981

Reynolds P, Smith R, Frenkel E: The diagnostic dilemma of small round cell neoplasm. Cancer 48:2088, 1981

Robbins S, Cotran R: Pathologic Basis of Disease. Philadelphia, WB Saunders, 1979

Roholl PJM, De Jong ASH, Ramaekers RCS: Application of markers in the diagnosis of soft tissue tumours. Histopathology 9:1019, 1985

Shields JA, Bakewell B, Augsburger JJ et al: Classification and incidence of space-occupying lesions of the orbit. Arch Ophthalmol 102:1606, 1984

Silva D: Orbital tumors. Am J Ophthalmol 65:318, 1968

Stout AP, Lattes R: Tumor of soft tissues. In Atlas of Tumor Pathology, 2nd series, Fascicle 1. Washington, DC, Armed Forces Institute of Pathology, 1966

Templeton AC: Orbital tumours in African children. Br J Ophthalmol 55:254, 1971

Triche T: Round cell tumours in childhood: The application of newer techniques to differential diagnosis. In Rosenberg HS, Bernstein J (eds): Perspectives in Pediatric Pathology, Vol 7, p 279. New York, Masson, 1982

Tsokos M, Linnoila R et al: Neuro-specific enolase in the diagnosis of neuroblastoma and other small, round cell tumours in children. Hum Pathol 15:575, 1984

Yanoff M, Fine BS: Ocular Pathology, 2nd ed. Philadelphia, Harper & Row, 1982

PART III

Diseases of the Orbit

CHAPTER 9

Inflammatory Diseases

Jack Rootman, William Robertson, and Jocelyn S. Lapointe

Clinical presentations of orbital inflammation based on differing pathologic infiltrations were discussed earlier. Individual case analysis can be done using patterns of acute, subacute, and chronic inflammation as a framework. This chapter will classify inflammatory disease from a clinical viewpoint into infective cellulitis, nonspecific inflammations, and specific inflammations.

The nonspecific inflammations can be divided into acute and subacute idiopathic inflammatory syndromes, sclerosing orbital inflammation, and noninfectious granulomatous inflammations of the orbit. The acute and subacute idiopathic inflammatory syndromes have the clinical and pathologic hallmarks of inflammatory disease. These disorders respond dramatically to anti-inflammatory therapy, and can be divided on the basis of location into anterior, diffuse, lacrimal, myositic, and apical. The remaining nonspecific inflammations tend to have a more chronic clinical onset and development with underlying pathology of sclerosing or granulomatous inflammation.

The specific inflammations are also largely idiopathic, but can be classified arbitrarily on the basis of histologically distinct patterns or clinical associations. They include sarcoidosis, Sjögren's disease, and a wide variety of vasculitic inflammations of the orbit. Finally, ocular inflammations may extend beyond the confines of the globe and produce orbital signs.

Thyroid orbitopathy is the most common orbital inflammatory disease. In our experience it constituted 48% of cases seen in the orbital clinic. Because of its incidence and unique character it will be dealt with separately. The remaining disorders, including infective cellulitis, nonspecific inflammatory syndromes, and specific orbital inflammations, account for 14% of all orbital cases in our series (132 cases). They were divided further on the basis of incidence into infective orbital cellulitis (infective, 43%), nonspecific inflammations (40%), and specific inflammations (17%).

■ ORBITAL CELLULITIS

Microbial

Infective cellulitis is a major cause of orbital inflammation. It may develop from contiguous inflammatory disease of the sinuses, face, and oropharynx; from foreign bodies; or secondary to septicemia. The causes include a variety of bacterial, viral, fungal, and parasitic pathogens that vary with regional epidemiology. In our experience most cases of orbital cellulitis arise from bacterial infections of the sinuses. The causes we encountered are outlined in Table 9-1.

The specific causes of infective orbital cellulitis tend to vary depending on the series studied, but the sinuses remain the most common source, particularly in adults. Schramm and co-workers, in a series of 303 patients with orbital cellulitis, described sinus origin in 85% and cutaneous origin in 10%, whereas the remaining 5% were due to lacrimal infection, facial fractures, dental sources, and surgical wounds. In children, periorbital (preseptal) cellulitis (87%) was more frequent than orbital cellulitis and sinusitis (13%) in a large series described by Weiss.

ORBITAL CELLULITIS AND SINUSITIS

In our experience sinusitis is the most frequent cause of orbital cellulitis, yet its rarity in an individual ophthalmic practice often produces quandaries in diagnosis and management, leading to late complications and inadequate or inappropriate treatment. Pathophysiologically, infection originating within the sinuses can spread readily to the orbit through the thin and often incomplete bony walls and its many foramina, or in a retrograde fashion by means of the interconnecting valveless venous system of the orbit and sinuses. The process develops through a sequence of edema and cellulitis to local and contiguous

TABLE 9-1.
**ETIOLOGY OF INFECTIVE ORBITAL CELLULITIS,
UNIVERSITY OF BRITISH COLUMBIA ORBITAL CLINIC**

Causes	Subtotal (%)	Total (%)
Sinusitis		58
Contiguous spread		28
Lid and facial	16	
Herpes zoster	7	
Conjunctiva	5	
Pyemic		3.5
Foreign body		10.5
Orbital implant	7	
Traumatic foreign body	3.5	

pyemic destruction of tissue planes with subperiosteal, orbital, and intracranial abscess formation and thrombophlebitis. Clinically, cellulitis is generally associated with axial displacement of the globe, whereas formation of an abscess, particularly in the subperiosteal space, usually causes nonaxial displacement and may ultimately track forward causing subcutaneous induration or fistulization. Posterior subperiosteal tracking may lead to rapid and catastrophic visual loss and neurosensory compromise due to apical compression.

Permanent visual loss can result from profound increased intraorbital tension associated with abscess leading to compromise of ocular and optic nerve function. In addition, visual loss may result from direct optic neuritis or vasculitis causing both inflammatory and ischemic damage to the globe and anterior visual pathway. A more devastating complication is spread of the infection by means of vascular emissaria to the cavernous sinus, leading to cavernous sinus thrombosis. In addition, spread by diploic vessels to the intracranial cavity can lead to subdural empyema or intracranial abscess formation. The intracranial complications of orbital cellulitis remain significant and life threatening.

In general, progress is characterized initially by evidence of increasing malaise, fever, lid injection, proptosis, chemosis, pain, orbital tension, motor dysfunction, rising intraocular pressure, and congestion of the veins of the choroid and retina (with papilledema and periphlebitis). Cavernous sinus thrombosis is associated with the development of headache, nausea, vomiting, fever, varying levels of consciousness, increased chemosis, bilaterality, nerve palsies (third, fourth, and sixth motor; fifth sensory), decreasing extraocular movements, and the development of a blue-purple lid. Despite the availability of antibiotics, cavernous sinus thrombosis frequently has a fatal outcome. The ophthalmological danger signals of progression are decreased vision, reduction of extraocular movements (especially if out of proportion to the degree of cellulitis), dilated pupil or afferent defect, en-

gorged fundus vessels, papilledema, perivasculitis, evidence of spread to the other orbit, a violaceous lid, increasing proptosis, rising intraocular pressure, and decreasing sensation (hypesthesia).

Classification

The classification of orbital cellulitis includes five groups originally described by Chandler (Table 9-2).

- Group 1: inflammatory edema (preseptal cellulitis, periorbital cellulitis) (Fig. 9-1A) is characterized by swelling of the eyelids with mild orbital edema, usually involving the upper eyelid (especially medially) in the initial stages. It reflects slowing and congestion of venous outflow. A slightly more advanced stage includes chemosis.
- Group 2: orbital cellulitis (Fig. 9-1B). The orbit is infiltrated, leading to variable mass and functional defects (edema, congestion, proptosis, motor and visual impairment). This can be a feature of either bacterial or sterile cellulitis.
- Group 3: subperiosteal abscess (Fig. 9-2). Purulent foci within the adjacent subperiosteal space may lead to nonaxial displacement, local tenderness, and possible fluctuant masses depending on degree and location. The size of the abscess and speed of development may reflect virulence of the pathogen or the unique pathophysiology of the subperiosteal space. Abscess formation may be rapid, because destruction of tissue planes is not a requisite to accumulation of purulent material in this potential space. In fact, a clinical clue to the development of subperiosteal abscess may be profound proptosis with a functional deficit in the absence of striking concomitant inflammatory signs, such as chemosis and lid injection. Displacement of the globe is frequently nonaxial and reflects the site of the abscess.
- Group 4: orbital abscess (Fig. 9-3). Progression of intraorbital cellulitis or spread from the subperiosteal space leads to intraconal or extraconal loculation. Proptosis, inflammatory signs, ophthalmoplegia, visual deficit, and systemic toxicity are frequently severe at this stage.
- Group 5: cavernous sinus thrombosis (Fig. 9-4) is heralded by profound central nervous system deficits or changes in local inflammatory signs with functional impairment (previously outlined).

Although this classification suggests an orderly progression, sudden and catastrophic events may occur with virulent pathogens or as a result of acute pressure blowout from a sinus into subperiosteal or orbital spaces. In addition, spread of infection to the cavernous sinus or orbital apex (Fig. 9-5) from contiguous disease (especially

TABLE 9-2.
ORBITAL CELLULITIS AND SINUSITIS

	Cellulitis	Abscess	Cavernous Sinus Thrombosis
Clinical Features			
Ocular and orbital	Group 1: Inflammatory edema Lid edema Group 2: Orbital cellulitis Increasing lid swelling Injection Chemosis Axial proptosis Venous congestion (choroid and retina) Increasing pain ± Increasing intraocular pressure	Group 3: Subperiosteal abscess ± Induration and fluctuation Increased lid swelling Chemosis ± Nonaxial displacement Increased intraocular pressure Increased orbital tension Decreased extraocular movement Local tenderness ± Decreased vision ± Papilledema Motor and sensory signs out of proportion to inflammation May be sudden Group 4: Orbital abscess Increased proptosis Increased inflammatory signs Ophthalmoplegia Decreased vision; papilledema Palpable fluctuant mass ± Perivasculitis	Group 5: Cavernous sinus thrombosis Bilaterality Increased chemosis Increased orbital tension Increased intraocular pressure Cranial nerve palsies (III, IV, V, VI) Decreased sensation Decreased extraocular movement Decreased movements out of proportion to cellulitis Dusky colored lids Increased venous engorgement Papilledema
General	± Malaise and fever	Increasing malaise and fever ± Spiking	Headache Varying consciousness Nausea Vomiting Fever
Imaging			
CT	Groups 1 and 2 Swelling of lid Sinus opacification Mucosal thickening ± Obscuration and infiltration of orbital fat	Group 3 Homogeneous subperiosteal accumulation of pus with smooth border on orbital side Enhancing capsule ± Gas Group 4 Homogeneous or heterogeneous mass ± Contrast enhancing capsule ± Gas in orbit	Group 5 Increased size of superior orbital vein (bilateral) Increased size of extraocular muscle Expanded cavernous sinus ± Cerebral infarct ± Abscess in central nervous system—subdural/intracerebral
Ultrasonography	Clear spaces Change in fat densities	Irregular, poorly defined lesion of medium or low reflectivity	Increased orbital vein size Increased extraocular muscle
Radiography	Sinus opacity ± Air fluid level	Sinus opacification ± Air fluid level	Sinus opacity ± Air fluid level

sphenoid sinusitis; see Fig. 9-4) may cause rapid, early, profound deterioration. Another important and frequent cause of variation in this pattern is incomplete or inappropriate treatment.

The ocular complications of orbital cellulitis are exposure and neurotropic keratitis, conjunctival prolapse, secondary glaucoma, septic uveitis and retinitis, exudative retinal detachment, optic neuropathy (see Fig. 9-5), and panophthalmitis.

Diagnosis

The clinical diagnosis of orbital cellulitis with associated sinusitis is necessarily supplemented by orbital imaging methods, because there may not be a direct correlation between orbital signs and the development of complications such as abscess formation (Fig. 9-6), particularly if incompletely treated. Ultrasonography and computed tomography (CT) permit accurate staging and localization

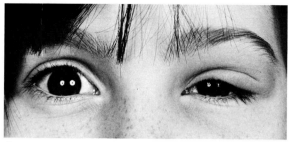

A

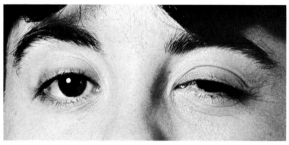

B

FIGURE 9-1. *(A)* This 10-year-old patient has the clinical features of group 1 orbital cellulitis or inflammatory edema (periorbital cellulitis) with mild edema (especially the upper lid) due to ethmoid sinusitis. *(B)* This 22-year-old woman presented with group 2 orbital cellulitis secondary to ethmoid sinusitis following an upper respiratory illness. She had 4 mm of proptosis, lateral displacement of the globe, pain, and tenderness associated with a slight decrease in vision. Both responded to intravenous antibiotic treatment.

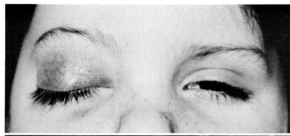

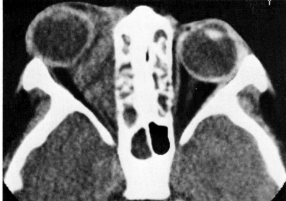

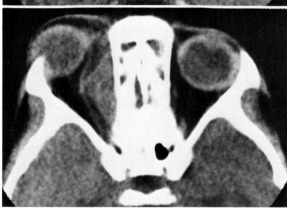

FIGURE 9-2. Group 3 subperiosteal abscess. This 10-year-old child presented with a 2-day history of sudden onset of right ptosis, injection of the lid, decreased vision (20/70), marked limitation of ocular movement, malaise, and anorexia following 7 days of lid swelling. He had mild papilledema and a tense orbit due to a medial subperiosteal abscess arising from ethmoid sinusitis, demonstrated on axial CT scans. Note slight tenting of the globe and bowing of the optic nerve *(middle)* and medial rectus *(bottom)*. He was treated with urgent drainage and systemic antibiotics, and recovered uneventfully.

of lesions. Routine sinus radiographs may show mucosal thickening, sinus opacification, or air fluid levels, but in our experience can fail to demonstrate early sinusitis and cellulitis that may be seen on CT scan. Ultrasonography is particularly sensitive in the anterior or medial orbit where abscess formation can appear as low or medium reflectivity of irregular or poorly defined lesions. Cellulitis may appear as clear or echolucent areas in the orbit on B scan.

CT scan will more clearly demonstrate the precise location and extent of the inflammatory process and can be used to follow improvement or worsening of the disease. Sinus pathology is reflected in mucosal wall thickening, opacification, and air fluid levels (Fig. 9-7). In chronic sinusitis, particularly of the maxillary or ethmoid sinuses, sclerotic thickening of the walls may be present. The inflammatory process may be secondary to a foreign body in the nasal passages (particularly in children), and this should be carefully sought after.

Preseptal cellulitis is readily recognizable clinically and radiographically by swelling of the soft tissues of the eyelid and face without involvement of the orbital tis-

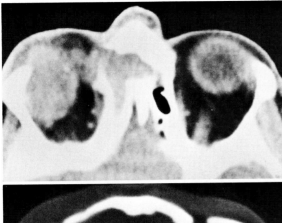

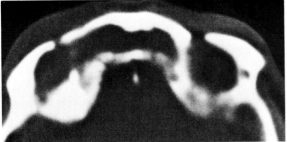

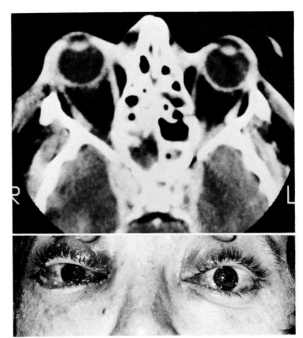

FIGURE 9-3. Group 4 orbital abscess is seen in axial CT scans of an abscess arising from the fronto-ethmoid complex (different window settings). The patient, a 70-year-old man, had a history of allergic rhinitis and recurrent papillomata removed from the sinus. This episode was preceded by a 3-week history of right supraorbital pain, inflammation, and swelling with intermittent drainage of purulent material "from the corner of the eye." He had developed a tense orbit with diplopia, ptosis, decreased vision (20/50), reduced extraocular movements, and downward displacement of the globe (5 mm). He was treated by drainage of the orbital abscess and sinuses and with intravenous antibiotics.

FIGURE 9-4. Group 5 cavernous sinus thrombosis. Axial CT scan of a patient who presented clinically with catastrophic onset of bilateral proptosis, chemosis, almost total limitation of ocular movement, ptosis, lid edema, profound decrease in vision, and varying level of consciousness. Note opacification of sphenoid sinus, engorgement of the cavernous sinus, and proptosis. This was preceded by a 2-week history of retrobulbar and frontal pain. The patient responded to systemic antibiotics, sinus drainage, and symptomatic therapy, but he had suffered a right cerebral infarct.

sues. Postseptal inflammatory disease or orbital cellulitis is usually associated with swelling of the preseptal tissues, chemosis, proptosis, and visual or oculomotor dysfunction. Depending upon the major location of the inflammatory process, the disease can be further subclassified radiologically into subperiosteal, extraconal, and intraconal.

Subperiosteal infection usually occurs secondary to contiguous sinus disease, most commonly ethmoiditis. Therefore, it is usually seen medially in the orbit. Following frontal sinusitis an abscess may accumulate beneath the orbital roof, and therefore is more readily visualized on coronal views. Fluid and pus that collect in the subperiosteal space may be seen on CT scan as a homogeneous or heterogeneous fluid collection. Because the orbital periosteum is relatively loose except at suture lines, it will be displaced away from the orbital wall as the abscess increases in size, leading to the development of a lesion with a convex configuration (see Figs. 9-2, 9-6, 9-7). Following contrast infusion, the periosteum may be

seen to enhance. As the lesion increases in size, it will displace the extraconal fat and extraocular muscles. Abscesses adjacent to the ethmoid sinuses displace the medial rectus and globe laterally, whereas those secondary to frontal sinusitis displace the superior rectus and globe anteriorly and inferiorly (Fig. 9-8).

When the inflammatory process involves the retrobulbar or intraconal space, the associated edema leads to an increase in the fat density (see Fig. 9-5). This is especially well noted in comparison with the contralateral orbit. Most commonly, inflammation begins in the extraconal space, then spreads to involve the intraconal compartment. If the intraconal space is predominantly involved and sinus disease is not present, a foreign body should be suspected. Inflammation here is also characterized by loss of the normal soft tissue planes that exist between the optic nerve, retrobulbar fat, and extraocular muscles. An abscess may be identified as a poorly defined mass lesion, and postcontrast infusion may present with one of three different patterns of enhancement: homoge-

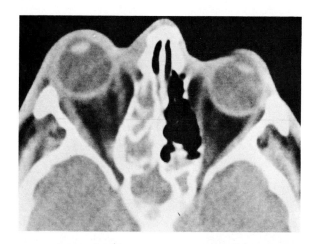

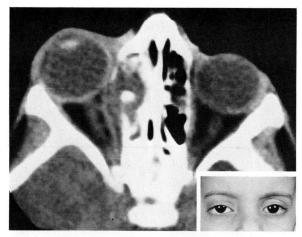

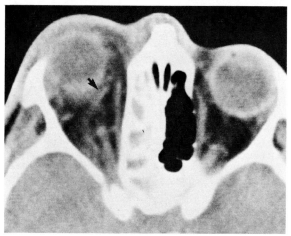

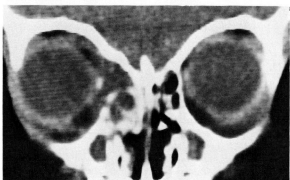

FIGURE 9-5.   Axial CT scans of an 80-year-old patient with right orbital cellulitis secondary to chronic and recurrent ethmoid sinusitis. Note lid edema, apical infiltration of the orbit *(bottom)*, and dilatation of the right superior ophthalmic vein *(arrow)*. He had suffered profound visual deterioration due to the apical cellulitis.

FIGURE 9-6.   This 3-year-old boy presented with a 10-day history of slight swelling of the right upper lid and lateral displacement of the globe. Two months earlier, he had lid swelling associated with fever and vomiting, which was treated with antibiotics for a short time. On admission, he had normal ocular findings other than minimal proptosis and lateral displacement. Axial and coronal CT scans show a destructive lesion arising from the right ethmoid sinus and extending subperiosteally, displacing the globe. At surgical exploration, it proved to be an organizing abscess from incompletely treated sinusitis. This case demonstrates a poor correlation between clinical signs and symptoms as a result of iatrogenic influence.

neous, heterogeneous, or ring enhancement. A homogeneous pattern may indicate the lesion has not yet cavitated. Orbital abscesses are most commonly located in the retrobulbar space or superiorly. Involvement of the globe is recognized by uniform or nodular thickening of the scleral uveal rim that demonstrates a uniform homogeneous enhancement. Even with the most accurate orbital imaging, a small percentage of cases may fail to show a lesion corresponding to the clinical findings.

The differential diagnosis has been outlined under the pathophysiology of acute inflammation. Basically, it includes ocular (uveitis, scleritis, and panophthalmitis) and orbital causes (nonspecific and specific inflammations, Graves' orbitopathy, and an untoward event in a primary or secondary neoplasm or cyst). Cavernous sinus thrombosis could be confused with arteriovenous shunting, but the absence of clinical inflammatory signs along with the distinct investigative features outlined in the section on vascular diseases would rule this out.

Epidemiology

There are differences in presentation, epidemiology, history, and prognosis in childhood and adult populations

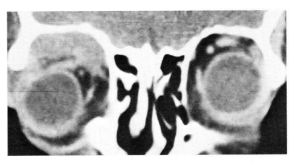

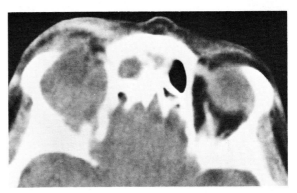

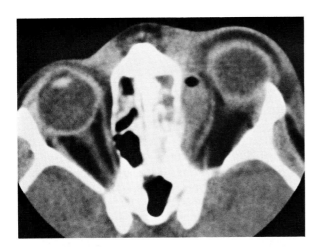

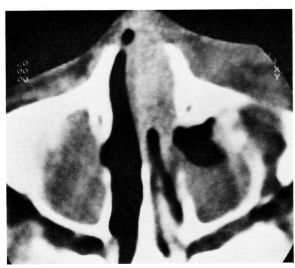

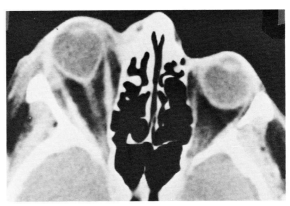

FIGURE 9-7. The patient, a 9-year-old boy, presented with progressive left upper lid swelling and injection, decreased vision (20/60), limited upgaze, and chemosis. Axial CT scans show a subperiosteal abscess with bilateral maxillary and left ethmoid sinusitis. Note air in the abscess, which is displacing the medial rectus and globe laterally, and the soft tissue swelling over the cheek. He was treated successfully with IV antibiotics, external ethmoidectomy with drainage, and antral lavage.

FIGURE 9-8.   Coronal *(top)* and axial *(middle, bottom)* CT scans of a 61-year-old woman who presented with an explosive onset of severe proptosis, downward displacement, and loss of vision as a result of an abscess in the right frontal sinus. There had been an antecedent history of progressive frontal pain for 2 weeks. The abscess penetrated into the right superior subperiosteal space, leading to massive and sudden proptosis. The marked posterior tenting of the globe is a result of severe orbital pressure and forward displacement from the tense abscess. In spite of rapid drainage, visual loss was permanent.

TABLE 9-3.
ORBITAL CELLULITIS AND SINUSITIS

	Child	Adult
Signs and symptoms	Lid edema, diplopia, decreased vision, proptosis	Lid edema, diplopia, decreased vision, proptosis, more frequent nonaxial displacement
General	More frequent malaise, fever, and anorexia	Less malaise, fever, and anorexia
Location	Ethmoid or pansinusitis	Frontoethmoid
History	Upper respiratory infection	Allergy, sinus problem, dental extraction
Bacteriology	May be no growth, gram-positive, gram-negative, *H. influenzae, S. aureus*	Frequent growth, gram-positive, gram-negative, *S. aureus,* mixed anaerobes
Management	Systemic antibiotics; drainage rarely necessary	Surgical drainage frequently necessary, plus antibiotics
Outcome	Recovery with few complications	More frequent complications including visual loss, central nervous system abscess, recurrent cellulitis, osteomyelitis

in children were of dominantly aerobic varieties, whereas polymicrobial and anaerobic growth was usual in adults. It is also suggested that long-term sinusitis in children, particularly those over the age of 6, is more commonly associated with preexisting allergic and local nasal problems, and may involve an anaerobic organism.

Symptomatically, both children and adults have similar frequency of decreased vision, diplopia, lid edema, proptosis, and facial pain with headache. Nonaxial displacement in adults is more common, reflecting abscess formation, whereas children tend to have more malaise, fever, and anorexia. In our series, bacteriology was successfully obtained in 62% of cases, more frequently in adults than in children. Bacteremia with positive culture is obtained in about one third of children, especially if there is leucocytosis and fever, whereas blood cultures are rarely positive in the adult. Direct nasopharyngeal, sinus aspiration, and abscess cultures are more frequently positive and clearly relevant.

The bacteriology of orbital cellulitis with sinusitis is as follows:

- Staphylococcal species (*S. aureus, S. epidermidis*)
- Streptococci
- Diphtheroids
- *H. influenzae* (children)
- *E. coli*
- *Pseudomonas* species
- Polymicrobial anaerobes and aerobes, especially in adults

(Table 9-3; Fig. 9-9). The differences reflect sinus development, predisposing diseases, response to specific organisms, and other factors. The ethmoid air cells begin to develop in the second trimester and the maxillary sinuses within the first 2 years of life. The frontal sinus develops between the fifth and seventh years, and continues to enlarge until adolescence. The locus of disease usually is ethmoidal and maxillary in children. The major predisposing cause of sinusitis in childhood is interference with flow of the normal mucosal secretions brought about by intercurrent (usually viral) illness. Children under 4 years of age are particularly prone to the development of infection with *Hemophilus influenzae* due to their inadequate humoral antibody response to polysaccharide-encapsulated bacteria. Hemophilus cellulitis is said to be associated with ecchymosis. Subperiosteal abscess formation occurs less frequently in children.

In contrast, adults typically develop disease in the fronto-ethmoid complex and have a predisposing history of sinusitis, polyps, allergy, trauma, and recent dental extraction. Recent evidence suggests that when adequate careful direct cultures are taken and promptly placed in anaerobic media, a high incidence of polymicrobial and anaerobic organisms are noted, particularly in the adult. This agrees with our findings that the organisms obtained

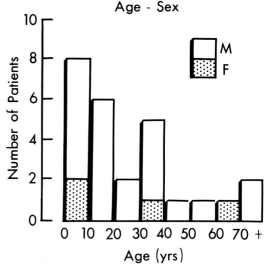

FIGURE 9-9. Age and sex distribution of patients with sinusitis and orbital cellulitis seen between 1976 and 1983 at the University of British Columbia Orbital Clinic.

The management and outcome of sinusitis and orbital cellulitis differs in adults and children. The literature suggests the overwhelming majority of children do not need sinus or abscess drainage with orbital cellulitis. In contrast, adults frequently require both sinus and abscess drainage. The need for drainage should be individualized and governed by the physiology of the particular case. We found that half of the children seen in our unit required sinus drainage, whereas 90% (13 of 15 patients) of adults required drainage. These percentages are vastly greater than stated in the literature (less than 5% in adults) and reflect the referral bias of severe cases in our series. Generally, few children (in some series none) need drainage.

Another major difference in the management of this disorder is underlined by the incidence of serious or persistent complications. In childhood most patients are successfully treated without long-term sequelae. Few childhood cases develop acute central nervous system signs, which generally resolve, and persistent or recurrent sinusitis is rare in children. In contrast, the adult patients in our series suffered severe and frequently frightening complications: six of the fifteen had permanent visual deficits, four had central nervous system damage (including abscess formation and epilepsy), one had cavernous sinus thrombosis, and two had recurrent cellulitis with osteomyelitis. This again is a reflection of referral bias, but overall the experience with adult orbital cellulitis secondary to sinusitis emphasizes the potential serious and permanent complications.

In summary, the differences between adult and childhood sinusitis with orbital cellulitis were more frequent antecedent sinus history in adults, fronto-ethmoid versus ethmoid involvement, a greater delay to diagnosis, frequent anaerobic growth, a need for sinus drainage, and a risk of serious complications. Another important factor in both adults and children is possible antecedent inadequate or inappropriate antibiotic treatment leading to persistence of an infective nidus.

Management

Treatment should reflect the serious nature of sinusitis and orbital cellulitis as well as differences in character, epidemiology, and complications that develop in adults and children. The role of the ophthalmologist is to establish the diagnosis and monitor ocular function during therapy. Staging of the disease is exceedingly important and may require extreme vigilance (every 2 hours if necessary), especially in the first 24 to 48 hours. One must observe and monitor changes in visual acuity, degree of proptosis, central nervous system function, horizontal and vertical displacement, extraocular movements, pupillary signs, and fundus. Careful orbital imaging studies are necessary in the presence of serious ocular dysfunc-

tion, marked proptosis, unexplained visual and motor signs (particularly when disproportionate to degree of cellulitis), or progression of cellulitis in the face of adequate treatment.

The principles of management are the prevention of complications, the use of antibiotics, surgical drainage (when necessary), symptomatic therapy, and follow up. They are elucidated below.

Prevention of Ocular and Nonocular Complications

Prevention of complications implies hospitalization, with careful monitoring of vision, systemic status, and central nervous system function as well as corneal protection with lubricants or moisture chambers. Severe orbital swelling may be associated with prolapse of the conjunctiva, which can perpetuate congestion if not properly managed. The swollen prolapsed conjunctiva can dry, ulcerate, and become inflamed, contributing to the orbital cellulitis. The conjunctiva should be carefully monitored and managed with antibiotic ointments and moisture chambers. In some instances when the orbit is not excessively tense, a temporary Frost suture attached to the lower lid and taped to the forehead can be used to elevate and partially close the lid, reinsert the conjunctiva, and allow for fluid absorption.

Use of Appropriate and Adequate Antibiotics

Cultures and Gram-stained smears should be taken from direct aspirates of the sinus or abscess and from the nasopharynx. Smears of sinus aspirates correlate with final growth in about two thirds of cases. Blood culture is more likely to be positive in the presence of leukocytosis and fever. Direct aspirates should be appropriately handled and placed in both aerobic and anaerobic culture media. Features of central nervous system involvement such as meningeal or bilateral orbital signs necessitate culture of spinal fluid.

Antibiotic Treatment of Periorbital Infection in Children.* The antibiotic of first choice for children with periorbital cellulitis or paranasal sinusitis is cefuroxime (Zinacef). This second-generation cephalosporin is effective against *S. aureus,* pneumococcis, group A streptococci, "oral" anaerobes, and *H. influenzae,* including strains that produce beta lactamase. Cefuroxime must be given parenterally; the dosage recommended for such patients is 100 mg/kg per day, divided in three or four doses. The drug penetrates well into soft tissues and bone and, unlike other second-generation cephalosporins, diffuses well into cerebrospinal fluid. The latter property adds a margin of safety in cases with unsuspected involvement of the cavernous sinuses or meninges. Adverse effects are infrequent and consist mainly of hypersensitivity

---

* Recommendations of Dr. Scheifele, Pediatric Infectious Disease Service, Children's Hospital, Vancouver, B.C.

reactions and occasional infusional thrombophlebitis. Cefuroxime is not available for oral administration; an oral agent with similar properties is cefaclor (Ceclor).

Alternative initial regimens include combinations of ampicillin and a penicillinase-resistant penicillin such as cloxacillin (100–150 mg/kg per day of each, divided in four doses) or cloxacillin and chloramphenicol (75 mg/kg per day, divided in four doses). The latter combination is more effective against beta lactamase-producing *H. influenzae,* an important consideration in patients thought to have cellulitis secondary to hemophilus bacteremia or sinusitis. For penicillin-allergic patients, clindamycin or a cephalosporin will provide adequate coverage for infections caused by skin bacteria, but cefuroxime should be considered or chloramphenicol added for infections originating in sinuses or blood.

The duration of antibiotic therapy is determined empirically. Most experts would continue antibiotic therapy until signs of periorbital inflammation have resolved fully. Associated bacteremia generally requires 7 to 10 days of intravenous therapy. If metastatic sites of infection are present, more prolonged treatment is required.

Antibiotic Treatment of Microbial Orbital and Periorbital Cellulitis (General). In adults, coverage should be with high-dose systemic antibiotics and aimed at gram-negative, anaerobic, and penicillin-resistant organisms (Table 9-4). Local epidemiologic differences should be taken into account and therapy altered depending on known resistances. Specific growth and resistances from cultures should alter therapy. When available, expert help in the area of infectious disease is advisable because of the complexity of organisms involved and changing antibiotic therapy. Empiric recommendations for treatment as suggested by Dr. A. Chow, Director of Infectious Diseases Services at the Vancouver General Hospital and the University of British Columbia, are listed in Table 9-4.

Surgical Drainage

In the event of demonstrable (clinical, CT, or ultrasonography) abscess formation or progressive deterioration and threat to ocular function, surgical drainage of the abscess or sinus is mandatory, because the organisms are in an avascular sanctuary. Ethmoid and frontal abscesses are best approached externally for drainage. A sinusotomy and antibiotic irrigation should also be performed, followed by insertion of a drain, which should be left in for about 7 days. In adults, sinus surgery should also aim to prevent recurrence by ensuring continued drainage or by obliteration of the sinus when necessary. A rough guideline for intervention can be based on the incidence of significant permanent visual deficit. It is suggested when vision drops below the 20/60 level the visual prognosis is poor, which may relate to either direct inflammatory effects or orbital tension. If an abscess is present and

vision is deteriorating, especially below 20/60, surgical drainage is mandatory. In addition, significant orbital tension that is not due to an abscess but has led to visual compromise may require removal and drainage of the sinus to aid in decompressing the orbit.

Symptomatic Therapy

Nasal decongestants and symptomatic therapy for pain, malaise, and fever should be instituted in cases of sinusitis and orbital cellulitis.

Follow Up

Careful and complete follow up is important to assure adequate treatment, because complications are frequently related to incomplete or inappropriate therapy. Noninvasive tests, such as ultrasonography and CT scan, may be useful to ensure adequate treatment. Resolution of inflammatory features with disappearance of the radiologic changes should be documented.

OTHER SOURCES OF MICROBIAL ORBITAL CELLULITIS

Other nonsinus sources for cellulitis include spread from contiguous structures (face, dental, intracranial); exogenous implantation secondary to wounds or foreign bodies; pyemia; and spread from infected intraorbital structures (dacryocystitis, dacryoadenitis, and panophthalmitis).

TABLE 9-4.
EMPIRIC ANTIMICROBIAL REGIMENS FOR ORBITAL CELLULITIS

Clinical Type	Predominant Organism	Recommended Regimens
Preseptal (periorbital)	*H. influenzae,* group A streptococci, *S. aureus*	Pen G + cloxacillin Chloramphenicol + cloxacillin Cefamandole or cefaclor
Orbital (sinusitis related)	Streptococci Pneumococci *H. influenzae* Bacteroides Fusobacterium Anaerobic cocci (coliforms are uncommon)	Penicillin or clindamycin Cefotaxime (Surgical drainage essential if abscess)
Trauma or foreign-body related	*S. aureus* *S. epidermidis* Streptococci	Cloxacillin, cefazolin, or vancomycin

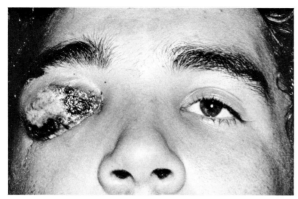

FIGURE 9-10. A 21-year-old patient with a severe necrotizing preseptal cellulitis 4 days after a minor lid laceration. He responded to systemic and local antibiotics with minimal scarring and no orbital involvement.

Contiguous Spread

The majority of infective cellulitides that spread from contiguous structures are preseptal. Involvement of the deeper orbital structures is rare (Fig. 9-10). In almost all instances, antecedent trauma with local infection has occurred. Hematomas and persistent subcuticular edema may predispose to bacterial colonization. Usually with infections there is a profound degree of swelling due to the loose subcutaneous tissues of the lid. Although swelling may give an impression of deeper orbital involvement, such spread is rare. However, in untreated or severe infections spread may occur into the deep orbit, resulting in catastrophic damage (Fig. 9-11). Preseptal cellulitis can usually be distinguished from orbital involvement by the absence of profound systemic malaise, fever, pain, chemosis, and proptosis, and the presence of normal vision and extraocular movements.

A large variety of organisms are encountered, but the most common are *S. aureus* and *Strep. pyogenes*. Staphylococcal infections are usually profusely purulent, and *Strep. pyogenes* may cause a gangrenous necrosis. Foul-smelling anaerobic infections may present as superinfections or in wounds contaminated by soil and bites, or in those associated with extensive trauma and necrosis. Infection with *Strep. pyogenes* group A may produce a distinctive but rare clinical picture of erysipelas. This usually starts with a well-defined erythematous leading edge and progresses to an intensely injected, firm, tender, hot lesion of the skin. There may be no known preexisting trauma. The infection can spread to the orbit. Generally, the patient has profound systemic malaise.

Management includes careful attempts at bacterial isolation, systemic and local antibiotics, and surgical drainage of abscesses. Direct culture and scraping of draining wounds will usually yield an organism. However, in the absence of drainage, careful limited aspiration of the subcuticular tissues can aid in isolation of bacteria. They can be obtained by direct aspiration or immediately following instillation in the tissue of a small amount (1/2 ml – 1 ml) of sterile saline.

Incision and drainage of the preseptal loculation is most effectively achieved over the lateral rim of the orbit or directly from a pointing site. If a preexisting wound is already draining, it may be enlarged. A small Penrose

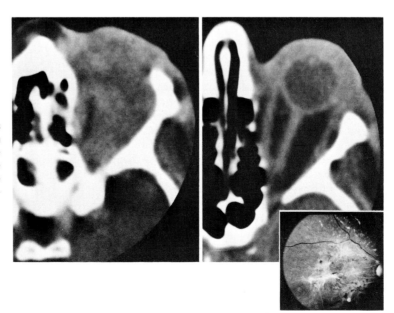

FIGURE 9-11. CT findings of orbital cellulitis resulting from an infected wound of the lid in a 34-year-old man. Note tenting of the globe due to severe orbital tension. In spite of drainage and systemic antibiotics, he remained blind due to retinitis and infarction. *(Inset)* Fundus photograph 3 months after cellulitis.

drain should be inserted and extracted slowly over several days to maintain drainage. Hot compresses promote exudation and aid in recovery. Antibiotics should be systemically administered and chosen by clinical features, initial smear, or likely organisms. Drugs effective against penicillin-resistant and gram-negative organisms should be instituted with demonstration of gram-positive cocci or gram-negative smears or following a negative Gram's stain. If the disease is localized and the patient systemically well, oral antibiotics will be sufficient. However, early intravenous antibiotics should be instituted in the presence of systemic malaise, orbital spread, and significant leucocytosis. Treatment should continue for 7 days or until drainage resolves. In the instance of streptococcal infections, a 10-day period of treatment is necessary to avoid late glomerulonephritis.

Contiguous (Exogenous) Cellulitis in Children

Infection of the skin and subcutaneous tissues, especially of the face, are common in children and warrant separate discussion. The immunologic and local predispositions are different in children, and produce several special syndromes, including impetigo, *H. influenzae* cellulitis and conjunctivitis, and maxillary osteomyelitis. Impetigo is a superficial mixed infection with *S. aureus* and group A *S. pyogenes*. Characteristically, impetigo involves the head and neck, starting as a reddish macule and progressing to vesicular eruptions that ultimately rupture and drain, producing yellow ocher crusts. When the lids are affected, profound injection and edema may occur. Treatment is with local hygiene, antibiotic ointment, and systemically administered antibiotic appropriate for penicillin-resistant organisms.

Children under 3 years of age are prone to a distinctive infection with *H. influenzae*. It is usually associated with an upper respiratory infection, systemic malaise, and fever. Involvement of the conjunctiva produces a mucopurulent discharge, and the lid is characteristically violaceous. The organism may also produce sinusitis and orbital cellulitis, as noted previously. Blood cultures are especially useful in this circumstance because bacteremia is common. Profound and rapid progression may occur, and intravenous systemic antibiotics are mandatory. Because *H. influenzae* organisms are frequently penicillin resistant, the drug of choice is ampicillin, or chloramphenicol if the organisms are ampicillin resistant. Chloramphenicol drops should be applied locally for the conjunctivitis.

A rare fulminant osteomyelitis of the superior maxilla may occur in children under the age of 9 months. The infection is due to *S. aureus* and associated with profound systemic symptoms and rapid progression. Because of rapid spread and potential intracranial, orbital,

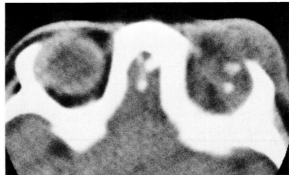
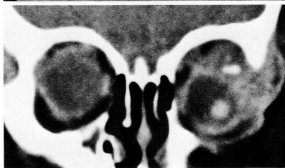

FIGURE 9-12. Axial and coronal CT scans show an orbital abscess secondary to a foreign body. This was seen in a 1 1/2-year-old girl who had a small stab wound of the upper lid 10 days earlier after falling on a lead pencil. She presented with a 2-day history of swelling of the lid and purulent drainage. There was no visible lid wound, but a small sinus was noted in the superior fornix. The abscess was drained and cultured mixed organisms *(Streptococcus viridans, Hemophilus influenza,* and anaerobic gram-negative rods).

and systemic involvement, high-dose antimicrobial intravenous therapy is indicated.

Other Contiguous Infections

Conjunctivitis rarely spreads to involve the deeper orbital tissues and has a characteristic conjunctival history. We have encountered several instances of orbital cellulitis progressing from severe conjunctivitis. Another common preseptal cellulitis we have encountered that masquerades as orbital cellulitis is that of herpes zoster. The older age group, lack of history, and development of sensory and vesicular signs (especially conjunctival and ocular) will point to this diagnosis.

Orbital Foreign Bodies

Orbital foreign bodies are another source of infection, the most common in our experience being infection from an eroding orbital implant. Generally, foreign bodies either induce a rapidly developing cellulitis or produce a

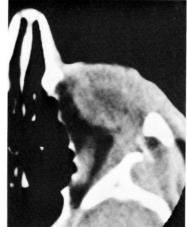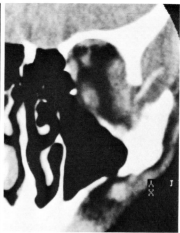

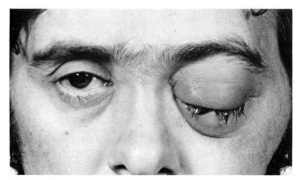

FIGURE 9-13.   This 55-year-old man presented with a chronic draining sinus and low-grade orbital cellulitis associated with trismus. He had fallen 3 months earlier into a thicket of branches. On axial and coronal CT scans, the wooden foreign body that had penetrated the left lateral orbital wall and temporalis fossa is identified as a linear density crossing the wall at right angles. At surgery, the branch that was extracted from the temporalis fossa had extended into the pterygopalatine fossa, accounting for the trismus.

localized abscess (Fig. 9-12) that may progress to fistulization. Vegetable foreign bodies may also induce a chronic granulomatous response with fistulization (Fig. 9-13). Treatment implies mandatory removal of the offending foreign body, local irrigation, and systemic antibiotics. Failure to remove the foreign body will ultimately result in a persistent cellulitis or draining fistula.

Pyemic Cellulitis

Pyemic orbital cellulitis is a rare but important occurrence, especially in the compromised host. In these circumstances local and systemic bacteriologic evaluation is important, because unusual organisms may be involved. We have seen two cases of panophthalmitis with orbital cellulitis secondary to bacteremia (Fig. 9-14). In both instances, the patients were compromised hosts; one was a chronic alcoholic, and the other an elderly patient with an intercurrent bladder infection.

Intraorbital Sources of Cellulitis

Dacryoadenitis, panophthalmitis (Fig. 9-15), and dacryocystitis are additional sources of orbital infection. In all these instances, the microbial infections may spread beyond the site of origin and into the orbit.

Fungus Infections

RHINO-ORBITAL MUCORMYCOSIS

Rhino-orbital mucormycosis is an aggressive opportunistic infection that occurs in debilitated patients. The ubiquitous fungal pathogen is from the class of Phycomycetes (order Mucoralis), which occur naturally in soil, air, skin, body orifices, manure, and food. Patients with uncon-

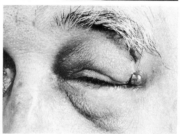

FIGURE 9-14.   This 33-year-old chronic alcoholic developed septic endophthalmitis and orbital cellulitis from a pulmonary infection. The organisms cultured from the anterior chamber were *Staphylococcus aureus* and betahemolytic *Streptococcus*.

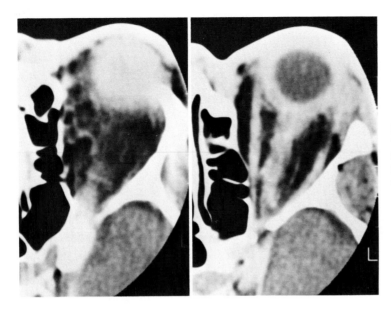

FIGURE 9-15. Axial CT scans demonstrate the features of severe endophthalmitis and orbital cellulitis following a posterior chamber lens implant. Note marked infiltration of the orbital fat and thickening of the uveoscleral envelope.

trolled diabetes with ketoacidosis and patients immuno-compromised by drugs or disease are particularly prone to infection, whereas healthy persons are rarely affected.

The sinus and nasopharyngeal tissues are inoculated by spores that are usually contained by phagocytes in persons with normal cellular and humoral defenses. Growth and spread of the organism into the tissues is associated with invasion by the hyphae. Histologically these large, nonseptate branching hyphae can readily be seen with routine staining methods (hematoxylin-eosin) (Fig. 9-16). This organism has a propensity to invade and occlude vascular lumina, leading to infarction, which compounds the inflammatory necrosis. The infarcted tissue forms a characteristic black eschar. Spread to adjacent tissues of the orbit and intracranial cavity lead to rapid and devastating progression and a fatal outcome.

Early diagnosis can allow for containment and successful therapy; thus, recognition of the characteristic pattern in a predisposed patient can save both sight and life. Orbital involvement is associated with antecedent sinusitis, pharyngitis, and nasal discharge. The earliest orbital sign is the presence of an apical boring pain. Progression is associated with the development of increasing cellulitis, proptosis, abrupt visual failure, and orbital apical neuropathies. The presence of a characteristic eschar of the skin, palate, or nasal mucosa in the early stages is rare. CT scan will show displacement of orbital structures adjacent to the opacified sinus, with and without bony destruction. In addition, increasing density of soft tissue and enlargement of the optic nerve with a central lucent area may be noted. Angiography may demonstrate obstruction of vessels.

Successful treatment implies a well-coordinated, prompt, and active multidisciplinary approach. An early definitive diagnosis is associated with a more favorable outcome. Tissues should be obtained for microscopic examination, fungal culture, and histopathology. Correction of the underlying metabolic disorder is mandatory: failure to respond metabolically may be a clue to diagnosis. Wide local excision of the involved tissues and adequate postoperative surgical drainage are also required. If caught sufficiently early, this need not imply exenteration. Systemic amphotericin B (optimum doses vary) as well as local irrigation of tissues with amphotericin B (1 mg/ml of irrigating solution) is the recommended antifungal therapy. The extent of surgical excision should be balanced against the threat to life and vision, and the expected deformity. A surgical clue to the line of excision is that little bleeding occurs in areas of significant involvement because of vascular occlusion caused by the organism. Some authors have suggested hyperbaric oxygenation may play a role in the management of this disorder. Although more patients are being successfully treated, the nature of the predisposing condition and the disease itself frequently militate against survival.

ASPERGILLOSIS

Aspergillus is a ubiquitous and usually harmless saprophyte best known as a source of opportunistic infections. In the environment, it exists as a conidiophore topped by a vesicle containing spores; the released spores constantly circulate in the atmosphere. It is the only fungus aside

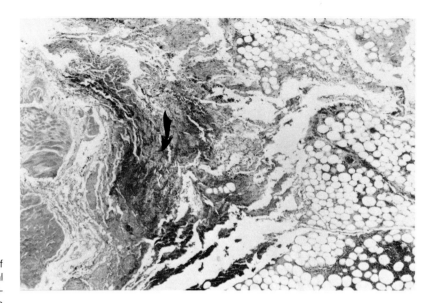

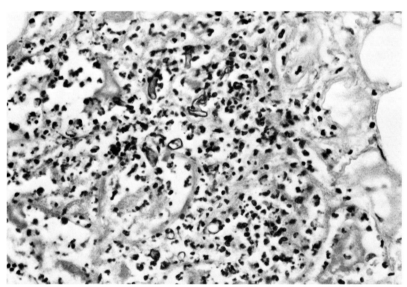

FIGURE 9-16. Histologic features of orbital mucormycosis. *(Top)* Note focal areas of necrosis and inflammatory infiltration *(arrow)*. *(Bottom)* Nonseptate branching hyphae of mucormycosis (H&E, original magnification × 2.5 *top*, × 25 *bottom*).

from *Rhizopus* that stains with hematoxylin-eosin in addition to the specific fungal stains. *Aspergillus*, however, is septate whereas *Rhizopus* is not. It is difficult to culture. This organism is becoming known to ophthalmologists as a cause of septic endophthalmitis, corneal ulcers, and orbital invasion. The increasing frequency is related to drug addiction, kidney transplants, and immunosuppressed hosts.

There are two clinical circumstances in which this organism presents. The first is a disseminated form that causes a widespread necrotizing angiitis due to microscopic foci of fungus in the small vessels, leading to thrombosis. Endophthalmitis is a common sequel to this. The disseminated form is no longer rare, with a 158% increase in the number of cases between 1970 and 1976; it is now the third most common systemic mycosis and the second most common mycotic infection of the central nervous system after candidiasis.

The second form of presentation in the orbit is a relatively slowly developing sclerosing, infiltrative mass, usually originating from an adjacent sinus. This local kind of infiltrative disease is more common in hot, humid climates. When anterior, it leads primarily to proptosis and displacement of the globe, but apical infiltrates may cause an orbital apex syndrome. This form of aspergillosis usually occurs opportunistically in healthy persons, but predisposition related to recurrent sinusitis and polyps is frequent. Although the usual infiltrate is a granulomatous fibrosing disease, focal abscess formation and fistulas may occur. Infiltration and damage to sensory and visual structures may lead to pain and amaurosis.

In disseminated aspergillosis, diagnosis may be difficult because the organism is seldom cultured before death. Local disease is probably best treated by surgical drainage and debridement. Amphotericin B and flucytosine may be used in nonneutropenic patients who have invasive aspergillosis.

OTHER MYCOTIC INFECTIONS

There are a number of other fungal organisms that have been rarely associated with orbital involvement, usually secondary to local extension from skin or sinus structures and, in some instances, with disseminated disease. Orbital involvement with North American blastomycosis, African histoplasmosis (H. duboisii), sporotrichosis, rhinosporidiosis, coccidioidomycosis, and candidiasis have been sporadically described.

Tuberculosis and Syphilis

TUBERCULOSIS OF THE ORBIT

In western countries, the decreasing incidence of tuberculosis has made its orbital manifestations a rare entity. Concomitant with this decrease has been a change in epidemiology such that extrapulmonary lesions are becoming proportionately more common. Orbital involvement occurs in two circumstances: either secondary to hematogenous spread or by direct extension from contiguous structures. Hematogenous dissemination of the disease can lead to two orbital manifestations. The first, and more common, is one of periostitis, which characteristically affects the malar bone of young people (first and second decade). Periostitis usually appears as an insidious localized inflammatory lesion that leads to cold abscess, sequestration, and fistula formation. Orbital tuberculoma is the other manifestation of hematologic spread. It is associated with the development of a cicatrizing infiltrative orbital mass, which may lead to neurosensory deficit. In both instances, active systemic tuberculosis is said to be rarely evident; however, strongly positive tuberculin skin tests are usually noted. In third world countries, concomitant evidence of active tuberculosis is said to be much more frequent.

The next major source of orbital tuberculosis is from direct spread from intraorbital structures (lacrimal gland) or more commonly from the adjacent sinuses. Sinus spread leads to a destructive necrotizing infiltrative lesion that can have cutaneous erosive fistulas.

In all of these circumstances, growth of acid-fast bacilli from direct biopsy material is rare, but caseating granulomas with considerable sclerosis are noted. Evidence of such a lesion in the presence of a strongly positive tuberculin skin test may warrant treatment on a presumptive basis while awaiting culture. Two cases have recently been described with positive response to antituberculous medication by Kahlil and co-workers. Recommended therapy is with systemic antituberculous drugs including INH, rifampin, or ethambutol.

SYPHILIS

Orbital involvement with syphilis is now uncommon compared to 100 years ago, when it accounted for 2% of syphilitic eye disease. Syphilitic periostitis may lead to diffuse or focal involvement of the orbital walls. It may appear as either an acute or chronic inflammatory process, which is characteristically painful. Fistulization, bone resorption, and secondary spread of syphilitic gummas into the orbit may occur. When the disease is apical, manifestations of a painful orbital apex syndrome are characteristic. Primary soft tissue gumma may also occur within the orbit, extraocular muscles, and lacrimal gland. Treatment with penicillin or broad-spectrum antibiotics should lead to resolution of local disease.

Parasitic Infestations

Parasitic infestations of the orbit have specific geographic prevalence, with the highest incidence seen in third world countries or in areas of endemic parasitoses. The most common orbital infestation is with echinococcosis but cysticercosis, microfilaremia, and trichinosis may also affect the orbit.

ECHINOCOCCOSIS (HYDATID CYST)

Echinococcus is a parasite infesting the intestines of dogs, sheep, pigs, cows, and other animals. It may parasitize man in its larval stage when it spreads to multiple sites of the body, forming cystic spaces. These cysts have a characteristic chitinous ectocyst and a cellular endocyst that may contain many scoleces in daughter cysts.

Orbital cysts are said to occur in 1% of infestations. Echinococcosis is common in temperate climates and the Middle East. The majority of cases are seen between the first and fourth decades. Lesions may occur anywhere in the orbit, but are particularly common in the superior and posterior portion. The onset of disease is usually insidious and dominated by mass effect. Rupture of a cyst may be associated with a more sudden and fulminant inflammatory course and may be a complication of either surgical incision or injury. Rarely, the cyst may erode through the orbit to the intracranial or sinus cavities or vice versa.

Diagnosis is made on the basis of the presence of a cystic lesion of the orbit. The lesion may have a calcified rim. The biological tests include an intradermal antigen reaction (Casoni reaction) and complement-fixating and hemagglutinating antibody tests. Results may be unreliable, making diagnosis difficult.

Treatment ideally is excision of the intact cyst by either a direct or lateral orbital route. Rupture of the cyst should be avoided, because a violent inflammatory reaction may ensue and the field become contaminated with daughter cysts. If complete excision is impossible, it is suggested that the cyst should be drained and sterilized with formalin or alcohol and irrigated with saline, following which the wall can be removed. If a violent inflammatory response results, it can be suppressed by local and systemic corticosteroid therapy.

CYSTICERCOSIS

Infestations with the larvae (*Cysticercus cellulosae*) of the tapeworm *Taenia solium* are rare in the orbit in spite of a preference for the eye and brain. The most common sites of occurrence are beneath the conjunctiva or in the eye itself. Orbital cases have generally been in the anterior orbit, and proptosis is unusual. The lesions tend to be small and may be quite inflamed. The presence of eosinophilia, positive complement fixation, and precipitin reactions are often inconclusive. Treatment is excision of the offending site.

Systemic cysticercosis has a propensity to deposit within muscles. We have recently encountered a case of extraocular muscle involvement with cysticercosis and are aware of another seen by Dr. Matas in San Francisco. The patient presented with limitation of abduction due to a mass lesion involving the lateral rectus muscle. This proved on extirpation to be an abscess containing a central scolex (Fig. 9-17).

TRICHINOSIS

Trichinae are derived from inadequately cooked pork containing encysted larvae, which escape in the intestinal tract and invade the bloodstream and tissues. Re-encystation occurs in striated muscle. The extraocular muscles are a site of preferential infestation.

Patients present with orbital manifestations of swelling of the lids, chemosis, visual disturbance, and a painful myopathy. Localized bulbar infestation may be recognized as a swelling over the insertions of the recti. Ocular muscle involvement is often antecedent to that of the generalized skeletal musculature.

The disease is diagnosed by eosinophilia, a serum reaction, positive skeletal muscle biopsy, or larvae in the blood. Treatment is with systemic thiabendazole and corticosteroids to reduce inflammatory signs and symptoms.

OTHER PARASITOSES

Rare microfilarial infection of the deeper orbit has been described, but the common infestation involves superficial tissues. Orbital onchocerciasis has also been noted, but is exceedingly rare. Other parasites, including Ascaris, Schistostoma, Entamoeba, and others, have been described in the orbit and lacrimal gland.

Other Infestations

Arthropodal infestation of the orbit is uncommon and usually occurs in conditions of chronic suppuration and debility, particularly in the tropics. Orbital myiasis can vary in degree from mild conjunctivitis with a localized larval infestation (*Oestrus ovis*) to full-blown, rapidly destructive lesions of the orbital soft tissues and bones (*Dermatobia noxialis* or *D. hominis*, *Hypoderma bovis*, *Wohlfahrtia magnifica*, and *Calliphora vomitoria*). Infestation with a single larva may produce a fistula and local inflammation that resolves on extrusion of the larva. Treatment consists of removal of the maggots and application of topical turpentine. Bacterial infections are treated with appropriate antibiotics and the tissues allowed to granulate. In severe cases, the dominant systemic debility usually leads to a fatal outcome.

■ NONSPECIFIC INFLAMMATIONS OF THE ORBIT

Acute and Subacute Idiopathic Inflammatory Syndromes

Traditionally, acute and subacute idiopathic inflammatory syndromes have been included with the polyglot of orbital "pseudotumors," a clinically and histologically confusing category of lesions. The described pathologic substrate for these myriad diseases ranges from nonspecific polymorphous lymphocytic and plasmacytic infiltrates to granulomatous disorders, depending on the spe-

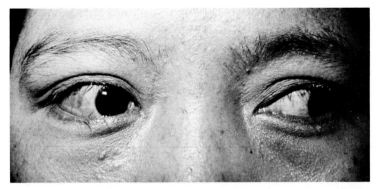

A

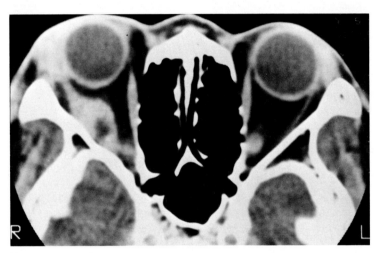

B

FIGURE 9-17.   *(A)* This 35-year-old Cambodian woman presented with a 1-week history of right ocular pain and swelling associated with diplopia on right and left gaze. She had pain on eye movement, 7 mm of right proptosis with restriction of abduction, and supraduction. In addition, the conjunctiva was injected with marked chemosis, mainly inferolaterally. White blood count was 8.1 with no eosinophils. *(B)* The axial CT scan shows a mass with a central lucency that was contiguous with and obscured the right lateral rectus muscle. Ultrasonographic examination suggested a solid mass in the right lateral rectus muscle. The patient underwent an orbitotomy for biopsy and at surgery an abscess was found within the right lateral rectus muscle, and was excised. *(C)* Histology reveals cysticercosis with scolex and cyst. Zonal inflammation of eosinophils, polymorphonuclear leucocytes, epithelioid cells, and occasional giant cells surround the organism (Masson, original magnification × 10).

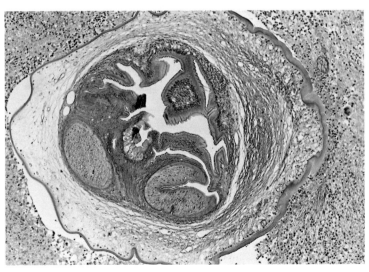

C

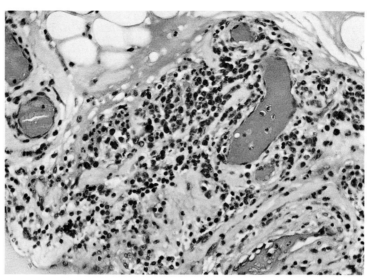

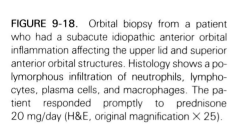

FIGURE 9-18. Orbital biopsy from a patient who had a subacute idiopathic anterior orbital inflammation affecting the upper lid and superior anterior orbital structures. Histology shows a polymorphous infiltration of neutrophils, lymphocytes, plasma cells, and macrophages. The patient responded promptly to prednisone 20 mg/day (H&E, original magnification × 25).

cific source in the literature. The full histologic spectrum, from truly inflammatory to pseudoneoplastic disease, has been described within this rubric. The histologic studies are confusing and may not correlate with the clinical features of the disease. Yet with improved orbital imaging and careful clinical analysis more specificity may be possible in defining the presentation and character of these diseases. The patterns of orbital involvement seen in these disorders may not point to pathogenesis, but do provide a clinical framework for diagnosis and management. They are a heterogeneous group etiologically, but in our opinion, their inclusion as inflammatory syndromes is more rational than a broader traditional framework. These entities probably include a number of different organ-specific immunologic disorders. Disease defined by the character of presentation and temporal sequence should form the essential diagnostic framework in this situation.

A common feature of these syndromes is that they have the clinical hallmarks of inflammatory disease, are generally acute or subacute in onset, and histologically are composed of polymorphous infiltrations of inflammatory cells, including neutrophils, lymphocytes, plasma cells, and macrophages, as well as some fibroblasts (Fig. 9-18). The rapidly developing inflammations are associated with an influx of cells and their chemical byproducts that produce pain, vascular dilatation, and edema with or without systemic malaise. In contrast, chronic or progressive infiltrative inflammations and granulomatous disease are usually characterized by mass effect associated with insidious destruction and desmoplasia; frequently they require biopsy to distinguish them from other entities.

Several clinical categories of acute and subacute nonspecific inflammations are defined by the location of the inflammation. All of these entities, although in differing orbital locations, have as a characteristic feature on orbital imaging an irregular margin adjacent to the primary focus. In addition, imaging suggests tissue swelling and enhancement with contrast media. We have divided the noninfectious inflammatory syndromes into nonspecific and distinct (specific) orbital inflammations. The specific inflammations are an extension of the nonspecific group, but are more clearly defined by histopathologic features suggestive of more precise etiologic relationships. The nonspecific acute and subacute idiopathic inflammatory syndromes can be divided into anterior, diffuse, apical, myositic, and lacrimal on the basis of differences in presentations and clinical findings. Although arbitrary, this division parallels the clinical situation and allows a framework for diagnosis, categorization, and management. In effect, most of the patients with acute and subacute idiopathic inflammatory syndromes are usually categorized as outlined and managed with nonspecific anti-inflammatory medication. The distinct and histologically defined group then derives from those who fail to respond to nonspecific anti-inflammatory treatment or those who have presented with features of a chronic onset or clinically distinct syndrome. Table 9-5 outlines the major features of acute and subacute idiopathic orbital inflammatory syndromes.

ACUTE AND SUBACUTE IDIOPATHIC ANTERIOR ORBITAL INFLAMMATION

In the anterior orbital group, the main focus of inflammation involves the anterior orbit and adjacent globe. The major features on presentation are pain, proptosis,

TABLE 9-5.
COMPARATIVE FEATURES OF ACUTE AND SUBACUTE NONSPECIFIC IDIOPATHIC INFLAMMATORY SYNDROMES OF THE ORBIT

	Anterior	Diffuse	Apical	Myositic	Lacrimal
Clinical					
Number	13	2	4	13	11
Onset	Acute and subacute	Subacute: remitting, progressive	Subacute: Chronic	Acute and subacute	Acute and subacute
Ages	14–77 (41)	6–13	18–61 (47)	18–70 (43)	16–83 (44)
M:F	8M:5F	1M:1F	2M:2F	7M:6F	9F:2M
Pain	+	+	++	On movement	With tenderness
Ocular and orbital features	Uveitis Retinal detachment Decreased extraocular movement Decreased vision Anterior inflammation Chemosis Diffuse injection and swelling of lid	Uveitis Retinal detachment Decreased extraocular movement Decreased vision Anterior inflammation Chemosis Diffuse injection and swelling of lid	Decreased vision Decreased extraocular movements Mild proptosis and chemosis	Painful Decreased extraocular movement Normal vision Localized injection and chemosis	Lateral swelling S-shaped deformity of lid Tenderness Pouting of lacrimal ducts Chemosis and injection localized
Visual outcome	Good	±	±	Good	Good
CT	Anterior: enhancing with irregular margins intimate to scleral envelope Variable extension along optic nerve Decreased fat density	Diffuse: enhancing with decreased fat density	Apical irregular infiltration Extends along muscle and optic nerve	Muscle irregularly enlarged Swelling of tendon Local scleral and Tenon's capsule swelling Fusiform enlargement of whole muscle	Irregular swelling of lacrimal gland and adjacent tissues
Ultrasonography	Sclerotenonitis with T sign	T sign	Negative	Increased extraocular muscle size	Local swelling with increased Tenon's space
Treatment	60–80 mg prednisone	60–80 mg prednisone	80 mg prednisone	40 mg prednisone	40 mg prednisone
Outcome	Generally resolve	Recurrent with residual	Clear 1–2 months May recur	Most clear dramatically May recur	Generally resolve

ptosis, lid swelling, injection, and decreased vision. Other findings may be ocular and include uveitis, sclerotenonitis, papillitis, and exudative retinal detachments (Fig. 9-19). The clinical pattern of presentation and severity correlates with the location and degree of involvement noted on CT scanning and ultrasonography.

In our 13 cases, the ages of patients ranged from 14 to 77 years with an average of 41 years. Eight of the thirteen patients were under 50 years of age. In the younger age group, the syndrome corresponds to that described by Mottow and Jakobiec as idiopathic inflammatory orbital pseudotumor in childhood. All of our patients presented with a history of onset over days or weeks. Thus, they could be categorized as either acute or subacute inflam-

mations. There were 8 males and 5 females. The characteristic CT pattern is one of a diffuse anterior orbital infiltration intimately related to the globe, producing scleral and choroidal thickening with obscuring of the junction of the globe and optic nerve and variable extension along its sheath. On ultrasonography, there is an irregular uniform density with anterior orbital infiltrate, sclerotenonitis with accentuation of Tenon's space, and doubling of the optic nerve shadow (T Sign) (Fig. 9-20). Systemic investigation may show an increased sedimentation rate and CSF pleocytosis, particularly in the younger age group.

The differential diagnosis of anterior nonspecific inflammation includes orbital cellulitis, a sudden event in a

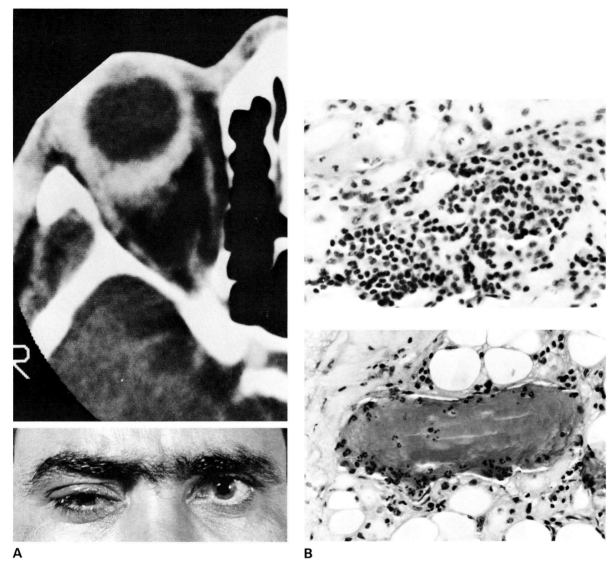

A

B

FIGURE 9-19. *(A)* This 37-year-old man presented with a painful, swollen right eye present for 2 days following a 2-week history of an upper respiratory ailment. He had lid swelling, injection, chemosis, and mildly restricted extraocular movements. On axial CT scan, there is a retrobulbar anterior orbital infiltration intimate to the sclera, without lid involvement. *(B)* Biopsy of the lesion shows vascular dilatation and sparse polymorphous inflammatory infiltrate (H&E, original magnifications, *top* × 25, *bottom* × 25). He responded promptly to prednisone 60 mg/day tapered rapidly over a 2- to 3-week period. There has been no recurrence in 3 years.

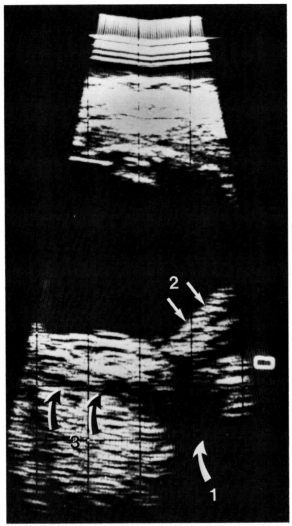

FIGURE 9-20. Ultrasonogram of a patient with an idiopathic anterior orbital inflammation. Doubling (squaring off, T sign) of the optic nerve shadow *(large white arrow),* peripapillary retinal detachment *(small white arrows),* and accentuation of Tenon's space *(black arrows)* are seen. (Rootman J, Nugent R: The classification and management of acute orbital pseudotumors. Ophthalmology 89:1040, 1982)

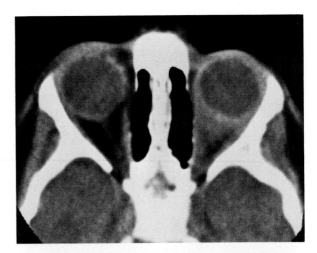

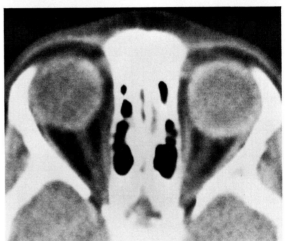

FIGURE 9-21. *(Top)* Axial CT scan (noncontrast) of left acute idiopathic anterior orbital inflammation. Note soft tissue density involving the posterior globe and anterior orbit with extension along the optic nerve. The soft tissue infiltration obscures the normal definition of the optic nerve and extraocular muscles in the plane just posterior to the globe. *(Bottom)* Noncontrast CT scan of the same patient 9 months after initiation of therapy. The globe, optic nerve, and anterior orbit are now well defined.

preexisting lesion (ruptured dermoid cyst or hemorrhage within a vascular lesion), local ocular inflammation (scleritis, uveitis), and systemic inflammatory syndromes (collagen vascular diseases). In young persons, rhabdomyosarcomas, metastatic neuroblastomas, or leukemic infiltration of the orbit can develop as sudden syndromes and may be confused clinically with idiopathic inflammation.

Treatment is with nonspecific anti-inflammatory drugs. We generally begin our patients on 60 to 80 mg of oral prednisone per day. This usually produces a dramatic reversal of signs and symptoms, particularly pain. In our series, the large majority (10 of 13) cleared within weeks, and a smaller number required several months of treatment. Three of our patients had recurrent episodes and two suffered from bilateral disease. As the disease resolves on steroid therapy, the junction of the optic nerve and globe can be visualized on CT scan and the infiltration disappears. Patients who have a satisfactory response are tapered off their steroids at a rate of 5 mg per week over a 2- to 3-month period (Fig. 9-21). Recurrence is handled by reinstituting the drug at a dose that controls the inflammation. Failure to respond suggests the need for specific definition by orbital biopsy and further treatment on the basis of findings. All of our patients in this group responded to nonspecific anti-inflammatory treatment; however, many authors suggest that failure of response followed by a biopsy confirming a benign process should be followed by low-dose orbital radiotherapy (between 1000 and 3000 rad). If the biopsy reveals a lymphoproliferative disease, treatment appropriate to the category is instituted (see Chapter 10).

ACUTE AND SUBACUTE IDIOPATHIC DIFFUSE ORBITAL INFLAMMATION

Diffuse idiopathic inflammation of the orbit is similar in many respects to acute anterior inflammation, with a greater severity of signs and symptoms including limitations of ocular movements, papillitis, and exudative retinal detachment (Fig. 9-22A and B). The severity correlates with CT scan findings, which show soft tissue infiltration involving the entire orbit, extending from the apex to the posterior margin of the globe (Fig. 9-22C). The optic nerve and extraocular muscles are obscured to a variable extent. With clinical resolution, the normal fat densities are restored and the extraocular muscles and optic nerves become well defined. Ultrasonography shows doubling of the optic nerve shadow (T sign), sclerotenonitis, and orbital infiltration.

Treatment is again with corticosteroids, and produces a rapid response (Fig. 9-22C and D). However, there is difficulty in tapering the patients off steroids because recurrence of the orbital or ocular inflammation is common in this group. Both of our patients have required intermittent steroids for years; however, one has resolved and is well controlled with an extremely low dose of steroids and adjuvant indomethacin. Our two patients with acute and subacute diffuse nonspecific inflammation were in childhood and adolescent years, and their course parallels that described for this age group.

ACUTE AND SUBACUTE IDIOPATHIC MYOSITIC ORBITAL INFLAMMATION (ORBITAL MYOSITIS)

In our series, this is the second most common group of nonspecific acute and subacute inflammations of the orbit. It is characterized by onset of painful extraocular movements, double vision, ptosis and swelling of the lid, localized chemosis and injection over the affected muscles, and limitation of extraocular movements (Fig. 9-23). The limitation of movement is in the direction of movement of the affected muscle. Pain is exacerbated by movement, and there may be a positive forced duction in the direction opposite to the movement of the muscle.

On CT scan these lesions present with relatively dif-

fuse enlargement of the extraocular muscles, which show slightly irregular margins. There may be localized adjacent infiltration of the orbital fat and thickening of the tendon of the involved muscle (Fig. 9-24). This disorder may affect more than one muscle, and may be bilateral (Fig. 9-25) or recurrent. The most frequently affected muscles are the superior complex (Fig. 9-26) and the medial rectus. The major differential diagnosis is Graves' orbitopathy (see Table 9-6). However, dysthyroid myopathy is usually painless in onset, asymmetric, slowly progressive, and associated with a systemic diathesis. Lid retraction, limitation of gaze in the direction opposite to the muscle involved, and deterioration of visual function (color vision, visual fields, and visual acuity) also may occur in thyroid orbitopathy in contrast to orbital myositis. On CT scan in thyroid orbitopathy, the extraocular muscle enlargement is usually fusiform and tapers towards the muscle insertion on the globe. Ultrasonographic examination will demonstrate enlargement of the extraocular muscle and local infiltration of surrounding structures (Fig. 9-27). Although these differences hold true for the overwhelming majority of cases, in our series of over 600 cases of thyroid myopathy, we have seen four documented instances of an acute onset of inflammation that parallels in every respect the idiopathic inflammatory myositis. Three of these cases were proven to have nonsuppressible thyroid function (TRH suppression, T_3 suppression tests) and one had biopsy proof suggestive of thyroid myopathy. All responded dramatically to corticosteroids.

Additional diseases that should be considered in the differential diagnosis include arteriovenous fistulas and malformations, orbital metastasis, Tolosa-Hunt syndrome, trichinosis, myasthenia gravis, and trochleitis. Arteriovenous fistula may be associated with injection of the globe and enlargement of extraocular muscles on CT scan. However, clinical signs vary considerably from acute myositis and are generally unassociated with pain or inflammatory features. Metastatic or locally infiltrative neoplasia to the extraocular muscles may mimic nonspecific inflammation. However, *sharp* pain is a rare clinical feature in metastatic tumors and enophthalmos is frequent. In addition, metastases are rarely characterized by an acute onset and CT and ultrasonographic findings tend to define a nodular infiltrative solid mass. Tolosa-Hunt syndrome usually has deeper, more constant, orbital pain and multiple neuropathies. CT scan evidence of either cavernous sinus enlargement or of no orbital findings will confirm this diagnosis. Trichinosis is usually associated with a dermatopathy. Trochleitis is associated with a very localized tenderness over the trochlea with limitation in elevation (an acute Brown's syndrome) and adduction. Myasthenia gravis is usually unassociated with inflammatory signs and has reversible ptosis follow-

(Text continues on p. 168)

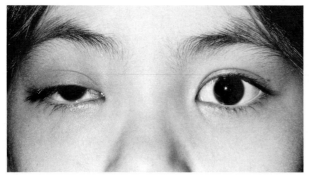

A

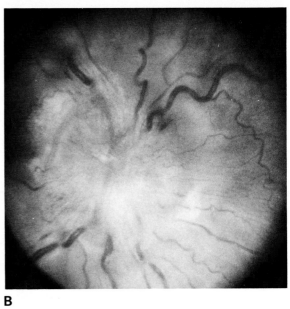

B

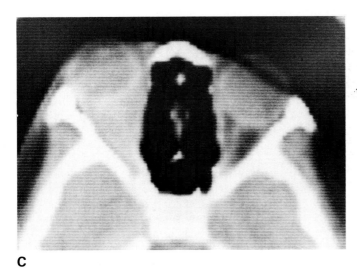

C

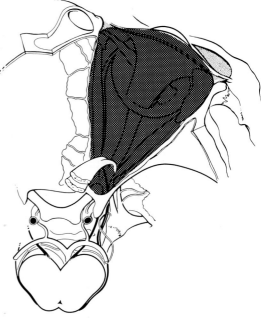

D

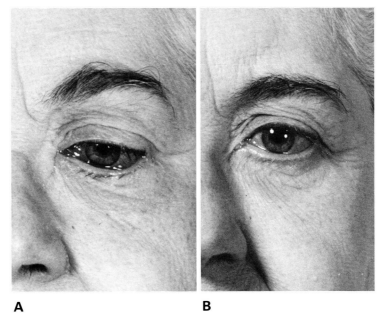

FIGURE 9-23. *(A)* Clinical features of a patient with acute medial and inferior idiopathic myositic inflammation. Note downward displacement with inferior and medial chemosis and injection. *(B)* The same patient after 1 week of steroid therapy. (Rootman J, Nugent R: The classification and management of acute orbital pseudotumors. Ophthalmology 89:1040, 1982)

A   B

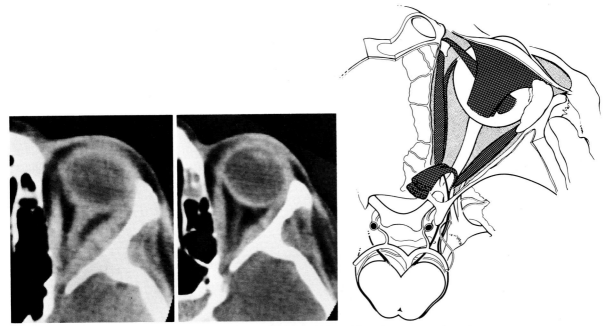

FIGURE 9-24. *(Left)* Axial CT scan shows orbital myositis. Note thickened lateral rectus muscle and tendon with fuzzy margins and increased orbital fat density. *(Middle)* CT scan of the same patient 2 months later following spontaneous clinical resolution. The lateral rectus has decreased in size. Since that time, the patient has had two episodes of orbital myositis.

FIGURE 9-22. *(A)* Clinical photograph of a 13-year-old patient with an idiopathic diffuse orbital inflammation and a 2-week history of uveitis followed 1 week later by ptosis, diplopia, proptosis, lid injection with edema, and signs of optic neuropathy (visual acuity 20/25, afferent pupillary defect, color desaturation), and papilledema. *(B)* Optic nerve photograph of the same patient with severe papilledema. *(C)* Axial CT scan (noncontrast, EMI 1010) of the patient shown in *A*. A soft tissue infiltrate involving the entire right orbit is noted. There is poor visualization of fat, muscles, and the optic nerve. *(D)* Axial CT scan (noncontrast, GE 8800) of same patient after intermittent steroid therapy. There is normal fat density and the extraocular muscles, globe, and optic nerve are now clearly defined. (Rootman J, Nugent R: The classification and management of acute orbital pseudotumors. Ophthalmology 89:1040, 1982)

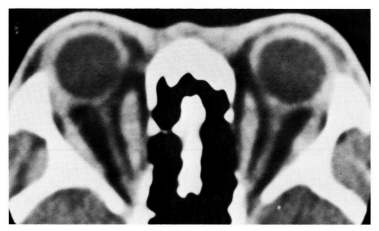

FIGURE 9-25. Axial CT scan of a 22-year-old man who presented with sudden onset of retrobulbar pain, swelling, ptosis, chemosis, and tenderness. He had restriction of extraocular movements in all directions of gaze. There is a bilateral diffuse mild enlargement of the extraocular muscles and tendons consistent with myositis. Systemic investigations were negative, and he responded to prednisone 20 mg/day.

ing edrophonium. However, it should be noted that a small percentage of patients with thyroid orbitopathy have concomitant myasthenia gravis. Anterior and diffuse nonspecific idiopathic orbital inflammations are characteristically associated with ocular findings and have distinctive CT scan and ultrasonographic features that allow categorization. Apical nonspecific idiopathic orbital inflammations may mimic myositis and, in fact, commonly involve the muscles at the apex. However, optic neuropathy is characteristic in contrast to myositis. Lacrimal nonspecific idiopathic orbital inflammations have a constellation of findings that point to the lacrimal gland.

The cause of orbital myositis is unknown, but immunologic mechanisms have been suggested. Cases of myositis have occurred secondary to upper respiratory tract infections and following flu-like viral illnesses. In addition, orbital myositis has been described in patients with the collagen vascular diseases including systemic lupus erythematosis, dermatomyositis, and periarteritis nodosa. Histologically, the inflammation consists of lymphocytic and polycellular infiltrations in myositis. All of these features suggest an underlying immunologic mechanism.

Idiopathic myositic inflammation is managed with corticosteroids and is almost pathognomonically responsive (Figs. 9-23 and 9-24). In our experience, 12 of 13 cases responded dramatically to a relatively low dose of steroids. We generally recommend a dosage of 40 mg per day and suggest tapering over 2 to 3 weeks depending on the response. Many authors have described the characteristic tendency of this condition to recur repeatedly,

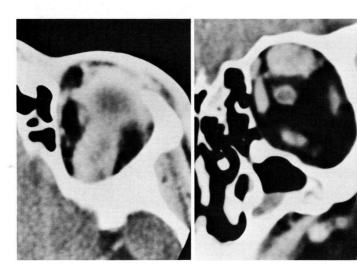

FIGURE 9-26. Axial and coronal CT scans of 58-year-old man with a 1-week history of left superotemporal headache, swelling of the upper lid, tenderness, slight limitation of elevation, abduction, and infraduction. There was injection and chemosis of the superior conjunctiva. Systemic investigation was negative, and he responded to low-dose steroids. The scans show enlargement of the superior rectus muscle.

TABLE 9-6.
DIFFERENTIAL DIAGNOSIS OF GRAVES' ORBITOPATHY VERSUS ORBITAL MYOSITIS

	Idiopathic Myositis	Graves' Orbitopathy
Clinical		
Onset	Rapid	Slow
Pain	Frequent especially on extraocular movement	Rare; generally gritty irritation
Lid		
Ptosis	Frequent	Rare, except in markedly congested orbits
Retraction		
Stare		
Lag	Absent	Frequent
Chemosis	Localized and injected	Generalized, but may be localized
Extraocular movements	Limitation and pain in field of movement of involved muscle	Limitation; painless in field of movement opposite to involved muscle
Visual function	Unimpaired	May be impaired
Response to steroids	Dramatic with complete resolution; may recur	Incomplete and slow
Orbital Imaging		
Bilaterality	Infrequent	Frequent
Number of muscles	More than one in up to 50%	Typically more than one
Muscle borders	Irregular	Regular
Extension into orbital fat	Frequent	Little or none
Tendon involvement	Frequent	None; rare
Scleral and Tenon's enhancement	Occasional and localized	None
Site	Any muscle especially superior and medial	Inferior and medial most frequent

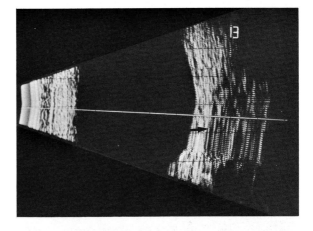

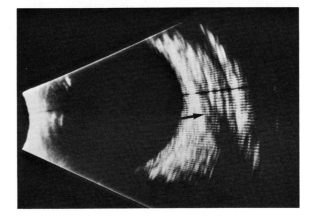

FIGURE 9-27. B scan ultrasonographic findings in orbital myositis. *(Top)* An irregular enlargement of the superior muscle complex (10 mm) *(arrow)*. The patient was a 49-year-old man who presented with left upper lid swelling, ptosis, injection, diplopia, and pain on extraocular movement. On physical examination, there was localized swelling and chemosis with downward displacement (2 mm), axial proptosis (1 mm), and limitation of upgaze. He responded dramatically to steroids within 1 week, and on investigation had a nonsuppressible thyroid gland on TRH stimulation, suggesting an underlying thyroid disorder. *(Bottom)* The scan demonstrates irregular echoes in the lateral rectus muscle *(arrow)* with slight infiltration of the adjacent fat. The patient was an 18-year-old boy who had pain on adduction of the right eye, injection, and chemosis over the lateral rectus muscle. He responded to prednisone 40 mg/day tapered over a 1-month period. Systemic investigations were negative.

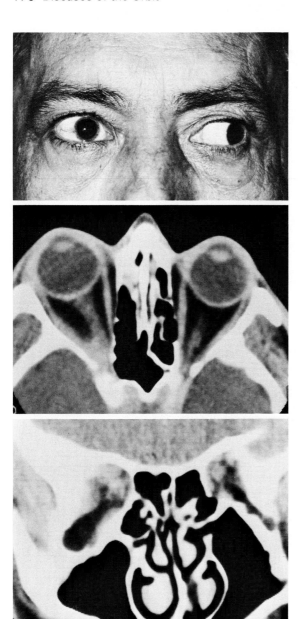

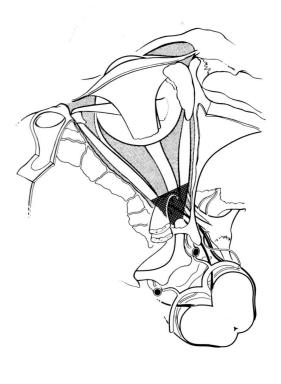

FIGURE 9-28. This 54-year-old man had a 5-week history of right superonasal and periorbital pain with mild injection and swelling of the lid. He had also noted a recent onset of double vision. On physical examination, he had hand movements vision on the right with a central and inferior visual field loss. In addition, there were decreased extraocular movements in all positions of gaze, 5 mm of proptosis, an afferent pupillary defect, and slight injection and chemosis of the conjunctiva. CT scan shows apical infiltration with involvement of adjacent muscle, optic nerve, and fat. He was diagnosed as having an idiopathic apical inflammatory process, and was treated with prednisone 80 mg/day. He responded dramatically, and within 1 week had 20/50 vision and increased extraocular movements. Systemic investigations were negative.

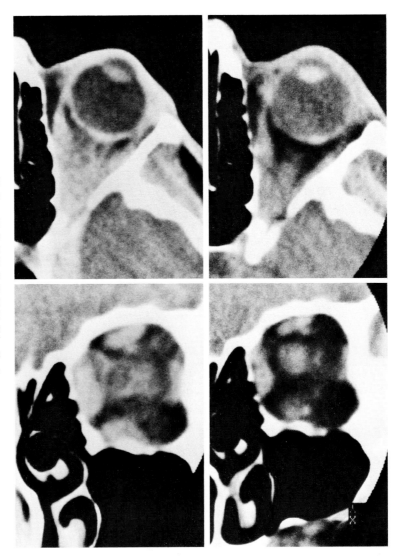

FIGURE 9-29. CT scans of a 57-year-old woman who presented with a 1 1/2 month history of redness and swelling of the left eye. She had complete ptosis for 3 to 4 days, and was aware of diplopia for 2 days with severe apical pain. On physical examination, the vision was 20/20. She had a 15-D hypertropia and left exotropia of 20 D with 4 mm of proptosis and was tender to ballottement. CT scans in both axial and coronal planes *(left)* show soft tissue infiltration of apex, fat, and adjacent muscles. She responded to 60 mg prednisone daily, tapered slowly over 2 months. The CT scans on the *right* show the orbit 3 1/2 months later when the patient was clinically normal. Systemic investigations were negative.

but in the long run, this remains a self-limited disorder in the majority of patients. A small number may not respond completely to steroids and, with persistence of the disorder, low-dose orbital radiotherapy with protection of the globe is recommended. Both recurrence and residual findings have been correlated with late diagnosis and prolonged inflammation prior to treatment.

ACUTE AND SUBACUTE IDIOPATHIC APICAL ORBITAL INFLAMMATION

Other nonspecific idiopathic orbital inflammations are those associated with infiltration of the apex. The cardinal features of this syndrome are a disproportionate functional abnormality compared to the degree of inflammatory signs. Patients present with a typical orbital apical syndrome of pain, minimal proptosis, and restricted extraocular movements (Fig. 9-28). On the other hand, they may occasionally present primarily with a decrease in vision when the infiltrate tends to be more perineuritic. The CT scan findings in apical nonspecific idiopathic orbital inflammation consist of an irregular infiltration of the apex of the orbit with extension along the posterior portion of the extraocular muscles or the optic nerve (Figs. 9-28, 9-29, 9-30). Localized infiltration of the orbital fat may be noted, and the involvement may be extensive enough to include the posterior half of the orbit. In one instance of apical infiltration extending anteriorly between the superior muscle complex and the

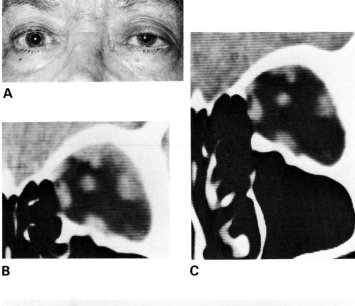

A

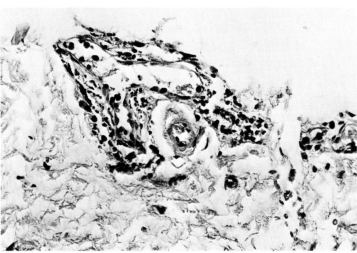

B

C

FIGURE 9-30. *(A)* This 73-year-old woman presented with swelling and ptosis of the left upper lid. It developed over a 2-week period and was associated with superotemporal pain and proptosis. She was aware of diplopia for 2 months and decreased vision for 1 week. On examination, she had counting fingers vision at 3 to 4 feet, had 2 mm of ptosis, 5 mm of proptosis, a left afferent pupillary defect, decreased elevation, and abduction of her eye. *(B)* The coronal CT scan shows a superolateral soft tissue density that extends to the superior orbital fissure and apex, and is intimate to the superior and lateral rectus muscles. Complete systemic investigation was negative. She was treated with prednisone 80 mg/day, and showed dramatic improvement. Within 1 week her vision was 20/70 and the extraocular movements were normal. Over the next 4 months her vision improved to 20/30 while the steroids were tapered. *(C)* A repeat coronal CT scan shows resolution of the lesion 2 months after steroids were discontinued. *(D)* Biopsy from the site shown in *A*. Note perivascular accumulations of lymphocytes and plasma cells consistent with a nonspecific inflammatory syndrome (H&E, original magnification *D* × 250).

D

lateral rectus, biopsy revealed angiocentric lymphocytic and plasmacytic infiltration (Fig. 9-30D). CT resolution is noted following treatment (Figs. 9-29, 9-30).

Because the visual, oculomotor, and optic nerve functions are affected early in this inflammation with corresponding minimal proptosis, ocular involvement, and lid involvement, the differential diagnosis includes optic neuritis, apical tumefactions, and Tolosa-Hunt syndrome.

We managed four such patients, all of whom resolved on prednisone therapy. Generally, treatment required 60 to 80 mg of prednisone per day tapered over a 6- to 8-week period depending on resolution of signs and symptoms. In one case, however, the disease recurred several times leading to a chronic infiltration of the orbit; biopsy was required, and apical orbital irradiation led to complete resolution.

IDIOPATHIC LACRIMAL INFLAMMATION

Nonspecific inflammations of the lacrimal gland represent a microcosm of inflammatory disease seen elsewhere in the orbit. They are easily divided into nonspecific and specific categories, because we advocate routine biopsy. Tumefactions of the lacrimal gland may be lymphoprolif-

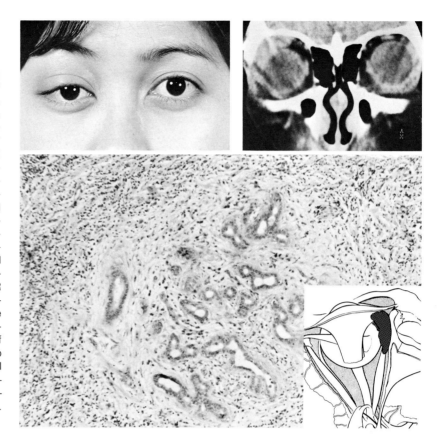

FIGURE 9-31. A 25-year-old woman had a 1-month history of swelling and slight tenderness of the right upper lid associated with 2-mm downward and 2-mm inward displacement of the globe. The coronal CT scan shows a mass in the lacrimal fossa. Biopsy shows a chronic polymorphous inflammatory infiltrate associated with sclerosis and destruction of the lacrimal gland and preservation of some ductal structures. She was treated with prednisone 40 mg/day tapered over a 3-month period, and showed rapid improvement. On systemic investigation, she had an elevated ESR (50 mm/h). She subsequently developed alopecia. The study at that time showed that she had decreased peripheral T lymphocytes, a high titer of cytomegalovirus antibody, and no other abnormalities (H&E, original magnification × 10). (Rootman J, Nugent R: The classification and management of acute orbital pseudotumors. Ophthalmology 89:1040, 1982)

erative, structural, or neoplastic disease and are frequently related to systemic syndromes. Thus, this category of nonspecific inflammation requires routine histologic confirmation as part of the management protocol, in contrast to the usual nonspecific inflammatory syndromes. Therefore, lacrimal inflammations nicely bridge the discussions of nonspecific and distinct (specific) orbital inflammatory disease.

In our experience, the lacrimal gland is the third most common location for nonspecific inflammation. Overall, the clinical pattern was equally divided between those categories and chronic presentations, rather than being dominantly acute and subacute. The age range was from 16 to 83 years with an average of 44 years. Of our 11 patients, 9 were females and 2 were males. The typical presentation of the acute and subacute disorder consisted of pain, tenderness, and injection of the temporal lid and conjunctival fornix with an associated palpable lacrimal gland, an S-shaped deformity of the upper lid, and pouting of the lacrimal ducts noted on biomicroscopy of the fornix (Fig. 9-31). This group showed minimal proptosis, and downward and inward displacement of the globe. Patients presenting with a more chronic onset had a relative absence of pain or significant inflam-

mation. None of the patients had major intraocular or extraocular orbital findings outside of those described for the lacrimal region. Two cases in this group had bilateral lesions, four had recurrent disease, and two had other immunologic problems (organ-specific inflammatory disease). The immunologic disorders encountered included alopecia and colitis.

On CT investigation, the infiltration was characteristically confined to the superolateral orbit, obscuring the lateral aspect of the globe and displacing it inferomedially (Fig. 9-32). On ultrasonography, a mass with internal reflectivity was noted superolaterally, with an echolucent area next to the scleral shell associated with thickening of the adjacent muscle anteriorly (Fig. 9-33).

Because the focus of the disease is lacrimal, the clinical syndrome is one of tumor, tenderness, and injection with pouting of the lacrimal ducts, lid swelling, and an S-shaped deformity of the lid. In contrast to the diffuse forms of pseudotumor, there was no ocular inflammatory component, and motility was involved in few and only minimally, with limitation in extreme abduction due to mass effect alone.

The differential diagnosis of nonspecific lacrimal inflammation includes viral and bacterial dacryoadenitis,

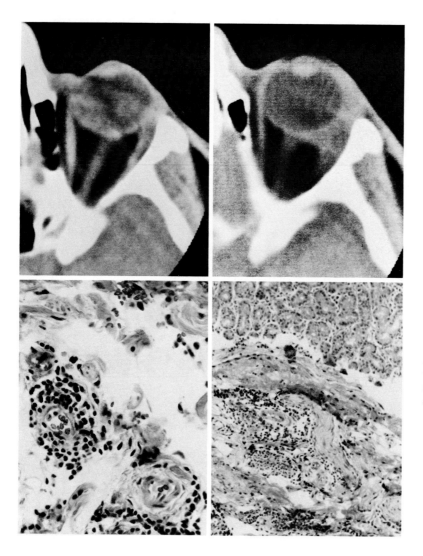

FIGURE 9-32. *(Top, right)* Axial CT scan shows an enlarged left lacrimal gland in a 33-year-old man with left mild superotemporal tenderness and swelling, pouting of the lacrimal ducts, diplopia in right gaze only, 3 mm of proptosis, 2 mm of inward and 2 mm of downward displacement, with a narrow interpalpebral fissure. Immunologic study was negative. *(Top, left)* Repeat CT scan shows the orbit 2 months after initiation of steroid therapy for an acute idiopathic inflammation of the lacrimal gland. Note slight prominence of the lacrimal gland, which has decreased in size. *(Bottom, left and right)* Biopsy shows a perivascular capsular lymphocytic infiltration of the lacrimal gland (H&E, original magnification *bottom left* × 10, *bottom right* × 25).

rupture of a dermoid cyst in the lacrimal gland region (rarely associated with significant acute or subacute inflammation in our experience; more typically only mass effect is noted), specific lacrimal inflammations such as sarcoidosis and Sjögren's disease, cysts, and neoplasia in this region. Because of the wide variety and incidence of the many different tumefactions, biopsy of this accessible site is necessary to define prognosis and management. In our experience, the biopsies in the nonspecific inflammatory group tended to produce five different pictures. Patients with acute inflammatory disorders tended to show on biopsy polymorphous cellular infiltration with edema and vascular dilatation, and did not have a striking degree of destruction of the lacrimal gland (see Fig. 9-32). The lesions in the subacute and chronic category included several that had a profound lymphocellular infiltration associated with glandular ablation (Fig. 9-34). The third pattern was one of sclerosing inflammatory infiltration

with gland destruction (see Fig. 9-31). The remaining histological findings on biopsy of the lacrimal gland included reactive lymphoproliferative disorders of the lacrimal gland or granulomatous inflammations (which will be discussed later). These were managed according to appropriate diagnosis. Reactive lymphoproliferation (benign lymphoepithelial lesion) with follicle formation, and islands of epithelial and myoepithelial cells (epimyoepithelial islands) replacing the interlobular ducts may occur independently as a distinct entity or may be a manifestation of rheumatoid or autoimmune disease. Furthermore, this histologic finding may imply a diagnosis of Sjögren's syndrome.

In our group of 11 patients, 7 were successfully treated with steroids (see Fig. 9-32) and 4 with milder inflammations were only observed. All of the lesions eventually resolved, but four patients had recurrent episodes. Steroid doses were generally in a moderate range

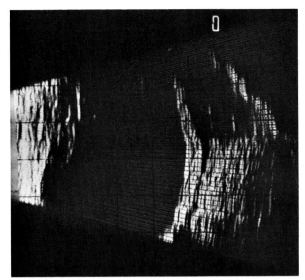

FIGURE 9-33. Ultrasonogram of the patient shown in Figure 9-32. Note superotemporal mass with internal reflectivity and an echolucent area adjacent to the scleral shell.

between 40 and 60 mg tapered over a 3- to 6-week period, depending on signs and symptoms. Overall resolution was generally over a 1- to 4-month period.

CONCLUSION

The five clinical syndromes of acute and subacute idiopathic orbital inflammation appear to correlate well with location and degree of disease identified on orbital imaging. Nonspecific anti-inflammatory treatment used in

these situations effect resolution that appears to be proportional to the length and amount of involvement. The rapid steroid responsiveness (especially as applied to pain) is almost pathognomonic. CT scanning is useful, particularly for assessing resolution with therapy. Failure of resolution should suggest alternative diagnoses, and a biopsy may become necessary. Management following biopsy for persistent, recurrent, or inconclusive disease will be governed by the histology of the lesion. In the clinical situation, acute cases often demand rapid action because the patients are frequently extremely uncomfortable, and there may be considerable threat to vision. Many authors have suggested that biopsy in acute anterior and diffuse inflammatory lesions may, in fact, be detrimental to the care of patients. Given the efficacy of current investigative techniques, we can now monitor the course of the diseases accurately. In all patterns, when patients have been appropriately investigated and treated and show little or poor response, biopsy may then become appropriate. In our experience, aside from lacrimal gland lesions, this is rarely necessary in acute and subacute inflammations, and the patients can be managed by categorization according to clinical presentation and location. Treatment can be monitored by clinical findings and follow-up orbital imaging.

Idiopathic Sclerosing Inflammation

Idiopathic sclerosing inflammation is characterized by insidious onset and progression of a chronic infiltrative process that leads to ocular and orbital dysfunction as the result of entrapment and inflammation. The distinguishing histologic features are desmoplasia and varying degrees of lymphocytic and plasmacytic inflammation that

FIGURE 9-34. Clinical photograph and biopsy of a 34-year-old man with tender, bilateral lacrimal masses. Histologically, there was an intense polymorphous lymphocytic and plasmacytic infiltrate. Clinically, the patient had multiple organ-specific immune disorders including ulcerative colitis, alopecia, parotitis, and vitiligo. He was treated with prednisone 30 mg/day, and the lacrimal masses resolved dramatically within 1 month. Systemic investigation was negative for rheumatoid factor and antinuclear antibodies.

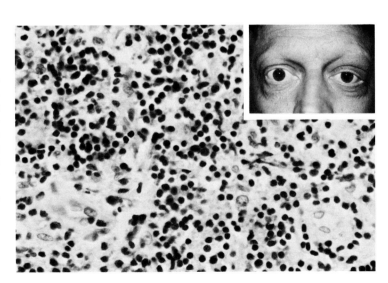

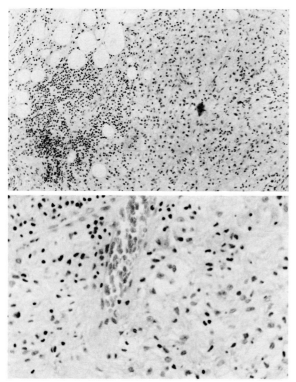

FIGURE 9-35. Histologic features of sclerosing orbital inflammation. Note scattered lymphocytes and intense desmoplastic response (H&E, original magnification *top* × 10, *bottom* × 25).

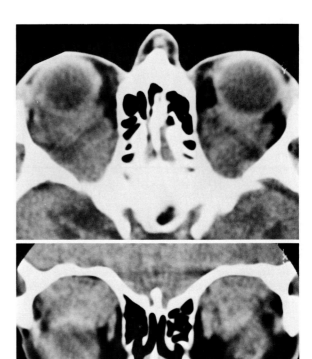

FIGURE 9-36. Axial and coronal CT scans of a 64-year-old man who had developed diplopia (especially on eye movement) 2 years earlier. It was intermittent and progressive for 1 year, but had become quiescent. Clinically, there was bilateral exophthalmos (OD, 21 mm; OS, 20 mm), reduced extraocular movements in all directions of gaze, positive forced ductions of the inferior medial and lateral rectus muscles, and an increase in the intraocular pressure on upgaze. The bilateral retrobulbar infiltrative masses proved on biopsy to be sclerosing orbital inflammation with a very sparse lymphocytic population. He has been observed for 1 1/2 year without further progression.

surround the orbital structures and cause fixation and damage (Fig. 9-35). This process can be relentless and unresponsive to therapy.

Clinically, we have experienced six cases in this category: four males and two females with an age range of 18 to 65 years. One of our cases was bilateral (Fig. 9-36), and they all occurred in different parts of the orbit. The onset was characteristically slow and the major symptoms were diplopia with muscle restriction, proptosis, mild persistent pain, and in two cases progressive visual loss (Fig. 9-37). Two patients, both with anteriorly located lesions, had mild inflammatory signs consisting of injection and lid edema. One was adjacent to the lacrimal sac and encompassed the inferior oblique muscle (see Fig. 5-12, p. 79). The other was next to and involved the levator muscle, causing unilateral lid retraction.

On CT examination these lesions appear as infiltrating, relatively homogeneous, dense lesions in the orbit. They may or may not have irregular margins and are usually contrast enhancing. They incorporate and infiltrate fat and adjacent orbital structures.

Histologically, the dominant feature is desmoplasia with evidence of various stages of scar formation. The inflammatory component is usually sparse, polymor-

phous, and distributed throughout the lesion, but does occur as larger focal collections of lymphocytes and plasma cells. In addition, several of the lesions showed collections of foamy macrophages (see Fig. 9-35; Fig. 9-38). It is our impression that more chronic and mature lesions have a denser collagen component and less inflammation.

Although these inflammations are typically responsive to steroids early in the disease, the general experience has been progression, incomplete response, and steroid resistance. Three of our cases were treated with combined steroids and radiotherapy, and in all cases the inflammatory progression was arrested (see Fig. 9-38). Functional damage occurring in five cases (two with optic atrophy, three with muscle restriction) either persisted or progressed due to cicatrization. One of our patients re-

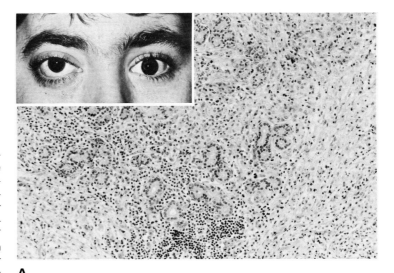

FIGURE 9-37. *(A)* An 18-year-old boy with progressive right proptosis over a 2-year period due to sclerosing inflammation, which started superolaterally in the right orbit. In addition, on presentation he had papilledema, reduced extraocular movements, reduced vision, a right afferent pupillary defect, and choroidal striae. *(B)* The CT scan shows extensive orbital involvement with encasement of the optic nerve and extraocular muscles *(inset)*. Histologically, it was a sclerosing inflammation that incorporated lacrimal structures *(A)* and invaded the orbit *(B)*. Review suggests it may have originated as a lacrimal gland ectopia. Systemically, he had increased circulating immune complexes, increased IgM levels, and a history of three bouts of aseptic arthritis. He responded clinically with arrest and improvement of proptosis, and extraocular movements following orbital radiotherapy (3000 rad over 10 days). His vision did not recover.

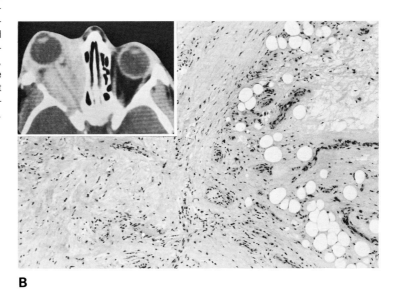

fused radiotherapy, and is only partially controlled by intermittent steroids; this patient has developed a second lesion in the orbit over a 1-year period. The remaining patient presented in the orbital clinic 2 years after the occurrence of his disease and following steroid therapy. He was in remission, but had evidence of bilateral infiltrative lesions with persistent oculomotor dysfunction and sclerosing inflammation proven by biopsy. The final patient is currently under treatment for her anteriorly located superior orbital infiltration.

A survey of the literature would suggest that the so-called "inflammatory pseudotumor or nonspecific inflammatory disease" groups fit in this category by passing from a dominantly inflammatory syndrome (lymphocyte rich) to scarring. However, we believe this is a distinct clinical disease process with an insidious, progressive, slow onset associated with a well-defined infiltration on orbital imaging and symptoms and histopathology as outlined. In contrast, among the nonspecific idiopathic orbital inflammations just described, the onset is usually acute or subacute dominated clinically by inflammatory features, and the CT findings are less distinct. In our experience, the nonspecific idiopathic acute and subacute inflammations have not progressed because they have responded to nonspecific anti-inflammatory therapy. We assume that, left untreated, some of the subacute nonspecific idiopathic inflammations of the orbit may indeed progress to the development of a reactive desmoplastic response. However, when managed as outlined, it appears that this is uncommon.

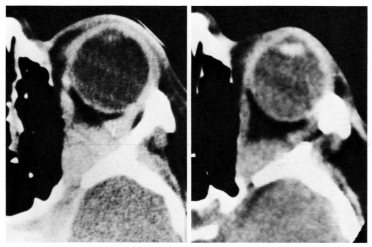

FIGURE 9-38. *(Left)* Axial CT scan of the left orbit of a 34-year-old woman who had a history of intermittent and progressive left temporal pain over a 3-year period. In the last 7 months she had noted intermittent diplopia, mild proptosis, and lid and conjunctival swelling. On physical examination, there was decreased visual acuity (20/40), a left afferent pupillary defect, reduced elevation and adduction, 2 mm of proptosis, a reduced forced duction, paresthesia involving nerves V1 and V2, and mild disc pallor. The lesion is an enhancing apical mass that extended into the superior orbital fissure and the optic foramen. Systemic investigation was negative. Biopsy revealed a sclerosing inflammatory lesion. *(Right)* CT scan 8 months after treatment with 3000 rad in ten fractions shows reduction in the size of the mass, with improvement in symptoms and signs. There has been no recurrence or progression of the lesion during a 3 1/2-year follow up.

The differential diagnosis of this entity is one of chronic inflammations (Wegener's granulomatosis, granulomatous orbital inflammations, and the like), metastatic and secondary cancers (especially sclerosing types), and lymphomas. Because of the relentless character of this disorder, early diagnosis and combined treatment (steroids and radiotherapy) is recommended. We usually deliver 2500 to 3000 rad to the orbit in ten fractions, and during therapy recommend use of steroids to prevent any rebound phenomenon. There are numerous references in the literature to the association of "idiopathic inflammatory pseudotumor" with retroperitoneal and mediastinal fibrosis. Histopathologically these resemble the inflammatory desmoplasia just described. One wonders whether the association is related to a similar fundamental pathologic mechanism.

Idiopathic Noninfectious Granulomatous Inflammation

Patients with idiopathic noninfectious granulomatous inflammation probably represent a heterogeneous group bound by similar inflammatory infiltration. The infiltrate is granulomatous, and affects the soft tissues of the orbit without specific localization or systemic associations. We had four patients in this category: three were female and one was male, and the age range was from 32 to 74 years. All four presented with evidence of mild inflammation, a palpable mass, and an onset of more than 1-month's duration in three instances and less than 1 month in one. Two of the patients presented with a superior anterior orbital mass and ptosis, whereas the other two had an upward displacement of the globe secondary to the presence of an inferolateral orbital mass. All four on biopsy had granulomatous inflammatory infiltration, which failed to reveal any specific related pathogen. Three lesions had the appearance of a naked nonnecrotizing granuloma (Fig. 9-39), and one had a lipogranulomatous response reminiscent of descriptions of lipogranulomatous pseudotumors (Fig. 9-40). All four patients failed to reveal any systemic associations on careful evaluation and appeared to have local orbital inflammatory disease. Two of these patients responded well to systemic corticosteroid treatment, although one had recurrent episodes, whereas the remaining two had relatively localized disease that responded to local corticosteroid injection, leaving a focal area of scarring. A thorough systemic investigation in patients with granulomatous disorders as well as careful assessment of the biopsy specimen for specific etiology is necessary before considering any form of treatment. These entities, although heterogeneous, appear to have a specific orbital focus and may be a unique category.

FIGURE 9-39. Coronal CT scan shows an anterior inferior orbital infiltrative lesion involving the lateral rectus, inferior rectus, and soft tissues. It was seen in a 74-year-old woman who presented with a firm, nontender mass of the right anterior inferior orbit. Histologically, it consisted of numerous focal collections of epithelioid and giant cells surrounded by lymphocytes. No other systemic abnormalities were identified, and the patient responded to local injection of corticosteroids. Local steroids were used because the patient had congestive heart failure, which contraindicated systemic steroids. This orbital granulomatous process suggested a localized sarcoid lesion; however, no systemic associations were identified, and we have classified it as an idiopathic noninfectious granulomatous orbital inflammation.

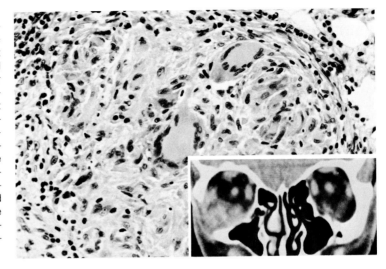

FIGURE 9-40. *(Top)* This 32-year-old man presented with right mild proptosis and elevation of the globe (3–4 mm) associated with minimal chemosis. There was a firm mass palpable just above the orbital rim on the right side, and he had 3 mm of proptosis. On CT scan there was an anterior infiltrative orbital mass. *(Bottom)* On biopsy, it proved to consist of an infiltrate of lymphocytes, plasma cells, epithelioid cells, giant cells *(arrows),* and fibroblasts. In addition, numerous lipid-laden macrophages were identified. The histologic picture was consistent with lipogranulomatous orbital inflammation. Treatment was with low-dose systemic corticosteroids, and the patient responded without recurrence to date (3-years' follow up).

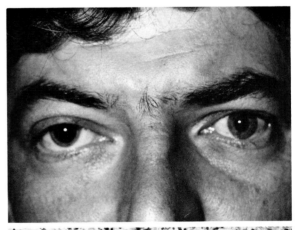

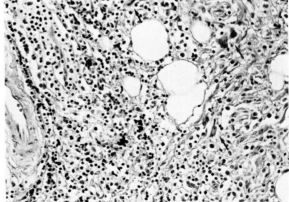

■ OTHER (SPECIFIC) ORBITAL INFLAMMATIONS

Specific orbital inflammations form an arbitrary collection; the disorders have in common either biopsy proof of identity or an association with a characteristic clinical syndrome (Table 9-7). This does not imply they have known or related etiologies, pathogenesis, or prognosis but that they are distinct enough to suggest separate categorization. Pathologically, they are heterogeneous with histology varying from desmoplastic to angiocentric, necrotizing, and granulomatous inflammatory processes. The separation is based on a practical concern for categorizing patients with inflammatory syndromes who either come to biopsy or have specific systemic associations. On the basis of these clinical and histologic findings, they can then be divided into these various groups and managed accordingly. Thus, we feel it rational to separate them from the previously described nonspecific orbital inflammatory syndromes. The different disorders in this category include sarcoidosis, Sjögren's disease, and the vasculitides. In addition, distinct ocular inflammations such as scleritis and sclerokeratitis with significant orbital findings have been included in this group on the basis of their unique diagnosable features.

Sarcoidosis

PATHOGENESIS, ETIOLOGY, AND PATHOLOGY

Sarcoidosis is a granulomatous multisystem disease of unknown cause. The noncaseating granulomas affect many tissues and organs, but in particular the hilar lymph nodes and pulmonary parenchyma. It is an immunologically mediated disease affecting delayed hypersensitivity.

TABLE 9-7.
OTHER ORBITAL INFLAMMATIONS, UNIVERSITY OF BRITISH COLUMBIA ORBITAL CLINIC, 1976–1986

Type of Inflammation	No. of Cases
Wegeners' granulomatosis	4
Other vasculitides	4
Systemic lupus erythematosis	2
Cogan's syndrome	1
Lacrimal	
Sjögren's syndrome	2
Sarcoid	3
Idiopathic Ocular Inflammation with Orbital Signs	
Scleritis	6

The granulomas develop by a combination of T lymphocyte, chemotactic and macrophage activation factors and are maintained by a T lymphocyte macrophage migration inhibition factor. These factors attract and retain blood monocytes and tissue phagocytes, which form epithelioid cells at the site of tubercles. The local infiltration appears to express an imbalance between T helper and suppressor cells with decreased suppressor cell function. Patients with this disorder demonstrate systemically deficient T-cell responses such as cutaneous anergy and a peripheral T-cell lymphopenia. In spite of this, they show hyperactive B-cells with enhanced humoral immunity and increased gamma globulin.

Histologically, the granulomas contain dense accumulations of polyhedral epithelioid cells surrounded by a sparse population of lymphocytes (naked tubercle) (Fig. 9-41). There is no central caseation and little evidence of fibrosis. These noncaseating granulomas have been identified in practically every organ or tissue site. The clusters of epithelioid cells often have giant cells of the Langhans' or foreign body type. They may also contain characteristic but not pathognomonic inclusions of three types: the conchoid Schauman body, the asteroid body, or colorless refractile inclusions. The histologic picture is not specific and identical lesions occur in tuberculosis, leprosy, berylliosis, hypersensitivity pneumonitis, fungal disease, Crohn's disease, and primary biliary cirrhosis as well as within lymph nodes draining inflammatory and neoplastic processes.

CLINICAL SYNDROME

Systemic

Sarcoidosis is commonly asymptomatic (4:1) and affects multiple systems. There is a racial and ethnic predilection (10 to 20 times more blacks than whites) and increased incidence in the southern United States, Sweden, Ireland, and the West Indies. Women are affected more frequently than men, and the disease occurs mainly in the second and third decades (two thirds of patients are under 40 years of age). The course of the disorder has been divided into acute, subacute, and chronic disease based on onset and development. About 10% to 15% of patients have a self-limited benign acute polyarthritis with erythema nodosum. The subacute and chronic diseases have durations greater or less than 2 years. The subacute disorder is the most common and is usually asymptomatic, whereas the chronic disorder is progressive, frequently extrathoracic, and occurs in an age group older than 30 years. When the lungs are affected, progressive pulmonary fibrosis is frequent in this group.

Intrathoracic disease is divided into three stages. Stage 1 consists of bilateral hilar lymphadenopathy, which is seen in 50% of patients. The majority of cases

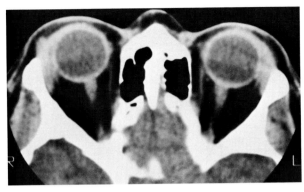

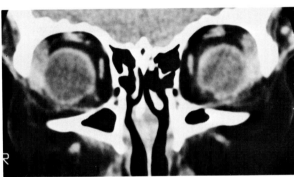

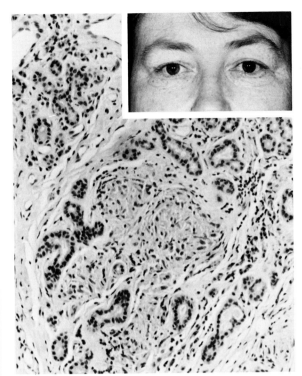

FIGURE 9-41. *(Left)* Axial and coronal CT scans demonstrate bilateral enlargement and protrusion of the lacrimal glands, which had been slowly progressive over a 2- to 3-month period. *(Right)* Histology demonstrates a naked tubercle within the lacrimal acini. The patient had bilateral hilar adenopathy, and the final diagnosis was sarcoidosis (H&E, original magnification × 25).

undergo spontaneous regression in 2 years. However, 10% persist, and 10% progress to stage 2, which is characterized by parenchymal and hilar involvement. Twenty-five percent of cases are first seen at this stage. Two thirds of these have a mild, self-limited disorder and one third persist or progress. Stage 3 is noted in 15% of patients at the time of diagnosis; they have pulmonary parenchymal involvement but no hilar involvement. These patients go on to severe pulmonary dysfunction.

Extrathoracic sarcoidosis is seen in 40% of patients. The incidence of thoracic and extrathoracic sarcoidosis is summarized in Table 9-8. The disease may involve the skin with erythema nodosum, cutaneous granulomas, and a distinctive involvement of the nose, cheeks, or ears with lupus pernio. The skin of the lids may be affected with these cutaneous granulomas. The disease may involve the liver, leading to hepatosplenomegaly and progressive dysfunction. The joints may be affected with an acute polyarthritis, which is often associated with central nervous system involvement affecting cranial nerves, hypothalamus, meninges, and pituitary gland. In particular, the facial nerve is affected, leading to a triad of facial palsy, parotid enlargement, and anterior uveitis (Heerfordt's syndrome). Nerve supply to the extraocular muscles is rarely affected. The chronic disorder may involve the nervous system, leading to multiple neuropathy. The subacute and chronic disease may affect the optic nerve with development of granulomas. A punched-out bony lesion of the phalanges may occur.

Ocular and Orbital Findings

The eye may be affected with uveitis, chorioretinitis, keratoconjunctivitis (sicca), and conjunctival inflammatory nodules. When acute uveitis is seen with arthritis, erythema nodosum, and hilar node enlargement, the course of ocular inflammation tends to be benign. In contrast, chronic uveitis is frequently associated with a progressive systemic and local course. The lacrimal gland is palpably enlarged and noted in 7% of patients, but shows functional abnormalities in 13% (decreased lacrimal secretion) (see Fig. 9-41; Fig. 9-42). The conjunctiva is affected either by focal nodules or a confluent infiltration, and positive biopsy can be obtained in 17% to 33%. Orbital soft tissue involvement is exceedingly rare in sarcoidosis; it usually affects the deep orbit or occurs secondary to contiguous bony involvement. A lesion histologically similar to those of sarcoidosis has been described as a

TABLE 9-8.
SARCOIDOSIS

Nature of Presentation	Features in Known Sarcoidosis	Ophthalmic Series
40% On routine chest X-ray	90% Radiographic bilateral hilar adenopathy	50% Ocular involvement
15% Acute polyarthritis (frequently associated with erythema nodosum and iridocyclitis)	40% Extrapulmonary manifestations	15% Present with ocular
11% Erythema nodosum	33%–50% Skin lesions	30% With posterior uveitis have CNS disease
6% Skin sarcoid	20% Hepatosplenomegaly	
7% Ocular sarcoid	20% Ocular	
0.6% Lacrimal	20% Bone change on X-ray	
	8% Salivary	
	7% Lacrimal mass	
	13% Reduced lacrimal secretions	
	17%–33% Positive conjunctival (on biopsy)	
	4% CNS	
	0.2% Orbital	
	Lung involvement Stage 1, 50% Stage 2, 25% Stage 3, 15%	

isolated orbital occurrence (sarcoid), but it should not be confused with the systemic syndrome of sarcoidosis and probably represents a different localized disorder.

DIAGNOSIS

Sarcoidosis is a diagnosis of exclusion, but there are a number of factors suggesting it. Patients with distinctive or typical bilateral hilar lymphadenopathy with and without erythema nodosum, uveitis, or arthritis are believed to have a specific syndrome. Biopsy findings from minor salivary glands (60%), liver (65%–75%), lung (60%–85%), and mediastinum (85%–90%) may aid in diagnosis. On laboratory study up to 10% of patients have increased serum calcium and 20% have hypercalciuria and hypersensitivity to vitamin D. The angiotensin-converting enzyme (ACE) is increased in the serum, particularly in active disease, reflecting an increase in T-cell activity. Gallium is preferentially taken up by granulomas of sarcoid in hilar nodes, lung, and specific extrapulmonary sites such as the lacrimal gland. The combination of increased ACE and a positive gallium scan is 99% diagnostic. Serum lysozyme may be increased in sarcoidosis, but this is not specific to the disease. Pulmonary function tests may demonstrate deteriorated function.

Lacrimal gland function may be abnormal with reduced tear secretion and increased tear lysozyme (a feature that distinguishes this disorder from Sjögren's disease). Angiotensin-converting enzyme levels are increased in sarcoidosis and diminish with treatment. These features may be used as a measure of response to systemic therapy.

MANAGEMENT

Treatment when indicated is with prednisone (30 mg daily) and is prolonged (6–12 months) with frequent relapse (over 50%). The indications for steroid therapy include progressive pulmonary disease, uveitis, and renal insufficiency and cardiac, central nervous system, or significant skin involvement. About 70% of patients recover with little dysfunction and 20% have permanent visual or pulmonary impairment. Even with steroid therapy 4% die of cardiac, pulmonary, CNS, and renal disease. Treatment for lacrimal sarcoid is with approximately 30 mg prednisone per day, tapered over an 8- to 10-week period depending on the response.

Sjögren's Syndrome

Sjögren's syndrome is defined by the presence of any two of the triad of keratoconjunctivitis sicca, xerostomia, and autoimmune disease. The primary or isolated form con-

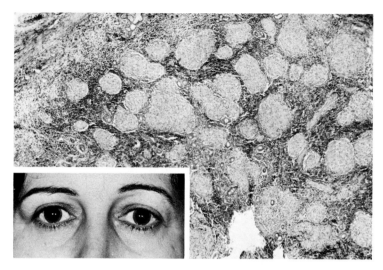

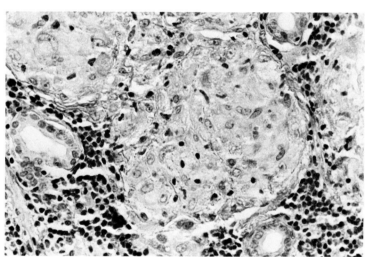

FIGURE 9-42. Histopathology and clinical features of a 50-year-old woman who presented with a progressive right superolateral mass. Histologically, the lacrimal gland was occupied by multiple focal granulomatous naked tubercles. The patient had bilateral hilar adenopathy, and the final diagnosis was sarcoidosis (H&E, original magnification *top* × 2.5, *bottom* × 40).

sists of the ocular and oral changes alone and is called the *sicca syndrome*. More commonly, however, patients have an associated autoimmune disease including rheumatoid arthritis (most common), systemic lupus erythematosus, polymyositis, vasculitis, scleroderma, mixed connective tissue disease, autoimmune liver disease, and hemolytic anemia.

PATHOGENESIS

Lymphocytic infiltration and sclerosis of the lacrimal and salivary glands account for the decrease in tears and saliva. The organ-specific damage may be due to both factors of cytotoxic T-cell infiltration and the presence of autoantibodies. Three quarters of patients have detectable rheumatoid factor even in the absence of clinical arthritis (50% of patients with sicca syndrome and almost all patients when they have the associated rheumatoid arthritis). In addition, about 70% have antinuclear antibody (ANA) and 25% a positive LE test. A multiplicity of organ-specific autoantibodies have been identified, including those to salivary duct cells, gastric parietal cells, and thyroid. There are two antinuclear antibodies associated with the syndrome, anti-SS-A and anti-SS-B. The SS-B antibodies are felt to be highly specific for Sjögren's syndrome, and are found in 60% to 70% of patients with the primary disorder. Anti-SS-A antibodies are seen in only 14% of patients and are not considered specific. The patients with associated autoimmune disorders appear to make up a distinctive subset with some difference in serologic and immunologic studies.

Pathologically, the glands (major and minor lacrimal and salivary, as well as other exocrine glands) are charac-

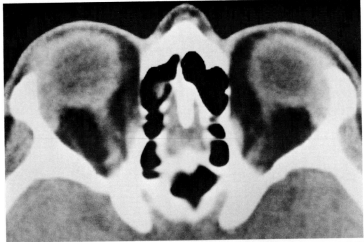

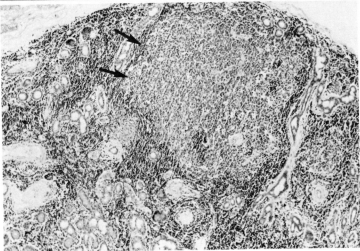

FIGURE 9-43. *(Top)* Axial CT scan demonstrates bilateral enlargement of the lacrimal glands in a 50-year-old woman with a 3-month history of nontender upper lid swelling associated with ocular grittiness. There was reduced tear secretion on Schirmer's test. *(Bottom)* Histopathology shows dense lymphocytic infiltration with partial destruction of the gland. Note large follicular center *(arrows)*. Systemically, the patient had bilateral modest effusions of her knees and a right submandibular salivary gland enlargement. The diagnosis was consistent with Sjögren's syndrome. The patient responded to systemic prednisone 30 mg/day with improvement in tear secretion and reduction in lacrimal swelling. The prednisone was tapered over a 3-month period and replaced by chloroquine (200 mg/day) for 6 months. There has been no recurrence during a 2-year follow up.

terized by early periductal lymphocytic infiltration (with and without lymphoid follicles) followed by atrophy of the acini, hyalinization, and fibrosis (Fig. 9-43). The ductal elements may undergo proliferation, forming epimyoepithelial islands. The early disappearance of lysozyme from the tears (versus an increase in sarcoidosis) may help in a diagnosis of Sjögren's syndrome.

CLINICAL FEATURES

The keratoconjunctivitis sicca is characterized by an insidious onset of burning, dryness, photophobia, and mucus secretion. This may lead to fluctuations in vision and blepharospasm. Clinically, it is associated with a filamentary keratopathy with multiple filaments and gray punctate lesions of the cornea. A thick mucus discharge may be noted in the fornix, and the keratitis is demon-

strable with rose bengal (1%) stain. Associated follicular or meibomian gland infection is frequent. There is a rapid breakup of the tear film and a reduced Schirmer test. Palpable enlargement of the lacrimal gland is rarely evident and may fluctuate when present. Clinically, lacrimal gland involvement may appear as a mild dacryoadenitis with decreased tear secretion and features of a sicca syndrome.

The salivary involvement leads to difficulty swallowing, reduction in taste, and thinning of the buccal mucosa. It may be associated with parotid gland enlargement (50%). The gland enlargement may fluctuate. Involvement of the nasopharynx and respiratory passages leads to epistaxis, reduced sense of smell, hoarseness, and recurrent bronchitis. In addition to the autoimmune disorders associated with sicca syndrome, patients may develop a lymphoproliferative disorder. It is usually a pseudolymphoma and may be difficult to differentiate from a malignant lymphoma. In fact, some patients go on to develop both salivary and extrasalivary malignant lymphomas (40-fold higher risk). In addition to the wide variety of autoimmune disorders, patients may suffer from Raynaud's phenomena, hypergammaglobulinemic purpura, hyperviscosity syndrome, and peripheral neuropathies. The neuropathies frequently affect the cranial nerves, in particular, the trigeminal nerve.

DIFFERENTIAL DIAGNOSIS

Inflammatory involvement of the lacrimal and salivary gland was once called Mikulicz's disease. The term now has been broadened to include all causes of lacrimal and salivary gland enlargement including sarcoidosis, Sjögren's syndrome, lymphoma, leukemia, tuberculosis, syphilis, and other specific and nonspecific inflammations. Therefore, Mikulicz's syndrome is a broad, nonspecific term incorporating a wide variety of diseases.

MANAGEMENT

The glandular disease appears to be resistant to treatment and is progressive. Systemic steroids and immunosuppressive agents are used in the presence of significant systemic disease. The mainstay of local management consists in the treatment of the keratoconjunctivitis sicca and xerostomia. We had a patient who responded to steroids followed by chloroquine therapy. Radiotherapy is contraindicated because of the high incidence of malignant lymphoma.

Vasculitis (Angiitides)

Vasculitis includes a wide variety of inflammatory angio-destructive processes. Vessels of varying caliber may be involved, while the inflammatory infiltrate ranges from polymorphonuclear leucocytic with leucocytoclasis (periarteritis nodosa, hypersensitivity angiitis) to granulomatous disease (Wegener's granulomatosis). The unifying histopathologic feature is evidence of destruction of vessels by the angiocentric inflammation. Blood vessel damage is characterized by any or all of the following: endothelial damage, vessel wall necrosis, and fibrin deposition within and around vessels. The vasculitides are thought to have an immunologic basis varying from immune-complex deposition to abnormalities of delayed hypersensitivity, but most evidence suggests that the major pathogenetic mechanism for vasculitis is an immune complex-mediated process. This is based on their resemblance to experimental immune-complex processes such as Arthus's phenomenon and serum sickness. In addition, immune complexes and complement have been noted in vasculitis associated with the collagen diseases and cryoglobulinemia. Hypersensitivity angiitis induced by drugs bears a strong resemblance to spontaneous vasculitis. Finally, there is a high incidence of hepatitis B antigen and immune complexes in patients with vasculitis.

Clinically, the vasculitides also express a continuum of features from acute and subacute to chronic inflammatory and vaso-obstructive signs and symptoms. The various entities are classified on the basis of the symptoms related to the organs or tissues affected, as well as their principal histopathologic features. However, it should be noted that some vascular inflammatory syndromes defy classification and may not fit neatly into a specific category. The entire group includes a wide variety of disorders, as outlined in Tables 9-9 and 9-10, but the major ophthalmic or orbital diseases include polyarteritis nodosa, Wegener's granulomatosis, giant cell arteritis (temporal arteritis), and hypersensitivity angiitis. More recently ocular findings (conjunctivitis, uveitis, or keratitis) have been documented with the mucocutaneous lymph node syndrome (Kawasaki's disease). Some of the connective tissue diseases may have a significant vasculitic component, including systemic lupus erythematosus, rheumatoid arthritis, scleroderma, and polymyositis.

Vasculitis deserves a special place in the description of orbital disease, because it reminds us of the protean nature of clinical inflammatory diseases and the important systemic associations many of them have. The necessity for careful initial and prospective systemic analysis and vigilance in orbital inflammations is underlined by

TABLE 9-9.
CLASSIFICATION OF VASCULITIS

Polyarteritis nodosa group of systemic necrotizing vasculitis
    Classic polyarteritis nodosa
    Allergic angiitis and granulomatosis (Churg-Strauss variant)
    Systemic necrotizing vasculitis "overlap syndrome"
Hypersensitivity angiitis
    Serum sickness and serum sickness-like reactions
    Henoch-Schönlein purpura
    Vasculitis associated with connective tissue disorders
    Essential mixed cryoglobulinemia with vasculitis
    Malignancy
Wegener's granulomatosis
Lymphomatoid granulomatosis
Giant cell arteritides
    Temporal arteritis
    Takayasu's arteritis
Mucocutaneous lymph node syndrome (Kawasaki's disease)
Thromboangiitis obliterans (Buerger's disease)
Miscellaneous (others)

(Robbins SL, Cotran RS, Kumar V: Pathologic Basis of Disease, p 520. Philadelphia, WB Saunders, 1984)

TABLE 9-10.
CHARACTERISTICS OF SOME SYSTEMIC VASCULITIDES

Angiitides	Vessels Involved	Organ or Tissue Affected	Principal Morphologic Features	Ocular and Orbital Findings
Polyartertis nodosa	Muscular arteries	Gastrointestinal tract, mesentery, liver, gallbladder, kidney, pancreas, lung, muscles, other sites	Lesions of varying ages; all layers of vessels with acute fibrinoid necrosis and extensive periarterial inflammation	Retinal and choroidal infarcts, sclerokeratitis, few with nonspecific orbital inflammation, with hypersensitivity angiitis may rarely have lid and anterior orbital inflammation
Allergic granulomatosis	Medium and small arteries, adjacent veins, arterioles, capillaries	Widespread, but lungs frequently involved	Necrotizing inflammation with extravascular granulomas, coexistence of acute and healing lesions, giant cells in granulomas, abundant eosinophils	Few with ocular findings including: episcleritis, uveitis, marginal corneal ulcer, lid swelling and conjunctival granuloma
Hypersensitivity angiitis	Small venules, capillaries, arterioles	All organs and tissues (skin, muscles, heart, kidneys, lungs)	Acute necrotizing vasculitis with fibrinoid necrosis of entire wall; often thrombosis of lumen	May rarely have lid and anterior orbital inflammation
Wegener's granulomatosis	Small arteries and veins	Lungs, kidneys, upper respiratory tract; occasionally systemic	Acute necrotizing vasculitis with fibrinoid necrosis of vessel wall; often proximate to granulomas in tissues	Ocular manifestations in 40%: (20%–38%) scleritis; (10%–20%) uveitis; (14%–28%) corneal gutter; (7%–18%) retinal vasculitis; (18%–22%) orbital involvement
Giant cell arteritis (temporal arteritis)	Muscular arteries	Usually temporal, ophthalmic, and cranial arteries; may be systemic	Disruption of elastic lamina with most intense reaction in intimal medial layers; giant cells engulf elastic fiber fragments, occasionally thrombosis of lumen	40% with ocular, chiefly visual problems

this group of entities. Although many of these disorders have relatively distinct systemic symptoms and signs, in early stages many are restricted to the orbit, making it difficult to diagnose and to differentiate them from nonspecific inflammatory diseases. Because these disorders have serious and even life-threatening consequences, we must be particularly careful in diagnosing and ruling them out in the face of nonspecific inflammations of the orbit.

PERIARTERITIS NODOSA (POLYARTERITIS NODOSA)

Classic periarteritis nodosa is a vasculitis of the medium and small arteries, adjacent veins, and occasionally arterioles and venules. The disease is segmental and has a predilection for involvement of bifurcations leading to nodular aneurysms. Lesions in a single patient may vary from active acute inflammation with fibrinoid necrosis to stages of both healing and healed vasculitis, suggesting that it is a multisystem process due to continuous antigenic insult. The major sites of predilection are kidney, heart, liver, and gastrointestinal tract. In addition, lesions of skin, peripheral nerves, pancreas, testes, and skeletal muscle occur.

The systemic syndrome has a predilection for males (2 to 3 : 1) in the second to fourth decade. The clinical manifestations are protean and the major symptoms are nonspecific low-grade fever, malaise, weakness, leucocytosis, and multisystem disease. Up to two thirds of untreated patients will die within 1 year as a result of renal, myocardial, and gastrointestinal involvement.

The major ophthalmologic manifestations are retinal and choroidal infarcts leading to exudative detachment and tissue necrosis. From an orbital point of view, a few cases with nonspecific orbital inflammation have been described; this may antecede the systemic syndrome. In addition, the ischemic inflammatory lesions may lead to corneal scleral necrosis and scleritis.

Definitive diagnosis requires biopsy proof of the segmental arteritis and is best obtained from clinically involved tissues such as muscle, skin lesions, and kidneys. The aneurysms may be demonstrated angiographically in up to 50% of cases, aiding in the diagnosis. The prognosis in the past has been grim, with death occurring as part of either a fulminant or more prolonged disease process. Systemic corticosteroids will modify and abate symptoms, and recent studies suggest that up to 80% of these patients will survive 5 years following treatment with corticosteroids and cyclophosphamide.

HYPERSENSITIVITY (LEUCOCYTOCLASTIC) ANGIITIS

Hypersensitivity angiitis resembles periarteritis nodosa microscopically, but affects smaller vessels and is more widely uniform in involvement. Pathologically the arterioles, venules, and capillaries are usually, but not necessarily, necrotic or may simply have perivascular infiltration with neutrophils undergoing karyolysis (leucocytoclasis). This is a frequent form of vasculitis and typically involves the skin, lungs, mucous membranes, heart, gastrointestinal tract, kidney, and muscle. In most instances drugs, microorganisms, or tumor antigens have been identified as precipitating the vasculitis. The angiitides associated with the collagen diseases and essential cryoglobulinemia are examples that also fit into this category. Because smaller vessels are involved, the signs and symptoms relate to hemorrhagic and microinfarctive lesions. The spectrum of clinical disease varies from widespread multisystem involvement to primary dermatologic lesions. Many patients may have a history of recent respiratory infection or drug ingestion. Patients may have arthralgia, arthritis, myalgia, pulmonary lesions with effusion, pericarditis, myocarditis, peripheral neuropathy, and encephalopathy. Gastrointestinal and renal involvement may also be noted.

Specific diagnosis is established by biopsy. The prognosis is difficult to predict for the group overall because of heterogeneity. Removal of the inciting cause, if related to drugs or toxins, will lead to reversal of the process. The signs and symptoms of the disease can be abated with corticosteroid therapy. It is important to rule out the possibility of underlying collagen diseases. We have divided our personal experience with leucocytoclastic vasculitis into three different groups: orbital vasculitis, vasculitis associated with connective tissue disorders, and Cogan's syndrome. All of these had similar histologic features consistent with a hypersensitivity angiitis, but had different associations.

Orbital Vasculitis

Henderson has described a series of cases in which patients presented with nonspecific orbital inflammatory disease proven on biopsy to be related to an arteritis involving small arteries and arterioles. The histology parallels that of hypersensitivity angiitis involving fibrinoid

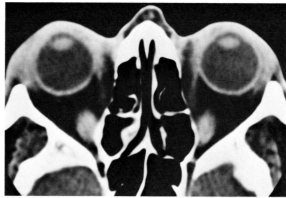

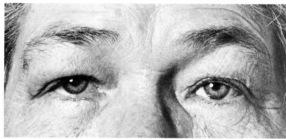

FIGURE 9-44.   This 39-year-old woman had noted swelling of the upper lids for a 2-month period, affecting the right more than the left. On axial CT scan, there was increased soft tissue of the lids and apparent enlargement of the lacrimal glands. On biopsy, the muscle and soft tissue were pale and thickened and the lacrimal structures appeared normal. Histologically, there was evidence of leukocytoclastic vasculitis.

change, disruption of the vessel with hemorrhage, necrosis, and adjacent fat destruction leading to replacement by connective tissue.

Symptomatically, the patients presented with nonspecific acute and subacute inflammation of the orbit leading to swelling of the lids, ptosis, chemosis, conjunctival injection, and discomfort. Half of the patients had proptosis. The clinical course and histology appeared to parallel each other and varied depending on degree of acute inflammatory infiltrate and fibrosis. At the time of diagnosis none had specific systemic associations and only a few of these patients subsequently developed them.

This appears to be a group of patients without a distinct systemic association that begs elucidation. We have also experienced two cases of primarily angiocentric leucocytoclastic idiopathic orbital inflammations without systemic association, which both involved the lid and anterior orbit and responded rapidly to systemic steroid treatment (Figs. 9-44 and 9-45).

When the dominant inflammatory infiltrate is acute, nonspecific anti-inflammatory therapy with steroids seems appropriate and in our experience was efficacious. However, Henderson has pointed out that some of these

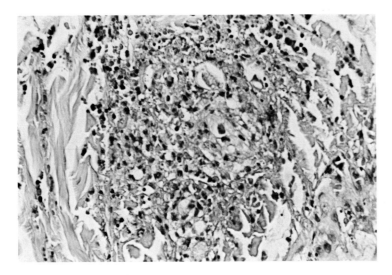

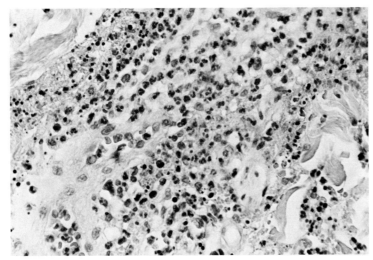

FIGURE 9-45. The vasculitis involves small vessels within skeletal muscle and adjacent connective tissue including capillaries, precapillary arterioles, and postcapillary venules (patient shown in Fig. 9-44). The inflammatory infiltrate in and surrounding the blood vessel wall consisted of a mixture of neutrophils associated with nuclear dusting consistent with leukocytoclastic vasculitis. Systemic investigation was negative, and the patient was treated with 25 mg/day of prednisone tapered over a 3-week period, with marked and complete improvement. There was no recurrence at 1-year follow up.

lesions may be recalcitrant to treatment and require low-dose radiotherapy. More recently, Kennerdell has suggested the use of immunosuppressives (cyclophosphamide [Cytoxan]) in the treatment of the resistant patient with this syndrome.

We have also seen two patients who had angiocentric orbital inflammation suggesting a vascular-related disease that did not fit into any of the above categories. They were clinically subacute or chronic in onset with mild inflammatory features. Both were anteriorly located in the orbit with pain, ptosis, lid swelling and injection on presentation. Histologically, there was a dense perivascular lymphocytic, and plasmacytic and monocytic infiltrate associated with endothelial swelling within the vascular channels. Complete immunological and systemic investigations in all of these circumstances yielded no

specific abnormalities. These patients responded well to systemic steroids within 3 months.

Vasculitis Associated with Connective Tissue Disorders

Any of the connective tissue disorders may be associated with systemic vasculitis; the most common include systemic lupus erythematosus, rheumatoid arthritis, and dermatomyositis. Histologically, the vasculitides resemble hypersensitivity angiitis and complicate the already protean manifestations of these autoimmune disorders.

Systemic lupus erythematosus is a relapsing chronic multisystem disease that primarily affects joints, skin, kidney, and the vascular system. It has a female:male ratio of 9:1 and occurs in the second and third decades.

FIGURE 9-46. This 22-year-old man with systemic lupus erythematosus and nephrotic syndrome presented with sudden onset of left central visual loss, profound lid edema, and chemosis. His vision was counting fingers at 6 feet OS, and he had marked reduction in extraocular movements. His exophthalmometry measurements were 20 OD and 22 OS, and he had marginal corneal infiltrates as well as multiple choroidal infarcts with a shallow exudative detachment. The axial CT scan shows marked left anterior orbital soft tissue swelling with a lateral component contiguous with the left lacrimal gland and insertion of the superior and lateral rectus muscles. In addition, there was evidence of thickening of the scleral envelope. The patient had small choroidal infarct on the right side; within 2 to 3 days he developed similar soft tissue findings. His local findings responded to intensive immunosuppressive therapy and plasmaphoresis.

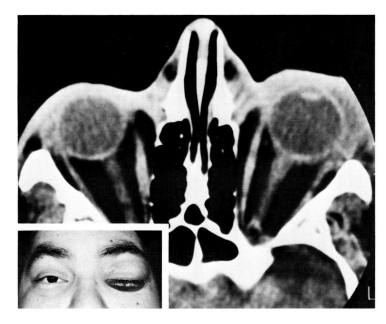

Laboratory evidence of antinuclear antibodies (ANA) is universally present in this syndrome. Although these antibodies may be found in other connective tissue disorders, antibody to double-stranded DNA is virtually diagnostic for lupus. Only 20% of cases have the pathognomonic feature of a positive LE cell test.

Twenty percent of patients have ocular involvement, primarily affecting the retinal vessels. The retinopathy is characterized by vasculitis or hypertensive changes. Orbital involvement is far less frequent and usually is secondary to conjunctival or ocular vasculitis. A few cases of orbital vasculitis have been described. We have had two patients with orbital manifestations secondary to systemic lupus. One patient presented with acute anterior orbital congestion secondary to vasculitis involving the scleral and intraocular structures. This responded to treatment of the systemic disease (Fig. 9-46). The second patient presented with idiopathic acute self-limited anterior inflammation that was associated with a systemic diagnosis of lupus erythematosus.

Dermatomyositis is an inflammatory myopathy with no known etiology. It is frequently associated with other connective tissue diseases and may be seen in association with malignancy. There may be several underlying causes. Orbital manifestations of dermatomyositis have only rarely been reported.

Cogan's Syndrome

Cogan's syndrome is divided into typical and atypical forms. Typical Cogan's syndrome was originally defined as interstitial keratitis associated with auditory symptoms and vertigo. The atypical form consists of ocular and orbital disease without corneal involvement. However, it has been suggested with careful study that many patients have a transient steroid-sensitive superficial (nummular) keratitis, which is typically in the peripheral cornea. The atypical syndrome may involve the sclera and periocular tissues leading to lid swelling, chemosis, injection, and anterior orbital inflammatory disease. Identifying this entity is important, because the systemic necrotizing vasculitis occasionally associated with it may be very severe and involve multiple sites, endangering life. We have seen one patient with this syndrome who presented with severe anterior orbital infiltration and inflammation as a primary symptom (Fig. 9-47). Within 1 week she developed the subepithelial nummular infiltrations and hearing problems. Biopsy of the conjunctiva revealed a perivascular infiltrate. This disorder will respond to systemic corticosteroids; however, in some instances, it can be fulminant and unresponsive.

WEGENER'S GRANULOMATOSIS

Wegener's granulomatosis is characterized by a triad of necrotizing granulomas in the upper and lower respiratory tract; necrotizing vasculitis of the lung, upper respiratory tract, and other sites; and glomerulonephritis. It is believed to involve abnormalities of the T cell system and perhaps immune complex formation due to hypersensitivity to an inhaled antigen. It may rarely be localized to the respiratory tract in a form of limited Wegener's granulomatosis. Pathologically, the cardinal features are a

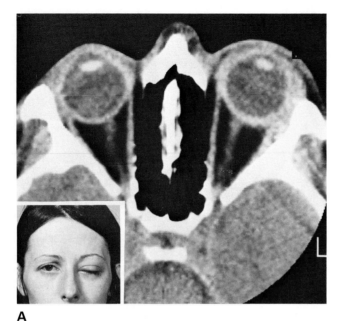

A

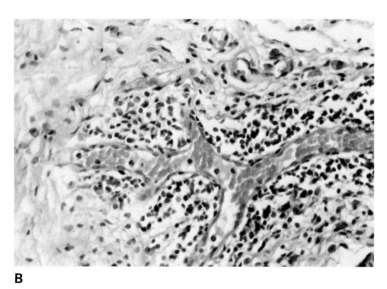

B

FIGURE 9-47. *(A)* This patient presented with severe left anterior orbital inflammation with lid edema, chemosis, ptosis, and superficial ocular inflammation associated with mild proptosis. Within 1 week, she developed subepithelial nummular infiltrations of the cornea and hearing problems. The axial CT scan shows thickening and enhancement of scleral coats on the left globe with increased anterior soft tissues. The patient was diagnosed as having Cogan's syndrome (atypical) and responded to high-dose corticosteroid therapy. *(B)* Biopsy of the conjunctiva showed an intense nonspecific perivascular lymphocytic and plasmacytic infiltrate.

combination of necrotizing vasculitis and granulomatous inflammation.

Although all ages may be affected, the peak incidence is in the fifth decade. Typically, males are affected two times more frequently than females. The major clinical features are pneumonitis, chronic sinusitis, mucosal ulcerations of the nasopharynx, and evidence of renal involvement. The respiratory symptoms may be mild to severe, and the mucosa is involved in 75% to 90% of cases. Adjacent bony destruction is associated with the development of a saddle-nose and fistula formation. Sinus and nasopharyngeal involvement may lead to ex-

tension into the orbit, mouth, and temporal fossa. Lower respiratory disease is seen in 90% and associated with cough and hemoptysis. Glomerulonephritis generally occurs late, but a small percentage (10%) of patients present with it. Remaining features of multisystem vasculitis include arthralgias (57%), dermatologic manifestations (48%), endocarditis (29%), and polyneuritis (24%). Hearing loss is common in Wegener's granulomatosis.

The limited form of Wegener's granulomatosis involves the upper and lower respiratory tract and is not associated with a glomerulonephritis. In the limited form there is a female dominance, milder course, and a high incidence of remission, with a suggestion that this may lead to underdiagnosis.

The ocular manifestations of Wegener's granulomatosis are seen in up to 40% to 45% of patients and may be divided into contiguous extension of necrotizing sinus and nasopharyngeal disease or isolated (focal) ocular involvement. The focal ocular lesions include scleritis and episcleritis (20%–38%), uveal disease (10%–20%), peripheral corneal ulceration and gutter formation (14%–28%), retinal vasculitis (7%–18%), and rare conjunctival involvement or exudative retinal detachment.

Orbital disease is seen in 18% to 22% of patients with Wegener's granulomatosis. The most common presentation is proptosis, usually with inflammatory features (acute, subacute, or chronic). The severity may vary from mild to profound involvement with reduction in ocular motility, chemosis, papilledema, and congestion leading to decreased vision. Fulminant disease may require urgent orbital decompression.

Characteristically, ocular and orbital involvement is bilateral and either nonresponsive or temporarily responsive to corticosteroids, providing a clue to diagnosis. Radiologically, sinus involvement is seen in the majority of these cases. Involvement of the ocular adnexa includes occasional dacryoadenitis, nasolacrimal obstruction, or eyelid fistula formation.

The diagnosis is based on evidence of any of the above lesions, particularly when bilateral and associated with systemic disease. The respiratory and systemic complex may occur subsequent to orbital disease; thus, patients with features of the ocular and orbital disease should be viewed with a high index of suspicion. There is a suggestion in the literature that isolated orbital involvement with a similar histologic entity may occur, but it is generally believed the diagnosis cannot be made without signs of systemic involvement, or distinctive histology.

We have encountered four patients with the diagnosis of Wegener's granulomatosis, and they demonstrated the spectrum of this disorder. Two of our patients presented with concomitant scleritis and subacute inflammatory orbital disease (Fig. 9-48). One had significant sinus disease, whereas the other had a more minor degree of involvement of these structures. The remaining two patients originally presented with relatively low-grade or chronic infiltrative orbital inflammation associated with destruction of the sinuses and nasopharyngeal structures, including a saddle-nose. One of these patients developed a sclerosing, destructive, progressive disease process involving the orbital apex and optic nerves on both sides, leading to visual loss over a 15-year period (Fig. 9-49).

Two of our patients went on to die of Wegener's granulomatosis. Both presented with relatively widespread systemic features and had a fulminant downhill course. Their systemic involvement was characterized by multisystem disease with clinical renal insufficiency in both and polyneuropathy. One patient discontinued her therapy and the second progressed despite treatment. Overall, three of the four patients developed an optic neuropathy that was responsive to therapy, but led to persistent optic nerve damage of varying degrees (see Fig. 9-49; Fig. 9-50).

Until recently the outcome was rapidly fatal. The introduction of combined corticosteroid-cyclophosphamide treatment has proven very successful in Wegener's granulomatosis, with up to a 90% remission rate. The ocular and orbital lesions respond to systemic therapy (see Figs. 9-48 and 9-49). Alternative immunosuppressives, especially azathioprine, may be used if the patient fails to respond to cyclophosphamide. Some authors have suggested that with progression of the disease, local radiotherapy and plasmaphoresis may play a role in treatment.

It should be noted that Wegener's granulomatosis is one of the entities that can develop a lethal midline granuloma. This may occur prior to systematization and recognition of the underlying Wegener's granulomatosis. Lethal midline granuloma is a clinical entity characterized by destructive processes involving the sinuses, nasopharynx, orbit, and central facial bones. The disorder may be caused by a number of different entities including: destructive inflammations such as syphillis and fungal disease; typical and atypical lymphomas; and Wegener's granulomatosis.

OTHER RESPIRATORY VASCULITIDES

Two other respiratory vasculitides are Churg-Strauss syndrome and lymphomatoid granulomatosis. Churg-Strauss syndrome (allergic granulomatosis and angiitis) more closely resembles polyarteritis nodosa histologically, but clinically is associated with lower respiratory disease and eosinophilia. Histologically, there may be a polymorphonuclear leucocytic vasculitis with or without granulomas. The systemic manifestations of Churg-Strauss syndrome are varied, and involve many organ systems. Peripheral eosinophilia is seen in up to 85% of cases.

The differentiation of Churg-Strauss syndrome from Wegener's granulomatosis is based on frequent association of allergy and asthma, eosinophilia, and responsiveness to corticosteroids alone in contrast to Wegener's granulomatosis.

The few cases of ocular involvement with Churg-Strauss syndrome consist chiefly of episcleritis, panuveitis, marginal corneal ulceration, lid swelling, and conjunctival granuloma. In addition, ischemic optic neuropathy has been described.

Management is usually with corticosteroids, and the

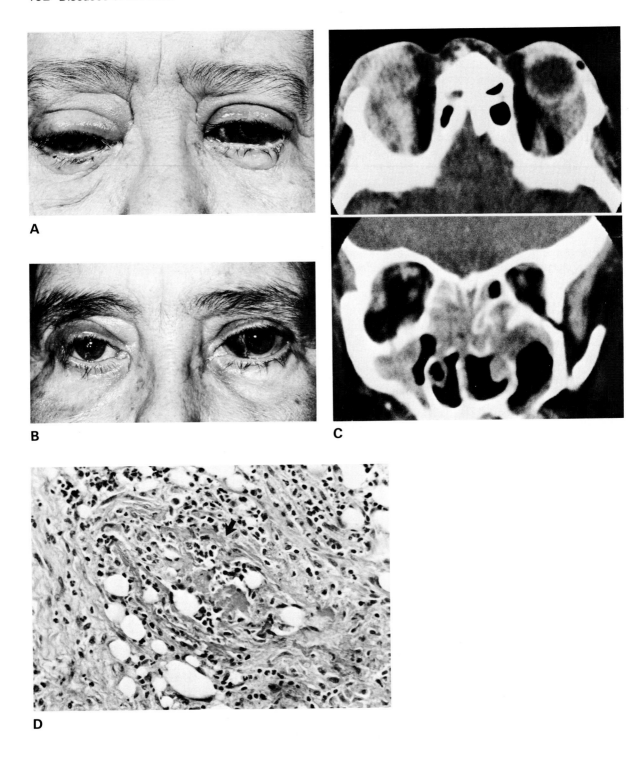

A

B

C

D

large majority of patients respond. Azathioprine or cyclophosphamide should be added for resistent cases.

Lymphomatoid granulomatosis is characterized by pulmonary involvement with lymphoid and plasmacytoid infiltrates, often demonstrating histologic atypia. The disorder is usually localized to the lungs initially and subsequently involves other organs. The pulmonary disease is seen in nearly all patients and systemic manifestations include neurologic symptoms in 30% of patients. Between 12% and 50% of patients subsequently develop malignant lymphoma. Ocular manifestations are chiefly related to cranial nerve involvement with occasional cases of uveitis, retinitis, and lid involvement. Fatality is common despite steroid and immunosuppressive therapy.

GIANT CELL (TEMPORAL) ARTERITIS

Temporal arteritis is the most common vasculitis and the best known to ophthalmologists. It is a focal granulomatous inflammation of medium and small arteries that primarily affects the cranial vessels (in particular the temporal artery) of the elderly. The average age of occurrence is 70 years and almost half of the patients have an onset characterized by systemic symptoms. The pathogenesis is thought to be a cell-mediated reaction to arterial wall antigens. Histologically, the lesions are granulomatous and associated with fragmentation of the internal elastic membrane. On the other hand, nonspecific inflammatory infiltration with or without intimal fibrosis and thrombosis may be noted. Clinically, a significant percentage of patients have negative arterial biopsies despite a typical syndrome. Although the ophthalmic, posterior ciliary, central retinal, and temporal arteries are commonly involved, the disease may be widespread and include aortic, coronary, and cerebral arteries.

The patients tend to present with headache, which may be insidious or sudden in onset and is often associated with generalized symptoms of malaise, fever, anorexia, weight loss, and muscular aching (polymyalgia rheumatica). There may be localized tenderness over the temporal artery and claudication of the jaw. About 40% of patients have ocular symptoms, which are usually visual due to vascular occlusions affecting the ophthalmic, central retinal, and posterior ciliary arteries. Occasionally, vasculitis involving orbital vessels may affect the ciliary ganglion and cause associated pupillary changes.

Temporal arteritis is diagnosed by the clinical syndrome in an elderly person with a high erythrocyte sedimentation rate (ESR). Biopsy may be negative, and given the typical syndrome and a known sensitivity to corticosteroids, a therapeutic trial may be justified.

Although the posterior ciliary and ophthalmic arteries are commonly involved with this disorder, strictly orbital manifestations are rare. Treatment is with high-dose corticosteroids to prevent involvement of the opposite side. The response is usually dramatic and can be monitored on the basis of reduced ESR and improvement symptomatically. Steroids can then be titrated downward.

Other Granulomatous and Histiocytic Lesions

There are a number of entities that could have been included with specific granulomatous inflammations, histiocytic disorders, or xanthomatous lesions including eosinophilic granuloma (histiocytosis-X), sinus histiocytosis with massive lymphadenopathy, juvenile xanthogranuloma, Erdheim-Chester disease, necrobiotic xanthogranuloma, pseudorheumatoid nodules, sarcoidosis, and fibrous histiocytoma. All of these lesions bear a

---

FIGURE 9-48. *(A)* This 67-year-old woman presented with a 6-month history of photophobia, tenderness, and inflammation of her eyes affecting the left more than the right. In addition, she had a mild increase in temperature and chronic sinus obstruction that was progressive for 6 months. On physical examination, she had severe bilateral scleritis with marginal corneal ulcers, reduced vision (20/400 OD, 20/200 OS), and scleral ectasia with periocular swelling, proptosis, and edema. *(B)* Physical appearance of the same patient 2 months after initiation of therapy, which consisted of cyclophosphamide and prednisone. At this time, her vision was 20/40 OD, and counting fingers at 6 feet OS. Systemic investigation was negative. The overall picture suggested a limited form of Wegener's granulomatosis. *(C)* CT scans show bilateral lateral orbital infiltration and extensive soft tissue changes with bone destruction of the paranasal sinuses and nasal airways. *(D)* Histopathology of orbital biopsy showed diffuse infiltration of the orbital tissue by lymphocytes, epithelioid cells, and occasional giant cells. Rare eosinophils and plasma cells were noted. Also, there were vessels *(arrow)* that showed necrotizing inflammatory changes with focal infiltration by neutrophils. Special stains with PTAH showed numerous areas of fibrinoid necrosis. The overall morphology was consistent with severe necrotizing angiitis of a granulomatous nature consistent with Wegener's granulomatosis (H&E, original magnification × 25).

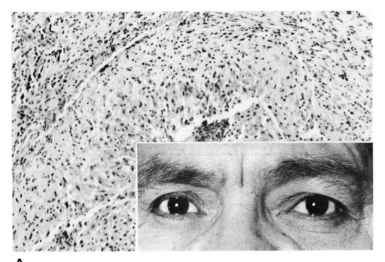

FIGURE 9-49. *(A)* This 48-year-old man had a 15-year history of progressive destructive granulomatous inflammatory lesions involving his nasopharyngeal and sinus structures. He had multiple sinus procedures, and had developed a saddlenose. Repeat biopsies demonstrated a necrotizing granulomatous process, which was negative on special stains for fungal or microbial infection. The patient had a history of pulmonary tuberculosis, but tubercle bacilli had never been identified in the nasopharyngeal or orbital infiltrates. The progressive orbital involvement had led to bilateral optic neuropathy.

A

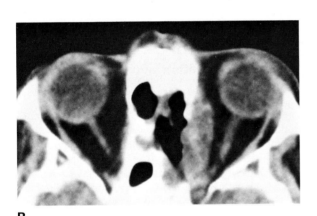

B

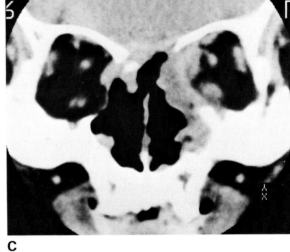

C

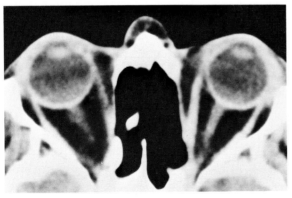

D

FIGURE 9-49 *(Continued).* *(B, C)* The overall clinical picture is a midline lethal granulomatous process without systemic association, and a presumptive diagnosis of Wegener's granulomatosis was made. The patient was treated with cyclophosphamide and prednisone. *(D)* The photograph demonstrates resolution of the orbital lesion after 6 months of therapy.

fundamental link based on local or systemic infiltration by histiocytes. We have discussed fibrous histiocytoma and nevoxanthogranuloma under mesenchymal lesions, and histiocytosis-X and sinus histiocytosis under lymphoproliferative and leukemic lesions of the orbit, but they could have been discussed within the context of the group of lesions just outlined. Erdheim-Chester disease, pseudorheumatoid nodules, and necrobiotic xanthogranuloma all have features suggesting an inflammatory basis; thus, they have been included in this section.

Erdheim-Chester disease is a systemic xanthogranulomatosis that occurs in adults; it may affect bones and viscera. This disease can lead to cardiac, kidney, and pulmonary infiltration with decompensation. Two cases of bilateral diffuse orbital involvement have been described. The infiltration and scarring led to compressive and restrictive effects on the orbital structures associated with a firm, subcuticular, xanthelasma-like lesion. Histologically, the infiltrate consists of bloated histiocytes, occasional Touton giant cells, and a mixture of lymphocytes and plasma cells with a background of fibrosis. These lesions may respond in part to steroids administered systemically.

Pseudorheumatoid nodules usually occur as focal masses in the dermis of children. They have been described in the periorbital region and occasionally affect the anterior orbit. These subcutaneous nodules consist of zonular granulomas surrounding necrobiotic collagen. These are thought to be more common in sites of previous trauma and are easily managed by simple excision.

Necrobiotic xanthogranuloma is a disorder characterized by the occurrence of multiple indurated xanthomatous subcutaneous nodules in patients with paraproteinemia. Ophthalmic manifestations are common and include xanthogranulomas involving the eyelid, orbit, and conjunctiva. In addition, episcleritis, scleritis, uveitis, and keratitis have been described. Many of the patients have had underlying systemic monoclonal gammopathies, B-cell lymphomas, or myeloma. The subcutaneous lesions may involve the anterior orbit and are characteristically waxy, firm, and injected. This disease usually occurs in the sixth decade. Pathologically, zonular granulomatous inflammatory infiltrate, with Touton giant and xanthoma cells, surrounds an area of necrobiosis. Bullock has suggested serum immunoglobulins complexed with lipid and deposited in the skin elicit the granulomatous response. These lesions may respond with treatment of the systemic lymphoma. Local injections of triamcinolone and excision may help local lesions but systemic steroids alone are not effective. In most instances, the local lesions tend to progress and ulcerate.

Differences in age, systemic association, distribution, histopathology, and character of these lesions help to differentiate the various histiocytic disorders.

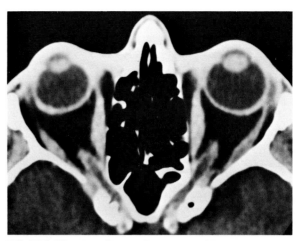

FIGURE 9-50. Axial CT scan demonstrates bilateral apical optic nerve swelling, mild medial and lateral rectus enlargement, and focal thickening of the scleral envelope. This was seen in a 64-year-old woman who had presented with bilateral scleritis and optic neuropathy (vision was hand movements bilaterally). Initial systemic investigations revealed no other abnormalities. A presumptive diagnosis of Wegener's granulomatosis with vasculitis was made, and the patient was treated with high-dose corticosteroids and cyclophosphamide. Vision on the left improved to 20/50, and remained at hand movements on the right. The patient refused to continue with therapy, and over the next several months developed multiple renal infarcts, bilateral pulmonary vasculitis, and pleural effusion. The patient died 8 months after the onset of scleritis and optic neuropathy due to Wegener's granulomatosis.

Ocular Inflammations with Orbital Signs

We have encountered a number of circumstances in which the differential diagnosis of orbital inflammatory disease is raised when patients present with relatively severe ocular inflammations affecting periocular tissues. This, of course, can occur in circumstances such as endophthalmitis and severe uveitis. The most common circumstances in which we experienced this differential were cases of scleritis. We had six cases of what were ultimately diagnosed as scleritis presenting as referrals to the University of British Columbia Orbital Clinic; four patients were females and two were males. All but one were unilateral and the characteristic features were chemosis (four), pain (four), swelling (three), and proptosis (three). One case was bilateral and three of the cases appeared to have other immunologically based diseases of the bowel. Five of the six cases presented as subacute inflammation, and one as chronic inflammation. Five of the six cases had severe anterior orbital inflammation with characteristic infiltration and thickening of the sclera. CT and ultrasonography (see Fig. 9-51) confirmed

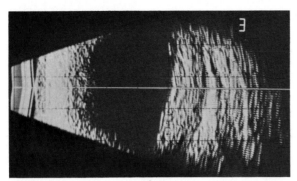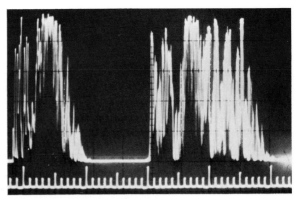

FIGURE 9-51. Ultrasonography demonstrates features of scleritis seen in a patient who presented with swelling and thickening in the medial portion of the right orbit. The ultrasonogram shows a thickening of the medial portion of the globe with an echolucent area between the sclera and orbital fat. The internal architecture of the lesion revealed high reflectivity with very little sound wave attenuation. The clinical and ultrasonographic findings were consistent with a scleritis. The patient was treated with oral prednisone, which led to resolution of the lesion.

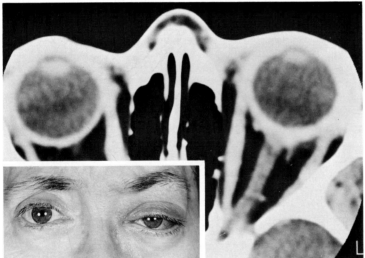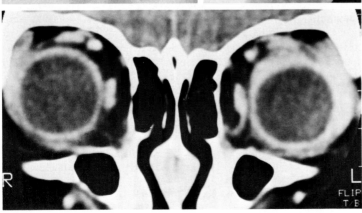

FIGURE 9-52. This 59-year-old woman presented with a history of a slowly developing left proptosis, ptosis, and injection of the globe. On physical examination she had proptosis (4 mm), an injected epibulbar surface, and some scleral thickening anteriorly. On enhanced CT scan, there was thickening of the scleral envelope and adjacent orbital infiltration, as well as proptosis and downward displacement of the left globe. Systemically, the patient had severe diabetes, hypertension, an organic brain syndrome, and myocardial insufficiency. While in the hospital, she died of acute coronary insufficiency. Autopsy study of the globe revealed nonspecific scleritis with anterior orbital inflammation.

essentially scleral involvement with some mild local infiltration of the orbit. One case presented in a patient with relatively diffuse features of anterior orbital inflammation and scleritis (see Fig. 9-52). She died of unrelated cardiovascular causes 2 weeks following initiation of treatment; autopsy findings on the globes and orbits showed a diffuse episcleral and anterior orbital inflammatory infiltration.

Cases of posterior scleritis may be extremely difficult to differentiate from some of the acute and subacute idiopathic anterior orbital inflammations, most particularly, those that are associated with relatively severe uveitis and choroiditis or exudative retinal detachment. However, the bulk of the anterior idiopathic orbital inflammations occur in a younger age group and are associated with other signs of orbital inflammation. In contrast, the posterior scleritis tends to occur in older persons, with fewer orbital inflammatory signs and some possible systemic associations.

Conclusion

The foregoing description of orbital inflammatory disease processes to some degree is arbitrary. The major rationale for it is that in a practical clinical situation, the division into these various categories ought to point to both investigative and therapeutic alternatives that appear to relate well to the clinicopathologic syndromes as described. With future improvements in diagnostic studies, a more specific characterization of these diseases may ultimately resolve many of the ambiguities.

Bibliography

GENERAL

Duke-Elder S, MacFaul PA: The Ocular Adnexa: Lacrimal, Orbital and Para-Orbital Diseases. In Duke-Elder S (ed): System of Ophthalmology, Vol 13, Part 2, p 876. London, Henry Kimpton, 1974

Henderson JW: Orbital Tumors, 2nd ed. New York, BC Decker, 1980

Jakobiec FA, Jones IS: Orbital inflammations. In Jones IS, Jakobiec FA (eds): Diseases of the Orbit. New York, Harper & Row, 1979

Jones DB: Microbial preseptal and orbital cellulitis. In Duane TD (ed): Clinical Ophthalmology, Vol 4, Chap 25. New York, Harper & Row, 1976

Petersdorf RG, Adams RD, Braunwald E et al: Harrison's Principles of Internal Medicine, 10th ed. New York, McGraw-Hill, 1983

Robbins SL, Cotran RS, Kumar V: Pathologic Basis of Disease, 3rd ed. Philadelphia, WB Saunders, 1984

ORBITAL CELLULITIS AND SINUSITIS

Amies DR: Orbital cellulitis. J Laryngol Otol 88:559, 1974

Aust R, Drettner B: Oxygen tension in the human maxillary sinus under normal and pathological conditions. Acta Otolaryngol 78:264, 1974

Bhandari YS, Sarkari NBS: Subdural empyema: A review of 37 cases. J Neurosurg 32:35, 1970

Bilaniuk LT, Zimmerman RA: Computer-assisted tomography: sinus lesions with orbital involvement. Head Neck Surg 2:293, 1980

Blumenfeld RJ, Skilnick EM: Intracranial complications of sinus disease. Trans Am Acad Ophthalmol Otolaryngol 70:889, 1966

Brook I, Friedman EM, Rodriguez WJ et al: Complications of sinusitis in children. Pediatrics 66:568, 1980

Brook I: Bacteriologic features of chronic sinusitis in children. JAMA 246:967, 1981

Carenfelt C, Lundberg C: Purulent and non-purulent maxillary sinus secretions with respect to pO_2, pCO_2 and ph. Acta Otolaryngol 84:138, 1977

Carenfelt C, Lundberg C, Nord CE et al: Bacteriology of maxillary sinusitis in relation to quality of the retained secretion. Acta Otolaryngol 86:298, 1978

Carenfelt C: Pathogenesis of sinus empyema. Ann Otol 88:16, 1979

Chandler JR, Langenbrunner DJ, Stevens ER: The pathogenesis of orbital complications in acute sinusitis. Laryngoscope 80:1414, 1970

Clairmont AA, Per-Lee JH: Complications of acute frontal sinusitis. Am Fam Physician 11:80, 1975

Clune JP: Septic thrombosis within the cavernous chamber. Am J Ophthalmol 56:33, 1963

El Shewy TM: Acute infarction of the choroid and retina. A complication of orbital cellulitis. Br J Ophthalmol 57:204, 1973

English GM: Sinusitis. In English GM (ed): Otolaryngology, Vol 2, Chap 21. Philadelphia, Harper & Row, 1980

Evans FO, Sydnor B, Moore WEC et al: Sinusitis of the maxillary antrum. N Engl J Med 293:735, 1975

Fernback SK, Naidich TP: CT diagnosis of orbital inflammation in children. Neuroradiology 22:7, 1981

Fleisher G, Ludwig S, Campos J: Brief clinical and laboratory observations. Cellulitis: Bacterial etiology, clinical features, and laboratory findings. Pediatrics 97, No. 4:591, 1980

Frederick J, Braude AI: Anaerobic infections of the paranasal sinuses. N Engl J Med 290:135, 1974

Galbraith JG, Barr VW: Epidural abscess and subdural empyema. Adv Neurol 6:257, 1974

Gellady AM, Shulman ST, Ayoub EM: Periorbital and orbital cellulitis in children. Pediatrics 61:272, 1978

Goldberg F, Berne AS, Oski FA: Differentiation of orbital cellulitis from preseptal cellulitis by computed tomography. Pediatrics 62:1000, 1978

Goodwin WJ, Jr, Weinshall M, Chandler JR: The role of high resolution computerized tomography and standardized ultrasound in the evaluation of orbital cellulitis. Laryngoscope 92:728, 1982

Grove WE: Septic and aseptic types of thrombosis of the cavernous sinus. Arch Otolaryngol 24:29, 1936

Gutman L: Appropriate antibiotics in orbital cellulitis. Arch Ophthalmol 95:170, 1977

Hamory BH, Sande MA, Sydnor A, Jr et al: Etiology and antimicrobial therapy of acute maxillary sinusitis. J Infect Dis 139:197, 1979

Harbour RC, Trobe JD, Ballinger WE: Septic cavernous sinus thrombosis associated with gingivitis and parapharyngeal abscess. Arch Ophthalmol 102:94, 1984

Harley MJ, Guerier TH: Orbital cellulitis related to an influenza: A virus epidemic. Br Med J 2:13, 1978

Harr DL, Quencer RM, Abrams GW: Computed tomography and ultrasound in the evaluation of orbital infection and pseudotumor. Radiology 142:395, 1982

Harris GJ, Syvertsen A: Multiple projection computed tomography in orbital disorders. Ann Ophthalmol 13:183, 1981

Harris GJ: Subperiosteal abscess of the orbit. Arch Ophthalmol 101:751, 1983

Haynes RE, Cramblett HG: Acute ethmoiditis: Its relationship to orbital cellulitis. Am J Dis Child 114:261, 1967

Holt R: The bacterial degradation of chloramphenicol. Lancet 1:1259, 1967

Hornblass A, Herschorn BJ, Stern K, Grimes C: Orbital abscess. Surv Ophthalmol 29, No. 3:169, 1984

Jarrett WH, II, Gutman FA: Ocular complications of infection in the paranasal sinuses. Arch Ophthalmol 81:683, 1969

Krohel GB, Krauss HR, Winnick J: Orbital abscess: Presentation, diagnosis, therapy, and sequelae. Ophthalmology 89, No. 5:492, 1982

Kronschnabel EF: Orbital apex syndrome due to sinus infection. Laryngoscope 84:353, 1974

Leo JS, Halpern J, Sachler JRL: Computed tomography in the evaluation of orbital infections. Comput Tomogr 4:133, 1980

Lerman SJ, Brunken JM, Bollinger M: Prevalence of ampicillin-resistant strains of Haemophilus influenzae causing systemic infection. Antimicrob Agents Chemother 18:474, 1980

Lew D, Southwick FS, Montgomery WW et al: Sphenoid sinusitis: A review of 30 cases. N Engl J Med 309, No. 19:1149, 1983

Londer L, Nelson DL: Orbital cellulitis due to Haemophilus influenzae. Arch Ophthalmol 91:89, 1974

Morgan PR, Morrison WV: Complications of frontal and ethmoid sinusitis. Laryngoscope 90:661, 1980

Nelson JD: Cefuroxime: A cephalosporin with unique applicability to pediatric practice. Pediatr Infect Dis 2:394, 1983

Noel LP, Clarke WN, Peacocke TA: Periorbital and orbital cellulitis in childhood. Can J Ophthalmol 16:178, 1981

Price CD, Hameroff SB, Richards RD: Cavernous sinus thrombosis and orbital cellulitis. South Med J 64:1243, 1971

Robie G, O'Neal R, Kelsey DS: Periorbital cellulitis. J Pediatr Ophthalmol Strabismus 14:354, 1977

Samson OS, Clark K: A current review of brain abscess. Am J Med 54:201, 1973

Schramm VL, Myers EN, Kennerdell JS: Orbital complications of acute sinusitis: Evaluation, management and outcome. Trans Am Acad Ophthalmol Otolaryngol 86:221, 1978

Schramm VL, Curtin HD, Kennerdell JS: Evaluation of orbital cellulitis and results of treatment. Laryngoscope 92:732, 1982

Shapiro ED, Wald ER, Brozanski BA: Periorbital cellulitis and paranasal sinusitis: a reappraisal. Pediatr Infect Dis 1, No. 2:91, 1982

Shopfner CE, Rossi JO: Roentgen evaluation of the paranasal sinuses in children. Am J Roentgenol Radium Ther Nucl Med 118:176, 1973

Smith BR, LeFrock JL: Cefuroxime: antimicrobial activity, pharmacology and clinical efficacy. Ther Drug Monit 5:149, 1983

Smith TF, O'Day D, Wright PF: Clinical implications of preseptal (periorbital) cellulitis in childhood. Pediatrics 62:1006, 1978

Teele DW: Management of the child with a red and swollen eye. Pediatr Infect Dis 2:258, 1983

Wald ER, Milmoe GJ, Bowen A et al: Acute maxillary sinusitis in children. N Engl J Med 304:749, 1981

Watters EC, Wallar PH et al: Acute orbital cellulitis. Arch Ophthalmol 94:785, 1976

Weiss A, Friendly D, Eglin K et al: Bacterial periorbital and orbital cellulitis in childhood. Ophthalmology 90, No. 3:195, 1983

Yarington CT, Jr: The prognosis and treatment of cavernous sinus thrombosis. Ann Otol Rhinol Laryngol 70:263, 1961

Yarington CT, Jr: Cavernous sinus thrombosis revisited. Proc R Soc Med 70:456, 1977

Yoshikawa TT, Chow AW, Guze LB: Role of anaerobic bacteria in subdural empyema: Report of four cases and review of 327 cases from the English literature. Am J Med 58:99, 1975

Zimmerman RA, Bilaniuk LT: CT of orbital infection and its cerebral complications. Am J Radiol 123:45, 1980

MUCORMYCOSIS

Baum JL: Rhino-orbital mucormycosis occurring in an otherwise healthy individual. Am J Ophthalmol 63:335, 1967

Best M, Obstbaum SA, Friedman B et al: Survival in orbital phycomycosis. Am J Ophthalmol 71:1078, 1971

Blodi FC, Hannah FT, Wadsworth JAC. Lethal orbito-cerebral phycomycosis in otherwise healthy children. Am J Ophthalmol 67:698, 1969

Bullock JD, Jampol LM, Fezza AJ: Two cases of orbital phycomycosis with recovery. Am J Ophthalmol 78:811, 1974

Burns RP: Mucormycosis of the sinuses, orbit and central nervous system. Trans Pac Coast Oto-Ophthalmol Soc 40:83, 1959

Ferry AP: Cerebral mucormycosis (phycomycosis): Ocular findings and review of the literature. Surv Ophthalmol 6:1, 1961

Ferry AP, Abedi S: Diagnosis and management of rhino-orbito-cerebral mucormycosis (phycomycosis): A report of 16 personally observed cases. Ophthalmology 90:1096, 1983

Fleckner RA, Goldstein JH: Mucormycosis. Br J Ophthalmol 53:542, 1969

Gass JDM: Acute orbital mucormycosis: Report of two cases. Arch Ophthalmol 65:214, 1961

Gass JDM: Ocular manifestations of acute mucormycosis. Arch Ophthalmol 65:226, 1961

Kohn R, Hepler R: Management of limited rhino-orbital mucormycosis without exenteration. Ophthalmology 92, No. 10:1440, 1985

Straatsma BR, Zimmerman LE, Gass JDM: Phycomycosis: A clinicopathologic study of fifty-one cases. Lab Invest 11:963, 1962

ASPERGILLOSIS

Bodey GP: Fungal infections complicating acute leukemia. J Chronic Dis 19:667, 1966

Chandra P, Ahluwalia BK, Chugh TD: Primary orbital aspergilloma. Br J Ophthalmol 54:693, 1970

Crivelli G, Riviera L: Unilateral blindness from aspergilloma at the right optic foramen. J Neurosurg 33:207, 1970

Elliott JH, O'Day DM, Gutow GS et al: Mycotic endophthalmitis in drug abusers. Am J Ophthalmol 88:66, 1979

Fraser DW, Ward JI, Ajello L et al: Aspergillosis and other systemic mycoses: The growing problem. JAMA 242:1631, 1979

Friedman AH, Chishty MI, Henkind P: Endogenous ocular aspergillosis. Ophthalmologica 168:197, 1974

Goldhammer Y, Smith JL, Yates B: Mycotic intrasellar abscess. Am J Ophthalmol 78:478, 1974

Green WR, Font RL, Zimmerman LE: Aspergillosis of the orbit: Report of ten cases and review of the literature. Arch Ophthalmol 82:302, 1969

Houle TV, Ellis PP: Aspergillosis of the orbit with immunosuppressive therapy. Surv Ophthalmol 20:35, 1975

Johnson R, Rootman J: Bilateral retinal infarction in disseminated aspergillosis. Can J Ophthalmol 17, No. 5:233, 1982

Jones DB: Fungal keratitis. In Duane T (ed): Clinical Ophthalmology, Vol 4, Chap 21, pp 1–13. Philadelphia, Harper & Row, 1976

Litricin O: Endogenous fungus endophthalmitis (probably Aspergillus). Ophthalmologica 179:42, 1979

MacCormick WF, Schochet SS, Jr, Weaver PR et al: Disseminated aspergillosis: Aspergillus endophthalmitis, optic nerve infarction, and carotid artery thrombosis. Arch Pathol 99:353, 1975

Miloshev B, Davidson CM, Gentles JC et al: Aspergilloma of the paranasal sinuses and orbit in Northern Sudanese. Lancet 1:746, 1966

Naidoff MA, Green WR: Endogenous Aspergillus endophthalmitis occurring after kidney transplant. Am J Ophthalmol 79:502, 1975

Tan K, Sugai K, Leong TK: Disseminated aspergillosis. Am J Clin Pathol 45:697, 1966

Wolter JR: Diagnosis and management of orbital aspergillosis. Ann Ophthalmol 8:17, 1976

Young RC, Bennett JE, Vogel CL et al: Aspergillosis: The spectrum of the disease in 98 patients. Medicine (Baltimore) 49:147, 1970

Zinneman HH: Sino-orbital aspergillosis: Report of a case and review of the literature. Minn Med 55:661, 1972

OTHER MYCOSES

Olurin O, Lucas A, Oyediran A: Orbital histoplasmosis due to Histoplasma duboisii. Am J Ophthalmol 68:14, 1969

Streeten B, Rabuzzi P, Jones D: Sporotrichosis of the orbital margin. Am J Ophthalmol 77:750, 1974

Vida L, Moel S: Systemic North American blastomycosis with orbital involvement. Am J Ophthalmol 77:240, 1974

TUBERCULOSIS OF THE ORBIT

Baghdassarian SA, Zakharia H, Asdourian KK: Report of a case of bilateral caseous tuberculous dacryoadenitis. Am J Ophthalmol 74:744, 1967

Farer LS, Lowell AM, Meador MP: Extrapulmonary tuberculosis in the United States. Am J Epidemiol 109:205, 1979

Glassroth J, Robins AG, Snider DE: Tuberculosis in the 1980's. N Engl J Med 302:1441, 1980

Jain MR, Chundawat HS, Batra V: Tuberculosis of the maxillary antrum and of the orbit. Indian J Ophthalmol 1:18, 1979

Khalil M, Lindley S, Matouk E: Tuberculosis of the orbit. Ophthalmology 92, No. 11:1624, 1985

Mortada A: Tuberculoma of the orbit and lacrimal gland. Br J Ophthalmol 55:565, 1971

Oakhill A, Shah KJ, Thompson AG et al: Orbital tuberculosis in childhood. Br J Ophthalmol 66:396, 1982

Spoor TC, Harding SA: Orbital tuberculosis. Am J Ophthalmol 91:644, 1981

Sheridan PH, Edman JB, Starr SE: Tuberculosis presenting as an orbital mass. Pediatrics 67:874, 1981

NONSPECIFIC ORBITAL INFLAMMATION

Aiello JS: Ocular findings in lupus erythematosus. Am J Ophthalmol 35:837, 1952

Bleeker GM, Wagenhaar SS, Peeters HJF et al: Orbital inflammatory pseudotumors. Immunologic aspects. Mod Probl Ophthalmol 14:393, 1975

Blodi FC: Orbital inflammation. Orbit 1:1, 1982

Blodi FC, Gass JDM: Inflammatory pseudotumor of the orbit. Br J Ophthalmol 52:79, 1968

Brenner EH, Shock JP: Proptosis secondary to systemic lupus erythematosus. Arch Ophthalmol 91:81, 1974

Burkhalter E: Unique presentation of systemic lupus erythematosus. Arthritis Rheum 16:428, 1973

Chavis RM, Garner A, Wright JE: Inflammatory orbital pseudotumor: A clinicopathologic study. Arch Ophthalmol 96:1817, 1978

Clay C, Bilanivk LT, Vignaud J: Orbital pseudotumors: Preliminary report on a new type of therapy. Neuro-ophthalmology 1:101, 1980

Contardo R: Evolution of the collagen diseases. Arch Ophthalmol 56:568, 1956

Coop ME: Pseudotumor of the orbit: A clinical and pathological study of 47 cases. Br J Ophthalmol 45:513, 1961

Cordes FC, Aiken SD: Ocular changes in acute disseminated lupus erythematosus. Am J Ophthalmol 30:1541, 1947

Donaldson SS, McDougall IR, Egbert PR et al: Treatment of orbital pseudotumor (idiopathic orbital inflammation) by radiation therapy. Int J Radiat Oncol Biol Phys 6:79, 1980

Enzmann D, Donaldson SS, Marshall WH et al: Computed tomography in orbital pseudotumor (idiopathic orbital inflammation). Radiology 120:597, 1976

Eshaghian J, Anderson RL: Sinus involvement in inflammatory orbital pseudotumor. Arch Ophthalmol 99:627, 1981

Font R, Yanoff M, Zimmerman L: Benign lymphoepithelial lesion of the lacrimal gland and its relationship to Sjögren's syndrome. Am J Clin Pathol 48:365, 1967

Gardner A: Pathology of pseudotumor of the orbit: A review. J Clin Pathol 126:639, 1973

Gordon DM: The eye in systemic disease. Postgrad Med 40:363, 1966

Harr DL, Quencer RM, Abrams GW: Computed tomography and ultrasound in the evaluation of orbital infection and pseudotumor. Radiology 142:395, 1981

Heersink B, Rodrigues MR, Flanagan JC: Inflammatory pseudotumor of the orbit. Ann Ophthalmol 9:17, 1977

Hollenhorst RW, Henderson JW: The ocular manifestations of the diffuse collagen diseases. Am J Med Sci 221:211, 1951

Jakobiec FA, McLean I, Font RL: Clinicopathologic characteristics of orbital lymphoid hyperplasia. Ophthalmology 86:948, 1979

Jakobiec FA, Mottow L: Pediatric orbital pseudotumor. In Jakobiec FA (ed): Ocular and Adnexal Tumors, p 654. Birmingham, Aesculapius, 1978

Jellinek EH: The orbital pseudotumor syndrome and its differentiation from endocrine exophthalmos. Brain 92:35, 1969

Kennerdell JS, Johnson BL, Deutsch M: Radiation treatment of orbital lymphoid hyperplasia. Ophthalmology 86:942, 1979

Kennerdell JS, Dresner SC: The nonspecific orbital inflammatory syndromes. Surv Ophthalmol 29, No. 2:93, 1981

Kenny AH, Halfner JN: Ultrasonic evidence of inflammatory thickening and fluid collection with the retrobulbar fascia: The T sign. Ann Ophthalmol 91:1557, 1977

Kim RY, Roth RE: Radiotherapy of orbital pseudotumor. Radiology 127:507, 1978

Knowles DM, Jakobiec FA: Ocular adnexal lymphoid neoplasms: Clinical, histopathologic, electron microscopic and immunologic characteristics. Hum Pathol 13:148, 1982

Knowles DM, II, Jakobiec FA, Halper JP: Immunologic characterization of ocular adnexal lymphoid neoplasms. Am J Ophthalmol 87:603, 1979

Manschot WA: The eye in collagen disease. Bibl Ophthalmol 58:1, 1961

Mottow LS, Jakobiec FA: Idiopathic inflammatory orbital pseudotumor in childhood. I. Clinical characteristics. Arch Ophthalmol 96:1410, 1978

Mottow-Lippa L, Jakobiec FA, Smith M: Idiopathic inflammatory orbital pseudotumor in childhood. II. Results of diagnostic tests and biopsies. Ophthalmology 88:565, 1981

Nugent RA, Rootman J, Robertson WD et al: Acute orbital pseudotumors: Classification and CT features. Am J Radiol 137:957, 1981

Rootman J, Nugent R: The classification and management of acute orbital pseudotumors. Ophthalmology 89:1040, 1982

Sergott RC, Glaser JS, Charyulu K: Radiotherapy for idiopathic inflammatory orbital pseudotumor: Indications and results. Arch Ophthalmol 99:853, 1981

Vail D: Diffuse collagen diseases with ocular complications. Trans Ophthalmol Soc UK 72:155, 1952

Van Wien S, Merz EH: Exophthalmos secondary to periarteritis nodosa. Am J Ophthal 56:204, 1963

Walton EW: Pseudotumor of the orbit and polyarteritis nodosa. J Clin Pathol 12:419, 1959

Wilkinson LS, Panusk RS: Exophthalmos associated with systemic lupus erythematosus. Arthritis Rheum 18:188, 1975

Young RSK, Hodes BL, Cruse RP et al: Orbital pseudotumor and Crohn disease. J Pediatr 99:250, 1981

Zimmerman LE: Pathology of diffuse collagen diseases. Arch Ophthalmol 56:548, 1956

MYOSITIC

Birch-Hirschfeld A: Handbuch der Gesamten Augenheilkunde, Vol 9, p 251. Berlin, Julius Springer, 1930

Blodi FC, Gass JDM: Inflammatory pseudotumor of the orbit. Br J Ophthalmol 52:79, 1968

Brenner EH, Shock JP: Proptosis secondary to systemic lupus erythematosus. Arch Ophthalmol 91:82, 1974

Bullen CL, Younge BR: Chronic orbital myositis. Arch Ophthalmol 100:1749, 1982

Divine RD, Anderson RL: Small cell carcinoma masquerading as orbital myositis. Ophthalmic Surg 13:483, 1982

Dunnington JH, Berke RN: Exophthalmos due to chronic orbital myositis. Arch Ophthalmol 30:446, 1943

Francois J, Rabaey M, Evens L: Myosites orbitaries chroniques. Ophthalmologica 131:105, 1956

Gleason JE: Idiopathic myositis involving the extraocular muscles. Ophthalmic Rec 12:471, 1903

Grimson BS, Simons KB: Orbital inflammation, myositis, and systemic lupus erythematosus. Arch Ophthalmol 101:736, 1983

Jellinek EH: The orbital pseudotumor syndrome and its differentiation from endocrine exophthalmos. Brain 92:35, 1969

Keane JR: Alternating proptosis: A case report of acute orbital myositis defined by the computerized tomographic scan. Arch Neurol 34:642, 1977

Mejlszenkier JD, Safran AP, Healy JJ: Myositis of influenza. Arch Neurol 29:441, 1973

Michail D, Rusu L: Les myosites des muscles périoculaires. Ann Ocul 177:97, 1940

Offret G: Les myosites chroniques dans le cadre des myosites orbitaires, valeur pathogénique des lésions vasculaires. Thesis. Paris, 1939

Purcell JJ, Jr, Taulbee WA: Orbital myositis after upper respiratory tract infection. Arch Ophthalmol 99:437, 1981

Sergott RC, Glaser JS: Graves' ophthalmopathy: A clinical and immunologic review. Surv Ophthalmol 26:1, 1981

Sergott RC, Glaser JS, Charyulu K: Radiotherapy for idiopathic inflammatory orbital pseudotumor: Indications and results. Arch Ophthalmol 99:853, 1981

Slavin ML, Glaser JS: Idiopathic orbital myositis: A report of six cases. Arch Ophthalmol 100:1261, 1982

Svane S: Peracute spontaneous streptococcal myositis: A report on 2 fatal cases with review of literature. Acta Chir Scand 137:155, 1971

Trokel SL, Hilal SK: Recognition and differential diagnosis of enlarged extraocular muscles in computed tomography. Am J Ophthalmol 87:503, 1979

Weinstein GS, Dresner SC, Slamovits TL et al: Acute and subacute orbital myositis. Am J Ophthalmol 96:209, 1983

Wolter JR, Hoy JE, Schmidt DM: Chronic orbital myositis: Its diagnostic difficulties and pathology. Am J Ophthalmol 62:292, 1966

IDIOPATHIC NONINFECTIOUS GRANULOMATOUS ORBITAL INFLAMMATION

Krohel GB, Carr EM, Webb RM: Intralesional corticosteroids for inflammatory lesions of the orbit. Am J Ophthalmol 101:121, 1986

SARCOIDOSIS

Avisar R, Menache R, Shaked P et al: Lysozyme content of tears in patients with Sjögren's syndrome and rheumatoid arthritis. Am J Ophthalmol 87:148, 1979

Bronson L, Fisher T: Sarcoidosis of the paranasal sinuses with orbital extension. Arch Ophthalmol 94:243, 1976

Cook JR, Brubaker RF, Savell J et al: Lacrimal sarcoidosis treated with corticosteroids. Arch Ophthalmol 88:513, 1972

Crick RP, Hoyle C, Smellie H: The eyes in sarcoidosis. Br J Ophthalmol 45:461, 1961

Crystal RG et al: Pulmonary sarcoidosis: A disease characterized and perpetrated by T lymphocytes. Ann Intern Med 94:73, 1981

Daniele RP: Sarcoidosis: Diagnosis and management. Hosp Pract 18:113, 1983

deLuise VP, Tabbara KF: Quantitation of tear lysozyme levels in dry-eye disorders. Arch Ophthalmol 101:634, 1983

Fanburg BC (ed): Sarcoidosis and other granulomatous diseases. New York, Marcel Dekker, 1983

Fisher O et al: Sarcoidosis involving the lacrimal sac. Am Rev Respir Dis 103:708, 1971

Hunninghake GW, Crystal RG: Pulmonary sarcoidosis. A disorder mediated by excess helper T-lymphocyte activity at sites of disease. N Engl J Med 305:429, 1981

James DG: The diagnosis and treatment of ocular sarcoidosis. Acta Med Scand 176 [Suppl] 425:203, 1964

James DG et al: Papilledema in sarcoidosis. Br J Ophthalmol 51:526, 1967

James DG, Neville E, Langley DA: Ocular sarcoidosis. Trans Ophthalmol Soc UK 96:133, 1976

Jampol LM et al: Optic nerve sarcoidosis. Arch Ophthalmol 87:355, 1972

Jensen VJ: Sarcoidosis of the orbit. Acta Ophthalmol [Kbh] 35:416, 1957

Karma A: Ophthalmic changes in sarcoidosis. Acta Ophthalmol [Suppl]:141, 1979

Karma A: Diagnosing sarcoidosis by transconjunctival biopsy of the lacrimal gland. Am J Ophthalmol 98:640, 1984

Karma A, Poukkula A, Ruokonen A: Gallium[67] citrate scanning in patients with lacrimal gland and conjunctival sarcoidosis: A report on three cases. Acta Ophthalmol 62:549, 1984

Katz P et al: Serum angiotensin-converting enzyme and lysozyme in granulomatous diseases of unknown cause. Ann Intern Med 94:359, 1981

Khan F, Wessely Z, Chazin SR et al: Conjunctival biopsy in sarcoidosis. Ann Ophthalmol 9:671, 1977

Lauttman RJ, et al: Biopsy of minor salivary glands in the diagnosis of sarcoidosis. N Engl J Med 301:922, 1979

Lauver JW, Gooneratne NS: Lacrimal, parotid and mediastinal uptake of gallium 67 in sarcoidosis. Br J Radiol 52:582, 1979

Mayock RI et al: Manifestations of sarcoidosis analysis of 145 patients with a review of nine series selected from the literature. Am J Med 35:67, 1963

Melmon K, Goldberg J: Sarcoidosis with bilateral exophthalmos as the presenting symptom. Am J Med 33:158, 1962

Neault R, Riley FC: Report of a case of dacryocystitis secondary to Boeck's sarcoid. Am J Ophthalmol 70:1011, 1970

Nichols CW, Mishkin M, Yanoff M: Presumed orbital sarcoidosis: Report of a case followed by computerized axial tomography and conjunctival biopsy. Trans Am Ophthalmol Soc 76:67, 1978

Nosal A, Schleissner LA, Mishkin FS et al: Angiotensin-1-converting enzyme and gallium scan in noninvasive evaluation of sarcoidosis. Ann Intern Med 90:328, 1979

Nowinski T, Flanagan J, Ruchman M: Lacrimal gland enlargement in familial sarcoidosis. Ophthalmology 90, No. 8:909, 1983

Obenauf CD, Shaw HE, Sydnor CF et al: Sarcoidosis and its ophthalmic manifestations. Am J Ophthalmol 86:648, 1978

Papo I, Beltrami CA, Salvoline U et al: Sarcoidosis simulating a glioma of the optic nerve. Surg Neurol 8:353, 1977

Scadding JG: Sarcoidosis. London, Eyre & Spottiswoode, 1967

Scharf JM, Obdenau N, Meshulam MD et al: Influence of bromhexine on tear lysozyme level in keratoconjunctivitis sicca. Am J Ophthalmol 92:21, 1981

Sharma OP, Bita JB: Determination of angiotensin-converting enzyme activity in tears: A noninvasive test for evaluation of ocular sarcoidosis. Arch Ophthalmol 101:559, 1983

Signorini E, Cianciulli E, Ciorba E et al: Rare multiple orbital localizations of sarcoidosis: A case report. Neuroradiology 26:145, 1984

Siltzbach L: Sarcoidosis: Clinical features and management. Med Clin North Am 51:483, 1967

Siltzbach LE: Sarcoidosis. In Fishman AP (ed): Pulmonary Diseases and Disorders p 889, New York, McGraw-Hill, 1980

Silverstein A et al: Neurologic sarcoidosis. Arch Neurol 12:1, 1965

Tabbara KF, Ostler HB, Daniels TE et al: Sjögren's syndrome: A correlation between ocular findings and labial salivary gland histology. Trans Am Acad Ophthalmol Otolaryngol 78:467, 1974

Thrasher DR, Briggs DD: Pulmonary sarcoidosis. Clin Chest Med 3:537, 1982

Weinreb RN, Barth R, Kimura SJ: Limited gallium scans and angiotensin converting enzyme in granulomatous uveitis. Ophthalmology 87:202, 1980

Weinreb RN, Yavitz EQ, O'Connor GR et al: Lacrimal gland uptake of gallium citrate Ga 67. Am J Ophthalmol 92:16, 1981

Wolk RB: Sarcoidosis of the orbit with bone destruction. AJNR 5:204, 1984

SJÖGREN'S SYNDROME

Adamson TC et al: Immunohistologic analysis of lymphoid infiltrates in primary Sjögren's syndrome using monoclonal antibodies. J Immunol 130:203, 1983

Alarcon-Segovia D, Ibanez G et al: Sjögren's syndrome in progressive systemic sclerosis. Am J Med 57:78, 1974

Bloch KJ, Buchanan WN, Wohl MJ et al: Sjögren's syndrome: A clinical, pathological and serological study of 62 cases. Medicine 44:187, 1965

Chisholm DM, Mason DK: Labial salivary gland biopsy in Sjögren's disease. J Clin Pathol 21:656, 1968

Fauci AS, Moutsopoulos HM: Polyclonally triggered B cells in the peripheral blood and bone marrow of normal individuals and in patients with systemic lupus erythematosus and primary Sjögren's syndrome. Arthritis Rheum 24:577, 1981

Feltkamp TE, vanRossum AL: Antibodies to salivary duct cells and other autoantibodies in patients with Sjögren's syndrome and other idiopathic auto-immune disease. Clin Exp Immunol 3:1, 1968

Heaton JM: Sjögren's syndrome and systemic lupus erythematosus. Br Med J 1:466, 1959

Kaltreider H, Talal N: The neuropathy of Sjögren's syndrome. Ann Intern Med 70:751, 1969

Moutsopoulos HM (moderator) NIH Conference: Sjögren's syndrome (sicca syndrome): Current issues. Ann Intern Med 92 (Part 1):212, 1980

Shearn MA: Sjögren's syndrome. Philadelphia, WB Saunders, 1971

Shearn MA: Sjögren's syndrome. Med Clin N Am 61:2, 1977

Talal N, Bunim JJ: The development of malignant lymphoma in the course of Sjögren's syndrome. Am J Med 36:529, 1964

Talal N, Sokoloff L, Barth W: Extrasalivary lymphoid abnormalities in Sjögren's syndrome (reticulum cell sarcoma, pseudolymphoma, macroglobulinemia). Am J Med 43:50, 1967

Tan EM: Antinuclear antibodies in diagnosis and management. Hosp Pract 18:79, 1983

VASCULITIS

Ammerman SD, Rao MS, Shope TC et al: Diagnostic uncertainty in atypical Kawasaki disease, and a new finding: Exudative conjunctivitis. Pediatr Infect Dis 4:210, 1985

Burns JC, Joffe L, Sargent RA et al: Anterior uveitis associated with Kawasaki syndrome. Pediatr Infect Dis 4, No. 3:258, 1985

Cupps TR, Fauci AS: The Vasculitides. Philadelphia, WB Saunders, 1981

Cupps TR, Fauci AS: The vasculitic syndromes. Adv Intern Med 27:315, 1982

Garrity JA, Kennerdell JS, Johnson BL et al: Cyclophosphamide in the treatment of orbital vasculitis. Am J Ophthalmol 102:97, 1986

Zeek P: Periarteritis nodosa: A critical review. Am J Clin Pathol 22:777, 1952

Zeek P: Periarteritis nodosa and other forms of necrotizing angiitis. N Engl J Med 248:764, 1953

PERIARTERITIS NODOSA

Astrom K, Lidholm S: Extensive intracranial lesions in a case of orbital non-specific granuloma combined with polyarteritis nodosa. J Clin Pathol 16:137, 1963

Boeck J: Ocular changes in periarteritis nodosa. Am J Ophthalmol 42:567, 1956

Cogan DG: Corneoscleral lesions in periarteritis nodosa and Wegener's granulomatosis. Trans Am Ophthalmol Soc 53:321, 1965

Goar EL, Smith LS: Polyarteritis nodosa of the eye. Am J Ophthalmol 35:1619, 1952

Harbert F, McPherson SD, Jr: Scleral necrosis in periarteritis nodosa: A case report. Am J Ophthalmol 30:727, 1947

Harcourt RB: Orbital granulomata associated with widespread angiitis. Br J Ophthalmol 48:673, 1964

Hope-Robertson WJ: Pseudo-tumour of the orbit as a presenting sign in periarteritis nodosa. Trans Ophthalmol Soc NZ 8:56, 1956

Ingalls RG: Bilateral uveitis and keratitis accompanying periarteritis nodosa. Trans Am Acad Ophthalmol Otolaryngol 55:630, 1951

Kielar RA: Exudative retinal detachment and scleritis in polyarteritis. Am J Ophthalmol 82:694, 1976

Rose GA, Spencer H: Polyarteritis nodosa. Q J Med 26:43, 1957

Van Wien S, Merz EH: Exophthalmos secondary to periarteritis nodosa. Am J Ophthalmol 56:204, 1963

Walton EW: Pseudo-tumour of the orbit and polyarteritis nodosa. J Clin Pathol 12:419, 1959

COLLAGEN DISEASE

Brenner E, Shock J: Proptosis secondary to systemic lupus erythematosus. Arch Ophthalmol 91:81, 1974

Gold D, Morris D, Henkind P: Ocular findings in systemic lupus erythematosus. Br J Ophthalmol 56:800, 1972

Hollenhorst R, Henderson J: The ocular manifestations of the diffuse collagen diseases. Am J Med Sci 221:211, 1951

Zimmerman LE, Rogers JB: Idiopathic thrombophlebitis of orbital veins simulating primary tumor of the orbit. Trans Am Acad Ophthalmol Otolaryngol 61:609, 1957

OTHER GRANULOMATOUS AND HISTIOCYTIC LESIONS

Alper MG, Zimmerman LE, LaPiana FG: Orbital manifestations of Erdheim-Chester disease. Trans Am Ophthalmol Soc 81:64, 1983

Bullock JD, Bartley GB, Campbell RJ et al: Necrobiotic xanthogranuloma with paraproteinemia. Ophthalmology 93:1233, 1986

Codere F, Lee RD, Anderson RL: Necrobiotic xanthogranuloma of the eyelid. Arch Ophthalmol 101:60, 1983

Floyd BB, Brown B, Isaacs H et al: Pseudorheumatoid nodule involving the orbit. Arch Ophthalmol 100:1478, 1982

Kossard S, Winkelmann RK: Necrobiotic xanthogranuloma with paraproteinemia. J Am Acad Dermatol 3:257, 1980

Robertson DM, Winkelman RK: Ophthalmic features of necrobiotic xanthogranuloma with paraproteinemia. Am J Ophthalmol 97:173, 1984

Ross MJ, Cohen KL, Peiffer RL et al: Episcleral and orbital pseudorheumatoid nodules. Arch Ophthalmol 101:418, 1983

COGAN'S SYNDROME

Bennett FM: Bilateral recurrent episcleritis associated with posterior corneal changes, vestibulo-auditory symptoms and rheumatoid arthritis. Am J Ophthalmol 55:815, 1963

Cobo LM, Haynes BF: Early corneal findings in Cogan's syndrome. Ophthalmol 91, No. 8:903, 1984

Cogan DG: Syndrome of nonsyphilitic interstitial keratitis and vestibuloauditory symptoms. Arch Ophthalmol 33:144, 1945

Cogan DG: Nonsyphilitic interstitial keratitis with vestibuloauditory symptoms: Report of four additional cases. Arch Ophthalmol 42:42, 1949

Cogan DG, Dickersin GR: Nonsyphilitic interstitial keratitis with vestibuloauditory symptoms: A case with fatal aortitis. Arch Ophthalmol 71:172, 1964

Fisher ER, Hellstrom HR: Cogan's syndrome and systemic vascular disease: Analysis of pathologic features with reference to its relationship to thromboangiitis obliterans (Buerger). Arch Pathol 72:572, 1961

Gilbert WS, Talbot FJ: Cogan's syndrome: Signs of periarteritis nodosa and cerebral venous sinus thrombosis. Arch Ophthalmol 82:633, 1969

Haynes BF, Kaiser-Kupfer MI, Mason P et al: Cogan's syndrome: Studies in thirteen patients, long-term follow-up, and a review of the literature. Medicine 59:426, 1980

Haynes BF, Pikus A, Kaiser-Kupfer M et al: Successful treatment of sudden hearing loss in Cogan's syndrome with corticosteroids. Arthritis Rheum 24:501, 1981

Ingalls RG: Bilateral uveitis and keratitis accompanying periarteritis nodosa. Trans Am Acad Ophthalmol Otolaryngol 55:630, 1951

McGavin DD, McNeill J: Scleritis and perceptive deafness: case report. Ann Ophthalmol 9:1287, 1977

McNeil NF, Berke M, Reingold IM: Polyarteritis nodosa causing deafness in an adult: Report of a case with special reference to concepts about the disease. Ann Intern Med 37:1253, 1952

Norton EWD, Cogan DG: Syndrome of nonsyphilitic interstitial keratitis and vestibuloauditory symptoms: A long-term follow-up report. Arch Ophthalmol 61:695, 1959

Oliner L, Taubenhaus M, Shapira TM et al: Nonsyphilitic interstitial keratitis and bilateral deafness (Cogan's syndrome) associated with essential polyangitis (periarteritis nodosa): Review of the syndrome with consideration of a possible pathogenic mechanism. N Engl J Med 248:1001, 1953

Peitersen E, Carlsen BH: Hearing impairment as the initial sign of polyarteritis nodosa. Acta Otolaryngol 61:189, 1966

WEGENER'S GRANULOMATOSIS

Ashton N, Cook C: Allergic granulomatous nodules of the eyelid and conjunctiva. The 35th Edward Jackson Memorial Lecture. Am J Ophthalmol 87:1, 1979

Austin P, Green WR, Sallyer DC et al: Peripheral corneal degeneration and occlusive vasculitis in Wegener's granulomatosis. Am J Ophthalmol 85:311, 1978

Brady HR, Israel MR, Lewin WH: Wegener's granulomatosis and corneo-scleral ulcer. JAMA 193:248, 1965

Brubaker R, Font RL, Shepherd EM: Granulomatous sclerouveitis: Regression of ocular lesions with cyclophosphamide and prednisone. Arch Ophthalmol 86:517, 1971

Bullen CL, Liesegang TJ, McDonald TJ et al: Ocular complications of Wegener's granulomatosis. Ophthalmology 90: 279, 1983

Carrington CB, Liebow AA: Limited forms of angiitis and granulomatosis of Wegener's type. Am J Med 41:497, 1966

Cassan SM, Coles DT, Harrison EG, Jr: The concept of limited forms of Wegener's granulomatosis. Am J Med 49:366, 1970

Cassan SM, Divertie MB, Hollenhorst RW et al: Pseudotumor of the orbit and limited Wegener's granulomatosis. Ann Intern Med 72:687, 1970

Coutu RE, Klein M, Lessell S et al: Limited form of Wegener's granulomatosis: Eye involvement as a major sign. JAMA 233: 868, 1975

Cutler WM, Blatt IM: The ocular manifestations of lethal midline granuloma (Wegener's granulomatosis). Am J Ophthalmol 42:21, 1956

DeRemee RA, Weiland LH, McDonald TJ: Respiratory vasculitis. Mayo Clin Proc 55:492, 1980

Drachman DA: Neurological components of Wegener's granulomatosis. Arch Neurol 8:145, 1963

Fahey JL, Leonard E, Churg J et al: Wegener's granulomatosis. Am J Med 17:168, 1954

Fauci AS, Haynes B, Katz P: The spectrum of vasculitis: Clinical, pathologic, immunologic, and therapeutic considerations. Ann Intern Med 89:660, 1978

Fauci AS, Haynes BF, Katz P et al: Wegener's granulomatosis: Prospective and therapeutic experience with 85 patients for 21 years. Ann Intern Med 88:76, 1977

Fauci AS, Wolff SM: Wegener's granulomatosis: Studies in eighteen patients and a review of the literature. Medicine 52:535, 1973

Faulds JS, Wear AR: Pseudotumor of the orbit and Wegener's granuloma. Lancet 2:955, 1960

Ferry AP, Leopold IH: Marginal (ring) corneal ulcer as presenting manifestation of Wegener's granuloma: A clinicopathologic study. Trans Am Acad Ophthalmol Otolaryngol 74:1276, 1970

Foster CS: Immunosuppressive therapy for external ocular inflammatory disease. Ophthalmology 87:140, 1980

Godman GC, Churg J: Wegener's granulomatosis: Pathology and review of the literature. Arch Pathol 58:533, 1954

Harcourt RB: Orbital granulomata associated with widespread angiitis. Br J Ophthalmol 48:673, 1964

Haynes BF, Fishman ML, Fauci AS et al: The ocular manifestations of Wegener's granulomatosis: Fifteen years experience and review of the literature. Am J Med 63:131, 1977

Henkind P, Gold DH: Ocular manifestations of rheumatic disorders: natural and iatrogenic. Rheumatology 4:13, 1973

Hoekstra JA, Fauci AS: The granulomatous vasculitides. Clin Rheum Dis 6:373, 1980

Leveille AS, Morse PH: Combined detachments in Wegener's granulomatosis. Br J Ophthalmol 65:564, 1981

Liebow AA: The J. Burns Anderson lecture: Pulmonary angiitis and granulomatosis. Am Rev Respir Dis 108:1, 1973

McDonald JB, Edwards RW: "Wegener's granulomatosis:" a triad. JAMA 173:1205, 1960

McIlvanie SK: Wegener's granulomatosis: Successful treatment with chlorambucil. JAMA 197:90, 1966

Novack SN, Pearson CM: Cyclophosphamide therapy in Wegener's granulomatosis. N Engl J Med 284:938, 1971

Pearson CM, Novack SN: Successful treatment of four cases of Wegener's granulomatosis with cyclophosphamide. Arthritis Rheum 14:408, 1971

Robin JB, Schanzlin DJ, Meisler DM et al: Ocular involvement in the respiratory vasculitides. Surv Ophthalmol 30, No. 2:127, 1985

Sevel D: Necrogranulomatous keratitis associated with Wegener's granulomatosis and rheumatoid arthritis. Am J Ophthalmol 63:250, 1967

Spalton DJ, Graham EM, Page NGR et al: Ocular changes in limited forms of Wegener's granulomatosis. Br J Ophthalmol 65:553, 1981

Straatsma BR: Ocular manifestation of Wegener's granulomatosis. Am J Ophthalmol 44:789, 1957

Thawley SE: Wegener's granulomatosis: Unusual indication for orbital decompression. Laryngoscope 89:145, 1979

Tyner GS: Wegener's granulomatosis: A case report. Am J Ophthalmol 50:1203, 1960

Weiter J, Farkas TG: Pseudotumor of the orbit as a presenting sign in Wegener's granulomatosis. Surv Ophthalmol 17:106, 1972

Wolff SM, Fauci AS, Horn RG et al: Wegener's granulomatosis. Ann Intern Med 81:513, 1974

Zeek PM: Periarteritis nodosa: A critical review. Am J Clin Pathol 22:777, 1952

Zeek PM: Periarteritis nodosa and other forms of necrotizing angiitis. N Engl J Med 248:764, 1953

CHURG-STRAUSS SYNDROME

Chumbley LC, Harrison EG, Jr, DeRemee RA: Allergic granulomatosis and angiitis (Churg-Strauss syndrome): Report and analysis of 30 cases. Mayo Clin Proc 52:477, 1977

Churg J: Allergic granulomatous and granulomatous-vascular syndromes. Ann Allergy 21:619, 1963

Churg J, Strauss L: Allergic granulomatosis, allergic angiitis, and periarteritis nodosa. Am J Pathol 27:277, 1951

Cury D, Breakey AS, Payne BF: Allergic granulomatous angiitis associated with uveoscleritis and papilledema. Arch Ophthalmol 55:261, 1966

Fauci AS: Vasculitis. J Allergy Clin Immunol 72:211, 1983

Hardyt WR, Anderson RE: The hypereosinophilic syndromes. Ann Intern Med 68:1220, 1968

Lanham JG, Eldon KB, Pusey CD et al: Systemic vasculitis with asthma and eosinophilia: A clinical approach to the Churg-Strauss syndrome. Medicine 63:65, 1984

Meisler DM, Stock EL, Wertz RD, et al: Conjunctival inflammation and amyloidosis in allergic granulomatosis and angiitis (Churg-Strauss syndrome). Am J Ophthalmol 91:216, 1981

Nissim F, Von der Valde J, Czernobilsky B: A limited form of Churg-Strauss syndrome: Ocular and cutaneous manifestations. Arch Pathol Lab Med 106:305, 1982

Sokolov RA, Rachmaninoff N, Kaine HD: Allergic granulomatosis. Am J Med 32:131, 1962

Strauss L, Churg J, Zak FG: Cutaneous lesions of allergic granulomatosis: A histopathologic study. J Invest Dermatol 17:349, 1951

Wilson KS, Alexander HL: The relation of periarteritis nodosa to bronchial asthma and other forms of human hypersensitiveness. J Lab Clin Med 30:195, 1945

LYMPHOMATOID GRANULOMATOSIS

DeRemee RA, Weiland LH, McDonald TJ: Polymorphic reticulosis, lymphomatoid granulomatosis. Two diseases or one? Mayo Clin Proc 53:634, 1978

Eichel BS, Harrison EG, Jr, Devine KD et al: Primary lymphoma of the nose including a relationship to lethal midline granuloma. Am J Surg 112:597, 1966

Fauci AS, Haynes BF, Costa J et al: Lymphomatoid granulomatosis. Prospective clinical and therapeutic experience over 10 years. N Engl J Med 306:68, 1982

Katzenstein AA, Carrington CB, Liebow AA: Lymphomatoid granulomatosis: A clinicopathologic study of 152 cases. Cancer 43:360, 1979

Liebow AA, Carrington CRB, Friedman PJ: Lymphomatoid granulomatosis. Hum Pathol 3:457, 1972

Nichols PW, Koss M, Levine AM et al: Lymphomatoid granulomatosis: A T-cell disorder? Am J Med 72:467, 1982

Waldron JA, Leech JH, Glick AD et al: Malignant lymphoma of peripheral T-lymphocyte origin: Immunologic, pathologic and clinical features in six patients. Cancer 40:1604, 1977

TEMPORAL ARTERITIS

Andrews JM: Giant cell (temporal) arteritis. Neurology 16:963, 1966

Chisholm J: Cortical blindness in cranial arteritis. Br J Ophthalmol 59:332, 1975

Cohen D: Temporal arteritis: An improvement in visual prognosis and management with repeat biopsies. Trans Am Acad Ophthalmol Otolaryngol 77:74, 1973

Davis R, Daroff R, Hoyt WF: Tonic pupil after temporal arteritis. Lancet 1:822, 1968

Fessel WJ, Pearson CM: Polymyalgia rheumatica and blindness. N Engl J Med 276:1403, 1967

Johnston AC: Giant cell arteritis: Ophthalmic and systemic considerations. Can J Ophthalmol 8:38, 1973

Ostberg G: Temporal arteritis in a large necropsy series. Ann Rheum Dis 30:224, 1971

Reinecke RD, Kuwabara T: Temporal arteritis. Arch Ophthalmol 82:446, 1969

Rootman J, Butler D: Ischaemic optic neuropathy: A combined mechanism. Br J Ophthalmol 64:826, 1980

Simmons RJ, Cogan DG: Occult temporal arteritis. Arch Ophthalmol 68:8, 1962

CHAPTER 10

Lymphoproliferative and Leukemic Lesions

Jack Rootman, William Robertson,
Jocelyn S. Lapointe, and Valerie White

No other area of orbital disease has undergone such profound redefinition as the lymphoproliferative lesions of the orbit. The primary impetus for this development has been the advent of increasingly more sophisticated and specific immunodiagnostic techniques in tissue pathology. In general, this has led to the recognition that lymphomas represent neoplasia derived from the immune system, and has resulted in a variety of classifications of lymphoid tumors. More recently, attempts have been made by an international group of pathologists to correlate these diverse classifications. Immunohistochemistry can identify B-cell, T-cell, and accessory cell origin, leading to more accurate diagnosis. Increasingly sensitive methods using DNA hybridization techniques promise improved sensitivity and suggest that even small populations of neoplastic cells may provide the drive for apparently polyclonal disorders.

For clinicians who are on the front line encountering patients with lymphoproliferative disorders, the new technological advances and classifications may seem somewhat intimidating. Yet in the practical clinical situation, diseases in this category tend to develop along relatively well-defined lines that allow for ease of categorization and management.

Some confusion in this area has resulted from the historical tendency to include a wide range of different disorders. Orbital lymphoproliferative lesions are generally uncommon, so it is difficult for both clinicians and pathologists to develop familiarity with the clinical presentation, pathologic interpretation, and subsequent course. Not only is the profusion of pathologic terminology confusing—pseudotumor, pseudolymphoma, sclerosing pseudotumor, inflammatory pseudotumor, atypical hyperplasia—but different authors have different definitions for the same term. Analogous problems exist in other mucosa-related extranodal sites, including the lung, salivary gland, thyroid, and gastrointestinal tract, where lymphoid infiltrates are difficult to evaluate. The histopathology is confusing, because most lymphomas of the orbit and conjunctiva are composed of small lympho-

cytes and thus can appear relatively benign. In addition, other inflammatory cells may be present, such as plasma cells, plasmacytoid lymphocytes, and histiocytes. It has been recognized that lesions labelled as benign reactive hyperplasia, atypical lymphoid hyperplasia, or malignant lymphoma may recur locally or the patients may develop disease in other sites, often with a somewhat similar frequency. Moreover, patients with lesions in all histologic categories may remain disease-free for many years and respond to minimal or local treatment, or may be simply observed and followed on a regular basis.

In spite of all of these problems, when such diseases do affect the orbit, they can usually be divided into three main categories: idiopathic inflammations, lymphoproliferative disorders (reactive and atypical), and frank lymphoma. We have discussed the idiopathic inflammatory diseases of the orbit in Chapter 9, and have divided them along pathophysiologic lines into acute, subacute, and chronic inflammations. The histopathology of these lesions parallels the clinical course and the disorders are generally responsive to corticosteroids. Histopathologically, they are distinguished on the basis of the predominant features that are clearly inflammatory, such as polymorphic infiltrate, fibrosis, or granulomatous inflammation. This approach to the separation of extranodal lymphomas from so-called "pseudotumors" has recently been emphasized by Colby and Carrington in a review of lymphocytic infiltrates of the lung and other extranodal sites.

In contrast to inflammatory disease, lymphoproliferative disorders represent a group with the basic unifying histopathologic feature being a densely cellular infiltrate consisting mostly of small lymphocytes. The lymphoproliferative disorders include benign, atypical, and lymphomatous lesions of the non-Hodgkin's variety. Some authors classify this spectrum even more broadly on the basis of histology into definitely malignant, apparently malignant, equivocal, apparently benign, and definitely benign. The apparently malignant category parallels the atypical lymphoproliferative lesions. The non-Hodgkin's lymphomas of the orbit tend to be in the low to intermediate grade categories.

The remaining group of lesions to be discussed include plasma cell tumors, Hodgkin's disease, and rarer entities including Burkitt's tumor. The other lymphoproliferative, hematopoietic, and histiocytic disorders that can affect the orbit include the chronic and acute leukemias, lymphoid tumors with primary macroglobulinemia, multiple myeloma, and some histiocytic and T-cell tumors.

■ BASIC CELLULAR CONCEPTS

Jack Rootman and Peter Dolman

Lymphocytes and macrophages are the principal players in the complex defense strategy of the immune system (Table 10-1). Lymphoid precursors arising in the fetal liver and later in adult bones migrate either to bursa-equivalent tissue (intestinal Peyer's patches) or to the thymus, where they differentiate into B and T lymphocytes, respectively. These virgin B and T cells circulate through the blood and seed the peripheral lymphoid tissue, including the spleen and lymph nodes. Macrophages and histiocytes of the mononuclear phagocytic (reticuloendothelial) system arise from blood monocytes derived from committed stem cells in the bone marrow.

B lymphocytes populate the white pulp of the spleen, follicles of lymph node cortex, and lymphoid tissue in skin, digestive tract, lungs, and bone, and account for 20% to 30% of lymphocytes present in the peripheral blood. After differentiation in bursa-equivalent tissue, virgin B cells express membrane-bound surface immunoglobulins and surface receptors for the Fc portion of IgG and for the third component of complement (C3b). The surface Ig is usually of the M or D class, which is determined by the heavy-chain polypeptide component of the immunoglobulin. When challenged by a foreign antigen (a complex process requiring the aid of macrophages and

TABLE 10-1.
CELLS OF THE IMMUNE RESPONSE

Ontogeny

Characteristics

Cell Type	B Cell	T Cell	Monocyte/Macrophage
Production site	Bursa-equivalent (bone marrow)	Thymus	Bone marrow histiocyte
	Per. lymphoid tissue	Per. lymphoid tissue	Per. tissues (histiocyte/macros)
Distribution of mature cells	Per. lymphoid Spleen Lymph node Skin, resp, GI	Per. lymphoid Spleen Lymph node Skin, resp, GI	Per. tissues Skin: histiocytes LN: tingible body Numerous other organs
Form in blood	B cell (20%)	T cell (80%)	Monocyte
Progeny cells	Plasma cell	T_{helper} $T_{suppressor}$ T_{killer}	Tissue specific histiocyte, Kuppfer tingible body, etc.
Function	Humoral immunity	Cellular immunity Immune regulator	Phagocytosis Immune effector, mediator
Surface markers	Surface Ig F_c receptor C_{3b} receptor	Sheep RBC receptor	F_c receptor C_{3b} receptor

Per. = peripheral; LN = lymph node

T lymphocytes) the B cell with surface immunoglobulin specific for that antigen undergoes blastic transformation. In lymph nodes this process occurs in the follicular centers, with intermediate follicular center cells undergoing a process of transformation from small and large cleaved to small and large noncleaved cells, which ultimately yield large cells with prominent nucleoli. During this process, the surface immunoglobulins are internalized and the cells develop the cytoplasmic apparatus necessary for immunoglobulin production. Immunoblasts differentiate into a population of memory B cells primed for subsequent challenge by the same antigen and into plasma cells, which secrete first IgM and later IgG and IgA of specificity identical to the progenitor B lymphocyte surface immunoglobulin.

T lymphocytes, morphologically identical to unchallenged B lymphocytes, are found in the perifollicular regions of lymph nodes, in the periarteriolar sheath of the spleen, and in other lymphoid tissue of the body, and account for 70% to 80% of lymphocytes circulating in the peripheral blood. Unlike B cells, T cells are long-lived. They can be identified and subclassified by surface differentiation antigens and by their ability to form rosettes with sheep red blood cells. They carry out cell-mediated immune responses (tumor and graft rejection, and delayed-type hypersensitivity) and regulate the humoral B-cell immune response.

Histiocytes and macrophages are widely distributed throughout peripheral lymphoid tissue and in blood (as monocytes). Their membranes contain two marker receptors for activated C3 and for the Fc portion of IgG. Apart from their important phagocytic function, they act as both inducers and effectors for both the humoral and cellular immune response.

Increasingly sophisticated cytochemical and immunologic methods are available for the identification of various cell types. These methods are becoming more specific and allow for characterization of lymphoproliferative, leukemic, and histiocytic lesions. The various common cytochemical and immunologic methods are outlined in Tables 10-2 and 10-3.

Lymphoproliferative diseases of the orbit and elsewhere probably represent disorders of immune regulation with abnormal proliferations of the immune cells and their progeny. Neoplastic transformation may result in blockade and replication at any stage along the differentiation pathway of B cell to plasma cell (resulting in B-cell lymphomas, immunoblastic lymphomas, multiple myeloma, solitary plasmacytoma, or Waldenstrom's macroglobulinemia), of T cells (resulting in T-cell lymphomas or immunoblastic lymphomas), or of histiocytes (resulting in rare true histiocytic lymphomas).

■ CLINICAL SPECTRUM

In spite of the diversity of these lesions, it has been our experience that four clinical syndromes can be recognized. The clinical syndromes and common disease processes included in these syndromes are summarized in Table 10-4 and illustrated in Figure 10-1. The most common syndrome (type 1) is characterized by insidious development of painless orbital masses (frequently anterior), which lead to little if any functional interference. This group is the dominant and collectively the largest in this category of diseases and is mainly made up of low-grade lymphoproliferative disorders (benign, atypical, and malignant). The major differential diagnosis relates to the insidious development of painless orbital masses with little functional interference. This differential diagnosis includes many well-differentiated and encapsulated tumors, as well as numerous noninfiltrative disorders in-

TABLE 10-2.
CELL IDENTIFICATION BY CYTOCHEMICAL METHODS

Cytochemical Reaction	Cell Types
Nonspecific esterase	Histiocytes, monocytes, megakaryocytes
Muramidase	Monocytes, histiocytes
Chloroacetate esterase	Neutrophils, promyelocytes, myeloblasts, mast cells
Peroxidase	Neutrophils, eosinophils, promyelocytes, myeloblasts, monocytes
Sudan black B	Neutrophils, promyelocytes, myeloblasts, monocytes
Methyl green-pyronine	Plasma cells, immunoblasts
Periodic acid-Schiff with diastase digestion	Plasma cells, immunoblasts
α-naphtyl acetate esterase	T lymphocytes
Terminal deoxynucleotidyl transferase	T lymphocytes
Tartrate-resistant acid phosphatase	Hairy cells

(Ioachim HL: Lymph Node Biopsy, p. 19. Philadelphia, JB Lippincott, 1982)

TABLE 10-3.
CELL IDENTIFICATION BY IMMUNOLOGIC METHODS

Immunologic Markers	Cell Types
Surface immunoglobulins	B lymphocytes
Polyclonal	Benign proliferations
Monoclonal	Malignant proliferations
Cytoplasmic immunoglobulins	Plasma cells, immunoblasts
Polyclonal	Benign proliferations
Monoclonal	Malignant proliferations
Receptor for sheep erythrocyte	T lymphocytes
E rosettes	
Receptor for complement (C3)	B lymphocytes
EAC rosettes (erythrocytes — IgM — complement)	
Receptor for Fc fragment	Monocytes, histiocytes
EA rosettes (erythrocytes — IgG)	
T-lymphocyte antigen	T lymphocytes
Anti T-lymphocyte heterologous antisera	

(Ioachim HL: Lymph Node Biopsy, p. 22. Philadelphia, JB Lippincott, 1982)

cluding other lymphoproliferations, localized granulomatous inflammation, isolated circumscribed tumors (such as neurofibroma, schwannoma, hemangioma, and hemangiopericytoma), ectopias, and cysts (dermoid, lacrimal, and mucoceles).

The type 2 group is characterized by a more fulminant (usually weeks to months) onset of orbital mass and infiltrative effect. This includes for the most part patients with lymphoproliferative or leukemic disorders, either in a late accelerated phase or of a more aggressive variety, such as poorly differentiated lymphomas, the acute leukemias, and rare histiocytic malignancies. In addition to these primary infiltrations, this patient population is prone to secondary infectious disorders due to immunoregulatory dysfunction related to their underlying disease or to treatment. This group includes the differential diagnosis of presumed inflammations of the orbit in an immunocompromised host. The most likely pathogen in this setting is bacterial, but the possibility of fungal infection must be considered. The distinction between pro-

TABLE 10-4.
COMMON OR TYPICAL CLINICAL SPECTRUM OF LYMPHOPROLIFERATIVE AND LEUKEMIC LESIONS OF THE ORBIT

Clinical Syndrome	Diseases
Type 1: Orbital mass	Lymphomas — B cell
	Atypical lymphoproliferations
	Reactive lymphoproliferations
	Soft tissue plasmacytomas
Type 2: Fulminant orbital infiltration	Leukemia (especially acute lymphoblastic or accelerated phases of hematopoietic malignancies)
	Secondary infection (immunocompromised host)
	Late Hodgkin's lymphoma
	Malignant histiocytosis
Type 3: Secondary orbital infiltration	
From bone	Plasma cell tumors
	Histiocytosis X
	Burkitt's lymphoma
	Myeloid leukemia
From skin	T-cell lymphomas
Type 4: Neuro-ophthalmic	Late disseminated leukemia
	Late disseminated lymphoma
	Histiocytic malignancies
	Late myeloma
	Late Burkitt's lymphoma

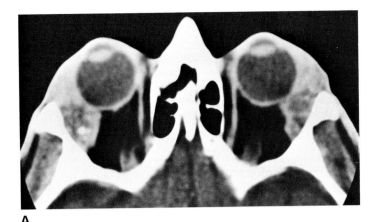

A

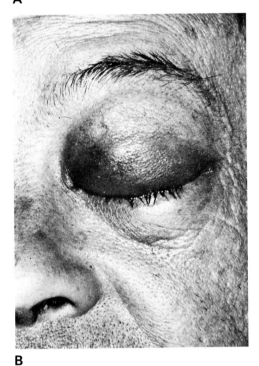

B

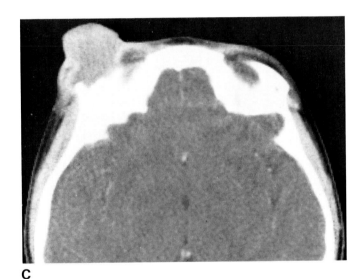

C

FIGURE 10-1. *(A)* Type 1 lymphoproliferative disease is demonstrated in this midorbit CT scan of bilateral orbital masses due to low-grade lymphoma of the lacrimal glands. The lesions are well defined, extraconal in location, and relatively symmetrical. They mold to the lateral margins of the globe and to the bony orbit. Punctate calcification, a rare finding, is present in the posterior portion of the right lesion. *(B)* Clinical photograph of a patient who developed a rapidly infiltrating lesion of the left orbit during a relapse of a poorly differentiated lymphocytic lymphoma. This demonstrates a type 2 clinical presentation of fulminant orbital infiltration due to lymphoma. It was responsive to reinstitution of systemic chemotherapy. *(C)* A CT scan through the superior orbit of a patient with type 3 clinical presentation (secondary orbital infiltration) demonstrates lid invasion from histiocytosis X arising in the underlying bone. *(D)* Midorbit CT scan demonstrates a subtle, soft tissue mass in the left anterior lateral extraconal space and left cavernous sinus expansion; the latter involvement represents a neuroophthalmic complication of a lymphoproliferative lesion (type 4 presentation). Clinically, the patient presented with associated cranial nerve palsies.

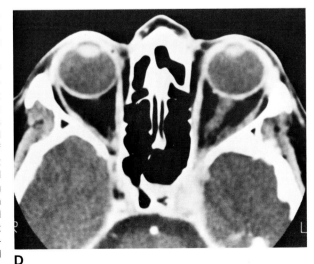

D

gression of disease and infection can be quite difficult, particularly when the patient is immunocompromised because of B-cell dysfunction.

The type 3 group includes patients who develop orbital manifestations of disease secondary to involvement of adjacent structures. The temporal nature and character of progression reflects the diversity of the underlying lesions. For the most part, these lesions represent tumors that have a propensity to involve bone, such as multiple myeloma or Burkitt's lymphoma, but may also arise from adjacent paranasal sinuses or skin. The secondary orbital infiltrations represent the problem of rapid onset of periorbital or orbital masses with bone destruction. Although multiple myeloma is well known to involve bone, other lesions to consider would include metastatic carcinoma (particularly derived from thyroid, kidney, prostate, lung, and breast), large arteriovenous malformation or fistula, aneurysmal bone cyst, or lytic meningioma.

The fourth clinical syndrome (type 4) is seen in patients who present with neuro-ophthalmic complications of either lymphoproliferative or leukemic disorders. By definition, this category includes end-stage lymphomas and leukemias that have invaded the central nervous system or the ocular structures, or both. Because of the increasing survival of patients with lymphomas and leukemias and the relative pharmacologic isolation of the central nervous system, ocular and neuro-ophthalmic complications are not infrequent.

The above clinical classification includes a wide variety of lymphoproliferative and hematopoietic lesions, all of which may produce signs and symptoms characteristic of any of the four syndromes outlined. The remainder of this chapter will address each of the disorders by dividing them along histopathologic lines into lymphocytic lesions, plasma cell tumors, and miscellaneous lymphoproliferative and leukemic lesions of the orbit.

■ LYMPHOCYTIC TUMORS

As stated earlier, the category of lymphocytic tumors includes purely lymphoproliferative rather than inflammatory disorders on the basis of clinical presentation, histopathology, evidence of systemic involvement, and prognosis. Clinically, the orbital manifestations of these disorders are strikingly similar and are characterized by an insidious onset of mass effect, typically in the anterior orbit. These lesions form a spectrum of diseases from benign through dysplastic to frankly malignant, as seen in similar lesions elsewhere in the body. For example, in squamous carcinoma of the lung there is considerable evidence for the evolution of a neoplastic process affecting the whole bronchial epithelium with varying stages of transformation potentially occurring in different sites or at different times in the same patient. Applying this con-

cept to orbital lymphocytic infiltrations makes them more comprehensible and helps to rationalize clinicians' experience with this spectrum of disorders. The fundamental pathophysiology may differ insofar as these lesions represent abnormalities of an immunoregulatory nature, but the concept of a benign, dysplastic, and malignant spectrum applies.

In many respects, the lymphoproliferative disorders of the orbit parallel the same kinds of lesions that are seen in extranodal and extramedullary sites. In addition, the pathogenesis may bear some identifiable relationship, because these extranodal sites are characterized by similar histopathology, course of disease, and prognosis. These lesions appear to be mucosally related or in sites of chronic antigenic stimulation. In addition, all of these sites are known to be affected by related disorders that may have an organ-specific autoimmune basis (abnormal immunoregulatory process) and are the site of diseases that may undergo systematization of either a polyclonal or monoclonal nature.

Reactive Lymphoid Hyperplasia

The truly benign disorders appear to have the hallmarks of reactive, non-neoplastic changes. These include such findings as lymphoid follicles, polyclonality, polymorphous infiltration, vascular hyalinization, hemosiderin deposition, and endothelial proliferation. Reactive lymphoid hyperplasias may display follicular organization with true germinal centers showing mitotic activity and tingible body macrophages. On the other hand, they may comprise a dense cellular infiltrate of mature lymphocytes along with a polymorphous population of plasma cells or histiocytes, or both, without a reactive stroma. The nature of these lesions can be clearly defined with immunologic tests, in which case they display polyclonality.

Clinically, these patients usually have an indolent course and the lesions appear as firm to rubbery, slightly nodular anterior orbital infiltrations (more rarely occurring in the posterior orbit). Not infrequently, there may be a subconjunctival component that has a fleshy appearance. If primarily conjunctival, without any orbital component, these lesions tend to be smaller, fleshy, and multinodular. They are usually painless and do not lead to any functional deficit. On CT scan, these lesions tend to mimic the appearance of atypical lymphoid hyperplasia and lymphomas of the orbit. However, it is our impression that these lesions may show slightly more infiltrative margins without the smooth nodularity of the lymphomas.

Patients with reactive lymphoid hyperplasia may not necessarily have isolated orbital disease. We have seen two patients with all the hallmarks of a polyclonal "reac-

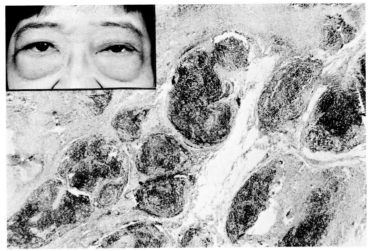

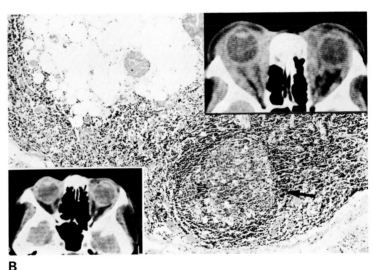

FIGURE 10-2. *(A, inset)* Clinical photograph of a 46-year-old woman with bilateral nodularity and thickening of her lids, which had been slowly developing for 16 years. She also had a history of a lesion of the right buttock and glandular enlargement of the iliac and lower paravertebral lymph nodes, diagnosed 17 years earlier as Hodgkin's disease. Retrospective review at this presentation led to a diagnosis of lymphoplasmacytosis within a hyperplastic lymph node. Histology of the orbital lesion shows a low-power view of reactive lymphoid hyperplasia with large collections of lymphocytes invading orbital tissue (H&E, original magnification × 2.5). *(B)* Higher power view of a reactive lymphoid follicle *(arrow)* (H&E, original magnification × 10). Immunopathology was polyclonal. *(Top inset)* CT scan demonstrates diffuse bilateral extraconal and intraconal orbital infiltration. *(Bottom inset)* CT scan after steroid treatment shows marked reduction of the bilateral orbital lesions. This case is an example of a reactive multisystem polyclonal disease. (Rootman J, Patel S, Jewell L: Polyclonal orbital and systemic infiltrates. Ophthalmology 91:1112, 1984)

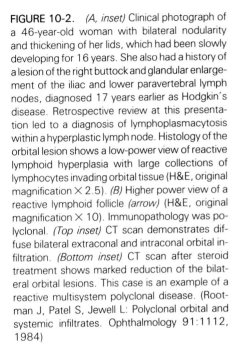

tive lesion" who have either presented with or developed multisystem polyclonal involvement (Fig. 10-2). The phenomenon is not unusual, because histologically similar lesions occurring in other tissues, such as the salivary gland, the gastrointestinal tract, and respiratory tract, have been noted to develop similar disorders that were truly polyclonal and disseminated. Indeed, a small percentage of benign lymphoreticular disorders may be capable of malignant transformation with time.

Therapeutically, two patterns of response are encountered. Many patients appear to be steroid sensitive, and have in our clinic responded to medium- to moderate-dose prednisone therapy (Fig. 10-3). On the other hand, those patients who fail to respond have widespread involvement, or achieve incomplete remission can usually be treated with good results either by the addition of a cytotoxic agent (*e.g.*, chlorambucil) or with local, relatively low-dose radiotherapy (2000 rad).

Atypical Lymphoid Hyperplasia (Dysplastic Category)

There has been a tendency to label lesions in the dysplastic category as localized with prognostic implications distinct from those in the clearly malignant category. Yet if one looks at histologically similar lesions in other organs,

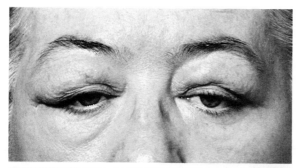
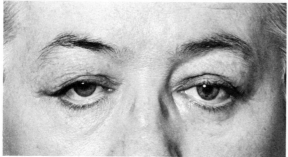

FIGURE 10-3. Upper photograph demonstrates bilateral diffuse swelling and nodular tumefaction of the lids. The patient had an 8-year history of progressive lid involvement, but retained normal tear secretion. Biopsy showed a reactive lymphoproliferative disease. Lower photograph of the same patient after 1 week of corticosteroid therapy (40 mg/day prednisone) demonstrates dramatic resolution. (Rootman J, Patel S, Jewell L: Polyclonal orbital and systemic infiltrates. Ophthalmology 91:1112, 1984)

Lymphomas

CLASSIFICATION

The understanding of non-Hodgkin's lymphoma has changed considerably over the last decade, and many different authors have attempted to develop classifications that would provide clear-cut clinical guidelines. The diversity of these classification schemes has led to a great degree of confusion as well as difficulty correlating results from various treatment centers. A recent comparative study of the various classifications has led to the development of a working formulation of the non-Hodgkin's lymphomas. This formulation constitutes in essence a composite of the various systems and allows cross-referencing from one classification to another. However, no matter what system is used, prognostically, non-Hodgkin's lymphomas are either low-grade, intermediate-grade, or high-grade lesions. Several classifications are outlined in Table 10-5.

CLINICAL FEATURES

Clinically, lymphomas form the largest group of lymphoproliferative disorders seen in the orbit. The onset is characteristically in the sixth and seventh decades of life; lymphomas occur rarely in children. Histologically, the orbital lymphomas are low to intermediate in grade with a predominance of the low-grade disorders. They usually occur in the anterior orbit and may be associated with pink, fleshy subconjunctival tumefaction, which tends to mold to the shape of the globe (Fig. 10-5). When there is no visible subconjunctival component, these lesions tend to be palpably nodular with relatively well-defined margins, and have a slightly friable texture at the time of surgery. They may have a rich, fine vascularity and can usually be encompassed surgically. However, nodular infiltrative edges may be noted intraoperatively.

On CT scan these lesions are usually fairly well defined and tend to mold to or encompass adjacent ocular and orbital structures (Fig. 10-6). They usually involve the anterior, superior, and lateral orbit and almost always have an extraconal component; an associated intraconal component may be seen, but rarely occurs alone. Lacrimal gland involvement is common and may be the only site of tumefaction (Figs. 10-7 and 10-8). The lesions are well defined, commonly with a lobulated or nodular edge, and are homogeneous in texture. They almost universally involve the orbital soft tissues, but rarely can be seen within an extraocular muscle (Fig. 10-9). They are isodense to the extraocular muscles both on noncontrast and contrast scans. Globe displacement, usually in an inferomedial direction, and mild proptosis may be seen.

such as the salivary gland, the gastrointestinal tract, or respiratory tract, it becomes apparent that dysplastic lesions represent a spectrum of disorders and can be part of a widespread lymphoreticular process. From a clinical point of view, these lesions tend to be resistant to corticosteroids, and treatments traditionally used in malignant disorders may be required. Half of our patients in this category showed evidence to support the concept of a spectrum of lymphoproliferative disorders. This included bilateral involvement and chronicity in one third, disseminated disease in another third, and evidence for either transformation or the development of a frankly malignant cell population in the remaining third.

In practical terms, patients with atypical hyperplasia differ very little in presentation and clinical course from patients with the low-grade lymphomas of the orbit (Fig. 10-4). Jakobiec and co-workers have suggested that the atypical polyclonal lesions and the well-differentiated group of monoclonal lesions both have an approximately 15% incidence of extraorbital manifestations. Also, lymphoproliferative diseases are not uncommonly seen in association with certain systemic disorders characterized by disturbed immunoregulation.

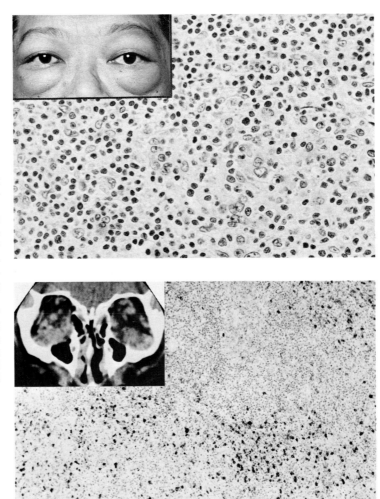

FIGURE 10-4. *(Top)* Clinical photograph *(inset)* of 50-year-old man with bilateral superior and inferior orbital masses, which had been present and progressive over an 8-year period. High-power view of the lesion demonstrates atypical lymphoid hyperplasia with mixtures of lymphoid and other inflammatory cells (H&E, original magnification × 40). *(Bottom)* Coronal CT scan *(inset)* of the patient demonstrates bilateral, predominantly inferior, infiltrating orbital lesions. Immunopathology was positive for cytoplasmic staining of lambda light chains in reactive plasma cells. Staining for kappa light chains showed a similar pattern. Note that not all cells are stained (peroxidase–antiperoxidase method; Mayer's hematoxylin counterstain, original magnification × 10). The patient developed atypical lymphoid hyperplasia of the cervical nodes 1 year after lid biopsy.

Orbital bony involvement and distortion of the globe are rare (Fig. 10-10). Roughly 75% of these lesions are unilateral and 25% bilateral. These findings are quite characteristic of the orbital lymphomas.

In our series of 37 lymphomas, 60% presented as localized lesions. The remaining 40% either had antecedent or concurrent evidence of involvement of other sites (Fig. 10-11). About 15% of patients with localized disease subsequently developed dissemination. All lesions of this type proved to be monoclonal B-cell proliferations. On the other hand, the less well-differentiated groups may show extraorbital manifestations in up to 50% of cases. Overall, the monoclonal B-cell extranodal lymphocytic lymphomas follow a relatively indolent clinical course associated with long-term survival, even with minimal therapeutic intervention. As stated earlier, underlying systemic disorders are not uncommon in patients with lymphoid lesions of the ocular adnexa and include chronic lymphocytic leukemia, Sjögren's syndrome, Waldenström's macroglobulinemia, collagen vascular disease, and various neoplasias.

Successful treatment of these patients rests upon obtaining an adequate orbital biopsy for histologic assessment, a proper staging workup, and a treatment strategy based upon the extent of involvement. The overall management of patients with lymphoproliferative disorders, especially lymphomas, is best provided by a multidisciplinary team with special interest in lymphomas. Those lesions that are localized to the orbit can be treated with orbital radiotherapy or observed until more widespread disease develops and requires intervention (Fig. 10-12). There is evidence to suggest that observation alone for

TABLE 10-5.
NON-HODGKIN'S LYMPHOMA CLASSIFICATIONS

Working Formulation of Non-Hodgkin's Lymphomas	Rappaport	Lennert	Lukes-Collins
Low Grade			
ML, small lymphocytic	Well-differentiated	ML, lymphocytic	Small lymphocyte (B or T cell)
Consistent with CLL	lymphocytic	CLL	
Plasmacytoid		LP, immunocytoma	Plasmacytoid lymphocytic (B cell)
ML, follicular			
Predominantly small cleaved cell	Nodular, poorly differentiated lymphocytic		
Diffuse areas		ML, centroblastic-centrocytic, follicular, with or without diffuse	Small cleaved FCC, follicular (B cell)
Sclerosis			
ML, follicular			
Mixed small cleaved and large cell	Nodular, mixed		
Intermediate Grade			
ML, follicular			Large cleaved FCC, follicular
Predominantly large cell	Nodular, histiocytic	ML, centroblastic-centrocytic, follicular, with or without diffuse	Large noncleaved FCC, follicular
Diffuse areas			
Sclerosis			
ML, diffuse			
Small cleaved cell	Diffuse, poorly differentiated lymphocytic	ML, centrocytic, small	Diffuse small cleaved FCC
Sclerosis			With sclerosis
ML, diffuse			
Mixed, small and large cell	Diffuse, mixed	ML, centroblastic-centrocytic, diffuse	
Sclerosis		(?)	Lymphoepithelioid cell
Epithelioid cell component			
ML, diffuse, large cell	Diffuse, histiocytic		
Cleaved cell		ML, centrocytic, large	Large cleaved FCC, diffuse
Noncleaved cell		ML, centroblastic	Large noncleaved FCC, diffuse
Sclerosis			
High Grade			
ML, large cell, immunoblastic	Diffuse, histiocytic	ML, immunoblastic (most cases)	Immunoblastic sarcoma
Plasmacytoid		T-zone lymphoma (some cases)	B-cell type
Clear cell			T-cell type
Polymorphous			
Epithelioid cell component			Lymphoepithelioid cell (T cell)
ML, lymphoblastic	Lymphoblastic		
Convoluted cell		ML, lymphoblastic, convoluted-cell type	Convoluted T cell
Nonconvoluted cell		ML, lymphoblastic, unclassified	
ML, small noncleaved cell	Diffuse, undifferentiated		Small noncleaved FCC, diffuse (B cell)
Burkitt's		ML, lymphoblastic, Burkitt type	Burkitt's variant (B cell)
Follicular areas			
Miscellaneous			
Composite			
Mycosis fungoides		Mycosis fungoides	Cerebriform, T cells
Histiocytic			Histiocytic (genuine)
Extramedullary plasmacytoma			
Unclassifiable			
Other			

ML = malignant lymphoma; CLL = chronic lymphocytic leukemia; LP = lymphoplasmacytoid; FCC = follicular center cell.
(Ioachim HL: Lymph Node Biopsy, p 210. Philadelphia, JB Lippincott, 1982)

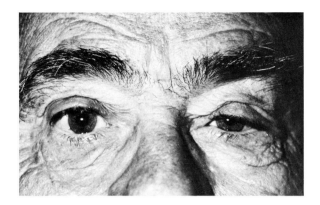

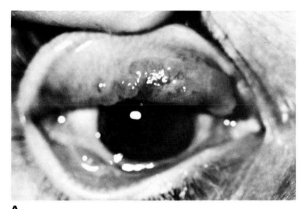
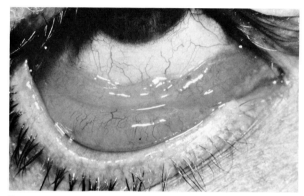

A   **B**

FIGURE 10-5. *(A)* This 73-year-old man first presented with a 1-year history of progressive left ptosis. In addition, he noted difficulty breathing due to lesions in the nasal passage. He was diagnosed and treated with systemic chemotherapy and nasopharyngeal radiotherapy for a diffuse lymphocytic lymphoma with bone marrow involvement. One year later he presented with 4 mm of inward displacement of the left globe and restricted upgaze associated with a superotemporal mass in the region of the lacrimal gland *(top)*. He had multiple salmon-pink sessile telangiectatic lesions of the conjunctiva *(bottom)*. *(B)* The large, confluent, salmon colored fleshy plaque in the inferior fornix is typical of a subconjunctival extension of lymphoma.

low-grade lymphomas does not alter the prognosis or affect institution of later treatment. Other patients are treated on the basis of age, overall systemic tumor load, and histological grade of the tumor. Generally speaking, the less well-differentiated tumors are treated with systemic chemotherapy or low-dose (1500 to 2500 rad) radiotherapy, or both. Overall, prognosis is excellent for these patients and any decision to give specific treatment should be weighed against the associated morbidity.

Summary

Patients with lymphoproliferative disease of the orbit typically present in the later stages of life with features of insidious onset, chronicity, or mass effect. Even when the lesions appear histologically nonmalignant (polyclonal),

they should be regarded as potentially multisystem disorders that may undergo transition to frank malignancy. Furthermore, lesions of this type are not uncommonly associated with underlying systemic disorders related to disturbed immunoregulation. Thus, management requires careful primary and prospective follow up for local spread and systemic involvement. Those lesions that are truly localized (whether polyclonal or well differentiated and monoclonal) can usually be observed, if no functional deficit occurs. If the lesions are bulky and clearly reactive histologically, they may respond to corticosteroid treatment. When atypical or low-grade localized lymphoma is large or associated with functional deficit, these lesions can be treated with local modalities, such as low-dose irradiation or resection. Patients who have orbital involvement as part of their systemic disease should be treated by an oncologist.

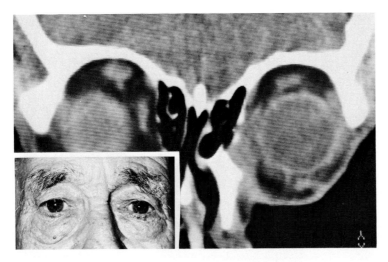

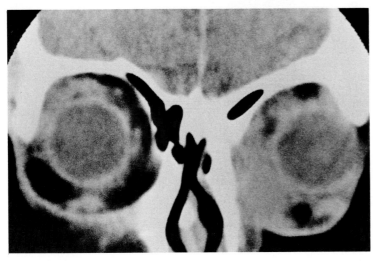

FIGURE 10-6. This 82-year-old man had a 1-year history of left ocular problems. Clinical examination revealed 1 mm lateral and 2 mm axial displacement of the left globe and a firm, nontender medial mass. Coronal CT scans demonstrate an anteromedial inferior left orbital mass that molds to the borders of the globe and orbit. Biospy led to a diagnosis of small cell lymphocytic lymphoma (low grade).

■ PLASMA CELL TUMORS

In many respects the plasma cell tumors parallel the lymphoproliferative lesions just described. In fact, the diffuse lymphomas of B-cell origin contain within their spectrum variants that possess B-cell surface markers and intracytoplasmic immunoglobulins, and display secretory activity. These so-called plasmacytoid lymphomas may secrete IgM paraprotein in sufficient quantities to cause a monoclonal peak in the serum; this is classically seen in Waldenström's macroglobulinemia. Plasma cell tumors, particularly as they affect the orbit and ocular structures, display the same spectrum of clinical involvement seen in the lymphoproliferative disorders. However, these lesions are far less frequent in and around the orbit and mainly comprise the myeloma end of the spectrum. Pa-

tients may present with solitary, well-defined soft tissue lesions (plasmacytoma and reactive plasmacytic granulomas), fulminant orbital infiltrations (as part of the manifestations of multiple myeloma, or supervening infection in an immunosuppressed host), or, most commonly, with an orbital tumor arising from within adjacent bone either as a solitary plasmacytoma or as part of generalized osseous involvement in multiple myeloma. Finally, certain ocular and neuro-ophthalmic complications are characteristic of multiple myeloma. The ocular lesions consist of features of the hyperviscosity state, including retinal venous engorgement, retinal hemorrhages, microaneurysms, retinal vein thrombosis, sludging, and peripheral pars plana ciliary body cysts. Furthermore, neuro-ophthalmic complications may be a manifestation of central nervous system involvement in multiple myeloma.

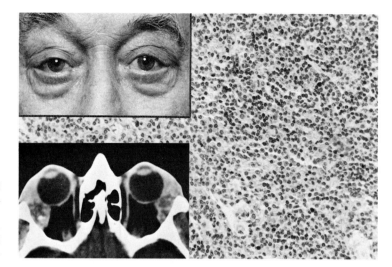

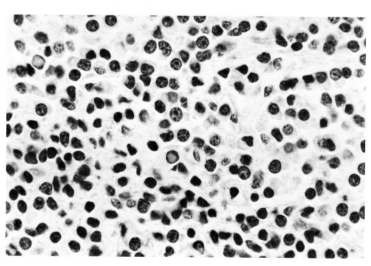

FIGURE 10-7. This 78-year-old man presented with a 2-month history of epiphora and superolateral orbital soreness with normal tear secretion. The clinical photograph demonstrates bilateral lacrimal masses. Axial CT scan at midorbit level reveals bilateral symmetrical inhomogeneous extraconal lesions that mold to the lateral margins of the globe and adjacent bone structures. Course punctate calcification is noted in the posterior portion of the right lacrimal lesion. Pathology revealed a diffuse plasmacytoid small cell lymphocytic lymphoma (low grade) (H&E, original magnification *top* × 25, *bottom* × 40).

The role of an ophthalmic physician encountering plasma-cell lesions parallels that defined for all lymphoproliferative disorders. That is, patients with a primary orbital or paraorbital presentation require a full clinical workup and biopsy to establish a histopathologic diagnosis. Further definition requires categorization into benign or reactive lesions, solitary plasma-cell tumors, or plasmacytomas associated with frank multiple myeloma. In some patients, orbital and ocular phenomena develop as a complication of an underlying systemic illness related to some disturbance in immunoregulation.

Plasma-cell neoplasia characteristically occur in the bone marrow as multiple focal lesions associated with a variable degree of marrow failure. In a minority of patients the neoplastic process is truly localized (solitary plasmacytoma). Soft tissue and extramedullary plasmacytomas without bony involvement also occur, of which three quarters are seen in the upper respiratory tract and oropharynx. Generally, the incidence of these presentations is 90% multiple myeloma, 10% solitary plasmacytoma of bone, and extramedullary plasmacytoma. Solitary osseous plasmacytomas appear to be an early form of multiple myeloma in the majority of patients, whereas extramedullary plasmacytomas tend to remain localized or spread to regional lymph nodes.

Histopathology

The plasma cell is characteristically oval to pear-shaped with an eccentric nucleus containing chromatin with a "cartwheel" distribution and a paranuclear halo or clear

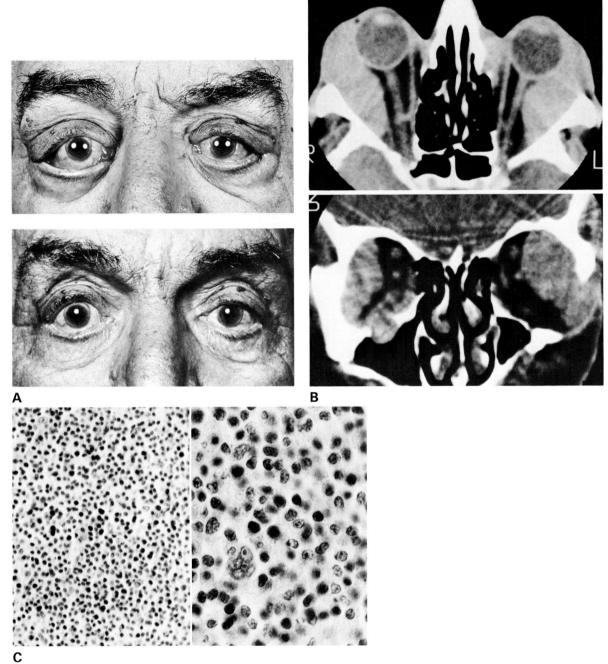

A

B

C

FIGURE 10-8. *(A, top)* This 78-year-old man presented with a 3-month history of uncomfortable gritty eyes with increasing proptosis and diplopia due to a small cell (well-differentiated) widespread lymphocytic lymphoma. He had bilateral masses in the lacrimal fossa with S-shaped deformities of the lid and downward inward displacement of the globes. In addition, salmon colored infiltrates of the conjunctiva were noted, along with dry eyes. *(Bottom)* After several months of systemic chemotherapy, the patient demonstrates a dramatic improvement. *(B)* Axial *(top)* and coronal *(bottom)* CT scans of the same patient demonstrate bilateral, homogeneous, predominantly extraconal smooth masses in the temporal portion of the orbits. Slight nodularity of the margins is noted, and the tumors mold to the shape of the globe. The coronal view shows expansion of the right inferior orbital fissure with soft tissue extension into the superior portion of the maxillary sinus. *(C)* Sections of the orbital biopsy from this patient show extensive replacement of the tissue by a small cell lymphoma with a diffuse pattern (low grade). On touch preparation, the cells had the morphology of small, mature, but slightly atypical lymphocytes, some with slight plasmacytoid features and a few with nuclear clefting. Occasional mitotic features were present. The immunoperoxidase stains were not specific, but showed changes suggestive of an IgG monoclonal pattern (H&E, original magnification × 25 *left,* × 40 *right*).

218

zone ("Hoff"). These cells can be binucleate and may contain intracytoplasmic inclusions (Russell bodies) or protein crystals (Fig. 10-13). Immunoperoxidase or immunofluorescent stains demonstrate these proteins to be immunoglobulins that are monoclonal in the malignant disorders and polyclonal in the reactive lesions. The cells are typically PAS-positive and diastase-resistant with a pyroninophilic cytoplasm. The electron microscopic features show numerous mitochondria, a characteristically stacked rough endoplasmic reticulum, and a prominent Golgi apparatus. In addition, membrane-bound crystals may be present (Fig. 10-14). The cytologic spectrum varies from this well-defined mature plasma cell to larger, immature plasma cells with increased mitotic activity and bearing only slight resemblance to the mature cell. Some lesions may show the full spectrum of differentiation.

Spectrum of Orbital Plasma Cell Tumors

Orbital involvement by plasmacytic lymphoproliferative disorders is rare. These lesions compose a spectrum of clinical involvement ranging from a reactive disorder to widespread multiple myeloma. The pathologic features of these tumors can be misleading and the use of ancillary diagnostic methods, such as electron microscopy and immunohistochemistry, may be necessary to define these lesions accurately. They may present as localized masses (type 1), fulminant orbital infiltrations (type 2), secondary orbital infiltrations particularly from bone (type 3), or neuro-ophthalmic complications of the disease (type 4). Each of these four categories can be further subdivided and discussed along two broad lines: solitary lesions and tumors associated with widespread involvement.

SOLITARY PLASMA CELL TUMORS

Clinically, solitary plasma cell tumors include slow-growing, circumscribed soft tissue tumors involving the orbit and solitary plasmacytomas of bone. The histopathologic groups are similar to those seen in lymphoproliferative diseases insofar as they may comprise polyclonal reactive lesions or monoclonal plasma cell tumors.

Polyclonal Plasma Cell Tumor

The polyclonal lesions consist of a heterogeneous population of plasma cells and lymphocytes associated with reactive changes. These lesions may display a follicular organization with varying morphologic features (including tingible body macrophages) in a more or less abundant reactive connective tissue stroma. A proliferation of capillaries and swollen endothelial cells is also seen. The

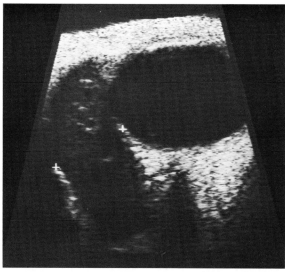

FIGURE 10-9. B-mode ultrasonogram of a patient with a low-grade orbital lymphoma involving the medial rectus muscle.

distinction between a plasma cell granuloma and a reactive plasma cell proliferation is vague in the literature, and these two entities probably represent the same lesion. With immunohistochemistry techniques, the presence of polyclonality will confirm the nature of this disorder. Electron microscopy can help differentiate monomorphic from polymorphic tumors. The reactive lesions may contain dense eosinophilic PAS-positive deposits of immunoglobulins that may include amyloid (a feature that may also be seen as part of the monoclonal disorders).

These lesions are more common in conjunctiva but have been described in the soft tissues of the orbit. We have encountered one such case, presenting as a well-defined, molding anterior superior orbital mass (Fig. 10-15). Therapy in these cases consists of excising as much of the tumor as possible. Regression of any residual tumor usually occurs. An inaccessible or extremely large tumor will respond to low-dose radiotherapy. Corticosteroids have been used, usually with only moderate responses.

Solitary Plasmacytoma

Solitary extramedullary plasmacytomas (SEMP) are rare monoclonal infiltrates of soft tissue or bone, and represent about 3% of all plasma cell neoplasms. The male to female ratio is around 3:1, and these lesions develop most frequently in the sixth and seventh decades. The majority occur in the upper respiratory tract or in the oronasopharynx. These tumors are associated with prolonged survival (mean 8.3 years), which has led Wiltshaw to consider this as a condition distinct from multiple myeloma.

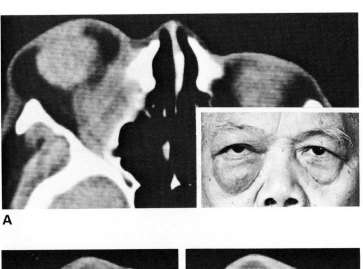

A

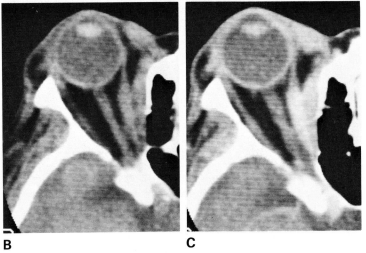

B   C

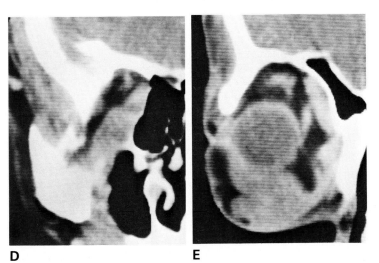

D   E

FIGURE 10-10. *(A)* This 73-year-old man had a mass of the right lower lid of 7 years' duration. He presented with increasing size of the lesion over the last year. A smooth, rubbery, inferior orbital mass caused 4 mm upward, 7 mm outward, and 5 mm axial displacement and slight limitation of up and down gaze. An axial CT scan through the lower orbit demonstrates proptosis and a well-defined inferior medial mass. Comparison of nonenhanced *(B)* and enhanced *(C)* axial CT scans at the level of the midorbit demonstrate an enhancing well-defined extraconal lesion in the medial portion of the right orbit. The lesion is displacing the mildly thickened medial rectus muscle laterally. Coronal CT scans *(D,* posterior orbit; *E,* anterior orbit) demonstrate the inferior medial location of the lesion with extension through the inferior orbital fissure into the maxillary sinus.

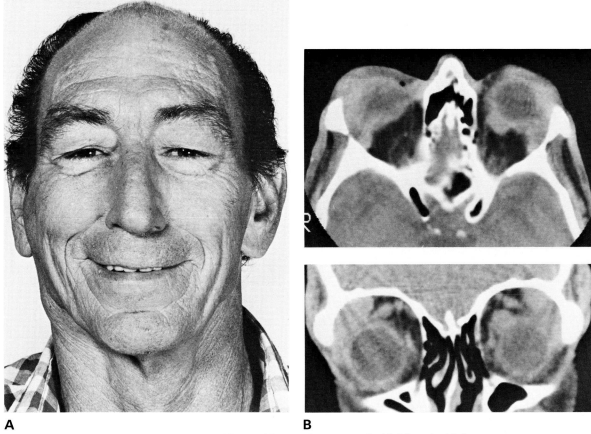

A **B**

FIGURE 10-11. *(A)* Clinical photograph of a 78-year-old man who presented with bilateral orbital masses 5 years after diagnosis and treatment of chronic lymphocytic leukemia. Note cervical adenopathy. *(B)* Axial and coronal CT scans of the same patient demonstrate bilateral, slightly nodular orbital masses that mold to and surround the globes and extend posteriorly into both intraconal and extraconal spaces. Biopsy showed a diffuse small cleaved cell lymphocytic lymphoma (intermediate grade).

Orbital involvement is exceedingly uncommon, with about 12 cases described in the world literature. Patients characteristically present with proptosis and ptosis. Other symptoms reflect a mass effect and include tearing and blurred vision, followed by diplopia and conjunctival congestion. Pain is rare, even though local bony erosion is present at the time of diagnosis in about half of the cases (Fig. 10-16). Orbital involvement may also develop secondary to a tumor of the paranasal sinuses.

Histologically, the lesions consist of a monomorphous cellular infiltrate of plasma cells that are somewhat larger than mature plasma cells (10 – 12 μm). Some variation and binucleate forms are common and the nuclei may show some irregularity with lobulation. Some of the nuclei may be vesicular with diffusely dispersed chromatin. There is usually a sparse delicate fibrous stroma with thin-walled vessels. The degree of differentiation has some bearing on prognosis, with less differentiated

tumors being more likely to disseminate, particularly to bone. Immunohistochemistry demonstrates monoclonality with rare tumors having a biclonal light chain.

On histologic grounds alone, solitary plasmacytoma cannot be distinguished from a well-differentiated multiple myeloma. The distinction is based on the absence of other findings on careful clinical evaluation, including skeletal survey and bone marrow biopsy. Paraproteinemia can be seen in association with solitary plasmacytomas and is, in part, a function of tumor size. Persistence of or increase in paraprotein levels after treatment indicates residual or recurrent disease and warrants reassessment and further therapy. These tumors may be locally invasive, leading to considerable bone destruction and pathologic fractures; rarely, these tumors are associated with osteosclerosis. The tumor usually spreads to the regional lymph nodes or, more rarely, to non-marrow containing bones. Progression to multiple myeloma is not

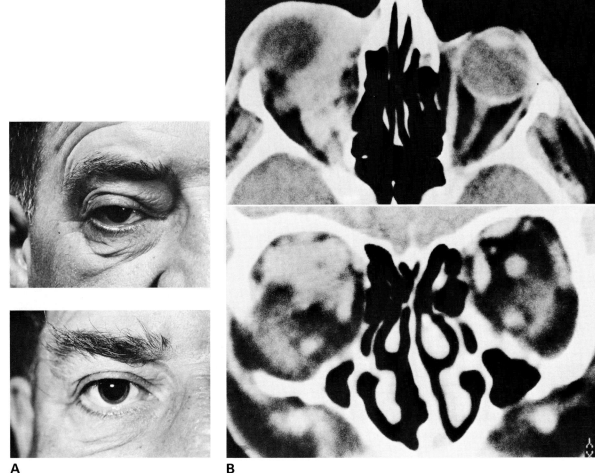

A   **B**

FIGURE 10-12. *(A)* This 54-year-old man had a 4-year history of a slowly progressive lesion in the superomedial right orbit *(top)*. *(Bottom)* The same man after radiotherapy (1500 rad in 5 fractions over 7 days with a 4 mV linear accelerator). Histologically, the lesion was a small cell lymphocytic lymphoma (low grade) with no systemic spread (follow up, 5 years since treatment). *(B)* Axial *(top)* and coronal *(bottom)* CT scans of the same patient demonstrate a superior, predominantly intraconal, nodular mass that molds to and obscures local structures and is displacing the globe anteriorly and inferiorly.

as common as previously believed. Initial bone involvement implies a poor prognosis.

Therapy consists of local irradiation at doses of 4000 to 5000 rad. Surgery and chemotherapy are reserved for persistent or recurrent disease.

ORBITAL INVOLVEMENT IN MULTIPLE MYELOMA

Multiple myeloma rarely involves the orbital tissues. When it occurs, however, in the majority of cases it is the initial presentation of the disease. Rodman and Font de-

scribed 30 cases presenting mostly with proptosis, although at the time of diagnosis all had some systemic manifestations, including bone pain, fatigue, recurrent infection, pathologic fractures, anemia, hyperglobulinemia, Bence Jones proteinuria, and abnormal immunoelectrophoresis (Fig. 10-17). In the latter stages of known myelomatosis, conjunctival involvement may be seen either as a discrete mass or, on occasion, as diffuse thickening or conjunctivitis.

Histologically, there may be a wide variation in the degree of differentiation and the nuclear chromatin may lack the cartwheel-like arrangement of mature plasma

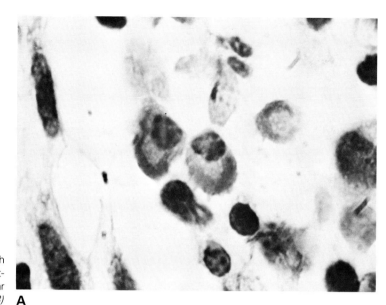

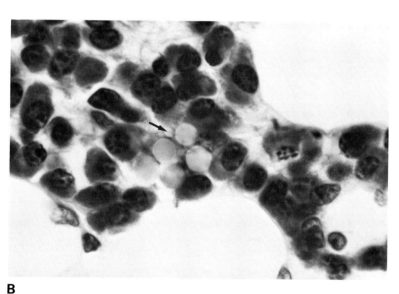

FIGURE 10-13. *(A)* Photomicrograph shows normal plasma cells with coarse "cartwheel" nuclear chromatin and paranculear halo (H&E, original magnification × 100). *(B)* Dense infiltrate of plasma cells that contain Russell's bodies *(arrow)* (Masson Trichrome, original magnification × 40).

A

B

cells. These tumors have been confused with idiopathic lymphoproliferative disorders, undifferentiated sarcoma, large-cell lymphomas, and amelanotic melanoma. In such cases, the diagnosis may be confirmed by electron microscopy or immunohistochemistry. Myeloma tumors generally show a strong monoclonal and occasionally biclonal staining pattern. Immunohistochemistry may be of prognostic significance, because longer remissions are seen in IgG and IgA myelomas, whereas IgD myeloma and light-chain disease have a much poorer prognosis.

Clinically, patients with orbital involvement related to multiple myeloma present at an older age than patients with solitary extramedullary plasmacytoma, usually in the seventh or eighth decade, with 60% being male. The median survival is around 20 months and death is usually due to infection or renal insufficiency. Particular care should be taken at the time of surgery, because these patients may develop acute renal failure as a result of anesthesia or as a result of CT scanning with contrast. Therapy consists of systemic chemotherapy and radiation for control of locally invasive lesions.

In disseminated multiple myeloma, soft tissue involvement often heralds the terminal stage of the disease. Because of the fulminant nature of this infiltration, it may

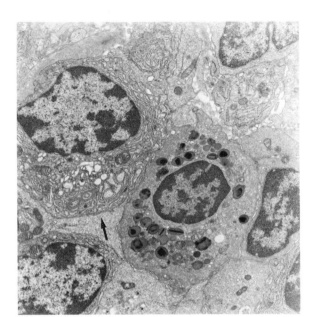

FIGURE 10-14. Electron micrograph showing an eosinophil and a lymphocyte in close proximity to a plasma cell *(arrow)*; the plasma cell is characterized by ''cartwheel'' nuclear clumping and cytoplasm filled with rough endoplasmic reticulum (original magnification × 7280).

be difficult to distinguish clinically between neoplastic infiltration and a supervening opportunistic infection. In one such case orbital involvement appeared to be part of a paranasal sinus infection, and the clinical picture was one of cellulitis (Fig. 10-18). However, biopsy proved the orbital infiltrate to consist of malignant plasma cells.

Finally, multiple myeloma is associated with certain ocular and central nervous system manifestations. Patients may show venous engorgement, focal ischemia with cotton-wool spots, retinal hemorrhages, microaneurysms, and cysts of the pars plana and ciliary epithelium. The cysts may be sufficiently large to cause anterior displacement of the lens. Central nervous system involvement (thrombosis, intracranial bleeding, meningeal involvement) can cause raised intracranial pressure with papilledema, or may lead to cranial nerve palsies involving the ocular and orbital nerve supply (type 4).

In summary, the spectrum of plasma cell tumors parallels that of the lymphoproliferative groups with disseminated myeloma having a much poorer prognosis. Clinically, these patients present with a variety of manifestations, including localized, well-defined orbital infiltration with tumefaction, periorbital bony involvement, fulminant orbital infiltrations, and central nervous system complications.

■ OTHER LYMPHOPROLIFERATIVE AND LEUKEMIC LESIONS

Undifferentiated Lymphoma, Burkitt's Type

Burkitt's lymphoma is a high-grade undifferentiated lymphocytic neoplasm endemic to Central Africa, but which also occurs sporadically worldwide. This disease is of great interest, because evidence exists for an oncogenic viral etiology involving the Epstein-Barr virus with a cofactor of chronic immune stimulation by malaria.

Clinically, this lymphoma can be multifocal, but usually presents as a solitary fulminant growth at a median age of 7 years in a dominant population of males (2:1). African Burkitt's lymphoma presents as a facial tumor in 60%, abdominal mass in 25%, and with paraplegia in 15% of cases. In younger patients (3 to 5 years of age) the maxillary and jaw tumor is a more frequent site of presentation. Although the orbit is ultimately involved in the majority of facial lesions, only 13% present with exophthalmos. Dissemination may occur to the central nervous system (meningeal) and bone marrow. In contrast, the non-African cases are seen in the first three decades (median age 11 years), and are more frequently abdominal with only one third of cases involving the jaw.

These lymphomas are believed to be of B-cell germinal center origin (small noncleaved follicular center cell). The dominant cell population consists of poorly differentiated, basophilic, highly mitotic lymphocytes. These cells commonly contain fat-filled cytoplasmic vacuoles. The sheets of lymphocytes are interspersed by phagocytic histiocytes, which give the characteristic "starry sky" pattern to the tumor.

Originally, the prognosis for this fulminant neoplasm was uniformly poor, but the introduction of chemotherapy and adjuvant radiotherapy has greatly improved the prognosis, with dramatic regressions and occasional cures. The major chemotherapeutic agents used are cyclophosphamide and methotrexate. Younger age and localized disease at onset are associated with a better prognosis.

Granulocytic Sarcoma and Leukemia

GRANULOCYTIC SARCOMA

Granulocytic sarcoma (chloroma) represents a localized, usually extramedullary, form of acute myeloblastic leukemia or of chronic granulocytic leukemia entering blast crisis. It occurs in about 3% of patients with myeloid leukemia. In children there is a characteristic predilection for the orbit and surrounding bone. It occurs usually as a rapidly expanding tumor. The mean age of onset is 7 years, with a male (3:2) and non-Caucasian predomi-

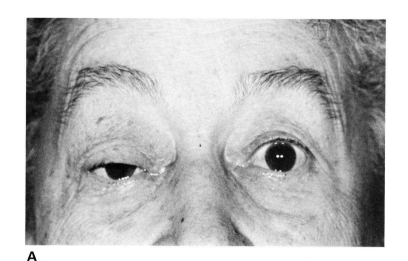

A

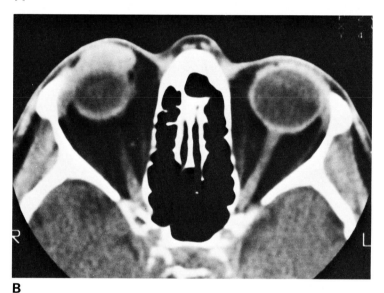

FIGURE 10-15. (A) This 71-year-old woman demonstrates ptosis (3 mm), downward displacement, and proptosis (3 mm) of the right globe due to a palpable superior orbital mass present for 4 months. (B) Unenhanced axial CT scan of the patient demonstrates an anterior superior homogeneous mass lesion with distinct borders that mold to the contours of the globe. (C) A magnified view of the histopathology from the same patient demonstrates the polymorphous cellular infiltrate and shows numerous plasma cells, lymphocytes, and a few macrophages, some of which contain tingible bodies (H&E, original magnification ×40). Immunocytochemistry was polyclonal.

B

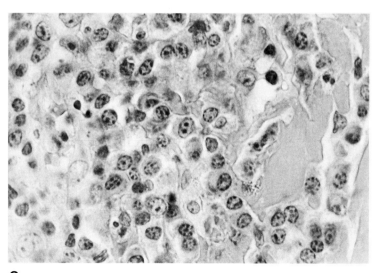

C

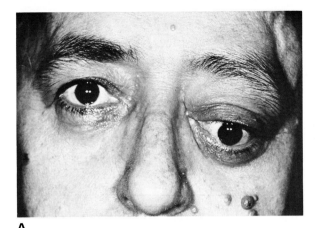

A

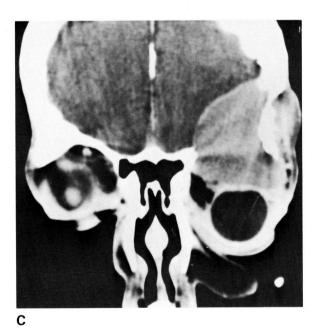

B

C

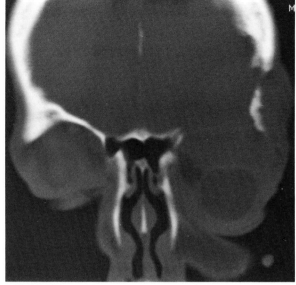

D

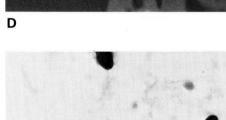

E

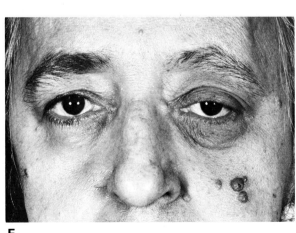

F

nance. In these cases the orbit is usually the site of initial presentation, but the disease ultimately progresses to full-blown acute myeloblastic leukemia 2 months to 3 years later.

The sites of orbital involvement may include the soft tissue, lacrimal gland, or orbital bones. In 10% of cases bilateral disease is present. Because the clinical presentation is fulminant, confusion with local inflammations and other malignant diseases is common. Biopsy reveals a poorly differentiated high-grade malignancy, which must be distinguished from other round cell tumors of childhood. In contradistinction to granulocytic sarcoma, true orbital lymphomas are exceedingly rare in childhood.

Histologically, the myeloid origin of the blast cell population can be confirmed by the presence of cytoplasmic granules or Auer rods, or both. The cytology is best assessed with Giemsa-stained imprints and smears. Characteristically, the presence of myeloperoxidase in the tissue imparts a green color to the tumor, accounting for the original designation of this tumor as a chloroma. Cells of myeloid origin can be identified in formalin-fixed tissue by the Leder stain for chloroacetate esterase (a neutrophil enzyme).

The prognosis for patients with this aggressive tumor is universally poor. Treatment consists of local irradiation and adjuvant chemotherapy, which, if instituted early, may prolong disease-free survival.

LEUKEMIA

There are a host of leukemic disorders, both acute and chronic, which fall mainly in the lymphoid and myeloid groups. The eye and adnexa are not infrequently involved, usually as a complication of late-stage disease. Generally, soft tissue involvement of the orbit is more frequent in acute (especially lymphoblastic) rather than in chronic leukemias. In childhood malignancies of the orbit acute leukemia and granulocytic sarcoma is a frequent cause of unilateral proptosis (11%), second only to

rhabdomyosarcoma in frequency. Bilaterality is seen in 2% of patients with orbital leukemia. Involvement may be due to soft tissue infiltration or hematoma and is characteristically sudden in onset. Soft tissue hemorrhage is more common in the myeloid group. Involvement of optic nerve (prelaminar and retrolaminar), meninges, uvea, and vitreous may also lead to ocular manifestations. In all of these circumstances involvement usually heralds a rapid demise, but local irradiation and local, intrathecal, and systemic chemotherapy may significantly prolong survival, thus emphasizing the importance of prompt recognition and management.

Hodgkin's Disease

CLINICAL FEATURES

Orbital manifestations of Hodgkin's disease are rare (about ten cases in the literature), but when they occur, it is (in 60% of cases) during the terminal phases of the disease. Four patients presented with orbital involvement before developing disseminated disease. The clinical syndrome consists of an orbital mass that develops relatively quickly in a patient with Hodgkin's disease. However, there are cases in which orbital tumors developed and the patient was subsequently discovered on further investigation to have either a mediastinal mass or regional lymphadenopathy, which on biopsy revealed Hodgkin's disease. We have reported a single case of nodular sclerosing Hodgkin's disease of the orbit associated with a long-standing, noninvasive mass effect with local bone involvement (Fig. 10-19).

PATHOLOGY

Histologically, Hodgkin's disease composes a spectrum of four subtypes with distinct prognostic implications. The central diagnostic feature is the presence of neoplas-

---

FIGURE 10-16. *(A)* This 56-year-old woman with a left temporal and brow mass demonstrated inferior (9 mm), medial (2 mm), and axial (12 mm) displacement of her eye. The masses, which developed over a 6- to 8-week period, demonstrated pulsation. Sharp, bony defects were palpated at their margins. *(B, C)* Enhanced axial and coronal CT scans demonstrate a large, soft tissue mass in the left superior orbit, invading the anterior cranial and temporalis fossa and displacing the globe inferiorly. Coronal views (*C*, soft tissue technique; *D*, bone technique) demonstrate destruction of the orbital roof and orbital process of the frontal bone. *(E)* Aspiration biopsy from this patient shows immature plasma cells with binucleate and multinucleated forms; several of the nuclei are irregular in shape (H&E, original magnification × 100). Cytoplasmic immunoperoxidase was strongly positive for IgG and monoclonal lambda light chain. Because systemic investigation showed no other lesions, the final diagnosis was plasmacytoma. *(F)* Four months after radiotherapy (3600 rad over a 3-week period), the patient shows marked reduction in the size of the mass. The bony defect has healed, and she shows only minimal proptosis.

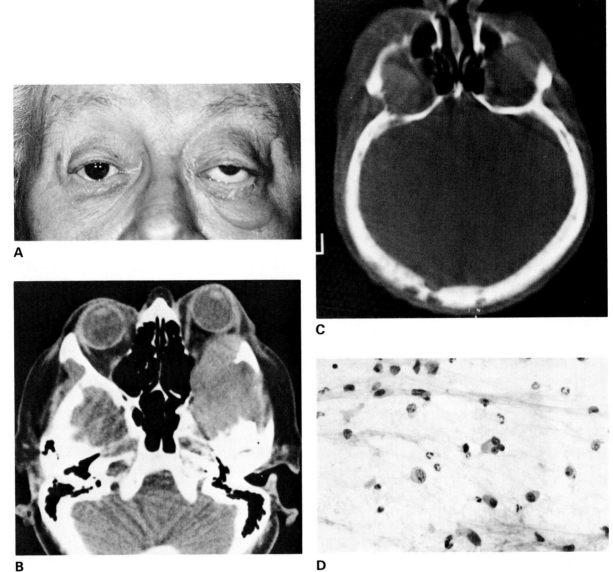

FIGURE 10-17. *(A)* This 60-year-old woman had a 1-year history of multiple myeloma, a 3-month history of progressive left-sided superotemporal and zygomatic numbness, left ptosis, downward displacement (5 mm), proptosis (8 mm), and edema of her lids. She had also noted diplopia. *(B)* An enhanced CT scan of this patient shows a large left posterior orbit and middle fossa homogeneous soft tissue mass that has caused partial destruction of the lateral wall of the orbit, the temporal bone, and the sphenoid bone. The globe is displaced anteriorly. *(C)* A coronal CT scan with bone setting demonstrates multiple lytic lesions in the cranial vault. *(D)* The aspiration smears demonstrated numerous scattered, individual polymorphonuclear leucocytes and numerous larger plasma cells. Some relatively mature-appearing plasma cells were present, whereas others had the appearance of plasmablasts. Binucleate and even multinucleate plasma cells were present (H&E, original magnification × 40).

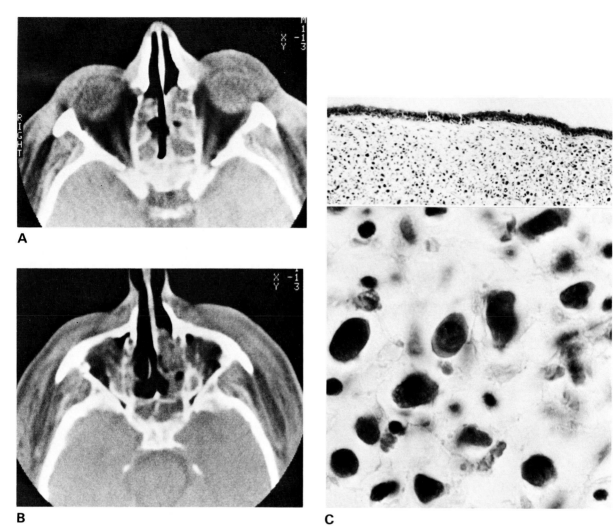

FIGURE 10-18. *(A, B)* An enhanced CT scan in this 57-year-old man with known myeloma for 2 years and a 6-week history of periorbital pain, swelling, stuffiness of his sinuses and nasopharynx, pyrexia, and fatigue demonstrates diffuse soft tissue swelling of the left upper lid. Note the opacification of the adjacent ethmoid and sphenoid sinuses. *(B)* Axial CT scan shows involvement of the maxillary sinuses. Some prominence of the left lower lid is also evident. *(C)* This photomicrograph shows numerous pleomorphic plasma cells. A few lymphocytes are visible. There is cellular invasion of nasal epithelial submucosa *(top)* (H&E, original magnification × 10 *top*, × 100 *bottom*).

tic mononuclear and multinucleated cells, which are believed to be either of macrophage or immunoblast derivation. The mononuclear cells are very large, indistinct cells with a vesicular nucleus and a large hyperchromatic nucleolus. The pathognomonic feature, however, relates to the presence of large multinucleated Reed-Sternberg cells. There are a number of variants of this cell, the classical one being the bilobed, mirror-image cell. In addition to the neoplastic cell, there is a background of mixed cellular infiltrates, including neutrophils, eosinophils, plasma cells, lymphocytes, histiocytes, and fibro-

blasts, which are felt to represent a reaction to the Hodgkin's lymphoma.

Patients with Hodgkin's disease are classified histologically into four subtypes, according to the Rye classification (Table 10-6). Prognosis is in part based on the amount of immune reaction to the tumor: the fewer the number of lymphocytes, the more aggressive the disease. Prognosis is also closely related to the staging of the tumor by anatomic involvement (see Table 10-6). The variable cellularity of this lesion makes it not infrequently a diagnostic conundrum for the pathologist, who must

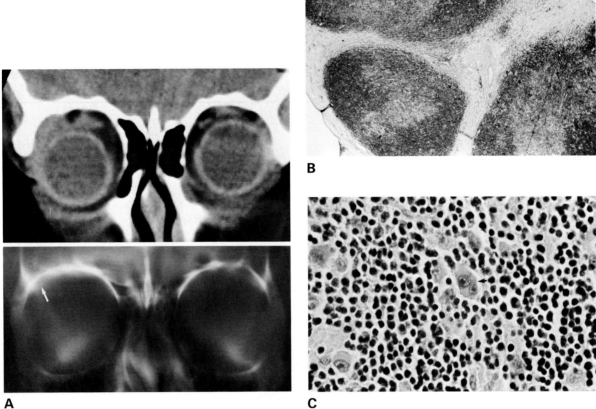

FIGURE 10-19. *(A, top)* This 27-year-old woman had a 29-month history of orbital asymmetry, recent onset of swelling of the right upper lid, and known systemic diagnosis of Hodgkin's disease. Coronal CT scan shows a soft tissue mass in the right lacrimal fossa. Note the localized smooth excavation of bone. *(Bottom)* AP polytomogram reveals localized expansion of bone adjacent to the right lacrimal fossa without evidence of bony destruction *(arrow)*. This suggested a long-standing lesion with pressure effect but no bony invasion. *(B)* Photomicrograph of tissue obtained at biopsy of this patient illustrates a lymphoproliferative lesion with dense septae (H&E, original magnification × 25). *(C)* A polymorphic population of lymphocytes, plasma cells, eosinophils, and diagnostic Reed–Sternberg cells *(arrow)* are present. The final diagnosis was nodular sclerosing Hodgkin's disease of the orbit (H&E, original magnification × 40). (Patel S, Rootman J: Nodular sclerosing Hodgkin's disease of the orbit. Ophthalmology 90:1433, 1983)

differentiate it from inflammatory and numerous neoplastic lesions.

MANAGEMENT

Overall, the management of Hodgkin's disease represents one of the therapeutic triumphs of modern oncology. Prognosis for low-stage tumors and prospects for cure are remarkably good. However, orbital involvement usually augurs poorly, because it is frequently a reflection of disseminated and aggressive disease. Treatment of orbital disease consists of local irradiation, to which the tumor is generally sensitive.

T-Cell Lymphomas

T-cell lymphomas represent a broad spectrum of disorders that have a predilection for cutaneous sites. There is often involvement of the viscera and paracortex of the lymph nodes, the classic site of T-cell populations. In contrast, B-cell lymphomas not uncommonly present as a primary orbital malignancy, and when disseminated involve bone marrow, lymph nodes, and the peripheral blood. The differences between these two types of lymphomas relates to their fundamental cytogenetic origin. T-cell lymphomas include mycosis fungoides, Sézary syndrome, lymphoma cutis, and adult T-cell leukemias.

TABLE 10-6.
RYE CLASSIFICATIONS FOR HODGKIN'S DISEASE

Histologic Types
Lymphocyte predominance
Nodular sclerosis
Mixed cellularity
Lymphocyte depletion

Staging*—Criteria for Evaluation
I: Disease limited to one anatomic region (stage I_1) or to two contiguous anatomic regions on the same side of the diaphragm (stage 1_2)
II: Disease in more than two anatomic regions or in two noncontiguous regions on the same side of the diaphragm
III: Disease on both sides of the diaphragm but not extending beyond the involvement of lymph nodes, spleen, or Waldeyer's ring
IV: Involvement of the bone marrow, lung parenchyma, pleura, liver, bone, skin, kidneys, gastrointestinal tract, or any tissue or organ in addition to lymph nodes, spleen, or Waldeyer's ring

* All stages will be subclassified as A or B to indicate absence or presence, respectively, of systemic symptoms (fever, night sweats, pruritus).

For the most part the orbital and ocular manifestations are a reflection of systemic disease or result from extension of local skin lesions, and usually present late in the course of the disease. The cutaneous T-cell lymphomas are subdivided according to major site of skin involvement into epidermotropic and nonepidermotropic stages. These lymphomas are more common in men and usually occur after the fourth decade of life.

Mycosis fungoides is the most well-described variant. This lesion develops in three progressive stages: erythematous, infiltrative plaque, and tumor stage (Fig. 10-20). The erythematous stage is the common feature of onset and consists of superficial, eczematous, psoriaform lesions of the skin. Biopsy at this stage reveals a polymorphic infiltrate and may be nonspecific, unless typical "mycosis" cells or epidermal involvement is noted. Biopsy at the plaque stage is usually diagnostic with evidence of convoluted lymphocytes and microabscesses in the epidermis (Pautrier microabscesses). The final stage is the development of ulcerating tumors, which may involve the eyelid, conjunctiva, and orbit. Rarely, this disorder may present in the tumor stage, as recently described by Meekins in a case involving the lid and invading the orbit.

Sézary syndrome, a variant of T-cell lymphoma, is associated with an exfoliative dermatopathy, lymphadenopathy, and circulating Sézary cells.

Histopathologic diagnosis rests on the identification of typical large and small "mycosis cells," which have markedly convoluted (serpentine) nuclei. Immunologic techniques confirm the T-cell origin (sheep erythrocyte and T-cell monoclonal markers). These cells do not bear B-cell markers.

Ocular and orbital involvement usually reflect extracutaneous spread and include deep lid, conjunctival, and caruncular lesions. Keratitis, uveitis, and optic nerve lesions have also been described.

Treatment is usually based on extent of involvement. When primarily dermal, radiotherapy, photochemotherapy, and topical antineoplastics can be used. In disseminated disease, systemic chemotherapy, leukapheresis, and antithymocyte globulin can be employed.

■ HISTIOCYTOSES

Histiocytosis X

Three disorders (Hand-Schüller-Christian disease, Letterer-Siwe disease, and eosinophilic granuloma) have traditionally been categorized as "histiocytosis X" because of their unknown etiology and the similarity of the observed histiocytes. Because they do not behave as true neoplasia, it has been suggested the pathogenesis may be related to abnormal immune regulation.

These disorders are rare (0.6 cases per million children under 15 years of age versus 42.1 cases per million for acute leukemia), occurring most commonly in children and typically encountered in the general pediatrics setting. Ophthalmologic manifestations are seen in about 10% of cases. Worldwide incidence and male predominance (2 : 1) have been noted. About one third of patients present with disseminated disease, which has a 50% mortality rate. The remaining two thirds have either unifocal or multifocal bone involvement, which can follow either an indolent or a progressive clinical course.

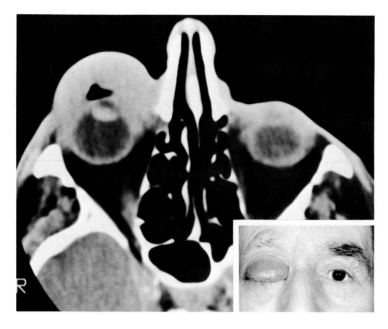

FIGURE 10-20. This 59-year-old man presented with a 6-week history of increased thickening of the right lid. On physical examination, it was associated with loss of brow hair and cilia. There were some typical salmon patches beneath the conjunctiva on the affected right side. He also had numerous raised, rather injected areas of skin throughout the head and neck region (note left brow). *(Top)* Axial CT scan demonstrates diffuse involvement of the lid and the anterior orbit. *(Bottom)* Biopsy shows infiltration of the subcuticular tissues by sheets of atypical lymphoid cells. The cells have large nuclei with a distinct nucleolus and a crenated or convoluted nuclear envelope. Immunoperoxidase staining was positive for a lymphoma of T-cell origin, and multiple patches of mycosis fungoides involving the head and neck region were noted.

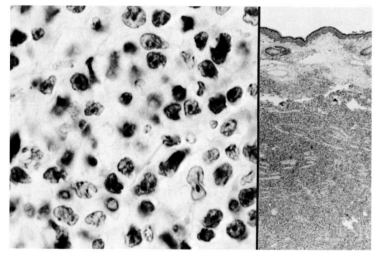

HISTOGENESIS AND PATHOLOGY

The histiocytosis X syndromes are thought to result from abnormal accumulations of specialized histiocytes of the dendritic cell family, specifically the Langerhans cell, of the epidermis. This cell can be identified by the presence of characteristic "racquet-shaped" cytoplasmic granules (Birbeck granules) on electron microscopy or by multiple immunohistochemical means. On routine microscopy, these relatively large mononuclear cells (12 mm) have a moderate amount of granular (occasionally vacuolated) eosinophilic cytoplasm and an indented, lobulated granular nucleus (Fig. 10-21).

The wide clinical disease spectrum is reflected in variations in the pathology and in the site and progression of the process. However, there is a characteristic granulomatous-histiocytic infiltrate, often associated with accumulations of granulocytes (especially eosinophils) and lymphocytes. The Langerhans cells may be identified by electron microscopy (Birbeck granules) and immunohistochemically. Typically, one sees histologic variation and progression through necrosis, xanthomatous change, and, ultimately, fibrosis in the late stage. Multinucleated giant cells may be present. Lesions often involve bone (especially the medullary cavity), whereas the disseminated form of the disorder may involve skin, lymph

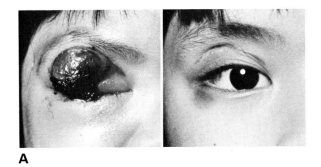

A

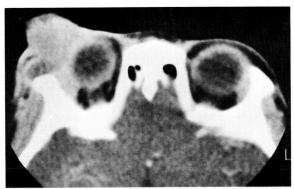

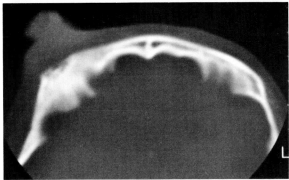

B

FIGURE 10-21. *(A)* This 7-year-old girl presented with a 3-month history of a right upper lid lesion characterized by a waxing and waning course with swelling of the lid. *(Left)* On presentation, she had a mass lesion that had eroded through the upper lid and appeared to be infiltrating the lower lid. *(Right)* The same patient a few months after radiotherapy (1200 rad in 4 fractions over 4 days with a 4 mV linear accelerator). *(B, top)* Axial CT scan shows the mass extending through the upper lid, surrounding the lateral margin of the globe, and displacing the globe posteriorly. *(Bottom)* Axial CT scan (bone setting) shows that the mass has caused erosion of the underlying bone. *(C)* Pathologic picture shows plump cells with abundant cytoplasm and vesicular nuclei with well-demarcated large nucleoli and an inflammatory background (H&E, original magnification × 40). *(D)* Electron micrograph shows C-shaped or indented nucleus and abundant X bodies, Birbeck or Langerhans' granules *(inset)* diagnostic for histiocytosis X (original magnification × 17,100; *inset* × 63,000).

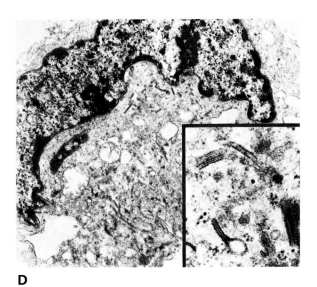

D

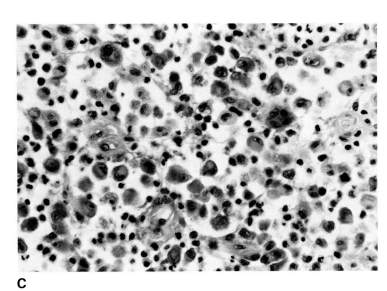

C

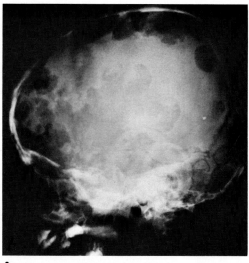

A

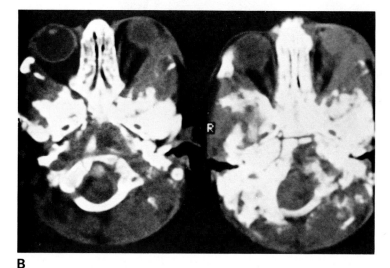

B

FIGURE 10-22. *(A)* Lateral skull radiograph of a 3-year-old boy with histiocytosis X shows multiple lytic lesions of the cranial vault. *(B)* Axial CT scans demonstrate extensive destruction of the orbit margins and cranial bones associated with soft tissue lesions of the left orbit and ethmoid sinuses. The patient was treated with radiotherapy and chemotherapy. When seen 3 years later, he had persistent proptosis and bilateral optic atrophy.

nodes, spleen, lung, liver, and bone marrow. An association with thymic failure and abnormal immunoregulation has been described.

CLINICAL SYNDROMES

The nature of involvement and prognosis seem to be related to age and rate of progression, as well as extent of disease. Several disorders have thus been described that vary significantly in terms of severity and rate of progression. Generally, younger patients have more aggressive disease. The classical spectrum comprises a fulminant systemic disorder (Letterer-Siwe), multifocal bone disease (Hand-Schüller-Christian), or localized bone involvement (eosinophilic granuloma). Generally, patients develop the character of their involvement at an early stage.

Localized disease usually involves bone and adjacent tissues, but is rarely seen in soft tissues alone. This presentation is more often encountered in older children (3 to 10 years). The skull (especially parietal and frontal bones) are preferentially involved and, when affected, the orbit characteristically demonstrates disease in the lateral superior quadrant. These lesions typically show focal, bony lysis, and soft tissue expansion (see Fig. 10-21).

Multifocal bone involvement may be relatively limited or quite extensive, with or without associated skin or visceral disease. Bone lesions have either a punched-out lytic or moth-eaten appearance with expansion of adjacent tissues (Fig. 10-22). Fibrosis may lead to local arrest of the process with sclerosis of the bone and failure of development (Fig. 10-23). This produces a characteristic shallow orbit and flattened forehead (Fig. 10-24). Radiologically, the sclerotic lesion must be distinguished from fibrous dysplasia, meningioma, dermoid cyst, lacrimal gland tumor, osteoblastic metastatic disease, or Caffey's disease. Skin involvement is characterized by pruritic eczematous yellow-red infiltration of the papillary dermis, especially of the scalp. The involvement of bone and surrounding tissues may lead to the well-described triad of diabetes insipidus, exophthalmos, and bony lesions. The acute spectrum of this disease affects infants and young children almost always under 3 years of age. It is usually associated with onset of fever and localized infections, skin lesions, otitis media, and hepatosplenomegaly. Lymphadenopathy and bony involvement are frequently seen. Bone marrow involvement may lead to anemia, thrombocytopenia, and leukopenia.

Prognosis is related to the age of the patient, extent, and progression of the disease. Children under 2 years of age have a mortality rate of 55% to 60% compared to 15% for older children. Disseminated disease correlates with poor survival. Patients with thrombocytopenia, jaundice, hepatosplenomegaly, anemia, and respiratory insufficiency have a high mortality rate. Overall, however, one observes considerable case-to-case variation without any clear-cut correlation between histopathology and prognosis.

Children with this disorder are treated with low-dose local irradiation, cytotoxic agents, and steroids. Treatment should be supervised by a pediatric oncologist and is usually effective in controlling local disease. The more fulminant and progressive forms of this disease fail to show significant response to any form of treatment. Lo-

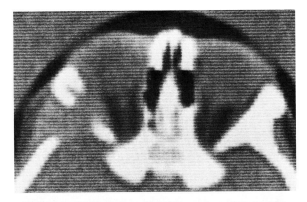

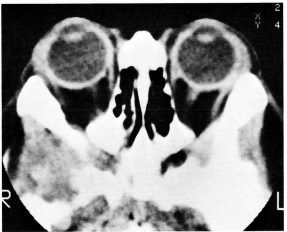

FIGURE 10-23.   *(Top)* Axial CT scan in this patient with histiocytosis X demonstrates destruction of the posterior lateral right orbital margin, temporal fossa, and a soft tissue mass in the orbit and temporalis fossa. *(Bottom)* Follow-up CT scan obtained 5 years later demonstrates regrowth and sclerosis of bone after treatment. Residual mass is still present.

FIGURE 10-24.   This patient demonstrates shallow orbits and exophthalmos due to the arrest of bony development following treatment for orbital histiocytosis X.

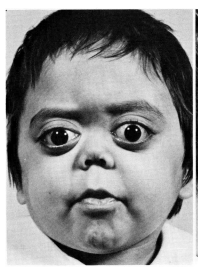
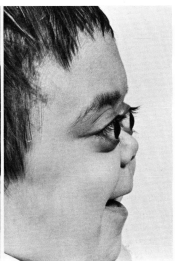

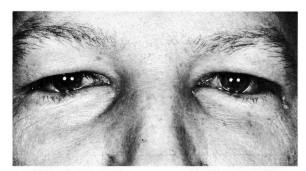

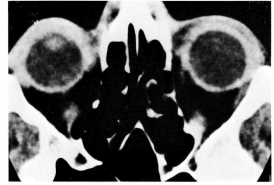

FIGURE 10-25. Clinical photograph of this 43-year-old man demonstrates periorbital swelling, chemosis, and subconjunctival hemorrhage of 1 month's duration. He also had respiratory difficulty and pedal edema secondary to widespread malignant histiocytosis diagnosed 2 months earlier. He died of his disease 6 months after onset. Axial CT scan demonstrates an irregular bilateral anterior infiltration and thickening of the lids and conjunctiva.

calized periorbital disease will generally respond to low-dose irradiation or local curettage.

Malignant Histiocytosis

Malignant histiocytosis represents a systemic neoplasm of histiocytic origin. This disorder has also been described under the term *histiocytic medullary reticulosis*. It is a fulminant neoplastic disorder affecting all age groups and is characterized by abrupt onset of fever, weakness, weight loss, hepatosplenomegaly, and generalized lymphadenopathy. The disease leads to progressive wasting, jaundice, purpura, anemia, leukopenia, and pleural effusions. Soft tissues and skin can also be involved, as was noted in a case we encountered (Fig. 10-25), where the patient developed orbital and periocular disease with cutaneous conjunctival and orbital soft tissue infiltrates. Histologically, the disease is associated with an infiltration of pleomorphic histiocytes showing evidence of ac-

tive erythrophagocytosis. Multinucleated giant cells and bizarre histiocytes are also seen.

Overall, the prognosis is poor and survival, when the disease is untreated, is less than 12 months. In some cases, the use of combination chemotherapy has resulted in remission.

Bibliography

GENERAL

Duke-Elder S, MacFaul PA: The Ocular Adnexa. In Duke-Elder S (ed): System of Ophthalmology, Vol 13. St Louis, CV Mosby, 1974

Henderson JW, Farrow GM: Orbital Tumors, 2nd ed. New York, Brian C Decker, 1980

Ioachim HL: Lymph Node Biopsy. Philadelphia, JB Lippincott, 1982

Jones IS, Jakobiec FA: Diseases of the Orbit. New York, Harper & Row, 1979

Lennert K: Malignant Lymphomas Other Than Hodgkin's Disease: Histology, Cytology, Ultrastructure, Immunology. New York, Springer-Verlag, 1978

Reese AB: Tumors of the Eye, 3rd ed. New York, Harper & Row, 1976

Robb-Smith AHT, Taylor CR: Lymph Node Biopsy. New York, Oxford University Press, 1981

LYMPHOCYTIC TUMORS

Abo W, Takada K, Kamada M et al: Evolution of infectious mononucleosis into Epstein-Barr virus carrying monoclonal malignant lymphoma. Lancet 1:1272, 1982

Astarita RW, Mincler D, Taylor CR et al: Orbital and adnexal lymphomas: A multiparameter approach. Am J Clin Pathol 73:615, 1980

Banerjee D, Ahmad D: Malignant lymphoma complicating lymphocytic interstitial pneumonia: A monoclonal B-cell neoplasm arising in a polyclonal lymphoproliferative disorder. Hum Pathol 13:780, 1982

Burke JS, Butler JJ, Fuller LM: Malignant lymphoma of the thyroid. Cancer 39:1587, 1977

Chavis RM, Garner A, Wright JE: Inflammatory orbital pseudotumor: A clinicopathologic study. Arch Ophthalmol 96:1817, 1978

Cleary ML, Chao J, Warnke R et al: Immunoglobulin gene rearrangement as a diagnostic criterion of B-cell lymphoma. Proc Natl Acad Sci USA 81:593, 1984

Cleary ML, Warnke R, Sklar J: Monoclonality of lymphoproliferative lesions in cardiac-transplant recipients: Clonal analysis based on immunoglobulin-gene rearrangements. N Engl J Med 310:477, 1984

Colby TV, Carrington CB: Lymphoreticular infiltrates and tumors of the lung: Part 1. Pathol Annu 18:27, 1983

Colby TV, Carrington CB: Pulmonary lymphomas: Current concepts. Hum Pathol 14:884, 1983

Compagno J, Oertel JE: Malignant lymphoma and other lymphoproliferative disorders of the thyroid gland. Am J Clin Pathol 74:1, 1980

Dorfman RF, Burke JS, Berard CW: A working formulation on non-Hodgkin's lymphomas: Background, recommendations, histological criteria and relationship to other classifications: In Rosenberg SA, Kaplan HS (eds): Malignant Lymphomas: Etiology, Immunology, Pathology, Treatment. Bristol-Myers Cancer Symposia, Vol 3, p 351. New York, Academic Press, 1982

Ellis JH, Banks PM, Campbell J et al: Lymphoid tumors of the ocular adnexa. Ophthalmology 92, No. 10:1311, 1985

Evans HL: Extranodal small lymphocytic proliferation: A clinicopathologic study. Cancer 49:84, 1982

Garner A, Rahi AHS, Wright JE: Lymphoproliferative disorders of the orbit: An immunological approach to diagnosis and pathogenesis. Br J Ophthalmol 67:561, 1983

Harris NL, Pilch BZ, Bhan AK et al: Immunohistologic diagnosis of orbital lymphoid infiltrates. Am J Surg Pathol 8:83, 1984

Isaacson P, Wright DH: Malignant lymphoma of mucosa-associated lymphoid tissue. Cancer 52:1410, 1983

Isaacson P, Wright DH: Extranodal malignant lymphoma arising from mucosal-associated lymphoid tissue. Cancer 53:2515, 1984

Jakobiec FA: Ocular inflammatory disease: The lymphocyte redivivus. Am J Ophthalmol 96:384, 1983

Jakobiec FA, Iwamoto T, Knowles DM: Ocular adnexal lymphoid tumors: Correlative ultrastructural and immunologic marker studies. Arch Ophthalmol 100:84, 1982

Jakobiec FA, Iwamoto T, Patell M et al: Ocular adnexal monoclonal lymphoid tumors with a favorable prognosis. Ophthalmology 93:1547, 1986

Jakobiec FA, Lefkowitch J, Knowles DM: B and T lymphocytes in ocular disease. Ophthalmology 91:635, 1984

Jakobiec FA, McLean I, Font RL: Clinicopathologic characteristics of orbital lymphoid hyperplasia. Ophthalmology 86:948, 1979

Knowles DM, Halper JP, Jakobiec FA: The immunologic characterization of 40 extranodal lymphoid infiltrates: Usefulness in distinguishing between benign pseudolymphoma and malignant lymphoma. Cancer 49:2321, 1982

Knowles DM, Jakobiec FA: Cell marker analysis of extranodal lymphoid infiltrates: To what extent does the determination of mono or polyclonality resolve the diagnostic dilemma of malignant lymphoma versus pseudolymphoma in an extranodal site? Semin Diagn Pathol 2:163, 1985

Knowles DM, Jakobiec FA: Ocular adnexal lymphoid neoplasms: Clinical, histopathologic, electron microscopic and immunologic characteristics. Hum Pathol 13:148, 1982

Knowles DM, Jakobiec FA: Orbital lymphoid neoplasms: A clinicopathologic study of 60 patients. Cancer 46:576, 1980

Knowles DM, Jakobiec FA, Halper JP: Immunologic characterization of ocular adnexal lymphoid neoplasms. Am J Ophthalmol 87:603, 1979

Koss MN, Hochholzer L, Nichols PW et al: Primary non-Hodgkin's lymphoma and pseudolymphoma of lung. Hum Pathol 14:1024, 1983

Morgan G: Lymphocytic tumors of the orbit. Mod Probl Ophthalmol 14:355, 1975

Morgan G, Harry J: Lymphocytic tumors of indeterminate nature: A 5-year follow-up of 98 conjunctival and orbital lesions. Br J Ophthalmol 62:381, 1978

Non-Hodgkin's Lymphoma Pathologic Classification Project: National Cancer Institute-sponsored study of classifications of non-Hodgkin's lymphomas: Summary and description of a working formulation for clinical usage. Cancer 49:2112, 1982

O'Connor NTJ et al: Rearrangement of the T cell receptor beta chain gene in the diagnosis of lymphoproliferative disorders. Lancet 1:1295, 1985

Papadimitriou CS, Muller-Hermelink V, Lennert K: Histologic and immunohistochemical findings in the differential diagnosis of chronic lymphocytic leukemia of B-cell type and lymphoplasmacytic/lymphoplasmacytoid lymphoma. Virchows Arch [A] 384:149, 1979

Patel S, Rootman J: Nodular sclerosing Hodgkin's disease of orbit. Ophthalmology 90:1433, 1983

Portlock CS, Rosenberg SA: No initial therapy for stage III and IV non-Hodgkin's lymphomas of favourable histologic types. Ann Intern Med 90:10, 1979

Rassiga AL: Advances in adult non-Hodgkin's lymphoma: Current concepts of classification, diagnosis, and management. Arch Intern Med 140:1647, 1980

Risdall R, Hoppe RT, Warnke R: Non-Hodgkin's lymphoma: A study of the evolution of the disease based upon 92 autopsied cases. Cancer 44:529, 1979

Rootman J, Patel S, Jewell L: Polyclonal orbital and systemic infiltrates. Ophthalmology 91:1112, 1984

Rosenberg SA: Current concepts in cancer: Non-Hodgkin's lymphoma–selection of treatment on the basis of histologic type. N Engl J Med 301:924, 1979

Sigelman J, Jakobiec FA: Lymphoid lesions of the conjunctiva: Relation of histopathology to clinical outcome. Ophthalmology 85:818, 1978

Taylor CR: An immunohistological study of follicular lymphoma, reticulum cell sarcoma and Hodgkin's disease. Eur J Cancer 12:61, 1976

Turner RR, Colby TV, Doggett RS: Well-differentiated lymphocytic lymphoma. Cancer 54:2088, 1984

Turner RR, Egbert P, Warnke RA: Lymphocytic infiltrates of the conjunctiva and orbit: Immunohistochemical staining of 16 cases. Am J Clin Pathol 81:447, 1984

Vogiatzis KV: Lymphoid tumors of the orbit and ocular adnexa: A long-term follow-up. Ann Ophthalmol 16:1046, 1984

Warnke R, Pederson M, Williams C et al: A study of lymphoproliferative diseases comparing immunofluorescence with immunohistochemistry. Am J Clin Pathol 70:867, 1978

Yeo JH, Jakobiec FA, Abbott GF et al: Combined clinical and computed tomographic diagnosis of orbital lymphoid tumors. Am J Ophthalmol 94:235, 1982

PLASMA CELL TUMORS

Azar HA: Pathology of multiple myeloma and related growths. In Azar H, Potter M (eds): Multiple Myeloma and Related Disorders, Vol 1, pp 1–85. New York, Harper & Row, 1973

Benjamin I, Taylor H, Spindler J: Orbital and conjunctival involvement in multiple myeloma. Am J Clin Pathol 63:811, 1975

Bush SE, Goffinet DR, Bagshaw MA: Extramedullary plasmacytoma of the head and neck. Radiology 140:801, 1981

Char DH, Norman D: The use of computed tomography and ultrasonography in the evaluation of orbital masses. Surv Ophthalmol 27:49, 1982

Clarke E: Plasma cell myeloma of the orbit. Br J Ophthal 37:543, 1953

Coppeto JR, Monteiro MLR, Collias J et al: Foster-Kennedy syndrome caused by a solitary intracranial plasmacytoma. Surg Neurol 19:267, 1983

Davis LE, Drachman DB: Myeloma neuropathy. Arch Neurol 27:507, 1972

Dolin S, Dewar JP: Extramedullary plasmacytoma. Am J Pathol 32:83, 1956

Fine RS, Amjad H, Schneider JR: Case report plasmacytoma presenting as unilateral proptosis. Postgrad Med 64:178, 1978

Hamburger HA: Orbital involvement in multiple myeloma a new angiographic presentation. J Clin Neuro Ophthalmol 4:25, 1984

Harwood AR, Knowling MA, Bergsagel DE: Radiotherapy of extramedullary plasmacytoma of the head and neck. Clin Radiol 32:31, 1981

Hayes JG, Petersen M, Kakulas BA: Multiple myeloma with bilateral orbital infiltration and polyneuropathy. Med J Aust 2:276, 1980

Hellwig CA: Extramedullary plasma cell tumors as observed in various locations. Arch Pathol 36:95, 1943

Jonasson F: Orbital plasma cell tumors. Ophthalmologica 177:152, 1978

Kennerdell JL, Jannetta PJ, Johnson BL: A steroid sensitive intracranial plasmacytoma. Arch Ophthalmol 92:393, 1974

Khalil MK, Huang S, Viloria J et al: Extramedullary plasmacytoma of the orbit: Case report with results of immunocytochemical studies. Can J Ophthalmol 16:39, 1981

Kim H, Heller P, Rappaport H: Monoclonal gammopathies associated with lymphoproliferative disorders: A morphologic study. Am J Clin Pathol 59:282, 1973

Kincaid MC, Green WR: Diagnostic methods in orbital diseases. Ophthalmology 91:719, 1984

Knowles DM, Halper JA, Trokel S et al: Immunofluorescent and immunoperoxidase characteristics of IgD myeloma involving the orbit. Am J Ophthalmol 85:485, 1978

Knowling MA, Harwood AR, Bergsagel DE: Comparison of extramedullary plasmacytomas with solitary and multiple plasma cell tumor of bone. J Clin Oncol 1:255, 1983

Kurzel RB, Mausolf R: Orbital involvement of an extramedullary plasmacytoma. Ophthalmologica 176:241, 1978

Kyle RA: Multiple myeloma review of 869 cases. Mayo Clin Proc 50:29, 1975

Levin SR, Spaulding AG, Wirman JA: Multiple myeloma: Orbital involvement in a youth. Arch Ophthalmol 95:642, 1977

Lewiski UH, Klein B, Gafter U et al: Acute plasma cell leukemia followed by extramedullary plasmacytoma. Br J Haematol 24:131, 1980

Macfadzean RM: Orbital plasma cell myeloma. Br J Ophthal 59:164, 1975

Maeda Y, Tani E, Nakano M et al: Plasma cell granuloma of the fourth ventricle. J Neurosurg 60:1291, 1984

Mewis-Levin L, Garcia CA, Olson JD: Plasma cell myeloma of the orbit. Ann Ophthalmol 17:477, 1981

Mill WB, Griffith R: The role of radiation therapy in the management of plasma cell tumors. Cancer 45:647, 1980

Mustoe TA, Fried MP, Goodman ML et al: Osteosclerotic plasmacytoma of maxillary bone (orbital floor). J Laryngol Otol 98:929, 1984

Nikoskelainen E, Dellaporta A, Rice T et al: Orbital involvement by plasmacytoma report of two cases. Acta Ophthalmol 54:755, 1976

Pasmantier MW, Azar HA: Extraskeletal spread in multiple plasma cell myeloma. Cancer 23:167, 1969

Rodman HI, Font RL: Orbital involvement in multiple myeloma review of the literature and report of three cases. Arch Ophthal 87:30, 1972

Rowan, RM: Multiple myeloma: Some recent developments. Clin Lab Haematol 4:211, 1982

Sayre RW, Castellino RA: Extramedullary plasmacytoma: Angiographic findings. Radiology 99:329, 1971

Schreiman JS, McLeod RA, Kyle RA et al: Multiple myeloma: Evaluation by CT. Radiology 154:483, 1985

Seddon JM, Corwin JM, Weiter JJ et al: Solitary extramedullary plasmacytoma of the palpebral conjunctiva. Br J Ophthalmol 66:450, 1982

Tong D, Griffin TW, Laramore GF et al: Solitary plasmacytoma of bone and soft tissues. Radiology 135:195, 1980

Vaquero J, Areito E, Martinez R: Intracranial parasellar plasmacytoma. Arch Neurol 39:738, 1982

Wiltshaw E: The natural history of extramedullary plasmacytoma and its relation to solitary myeloma of bone and myelomatosis. Medicine 55:217, 1976

Woodruff RK, Whittle JM, Malpass JS: Solitary plasmacytoma 1: Extramedullary soft tissue plasmacytoma. Cancer 43:2340, 1979

Yee RD, Savage DD, Cogan DG et al: Plasma cell infiltration of the conjunctiva associated with pancytopenia, dermatitis and polyclonal gammopathy. Am J Ophthalmol 82:486, 1976

BURKITT'S LYMPHOMA

Banks PM, Arseneau JC, Gralnick HR et al: American Burkitt's lymphoma: A clinicopathologic study of 30 cases. II. Pathologic correlations. Am J Med 58:322, 1975

Berard CW, O'Conor GT, Thomas LB et al (eds): Histopathological definition of Burkitt's tumor. Bull WHO 40:601, 1969

Burkitt D: A sarcoma involving the jaws in African children. Br J Surg 46:2018, 1958

Burkitt D, O'Conor GT: Malignant lymphoma in African children. I. A clinical syndrome. Cancer 14:258, 1961

De Thé G: Role of Epstein-Barr virus in human diseases: Infectious mononucleosis, Burkitt's lymphoma and nasopharyngeal carcinoma. In Klein G (ed): Viral Oncology, Vol 2, p 769. New York, Raven Press, 1980

Feman SS, Niwayana G, Hepler RS et al: "Burkitt tumor" with intraocular involvement. Surv Ophthalmol 14:106, 1969

Flandrin G, Brouet JC, Daniel MT et al: Acute leukemia with Burkitt's tumor cells: A study of six cases with special reference to lymphocyte surface markers. Blood 45:183, 1975

Henle W, Henle G: Evidence for an oncogenic potential of the Epstein-Barr virus. Cancer Res 33:1419, 1973

Lukes RJ, Collins RD: New approaches to the classification of the lymphomata. Br J Cancer [Suppl 2] 31:1, 1975

Mann RB, Jaffe ES, Berard CW: Malignant lymphomas: A conceptual understanding of morphologic diversity. Am J Pathol 94:105, 1979

Mann RB, Jaffe ES, Braylan RC et al: Non-endemic Burkitt's lymphoma: A B-cell tumor related to germinal centers. N Engl J Med 295:685, 1976

O'Conor GT, Rappaport H, Smith EB: Childhood lymphoma resembling "Burkitt's tumor" in the United States. Cancer 18:411, 1965

Wright DH: Burkitt's lymphoma: A review of the pathology, immunology and possible etiologic factors. Pathol Annu 6:336, 1971

Ziegler JL: Treatment results of 54 American patients with Burkitt's lymphoma are similar to the African experience. New Engl J Med 297:75, 1977

Ziegler JL, Magrath IT: Burkitt's lymphoma. Pathobiol Annu 4:129, 1974

LEUKEMIA: GRANULOCYTIC SARCOMA

Brugo EA, Larkin E, Molina-Escobar J et al: Primary granulocytic sarcoma of the small bowel. Cancer 35:1333, 1975

Cavdar AO, Arcasoy A, Gozdaxoglu S et al: Chloroma-like ocular manifestations in Turkish children with acute myelomonocyte leukemia. Lancet 1:680, 1971

Edgerton AE: Chloroma: Report of a case and a review of the literature. Trans Am Ophthalmol Soc 45:376, 1947

Krause JR: Granulocytic sarcoma preceding acute leukemia. Cancer 44:1017, 1979

Leder LD: Ueber die selektive Ferment cytochemische Darstellung von neutrophilen myeloischen Zellen und Gewebsmastzellen im Paraffinschnitt. Klin Wochenschr 42:553, 1964

Liu PI, Ishimaru T, McGregor DH et al: Autopsy study of granulocytic sarcoma (chloroma) in patients with myelogenous leukemia, Hiroshima-Nagasaki 1949–1969. Cancer 31:948, 1973

Long JC, Berard CW: Short Course 42: The Pathology of Lymph Nodes. New Orleans, International Academy of Pathology, 1980

Mason TE, Demaree RS Jr, Margolis CI: Granulocytic sarcoma (chloroma) two years preceding myelogenous leukemia. Cancer 31:423, 1973

Wiernik PH, Serpick AA: Granulocytic sarcoma (chloroma). Blood 35:361, 1970

Zimmerman LE, Font RL: Ophthalmologic manifestations of granulocytic sarcoma (myeloid sarcoma or chloroma). Am J Ophthalmol 80:975, 1975

HODGKIN'S LYMPHOMA

Consul BN, Kulshrestha OP: Hodgkin's disease and bilateral exophthalmos. Am J Ophthalmol 56:462, 1963

Fratkin JD, Shammas HF, Miller SD: Disseminated Hodgkin's disease with bilateral orbital involvement. Arch Ophthalmol 96:102, 1978

Patel S, Rootman J: Nodular sclerosing Hodgkin's disease of the orbit. Ophthalmology 90:1433, 1983

Sen DK, Mohan H, Chatterjee PK: Hodgkin's disease of the orbit. Int Surg 55:183, 1971

T-CELL LYMPHOMAS

Bunn PA Jr, Carney DN: Treatment of cutaneous T-cell lymphoma. J Dermatol Surg Oncol 6:383, 1980

Chu AC: The use of monoclonal antibodies in the in situ identification of T-cell subpopulations in cutaneous T-cell lymphoma. J Cutan Pathol 10:479, 1983

Edelson RL: Cutaneous T cell lymphoma: Mycosis fungoides, Sézary syndrome, and other variants. J Am Acad Dermatol 2:89, 1980

Edelson RL: Cutaneous T cell lymphoma. J Dermatol Surg Oncol 6:358, 1980

Edelson RL, Raafat J, Berger CL et al: Antithymocyte globulin in the management of cutaneous T cell lymphoma. Cancer Treat Rep 63:675, 1979

Epstein EH, Jr: Mycosis fungoides: Clinical course and cellular abnormalities. J Invest Dermatol 75:103, 1980

Epstein EH, Jr, Levin DL, Croft JD, Jr et al: Mycosis fungoides: Survival, prognostic features, response to therapy, and autopsy findings. Medicine 51:61, 1972

Haynes BF, Metzgar RS, Minna JD et al: Phenotypic characterization of cutaneous T cell lymphoma: Use of monoclonal antibodies to compare with other malignant T cells. N Engl J Med 304:1319, 1981

Levi JA, Wiernik PH: Management of mycosis fungoides: Current status and future prospects. Medicine 54:73, 1975

Lutzner M, Edelson R, Schein P et al: Cutaneous T cell lymphomas: The Sézary syndrome, mycosis fungoides, and related disorders. Ann Intern Med 83:534, 1975

Meekins B, Proia AD, Klintworth GK: Cutaneous T cell lymphoma presenting as a rapidly enlarging ocular adnexal tumor. Am Acad Ophthalmol 92:1288, 1985

Rappaport H, Thomas LB: Mycosis fungoides: The pathology of extracutaneous involvement. Cancer 34:1198, 1974

Safai B, Good RA: Lymphoproliferative disorders of the T cell series: A review. Medicine 59:335, 1980

Stenson S, Ramsay DL: Ocular findings in mycosis fungoides. Arch Ophthalmol 99:272, 1981

Vonderheid EC: Evaluation and treatment of mycosis fungoides lymphoma. Int J Dermatol 19:182, 1980

HISTIOCYTOSIS X

Avery ME, McAfee JG, Guild HG: The course and prognosis of reticuloendotheliosis (eosinophilic granuloma, Schuller-Christian disease and Letterer-Siwe disease): A study of forty cases. Am J Med 22:636, 1957

Baghdassarian SA, Shammas HF: Eosinophilic granuloma of orbit. Ann Opthalmol 9:1247, 1977

Chawla HB, Cullen JF: Eosinophilic granuloma of the orbit. J Pediatr Ophthalmol 5:93, 1968

Crocker A: The histiocytosis syndromes. In Fitzpatrick T, Arndt K, Clark WH et al (eds): Dermatology in General Medicine, 1st ed, p 1328. New York, McGraw-Hill, 1971

Enriquez P, Dahlin DC, Hayles AB et al: Histiocytosis X: A clinical study. Mayo Clin Proc 42:88, 1967

Favara BE, McCarthy RC, Mierau GW: Histiocytosis X. Hum Pathol 14:663, 1983

Heuer HE: Eosinophilic granuloma of the orbit. Acta Ophthalmol 50:160, 1972

Lichtenstein L: Histiocytosis X: Integration of eosinophilic granuloma of bone, "Letterer-Siwe disease," and "Schuller-Christian disease" as related manifestations of a single nosologic entity. Arch Pathol 56:84, 1953

Lichtenstein L, Jaffe HL: Eosinophilic granuloma of bone: With report of a case. Am J Pathol 16:595, 1940

Nesbit ME, Wolfson JJ, Kieffer SA et al: Orbital sclerosis in histiocytosis X. Am J Roentgenol 110:123, 1970

Oberman HA: Idiopathic histiocytosis: A correlative review of eosinophilic granuloma, Hand-Schuller-Christian disease and Letterer-Siewe disease. J Pediatr Ophthalmol 5:86, 1968

Straatsma BR: Eosinophilic granuloma of bone. Trans Am Acad Ophthalmol Otolaryngol 62:771, 1958

MALIGNANT HISTIOCYTOSIS

Ballard J, Binder R, Rath C et al: Malignant histiocytosis in a patient presenting with leukocytosis, eosinophilia, and lymph node granuloma. Cancer 35:1444, 1975

Henderson DW, Sage RE: Malignant histiocytosis with eosinophilia. Cancer 32:1421, 1973

Ho FCS, Todd D: Malignant histiocytosis. Cancer 42:2450, 1978

Lampert IA, Catovsky D, Bergier N: Malignant histiocytosis: A clinico-pathological study of 12 cases. Br J Haematol 40:65, 1978

Scott RB, Robb-Smith AHT: Histiocytic medullary reticulosis. Lancet 2:194, 1939

Stein RS, Moran EM, Byrne GE, Jr: Malignant histiocytosis: complete remission with combination chemotherapy. Cancer 38:1083, 1976

Vilpo JA, Klemi P, Lassial O et al: Cytological and functional characterization of three cases of malignant histiocytosis. Cancer 46:1795, 1980

Warnke RA, Kim H, Dorfman RD: Malignant histiocytosis (histiocytic medullary reticulosis). Cancer 35:215, 1975

Zucker JM, Caillaux JM, Vanel D et al: Malignant histiocytosis in childhood. Cancer 45:2821, 1980

CHAPTER 11

Graves' Orbitopathy

Jack Rootman; Radiology by Robert Nugent

Graves' orbitopathy has been known for close to 200 years. The literature is replete with diverse nomenclature, diagnostic groupings, classifications, and eponyms, making it difficult in the practical situation to appreciate the nature of this disorder as it presents in the individual patient. We have chosen to refer to the orbital changes and ocular abnormalities of this disorder as *thyroid orbitopathy* or *Graves' orbitopathy* because it is an orbital rather than ophthalmic process. Not all cases are thyroid related, but the orbital process appears to be the same even in the absence of detectable thyroid abnormality. The ocular changes associated with thyroid disease were first published by Graves in 1835 and by Von Basedow in 1840, but were apparently noted in 1825 by Parry (published posthumously). It is the most common cause of unilateral or bilateral proptosis and, as such, has been the subject of a vast and exhaustive literature including two recent books by Char and by Gorman, Waller, and Dyer. It would be impossible in the context of this book to deal with the subject in such depth, but this chapter will attempt to highlight the major features of Graves' orbitopathy based on our experience of 675 cases to provide practical guidelines and our current management philosophy.

Graves' orbitopathy usually occurs in association with hyperthyroidism (frequently close to or within 18 months of hyperthyroidism), but the onset, course, severity, and relationship to the systemic disease is variable. In addition, subclinical thyroid abnormalities or even normal thyroid function may be noted in some patients with typical features of Graves' orbitopathy. It is best understood if the dynamics of the pathophysiologic situation are individualized and the physician attempts to deal with the patient on this basis. Management should consist of a coordinated multidisciplinary medical–surgical approach based on clinical–pathophysiologic inference, staging of the disease, and knowledge of its effects on the orbital and ocular structures. Broadly speaking, management is directed towards abatement or control of inflammation, prevention of ocular and psychovisual damage, redressing ocular motor abnormalities, and improving cosmetic disfigurement.

■ PATHOGENESIS, PATHOLOGY, AND PATHOPHYSIOLOGY

Graves' orbitopathy occurs in a genetically preselected population affecting females (usually middle-aged females) four to five times more frequently than males. The propensity for development of and, indeed, the severity of thyroid disorder and orbital disease may be related to immunogenetic predisposition. Patients with HLA-DR3 histocompatibility loci may be genetically predisposed to thyroid disease. The cause remains unknown, but an accumulating body of evidence links both the infiltrative orbitopathy and the thyroid disorder to immune mechanisms with both cell-mediated and humoral components. It may be initiated by a primary abnormality of immune surveillance or by an intrinsic cellular disorder with secondary autoimmune phenomena. Evidence suggests that the orbital disease is a very closely related but separate organ-specific autoimmune disorder with target autoantigens and circulating autoantibodies. Others have argued that both the thyroid disease and the orbitopathy have a uniform and singular etiology. The orbital and eye muscle antigens may be linked to thyroiditis by shared antigenicity. The extraocular muscles, connective tissue, and possibly the lacrimal gland are believed to be the target for cell-mediated immunologic reactions (involving T-, B-, and/or K- [killer] lymphocytes). The inherited defect in immunoregulation may lead to abnormalities of function of suppressor T-lymphocytes, which then fail to prevent proliferation of randomly mutating B-lymphocytes. These B-lymphocytes produce autoantibodies that target orbital tissues and extraocular muscle fibers. In addition, absent or poorly functioning T-suppressor lymphocytes allow influx of cytotoxic T-lymphocytes, which contribute to eye muscle damage and affect other orbital tissues. Pathologic study, orbital imaging, and clinical inference suggest the major target affected is the extraocular muscles. The immune-mediated process leads to inflammation and deposition of hydrophilic mucopolysaccharides and collagen, resulting in muscle injury and scarring.

Eighty percent of patients who develop thyroid orbi-

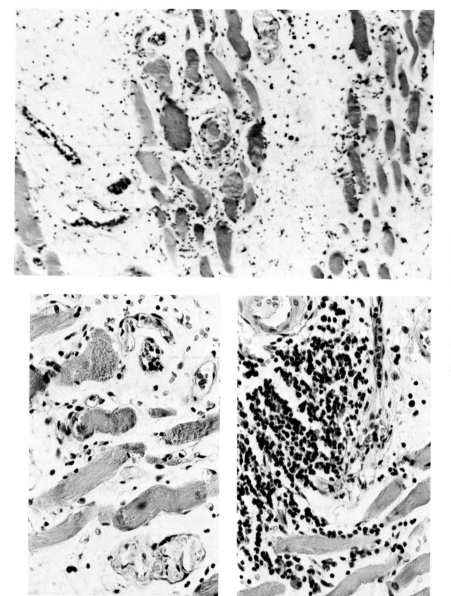

FIGURE 11-1. Histopathology of the typical features of thyroid orbitopathy. The scattered inflammatory infiltrate has some foci of more intense cellularity consisting of plasma cells, lymphocytes, and occasional mast cells. The muscle fibers appear distended and there is a loose, mucopolysaccharide-rich stroma (H&E, original magnifications *top* ×10, *bottom* ×2.5).

topathy do so either during or after an episode of hyperthyroidism. Nevertheless, it may present without evidence of hyperthyroidism, and on careful evaluation of the response to hormone stimulation the patient may show autonomous thyroid function (euthyroid Graves' disease). A small number of patients fail to demonstrate any thyroid abnormality even with T3 suppression or TRH stimulation tests (ophthalmic Graves' diseases). In addition, 10% of patients with thyroid orbitopathy suffer from hypothyroidism or autoimmune thyroiditis.

The pathology of orbital involvement reflects the immunopathogenic mechanism suggested. The extraocular muscles are infiltrated by lymphocytes, plasma cells, and mast cells; and deposition of hydrophilic mucopolysaccharides and formation of collagen cause degenerative changes in the extraocular muscles, reflecting target effects on the orbital myocyte and the endomysial fibroblast. The plasma cells mediate the release of mucopolysaccharides and the formation of collagen by the fibroblasts. The varying pathology reflects the intensity and stage of the disease when tissues are examined. There is usually a moderate inflammatory cell infiltration with plasma cells, lymphocytes, and mast cells surrounding blood vessels and muscle fibers (Fig. 11-1). This is associated with separation of the muscles fibers by a loose, mucopolysaccharide-rich stroma. With increasing severity and duration of inflammation, stromal collagen deposition and muscle degeneration may be noted (Fig. 11-2). Ultimately, as the disease passes into a more quiescent stage, the degenerated muscle tissues may be replaced by fat (Fig. 11-3).

The local pathophysiology reflects several interacting and variable factors that explain the broad spectrum of presentation. These factors include the degree and rapidity of inflammation, the mass effect, orbitoseptal relationships (compliance), absence of deep orbital lymphatics, and location of disease. Inflammation induces muscle swelling and contributes to chemosis, tearing, injection, and discomfort. It is the middle and posterior thirds of the muscles that are primarily affected by the disease process. The progressive swelling of the extraocular muscles (mass effect), collagen deposition, and damage contribute to the development of extraocular motor abnormalities, psychovisual defects, and exposure. The interaction of inflammation, mass effect, and orbital compliance (*i.e.*, tightness of the orbital septal complex or "box") govern the secondary effects of this disease, and lead to manifestations of venous obstruction, increased congestion, and progressive symptoms. The absence of deep orbital lymphatics in association with the venous obstruction tax the lymphatics of the lid and conjunctiva, and contribute to the disproportionate swelling of the anterior structures. Another major aspect governing the effects of this disease is the location of the process within the orbit. For example, apical muscle swelling is the major pathogenetic factor involved in the development of psychovisual deficit, which may be out of proportion to the degree of either inflammation or apparent overall mass effect but correlates well with myopathy. In addition, the degree and site of involvement of single or multiple muscles affects the clinical presentation of the myopathy.

■ CLINICAL CONSTELLATIONS

As noted, the dynamics of Graves' orbitopathy are variable and result in a spectrum of presentations that reflect the speed, nature, and severity of the specific orbital involvement. However, there are two major clinical groups: the mild or so-called noninfiltrative orbitopathy and the infiltrative or severe orbitopathy. Broadly speaking, those cases that appear to reflect either a minimal inflammatory reaction or slow alteration in orbital mass fall into the noninfiltrative category. Patients in this group usually present with evidence of lid retraction and minimal discomfort with or without a degree of exophthalmos, and they are often younger. In contrast, cases that have a more fulminant course with significant infiltration, inflammation, and scarring are categorized as infiltrative. These patients have disease with a disturbing spectrum of early ocular discomfort, swelling of the lids and conjunctiva, diplopia, corneal exposure, proptosis, and optic neuropathy. Clinically significant infiltrative orbitopathy is seen in 3% to 5% of patients with hyperthyroidism, but subclinical evidence of orbital disease is present in most patients with diffuse goiter and hyperthyroidism. Pretibial myxedema and the infiltrative orbitopathy are frequently seen in the same group of patients.

Werner's classification of ocular involvement has six classes, each with varying degrees of severity (Table 11-1). Basically, 90% of cases are noninfiltrative and fall into classes 0 or 1. Class 1 cases produce signs without symptoms including lid retraction, lid lag, and exophthalmos up to but not exceeding 22 mm (Figs. 11-4, 11-5). Classes 2 through 6 have infiltrative disease and account for 10% of all cases of Graves' hyperthyroidism. In these cases, the orbital volume may increase up to 400%.

Class 2 describes the soft tissue changes including lacrimation, fullness of the lids (with a tendency to diurnal variation), conjunctival injection, and a gritty, burning sensation (see Fig. 11-2). Van Dyk has suggested a modification of class 2 orbital changes, listing them as six soft tissue signs:

- Resistance to retrodisplacement of eye,
- Edema of conjunctiva and caruncle,
- Lacrimal gland enlargement,
- Injection of the conjunctiva,
- Edema, and
- Fullness of the lids.

The first letter of each sign forms the mnemonic "relief." Infiltrative orbitopathy tends to be associated with a characteristic pattern of swelling and fullness of the lids. Usually it starts in the upper lids, and often the patient is aware of swelling of the medial followed by a distinct fullness of the lateral portion of the lid. The lid usually has a slightly rosy appearance to it, particularly laterally. Patients are also aware of development of bagginess of the lower lids and a tendency for the lids to be more tense and edematous in the morning and after recumbency.

Class 3 delineates the degree of proptosis as minimal (21 mm – 23 mm), moderate (24 mm – 27 mm), or marked (28 mm or more).

Class 4 describes extraocular muscle involvement. This develops in a number of patterns that reflect the clinical incidence of muscle involvement with inferior rectus (hypotropia; Fig. 11-6) being most frequent, medial rectus (esotropia; Fig. 11-7) second most frequent, and superior (hypertropia; Fig. 11-8) and lateral rectus (exotropia) least frequent. The dynamic balance of muscles affected correlates with the specific clinical presentation.

Corneal affectations delineated by class 5 are due to multiple factors including the degree of exposure from proptosis, lagophthalmos, lid retraction, abnormal blinking, absence of a Bell's phenomenon related to inferior rectus tethering, and changes in tear film and secretion

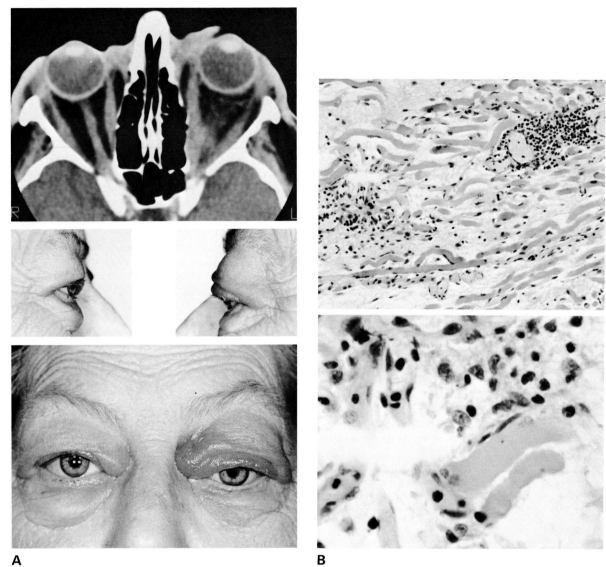

A   **B**

FIGURE 11-2.   *(A)* This 67-year-old woman was seen 6 months after the onset of a cryptogenic bilateral orbital inflammatory syndrome, which was worse on the left than on the right. It was characterized by chemosis, proptosis, marked lid edema, and injection of the skin and conjunctiva. She had exophthalmometry of 19 mm on the right and 22 mm on the left with 2 mm of downward displacement, and marked limitation of elevation, abduction, adduction, and infraduction on the left side, and limitation of abduction on the right. She had a 25-D left hypotropia due to a restrictive myopathy. Vision was 20/20 on the right and 20/40 on the left, and visually evoked response was delayed on the left, with an acquired red/green defect. She had been thoroughly investigated for thyroid disease, and all tests (including TRH stimulation test) were negative. The axial CT scan demonstrates bilateral myopathy, enlarged anteriorly displaced lacrimal glands, and some left apical crowding. On the left side there is also evidence of infiltration of orbital fat, an unusual (but not unknown) feature of thyroid orbitopathy. *(B)* Because of the unusual orbital infiltration, a perconjunctival biopsy of orbital muscle was done. It demonstrated infiltration by focal and scattered plasma cells and lymphocytes surrounding blood vessels and adjacent to some muscle fibers. Note the loose stroma with collagen deposition (H&E, original magnifications *top* ×10, *bottom* ×40).

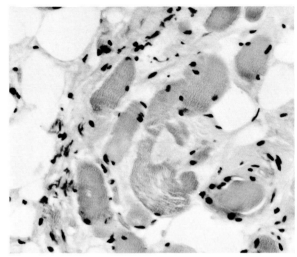

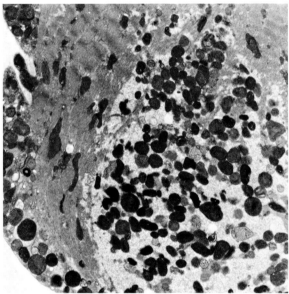

C

(C) Degenerative changes (swelling and disruption) of the muscle on light *(top)* and electron *(bottom)* microscopy. The electron micrograph shows massive accumulations of mitochondria (some swollen, others degenerating) within the disrupted muscle fiber (H&E, original magnifications *top* × 25, *bottom* × 11,750). Immunohistochemical stains using antithyroglobulin antibody did not show cross-reactivity with the muscle membranes. This case demonstrates a more severe stage of thyroid orbitopathy than that seen in Figure 11-1. The patient was treated with orbital radiotherapy. She recovered her vision, and the soft tissue signs and symptoms improved, but the restrictive component of her myopathy progressed.

(Fig. 11-9). Exposure may ultimately lead to clouding, necrosis, and even perforation in rare circumstances. The constant exposure and drying of the eye may lead to a secondary infection, which can sometimes be disastrous depending on the organism. Another unusual but not infrequent association with thyroid abnormality is the development of superior limbic keratoconjunctivitis (Fig. 11-10).

Class 6 is sight loss due to optic nerve involvement. Optic neuropathy is categorized on the basis of mild, moderate, or severe visual deficit (Figs. 11-11, 11-12).

The Werner classification allows us to record the clinical status of a patient, but does not reflect a continuum of disease or progression in an individual patient. In the practical situation one tends to define the ocular management protocol primarily on the basis of evidence of inflammaton (activity and progression), degree of myopathy, and threat to vision. Therefore, we prefer to categorize patients into major subgroups of noninfiltrative or infiltrative disease. Those whith infiltrative disease can be further categorized in terms of inflammation, degree of clinical myopathy, or the constellation of features that suggests apical orbital crowding and optic neuropathy.

Noninfiltrative Disease

Patients with noninfiltrative disease may simply have lid lag, stare, or retraction or all three as part of the overall manifestations of hyperthyroidism. This may regress in some patients with control of hyperthyroidism. On the other hand, there is a group, particularly those with adolescent or young adult onset, that is characterized by lid retraction, lid lag, and proptosis without significant manifestations of myopathy or functional visual deficit (see Fig. 11-4). In spite of the fact that patients may not have clinical evidence of a myopathy, the majority have subclinical orbital disease as suggested by a raised intraocular pressure on upgaze or ultrasonography and CT evidence of slightly enlarged extraocular muscles (see Fig. 11-5). These patients may have a significant degree of proptosis, but rarely encounter serious ocular problems. The CT findings in this group consist of mild extraocular muscle enlargement with a disproportionate degree of proptosis that may reflect some increase in the fat volume. The pathogenesis, differential diagnosis, and management of lid malposition will be discussed later.

Infiltrative Disease

Infiltrative disease manifests along three major lines, which may be independent or concurrent. These are frank soft tissue features, myopathy, and the crowded orbital apex syndrome.

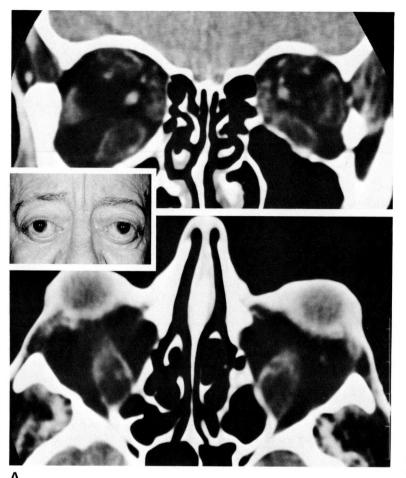

A

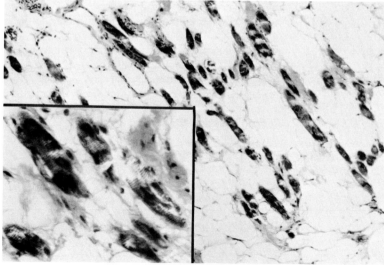

B

FIGURE 11-3. *(A)* This patient demonstrates the features of a long-standing thyroid orbitopathy with severe exophthalmos. It had been present for 35 years, and its onset was associated with hyperthyroidism. The axial and coronal CT scans demonstrate enlarged and multiple low-density foci within all of the muscles. He was referred with severe and acute corneal exposure. He underwent decompression, when a muscle biopsy was also done. *(B)* Photomicrograph demonstrates replacement of the degenerated muscle by bundles of fat (PTAH, original magnification × 10, *inset* × 25).

TABLE 11-1.
DETAILED CLASSIFICATION OF EYE CHANGES OF GRAVES' DISEASE

Grade	Suggestions for Grading
Class 0	No physical signs or symptoms
Class 1	Only signs (signs limited to upper lid retraction, stare, and lid lag)
Class 2	Soft-tissue involvement with symptoms and signs
0	Absent
a	Minimal
b	Moderate
c	Marked
Class 3	Proptosis 3 mm or more in excess of upper normal limits, with or without symptoms
0	Absent
a	3- to 4-mm increase over upper normal
b	5- to 7-mm increase
c	8 mm or more increase
Class 4	Extraocular muscle involvement (usually with diplopia, other symptoms, and other signs)
0	Absent
a	Limitation of motion of extreme gaze
b	Evident restriction of motion
c	Fixation of globe or globes
Class 5	Corneal involvement (primarily due to lagophthalmos)
0	Absent
a	Stippling of cornea
b	Ulceration
c	Clouding, necrosis, perforation
Class 6	Sight loss (due to optic nerve involvement)
0	Absent
a	Disc pallor or choking, or visual field defect; vision 20/20 to 20/60
b	Same, but vision 20/70 to 20/200
c	Blindness; i.e., failure to perceive light, vision <20/200

(Werner SC: Modification of the classification of the eye changes of Grave's disease: Recommendations of the Ad Hoc Committee of the American Thyroid Association. J Clin Endocrinol Metab 44:203, © by The Endocrine Society, 1977)

SOFT TISSUE FEATURES

As stated previously, the soft tissue features of infiltrative disease consist of conjunctival swelling (chemosis), vascular engorgement, injection, lid edema, tearing, lacrimal gland enlargement, and surface discomfort. In most circumstances, these signs appear to develop in a subacute or chronic pattern. That is, the onset and progression is over months and may be intermittent and variable in course. However, in a retrospective questionnaire to patients, we have found that they are usually aware of a relatively precise onset of the soft tissue signs and symptoms and are able to pinpoint a time of onset of lid swelling and ocular discomfort.

There are a number of practical tips with regard to early clinical diagnosis. The earlier manifestations are related to the effect of inflammation and pressure within the orbit. The patient often presents to the general practitioner with intermittent lid swelling that has a diurnal pattern, generally worse in the morning after lying prone all night, which may lead to a misdiagnosis of allergic disease. In contrast to allergy, these patients tend to be aware of some retrobulbar discomfort, intermittent asthenopia, and ocular fatigue (particularly with reading). Further, they do not have evidence of conjunctival follicle formation or seasonal relationships. It is also important to keep in mind that they frequently present with asymmetric disease, one orbit more involved than the other. The infiltration, edema, and proptosis affect the conjunctival structures and lead to burning, injection, grittiness, and an excessive outpouring of mucus with intermittent blurring of vision. This may be coupled with an abnormal lid position and chemosis, which may cause functional or physical obstruction of the lacrimal drainage system, leading to epiphora.

We have occasionally encountered some patients who have a disproportionate degree of lid swelling when compared to their epibulbar and myopathic symptoms. They usually evidence a rather pale, edematous, noninjected distention of the lower lids, which tends to be sensitive to anti-inflammatory intervention (steroids, radiotherapy) (Fig. 11-13).

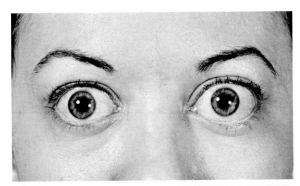

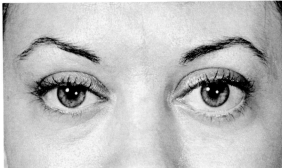

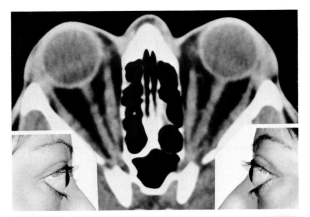

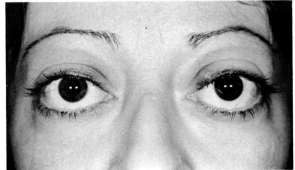

FIGURE 11-4. *(Top)* This 30-year-old woman demonstrates the features of noninfiltrative orbitopathy, consisting of very mild proptosis and lid retraction occurring concomitant to hyperthyroidism. *(Bottom)* Photograph taken 1 year later shows her postoperative appearance after a graded upper lid lengthening procedure (müllerectomy).

FIGURE 11-5. This 32-year-old woman demonstrates the features of noninfiltrative thyroid ophthalmopathy persisting 3 years after the onset and treatment of hyperthyroidism. Her major clinical features were exophthalmos (23 right, 24 left), normal ocular movements, and a 6-mm rise in intraocular pressure on upgaze. The axial CT scan shows mild bilateral swelling of the extraocular muscles with an apparent increase in fat volume and anterior displacement of the lacrimal glands.

MYOPATHY

Infiltration and scarring of the muscles generally manifest as diplopia with limitation of ocular movement that is classically intermittent in onset, occasionally sudden and permanent, progressive in many, and spontaneously reversible in rare instances. Myopathy is frequently associated with the soft tissue inflammatory signs, but it can occur in few muscle groups asymmetrically and with few inflammatory signs and symptoms.

When the patient begins to have oculomotor involvement, the early symptoms are frequently related to the apparent propensity of this disorder to affect the vertical muscles. Thus, the patients are more vulnerable in positions of gaze requiring use of these muscles and at times of day when orbital edema is maximal, that is, in the morning. They are often aware of diplopia when lying in bed, a position that forces use of the vertical muscles. This diplopia is characteristically present for the first few hours of the day in the early stages; however, with time it may become persistent throughout the day. In addition, patients with myopathy frequently become aware of an inability to read for extended periods of time (fatiguability and discomfort) early in the course of their disease. This is related to decreased convergence.

The frequency of clinical occurrence in myopathy in descending order is usually inferior rectus, medial rectus, superior rectus, and lateral rectus involvement (see Figs. 11-6 to 11-8). With progression, the degree of deviation increases, particularly in patients who have asymmetrical disease. In contrast, patients with symmetrical disease affecting the vertical muscles often show lesser degrees of

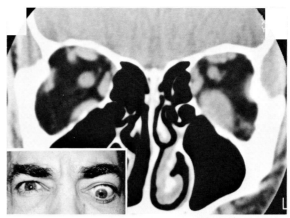

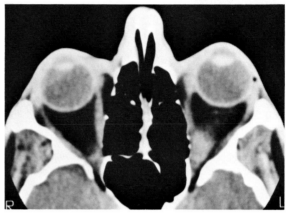

FIGURE 11-6. Although thyroid orbitopathy is usually characterized by involvement of more than one muscle, this 47-year-old man demonstrates a striking unilateral left inferior rectus myopathy (30-D left hypotropia). Complete investigations, including TRH stimulation test, revealed normal thyroid function. He subsequently developed mild disease affecting the right eye. The coronal and axial CT scans demonstrate the enlarged inferior rectus. The axial scan has an appearance that may be mistaken for an apical orbital mass (lollipop sign). After stabilization, he underwent a left inferior rectus and right superior rectus adjustable recession and achieved orthophoria in the primary position and to 20 degrees upgaze and 50 degrees downgaze. He subsequently underwent bilateral müllerectomies and a left lower lid elevation.

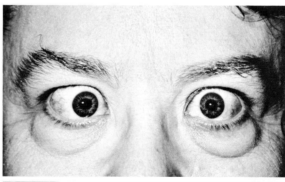

FIGURE 11-7. This 43-year-old woman originally presented 1 year after treatment of hyperthyroidism, at which time she had bilateral optic neuropathy associated with swelling of the optic nerve head and symmetrical severe limitation of ocular movements. CT scan at that time demonstrated apical orbital crowding. She underwent bilateral ethmoidal decompression with recovery of vision. *(Top)* Her appearance is shown 6 months after decompression, when she had developed a 30-D esotropia. *(Bottom)* Her postoperative appearance is shown following a bimedial rectus recession with a right adjustable suture.

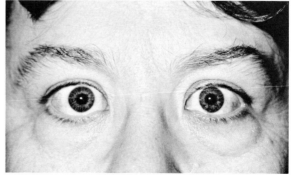

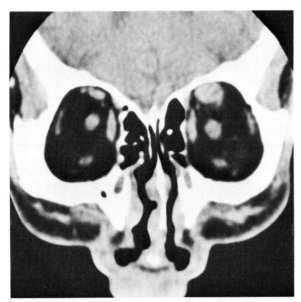

FIGURE 11-8. Coronal CT scan demonstrates an unusual appearance of thyroid-related myopathy with predominant enlargement of the left superior rectus muscle. It was seen in a 67-year-old man who presented with a left hypertropia 2 years after being diagnosed as hypothyroid. He had a 30-D left hypertropia and a positive forced duction test involving the left superior rectus.

vertical deviation because of commitant degrees of involvement. On the other hand, increasing medial myopathy is associated with progressive esodeviation. The majority of patients have some degree of asymmetry in the onset and progression of their myopathy. With increasing involvement of the muscle, the anterior radicals of the muscular vessels become engorged, producing characteristic dilated and visible vessels subconjunctivally over the insertions (see Fig. 11-12). As the muscles tether, they become ridgid on forced duction testing and the degree to which the intraocular pressure rises on movement opposite to the field of action of the muscle is greater.

There is an unusual and small subcategory of patients who present with a fulminant inflammatory and myopathic syndrome. We have seen four patients in this category out of 675 thyroid orbitopathies (Fig. 11-14). They had an acute myositis characterized by a very rapid (acute —days) onset of orbital inflammation, congestion, chemosis, injection, and *painful* limitation of ocular movements. In every respect, they parallel the nonspecific orbital inflammatory myositic syndromes except that they demonstrate an association with an underlying thyroid disorder (*i.e.*, a nonsuppressible thyroid gland). This particular subcategory is exquisitely sensitive to treatment with corticosteroids, and emphasizes the need to rule out thyroid disorders in acute myositis. The differential features of thyroid myopathy and orbital myositis have been discussed in Chapter 9. In fact, the majority of patients with myositis do not have thyroid abnormalities.

It should be noted that thyroid orbitopathy has an infrequent association with myasthenia gravis. We have had three such cases. This should be suspected when the patient demonstrates a variable ptosis, a changing or unusual deviation, and a negative or incongruous forced duction test.

DYSTHYROID OPTIC NEUROPATHY: THE CROWDED ORBITAL APEX SYNDROME

Jack Rootman and Janet M. Neigel

Optic neuropathy in patients with Graves' orbitopathy has long been recognized as a serious and often alarming complication of Graves' disease. The pathogenesis has been ascribed to many different causes including toxic optic neuropathy, but more recently has been attributed to apical orbital crowding. We have reviewed the clinical and computed tomographic findings for 95 eyes with dysthyroid optic neuropathy and compared them to the control thyroid orbitopathy group (119 eyes) without optic neuropathy (Table 11-2). Our experience confirmed orbital crowding as the major mechanism and identified clinical signs and symptoms that reflect crowding of the orbital apex leading to a specific psychovisual and motor syndrome (Fig. 11-15). This syndrome affected 58 (8.6%) of a total of 675 patients with thyroid orbitopathy.

Clinically the major manifestation of this insidious disease is optic neuropathy, but it has other features of orbital crowding such as proptosis, palpable lacrimal glands, increased intraocular pressure in upgaze, marked oculomotor limitation, and soft tissue components. In short, this group of patients has physical findings that reflect a more severe degree of myopathy when compared to a control group of patients with thyroid orbitopathy. In addition, these features may obscure that diagnosis and dominate the symptoms, leading to a failure of physician and patient to recognize the insidious onset of optic neuropathy. In fact, in half of the instances on referral, neither the physician nor the patient was aware of the early signs of optic neuropathy. This situation implies a need to be particularly vigilant in patients who have the constellation of findings suggesting predisposition to optic neuropathy.

The optic neuropathy patients are older at the time of examination and are more likely to be male (Fig. 11-16). Diabetics seem to have a greater risk for optic neuropathy, a stormier and more recalcitrant course, and, overall, tend to have more severe optic neuropathy. The chief (Text continues on p. 254.)

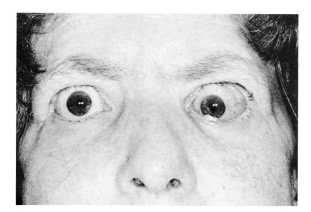

FIGURE 11-9. The features of corneal exposure in thyroid orbitopathy. *(Top)* This 54-year-old woman was seen 3 years after the concomitant development of hyperthyroidism and orbital disease. She had bilateral corneal exposure due to lid retraction, exophthalmos, and marked restriction of upgaze. On the left side, she had a hypotropia with trichiasis. *(Center)* Corneal drying secondary to marked chemosis is shown. *(Bottom)* This patient presented with a right *Pseudomonas* corneal ulcer secondary to severe exophthalmos, lagophthalmos, and bilateral inferior rectus restrictive myopathy.

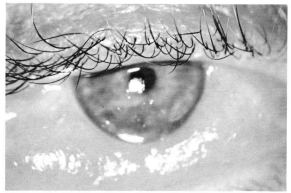

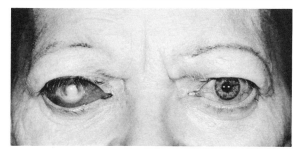

FIGURE 11-10. The features of superior limbic keratoconjunctivitis. This nonspecific condition has no known cause, but when bilateral, it is frequently associated with dysthyroid states. This patient is a 41-year-old woman who had developed mild thyroid orbitopathy associated with hyperthyroidism 1 year prior to this presentation.

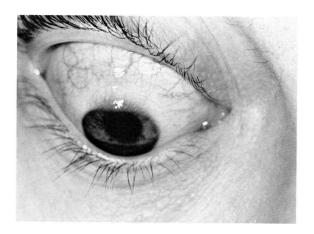

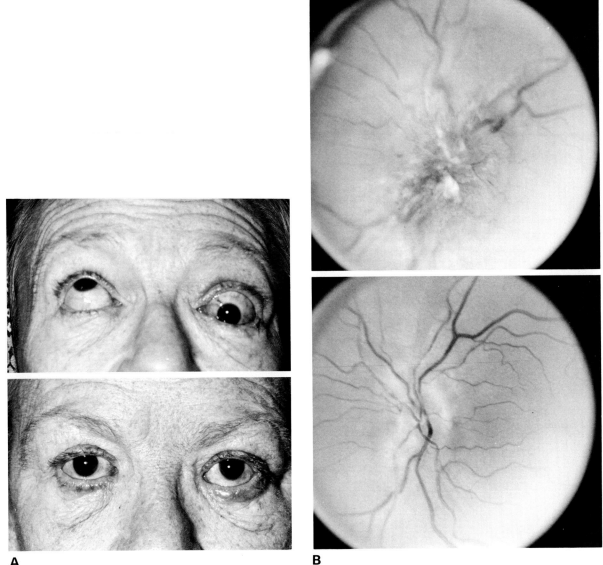

A   **B**

FIGURE 11-11. *(A, top)* This 65-year-old woman was referred with severe thyroid ophthalmopathy some months after a right inferior rectus recession. On presentation, she had a marked right hypertropia with tethering of the left inferior and right superior rectus associated with a weakness of the right inferior rectus secondary to over-recession. She had a history of thyroid orbitopathy that presented 25 years earlier and 3 years before the onset of thyrotoxicosis. *(B, top)* Photograph of the left fundus at the time of presentation shows papilloedema and venous engorgement. The patient's vision was 20/50. *(A and B, bottom)* The patient is shown following bilateral orbital decompression combined with a short course of corticosteroids and followed by strabismus surgery. Her vision recovered to 20/25.

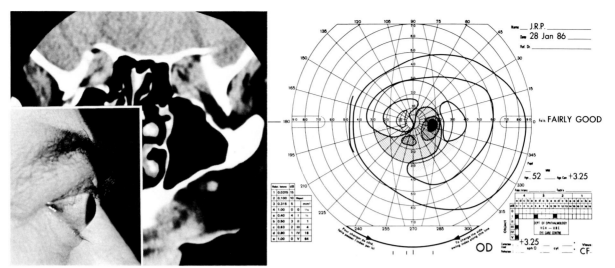

FIGURE 11-12. This patient first presented in 1976 at age 43, 10 years after an episode of hyperthyroidism, with progressive thyroid orbitopathy present for 1 year. He had 23 mm of proptosis on the right and 20 mm on the left. He was treated with systemic steroids, which led to gradual improvement over the next 6 months. He underwent bilateral müllerectomy in 1979 and was stable until 1985, when he again presented with progressive proptosis that developed over a 9-month period and measured 28 mm bilaterally. It was associated with a marked diminution in vision occurring over a 3-week period. He had counting fingers vision at 8 feet on the right and was 20/20 on the left. *(Left)* The lateral view demonstrates engorgement of the vessels over the lateral rectus muscle, and the coronal CT scan shows marked apical orbital crowding. *(Right)* The right visual field shows an inferior arcuate scotoma. The patient underwent bilateral three-wall orbital decompression with a short course of steroids. Within 1 month his vision returned to 20/25 right and 20/20 left, and exophthalmometry measured 22 mm bilaterally. Postoperatively, he developed an esotropia. During follow up 8 months later, he had a recurrence of right optic neuropathy. His vision dropped to 20/40, and he developed a paracentral scotoma in spite of adequate decompression visualized on CT scan. He underwent orbital radiotherapy (2000 cGy in ten fractions) combined with a short term of corticosteroids, and his vision returned to 20/20 within 1 month. He subsequently underwent successful strabismus surgery after having been stable for 1 year. His case demonstrates the characteristic features of apical orbital crowding and the sometimes variable and recalcitrant course of infiltrative thyroid orbitopathy.

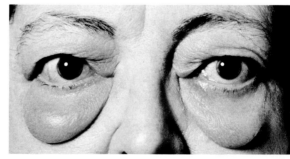
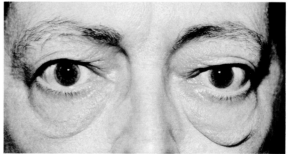

FIGURE 11-13. This 61-year-old woman with thyroid orbitopathy demonstrates a disproportionate swelling of the anterior soft tissues. It was exquisitely sensitive to steroids, as shown in the lower photograph taken 2 weeks after induction of steroid treatment (30 mg/day tapered to 15 mg/day). In spite of the marked lid swelling, she had 20 mm of proptosis, mild muscle enlargement, and normal extraocular movements. Withdrawal of steroids caused recurrence of the marked lid swelling.

253

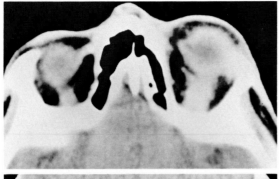

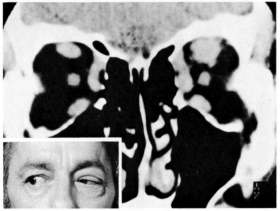

FIGURE 11-14. This 49-year-old man presented with a 3-week history of painful, tender swelling of the left upper lid, and injection and chemosis associated with ptosis. He had pain on ocular movement and was becoming aware of diplopia on upgaze. Physical examination revealed a left ptosis with 2 mm of downward displacement and 1 mm of proptosis. CT scans demonstrate an enlarged left superior rectus muscle with infiltration of the adjacent orbital fat. From a medical point of view, he had a history of ankylosing spondylitis and on investigation had a normal free thyroxine level, a low TSH level, and did not respond to TRH stimulation. These findings were compatible with euthyroid Graves' disease. The orbital myositis responded dramatically to oral steroids. This patient demonstrates the unusual association of acute myositis with abnormality of thyroid function.

presenting symptom that differentiates optic neuropathy patients from others with thyroid orbitopathy is graying of vision or desaturation of colors. Patients rarely volunteered this information unless specifically questioned. They frequently have a tight orbital septum and often complain of an aching fullness or pressure like sensation behind the eyes, suggesting apical orbital crowding.

In our experience, the orbital physical findings that should alert the clinician to optic neuropathy are more marked proptosis; palpable lacrimal glands; a greater increase in intraocular pressure on upgaze; a greater restriction of extraocular muscles, particularly in superduction and abduction; and a greater incidence of vertical tropia (see Table 11-2 and Fig. 11-11). We noted that the muscle restriction is often bilateral but asymmetrical, in contrast to Trobe and co-workers, who noted symmetry. Others have suggested that proptosis was not helpful in assessing the risk of optic neuropathy; however, we found that, overall, patients with optic neuropathy had greater degrees of proptosis. The most significant physical features correlate with *severity of myopathy,* suggesting that the risk of optic neuropathy is related to increase in extraocular muscle volume.

Visual acuity was poorer in the optic neuropathy group, but was certainly not as poor as might be expected with some patients still able to read 20/20. Ophthalmo-

scopy of the optic nerve head was also a less consistent indicator; slightly less than half of the patients had normal-appearing discs. Nevertheless, elevation and hyperemia or pallor are significant signs. Afferent pupillary defect was not a consistent finding and its absence usually reflects bilateral compression. Visual field abnormalities included increased size of blind spot, paracentral scotoma, nerve fiber bundle defect, central or centrocecal scotoma, and generalized constriction. These defects appeared in isolation or in varying combinations. As noted by others, six out of seven nerve fiber bundle defects were inferior (Figs. 11-17, 11-18; also see Figs. 11-12 and 11-16). We had also noted a vertical step in four visual fields, including one that was bilateral. In our experience, color vision is a relatively sensitive indicator of optic nerve dysfunction and is a simple and reliable test that can be routinely applied in the clinical setting. The most sensitive test was visually evoked potential, which serves as a good indicator of optic nerve dysfunction and a means of following patients, especially after treatment. A number of patients with severe apical crowding may have an associated congestion of the choroid that leads to striae in the posterior pole.

In summary, from a clinical point of view, optic neuropathy is frequently insidious, may be masked by other symptoms, and may be missed unless specifically elicited.

TABLE 11-2.
DYSTHYROID OPTIC NEUROPATHY VERSUS THYROID ORBITOPATHY CONTROL, UNIVERSITY OF BRITISH COLUMBIA ORBITAL CLINIC, 1976–1986

	Dysthyroid Optic Neuropathy	Thyroid Orbitopathy Control
Sex	F:M, 1.6:1	F:M, 3.3:1
Age		
At diagnosis	57.5 years	49.2 years
At onset of thyroid orbitopathy	53.6 years	46.4 years
Systemic associations		
Diabetes	15.5%	1.7%
Physical findings		
Average proptosis	23.2 mm	20.5 mm
Palpable lacrimal gland	33.3%	12.9%
Intraocular pressure		
Primary position	20.9 mm Hg	17.6 mm Hg
Upgaze	30.2 mm Hg	21.5 mm Hg
Difference	9.5 mm Hg	4.5 mm Hg
Extraocular movements		
Restriction	Greater in all fields	Less in all fields
	Less symmetrical ductions	More symmetrical ductions
	Worse tropias	Less severe tropia
	More vertical tropia	Less vertical tropia
	Vertical, 67.3%	Vertical, 33%
	Esotropia, 26.9%	Esotropia, 13.3%
	Exotropia, 13.5%	Exotropia, 13.3%
Abnormal Disc	52.6%	2.5%
Elevation and hyperemia	28.6%	1.7%
Pallor	24.2%	0.8%
Visual function		
Vision 20/40 or better	52.6%	96.6%
Afferent pupillary defect	34.8%	1.7%
Abnormal VEP	94.0%	9.1%
Visual field defect	63.7%	0
Color vision	64.0%	22.0%

Our observations suggest the group of patients to suspect are older, more frequently male, have a later onset of thyroid disease, and are more frequently diabetic. The most sensitive indicator of incipient neuropathy was abnormality of visually evoked potentials. On physical examination, these patients have more proptosis, a higher incidence of significant vertical deviation, and more severe limitation of extraocular movements. In addition, this greater severity of myopathy was reflected in higher increases in intraocular pressure on upgaze. In effect, the more severe the disease in terms of the myopathy, the greater the index of suspicion for optic neuropathy.

CT scan is perhaps the single most important laboratory test when optic neuropathy is suspected. The findings of apical crowding, increased proptosis, enlarged muscle diameter, increased superior ophthalmic vein diameter, and anterior displacement of the lacrimal gland should alert the clinician to a possible optic neuropathy, and appropriate psychophysical and electrophysiologic testing should be done. Another feature that may indicate apical crowding is evidence of a realtively sudden angulation of the posterior third of the muscle as it abuts on the optic nerve (see Fig. 11-15). In particular, coronal scans are most useful in assessing the degree of crowding of the apex and the relief of this following operative decompression (Fig. 11-19). This crowding, along with inflammation, is the physiological basis for the compromised venous outflow, neuropraxia, reduced axonal transport, and restricted ocular movements that constitute this syndrome. All muscle indices (extraocular muscle diameters; muscle diameter index, *i.e.*, the sum of all mean muscle diameters) were significantly increased in optic neuropathy orbits as opposed to non-neuropathy orbits. Examination of muscle enlargement ratios (*i.e.*, the ratio of maximum muscle diameter of each muscle compared to the same muscle in a group of normals) showed a portional enlargement of the major muscle groups in neuropathy and non-neuropathy thyroid orbi-

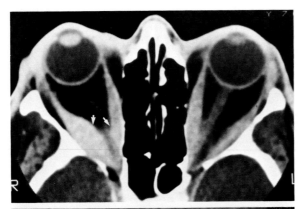

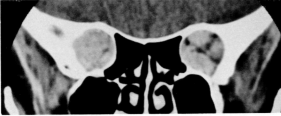

FIGURE 11-15. Axial and coronal CT scans demonstrate the features of apical orbital crowding in dysthyroid optic neuropathy. Note the dramatic involvement of the posterior half of the muscle belly and the acute angulation *(arrows)* of the right medial and lateral rectus in the axial CT scan, as well as obliteration of the perineural fat on the coronal scan.

topathies. However, the degree of enlargement was greater in those patients with optic neuropathy. This suggests that no specific muscle or group of muscles was enlarged out of proportion in neuropathy orbits. Increases in superior ophthalmic vein diameter and retrobulbar optic nerve sheath diameters (due to expansion of the subarachnoid space) were noted in optic neuropathy orbits as opposed to those without. The overall constellation of symptoms, signs, psychophysical findings, and CT investigations outlined should raise the clinical index of suspicion and lead to prompt recognition and management of optic neuropathy.

Lid Malposition in Thyroid Orbitopathy

Lid malpositions, particularly upper lid retraction, are probably the most common ocular features of thyroid orbitopathy. However, lower lid retraction, ptosis, and entropion may occur. The lid malpositions contribute to the exposure, tearing, and cosmetic deformity of Graves' orbitopathy. The major pathophysiologic mechanisms for lid retraction are fibrosis and contracture of the upper or lower musculoaponeurotic complexes, and possibly

sympathetic stimulation or increased sympathetic tone. In addition, proptosis contributes to lid retraction and exposure. The degree of lid retraction may be variable as a manifestation of sympathetic stimulation, overmedication (thyroid replacement), or natural anxiety level. Upper lid retraction is often worse in acute thyrotoxicosis or when the patients are anxious at the time of examination (a factor that should be taken into account when assessing lid retraction).

Some acute upper lid retraction has been ascribed to sympathetic stimulation or increased sensitivity to circulating catecholamines. However, in a clinical, CT, and pathologic study of patients undergoing müllerectomy for lid retraction, we have found that features of smooth muscle damage were not evident and the factor that best correlated with lid retraction was evidence of involvement of the superior striated muscle complex (Fig. 11-20). In his extensive review of thyroid orbitopathy, Surgott supports this concept as the major mechanism of lid retraction.

Upper lid retraction is often the first sign, and may be asymmetrical and intermittent in onset. It is often associated with some evidence of swelling of the lid, but this need not necessarily be the case. There is a tendency for the upper lid to show some lateral arching, and on downward pursuit, lid lag or a staccato-like delayed movement is noted. Exact quantification of upper lid retraction can be difficult, so it is probably best classified in terms of a mild, moderate, or severe degree of retraction. Mild lid retraction usually implies intersection of the lid with the upper limbus; moderate suggests 3 mm to 4 mm of scleral show; and severe suggests more than 4 mm of scleral show.

The patient with only lid retraction invokes the differential diagnosis outlined in Table 11-3. The major causes are neurologic abnormalities, cicatricial processes, and ocular and orbital malposition.

In addition to lid retraction, a small percentage of patients with thyroid orbitopathy are prone to the development of ptosis. The major cause is stretching of the capsulo palpebral structures and infrequently an association of thyroid orbitopathy with myasthenia gravis. Patients with Graves' disease have a higher incidence of other autoimmune-related diseases including myasthenia gravis. Concurrent myasthenia gravis should be suspected in patients who have ptosis, an unusual strabismus (*e.g.,* exodeviation), markedly variable diplopia, or fluctuating lid retraction. Thus, care should be taken to assess patients for a nonsclerotic component to their myopathy (*i.e.,* negative forced duction or failure of the forced duction to correlate with degree of deviation). Long-standing and severe proptosis may lead to ptosis as a result of stretching of the levator structures, wherein there is evidence of thinning of the aponeurosis, absence of an upper lid fold, and general lengthening of the lid. Finally,

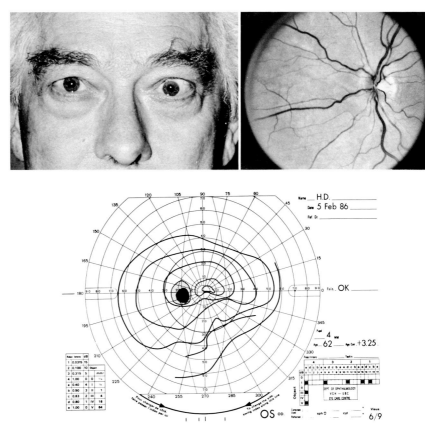

FIGURE 11-16. This 62-year-old man was referred with diplopia, proptosis, and lid swelling of 1-month's duration, and desaturation of left color vision for 3 months. He had been treated for hyperthyroidism at the onset of his orbitopathy. On physical examination his vision was 20/20 right, 20/25 left. Exophthalmometry was 18.5 right and 20 left, and there was an 8-D right hypertropia and 12-D esotropia with marked limitation of ductions bilaterally. On fundus examination he had slightly hyperemic discs with minimal blurring of the nasal margin. He had been treated with high-dose steroids and had failed to respond visually. His VEP showed a large delay in implicit times from the left eye, and Goldmann visual fields demonstrated an inferior nasal depression with a small relative paracentral defect. CT scan demonstrated severe apical crowding bilaterally. He underwent bilateral apical decompressions with full recovery of vision and an increase in esotropia to 30-D. He subsequently had bimedial recession with adjustable sutures, and is currently orthophoric.

it should be noted that in our experience, ptosis can be a feature of severe apical orbital crowding in a particularly tight orbit. We have noted in such instances that following decompression, lid retraction usually replaces the ptosis.

Lower lid retraction reflects the same pathogenetic mechanisms as the upper, but tends to be more constant in appearance. In combination with proptosis and chemosis, it may significantly increase epiphora—a common feature of thyroid orbitopathy. The poor lid position interferes with the normal flow of tears and the chemosis may act as an obstructive element in the punctal region.

Entropion and lateral lid elevation are more commonly seen as a complication of decompressive or lid surgery.

A particularly striking eyelid malposition phenomenon that we rarely noted is the tendency for the lower lid to contract in a peculiar manner in circumstances of severe proptosis. These patients demonstrate a horizontal shortening of the lower lid associated with blinking, rather than a relaxation. This contraction of the lid may occasionally be associated with retroplacement behind the equator and an alarming, acute proptosis that can be reversed by relaxation of the lid and gently applying pressure to the globe.

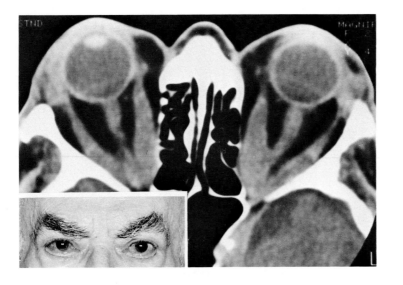

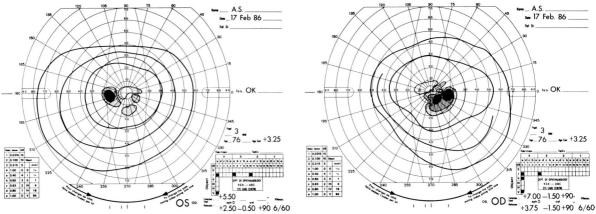

FIGURE 11-17. This 76-year-old man was referred with Graves' orbitopathy that began 4 months after treatment for hyperthyroidism. He had developed progressive proptosis, soft tissue signs, chemosis, and reduction of vision to counting fingers bilaterally. In spite of treatment with 100 mg prednisone when referred, his vision was 20/400 right and 20/200 left. Exophthalmometry was 21 bilaterally, and he had marked symmetrical limitation of ocular movements. Fundus examination revealed choroidal striae. Axial CT scan demonstrates apical compression, proptosis, and anterior displacement of the lacrimal gland. Visual fields showed bilateral inferior scotomata that are worse on the right than on the left. He underwent bilateral apical decompression with removal of the medial wall and floor by means of an ethmoidal incision. At follow up 2 months later, his vision was 20/40 bilaterally with retention of a small paracentral scotoma on the left side.

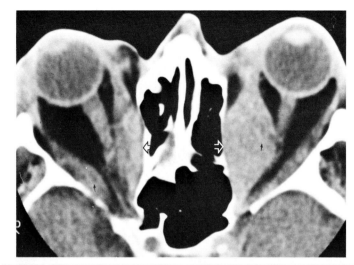

FIGURE 11-18. This 76-year-old man developed hyperthyroidism 13 years prior to referral. His initial orbitopathy was noted 5 years after treatment with radioactive iodine. On presentation he was aware of deteriorating vision (worse on the left than on the right), increasing proptosis, and fading of color vision. On physical examination he had vision of 20/20-1 right, and 20/40 unimprovable on the left. He had palpable lacrimal glands, markedly widened interpalpebral fissures, and 27 mm of exophthalmos bilaterally. There was bilateral limitation of elevation and inferior punctate keratopathy. CT scans demonstrated apical crowding that was worse on the left than on the right with medial bowing (Coca-Cola sign; *large arrows*) into the ethmoids, marked proptosis, anterior displacement of lacrimal glands, and low-density areas within muscles *(small arrows)*. Visual field showed an inferior arcuate scotoma on the left, and VEP demonstrated bilateral optic neuropathy more severe on the left. In view of the degree of proptosis and the apical orbital crowding, the patient underwent a left three-wall decompression and a right two-wall decompression. Postoperatively his vision improved to 20/25 left, and exophthalmometry was 20 bilaterally with recovery of fusion.

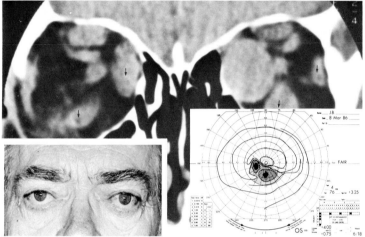

■ DIAGNOSIS OF GRAVES' ORBITOPATHY

Although most cases of Graves' orbitopathy occur during or after a hypermetabolic state (80%), this is not necessarily true for all patients. As noted earlier, subclinical thyroid abnormalities or even a euthyroid status may be associated with the typical orbital disorder. There are a number of methods that help in the diagnosis of euthyroid orbitopathy (Table 11-4). In the realm of laboratory testing, autonomy of glandular function can be demonstrated in 86% of euthyroid patients with progressive or active orbital disease. The classic T_3 suppression or Werner test will identify 75% of these cases. Thyrotropin-releasing hormone (TRH) can also be used to demonstrate thyroid autonomy. The recently described immunoradiometric assay of thyrotropin may aid in the diagnosis of borderline hyperthyroidism. In spite of this, a small group of patients may not demonstrate any identifiable laboratory abnormality, yet have the features of thyroid orbital disease, suggesting a clinically distinct disorder of isolated Graves' orbitopathy. In addition, a wide range of immunological tests are being studied that may help to elucidate the character and pathogenesis of this disorder. These include a search for thyroid-stimulating immunoglobulins and thyroid antibodies. Wall, in a review of humoral mechanisms in Graves' orbitopathy, has noted circulating autoantibodies against an eye muscle-derived soluble antigen that appears to correlate with active Graves' orbitopathy, its clinical severity, and the effect of treatment.

In the last few decades improvements in orbital imaging have allowed for identification, diagnosis, and characterization of patients who may be clinically or chemi-

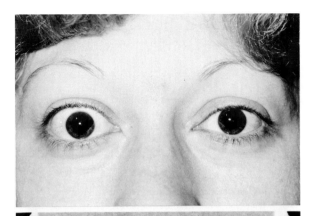

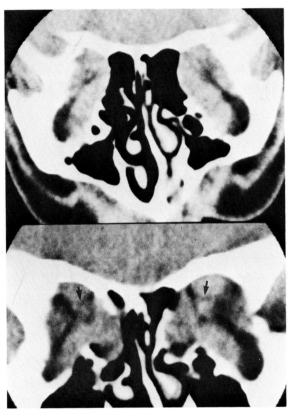

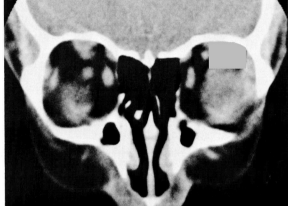

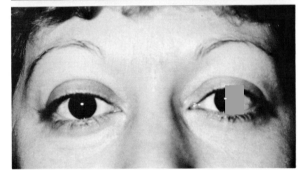

FIGURE 11-19.   Coronal CT scans before *(top)* and after *(bottom)* decompression demonstrate relief of crowding of the apex of the orbit following medial decompression for optic neuropathy. Note reappearance of fat zone around the optic nerve *(arrows)*.

FIGURE 11-20.   *(Top)* This 30-year-old woman presented 4 years after an episode of hyperthyroidism with right lid retraction. *(Center)* The coronal CT scan demonstrates a very slight enlargement of the superior muscle complex. *(Bottom)* The patient's appearance is shown after a graded right müllerectomy.

cally diagnosed and those who cannot. Again, it should be noted that a significant increase (more that 3 mm Hg) in intraocular pressure related to positional change (upward gaze) usually suggests thyroid-related orbital disease. Ultrasonography can demonstrate subtle changes occurring in extraocular muscles and the orbital fat. These changes are reflected in an irregular posterior outline of the retrobulbar fat pattern, quantifiable enlargement of the extraocular muscles, and accentuation of the orbital walls. The enlarged muscles show intramuscular echoes due to separation of the muscle bundles (Fig. 11-21). Optic neuropathy may be associated with expansion and reduplication of the distal portion of the optic nerve sheath due to expansion of the subarachnoid space. A-scan demonstrates high acoustic reflectivity in the muscle bellies due to separation of the muscle fibers.

The CT findings classically consist of enlargement of the extraocular muscles. In our experience, about 90% of patients with thyroid orbitopathy will have bilateral CT abnormalities, even if the clinical involvement is unilateral. Relatively symmetrical CT findings are seen in 60% to 70% of patients, and any of the extraocular muscles can be involved. CT evidence of enlargement is most frequently and easily identified in the inferior rectus, followed closely by the medial rectus, and less frequently by involvement of the superior and lateral recti, which parallels the clinical oculomotor manifestations. When assessing the extraocular muscle size on CT scan and comparing it to the normal size of muscle, we have noted that the superior muscle group is more frequently involved than has heretofore been suspected. This feature helps to explain the almost universal presence of lid retraction in thyroid orbitopathy, and reflects the normal gradation and size relationships of the extraocular muscles on coronal CT scan. Superior oblique muscle enlargement can be readily identified but appears to occur less often. The inferior oblique muscle, because of its anterior position relatively close to the globe, is difficult to assess. Typically, enlargement involves the muscle belly, from the annulus to the origin of the tendon, and so occurs primarily behind the posterior margin of the globe. However, in our experience there are rare patients who show thickening of the tendinous portion. Also noted early in the development of thyroid myopathy are areas of low density within the muscle bellies. These areas may represent lymphorrhages (focal accumulation of lymphocytes) or mucopolysaccharide deposition. These low-density areas can measure up to one cm, but are more commonly only a few millimeters in size. With long-standing disease, larger low-density areas may appear in the muscle, probably representing fatty replacement (see Fig. 11-3). The CT features that suggest optic neuropathy have been previously outlined and are best noted in coronal views, although the reduced size of the space surrounding the posterior portion of the optic nerve and the previously

TABLE 11-3.
DIFFERENTIAL DIAGNOSIS OF EYELID RETRACTION IN THYROID EYE DISEASE

Graves' disease

Neurologic disease
  Marcus Gunn phenomena
  Midbrain disease
  Hydrocephalus
  Parinaud's syndrome
  Trauma to cranial nerve III
  Aneurysm involving cranial nerve III

Sympathomimetic drugs

Cirrhosis

Congenital

Postsurgical retraction
  Ptosis surgery
  Lid reconstruction

(Waller RR, Samples JR, Leatts RP: Eyelid malpositions in Graves' disease. In Gorman CA, Waller RR, Dyer JA: The Eye and Orbit in Thyroid Disease, p 263. New York, Raven Press, 1984)

TABLE 11-4.
SEQUENTIAL LABORATORY APPROACH FOR THE DIAGNOSIS OF THYROID ORBITOPATHY

1. Serum T_4
2. Serum T_3
3. Resin T_3 uptake test
4. Calculated free T_4 index (thyroxine), free T_3 index
5. Thyrotropin receptor antibodies (TSI)
6. Antithyroid antibodies
7. Sensitive serum TSH test
8. TRH stimulation test
9. Thyroid (T_3 or Werner) suppression test

(Modified from Char DH: Thyroid Eye Disease. Baltimore, Williams & Wilkins, 1985; © 1985, the Williams & Wilkins Co., Baltimore)

mentioned sharp angulation of the posterior belly of the medial and lateral rectus muscles may be better appreciated on an axial view.

Generally, in infiltrative disease the extent of proptosis correlates with the degree of muscle enlargement, although there are exceptions. In noninfiltrative disease, there may be more evidence of increased fat than increased muscle bulk (Fig. 11-22). Infrequently, Graves' orbitopathy can be associated with changes in the bony orbit, particularly in patients with very long-standing and significant orbital crowding. This usually involves bowing of the medial wall and reduction in the size of the adjacent ethmoid sinuses (Coca-Cola sign; see Fig. 11-18). In addition, rare focal bony erosion of the roof has been described, but the bone here can be so thin as occasionally to appear deficient even in normal patients.

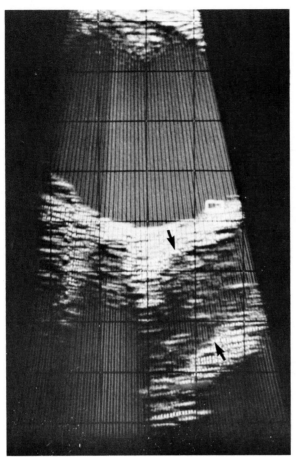

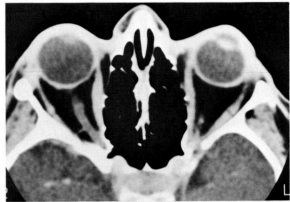

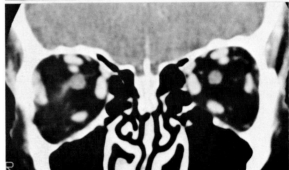

FIGURE 11-21. B-scan ultrasonography demonstrates enlargement of the lateral rectus muscle *(arrows)*, accentuation of the orbital wall, and intramuscular echoes in thyroid orbitopathy.

FIGURE 11-22. CT findings in a patient with moderate proptosis and clinically mild noninfiltrative orbitopathy. Note the relatively minor changes in muscle mass with significant proptosis.

Therefore, we believe that in most circumstances of thyroid orbitopathy focal erosion represents an artifact. The fat is usually lucent, but increased density of the orbital fat may be infrequently noted on CT (Fig. 11-23; also see Fig. 11-2). An additional finding that correlates with proptosis and crowding is forward displacement and slight enlargement (engorgement) of the lacrimal gland. The optic nerve may appear on occasion somewhat thin. In patients with rapid or severe proptosis, there may be traction on the globe producing "tenting" of the posterior globe.

■ MANAGEMENT

The categorization and management of the individual patient requires that the ophthalmologist bring to bear a broad range of expertise with definitive assessment of visual function, extraocular movement, visual fields, color vision, fluorescein angiography, and electrodiagnostic tests. Prospective observation of the intraocular pressure is important because many patients develop raised pressures, usually related to ocular position. The resting position of the eye is usually 5 to 10 degrees below the primary, and is the best position for accurate measurement of intraocular pressure. In patients who have significant inferior rectus tethering, the resting position may be even more inferior. It should also be noted that a number of patients with thyroid orbitopathy are already receiving topical steroids, which may exacerbate a rise in intraocular pressure.

Specific management or prevention awaits clearer elucidation of the pathogenesis of this disorder. For the most part, treatment is preventive and expectant because spontaneous remission and subsidence is characteristic. In addition, recurrence of Graves' orbitopathy is extremely rare; we have seen only a handful of patients with an apparent resurgence of orbitopathy. In most instances, it is more likely a low-grade progression.

From a practical point of view, it is very important to emphasize to the individual patient that the disease does remit, because they often feel that it will not abate, and they are distressed by the marked cosmetic disfigurement and the potential for visual loss. In our experience, many of these very anxious people will not volunteer their true degree of concern about fear of visual loss or the extreme disfigurement they feel. Sensitivity is required in eliciting their real feelings and providing the considerable reassurance and friendship they need. It is also important to make them aware of the availability of therapies and procedures that can successfully address their concerns about the functional, physical, and cosmetic defects.

The general course of active disease is from 6 months to 2.5 years. It tends to fluctuate from day to day, but an overall trend can be discerned on periodic examination of the patients. From a medical point of view, there are a number of significant things to keep in mind. Close cooperation with an endocrinologist or internist is essential to ensure a stable metabolic state and to evaluate patients for other systemic diseases. It has been suggested that hyperthyroidism does have some concurrent effect on the orbitopathy. Effective treatment is usually associated with improvement in the orbital problem. Some authorities believe that rapid development of post-therapy hypothyroidism is generally to be avoided because it may worsen the orbital process; however, this view is controversial. In our experience, patients with more severe orbital disease at the time of treatment of hyperthyroidism are more likely to have progressive changes after metabolic control.

It has been noted that children and teenaged females tend to be spared the severe and progressive orbital problems, and generally have a significantly milder oribitopathy.

The general principles of management consist of careful evaluation and categorization, early patient education, medical intervention to abate and control the course of infiltrative disease, and repair of mechanical and physical dysfunction. Mild and noninfiltrative disease can be observed or managed conservatively for a time to ensure nonprogression, and the problems of lid retraction and cosmesis can be dealt with subsequently. Patients with sight-threatening infiltrative disease require urgent medical and surgical management, and motor and cosmetic problems should be redressed later. The majority of non-sight-threatening infiltrative disease can be dealt with either by conservative local measures and careful periodic observation or by medical intervention (anti-inflammatories or radiotherapy or both) followed by muscle, lid, and cosmetic surgery. Thus, the major treatment concerns include addressing problems of infiltra-

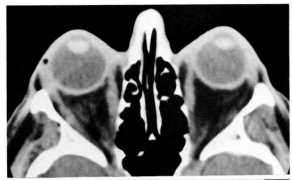

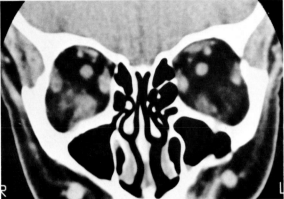

FIGURE 11-23. Axial and coronal CT scans demonstrate mild involvement of extraocular muscles with increased density of the orbital fat (a feature infrequently seen in thyroid orbitopathy) in a 65-year-old woman who developed thyroid orbitopathy 18 months after a thyroidectomy. Exophthalmometry was 21 bilaterally, and there was a 4-D esotropia with markedly widened interpalpebral fissures.

tive disease, exposure, and lid retraction, and the proper timing and choice of elective surgery.

Infiltrative Disease

Infiltrative disease can be sight threatening, and management requires careful judgment because treatment modalities are powerful and have significant side-effects. Medical measures for abating and controlling inflammation include the use of anti-inflammatory drugs, immunosuppressives, and radiotherapy. Several reports of the use of plasmapheresis for severe orbital disease have claimed improvement, but a large, controlled series has not yet been published. Wall and colleagues have detected a circulating antibody against eye muscle-derived soluble antigen, which may be useful in the diagnosis and management of patients with Graves' orbitopathy and bears some relationship to the severity of the eye disease.

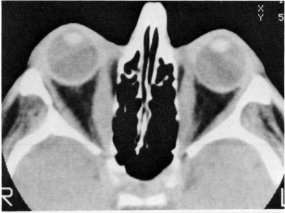

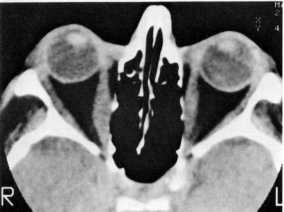

FIGURE 11-24. Improvement in the size of the extraocular muscles is demonstrated on axial CT scans taken before *(top)* and 1 month after *(bottom)* orbital radiotherapy for a euthyroid orbitopathy that was associated with significant soft tissue signs, exophthalmometry of 18 right and 17 left, and a 10-D esotropia. Clinically, the patient showed dramatic resolution of chemosis with improvement of lid edema and ocular comfort. The esotropia remained stable. He subsequently underwent a right medial rectus recession with adjustable suture.

Simple medical measures include elevating the head of the patient's bed to reduce periorbital edema, cool compresses, and ocular moisture chambers. Although diuretics are frequently prescribed by clinicians, we believe that they have little or no effect on the periorbital edema. The use of immunosuppressives such as cyclophosphamide and azathioprine (Imuran) have had questionable clinical value, as has the use of plasmaphoresis. In addition, there is not enough evidence to suggest that the benefits of any of these modalities clearly outweigh the risks. From a practical point of view, the two major antiinflammatory modalities in common clinical use are corticosteroids and orbital radiotherapy.

The role of corticosteroids in the treatment of this disorder is well established, but there are several tips and cautions in their use. These patients require titration because they clearly demonstrate critical dose levels to induce a response. Patients with primarily soft tissue signs require induction doses between 20 mg and 30 mg daily to be titrated downward or maintained on an alternate-day regimen at the lowest dose necessary to obtain and sustain relief. Those with severe congestion of the orbit and optic neuropathy may require heroic doses anywhere between 80 mg and 125 mg/day, titrated downward after evidence of response, which should be noted within 1 week or so. Steroids are effective in the sight-threatening situations and clearly reduce the degree of inflammation and swelling. It should be noted that as steroid dosage is brought down or discontinued, it is very common to experience rebound and resurgence of soft tissue signs and symptoms. Treatment of optic neuropathy may be plagued by recurrence following reduction of steroids. Patients with extraocular muscle involvement generally will have improvement in their soft tissue signs, but only about one third of them will show improvement in the extraocular movements on corticosteroids. One generally has to resort to use of prisms or surgery to deal with the final oculomotor abnormalities. Significant degrees of proptosis will also have to be dealt with surgically.

The efficacy of steroids should be balanced against the many systemic side-effects. In our experience, titrating the doses downward usually takes a long time, and to control soft tissue symptoms patients may be receiving intermittent steroids for anywhere between 3 months and 1 year. We have been impressed with the frequency with which patients receiving corticosteroids suffer side-effects, and even small doses can have serious side-effects. The severity varies from full-blown Cushing's syndrome to mild or minimal side-effects. These patients, who are already suffering major physical changes, now have the added problems of weight gain, acne, hirsutism, facial rubor, and weakness. We have also been impressed by the frequency with which patients complain of the effect of corticosteroids on personality, producing depression in some, and hyperactivity and sleeplessness in others. Aside from these side-effects one should be aware of the potential for osteoporosis, secondary infections, and glucose intolerance. Because of these many side-effects, we have developed a philosophy of avoiding the long-term use of steroids, using them in relatively low doses as an adjunctive measure or for short periods of time.

Orbital irradiation using modern techniques appears to be efficacious, and *careful limited irradiation* produces rapid palliative relief of congestion and enhances comfort and vision. Clinically, one can expect 70% of patients to have a good to excellent response (Figs. 11-24, 11-25). The best response is generally obtained in the abatement of soft tissue signs and symptoms. We have noted that about 20% of cases may show a transient worsening of

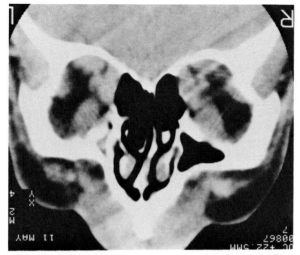

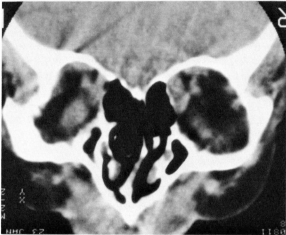

FIGURE 11-25.   Reduction in muscle mass is shown on coronal CT scans taken before *(top)* and 4 months after *(bottom)* orbital radiotherapy for marked soft tissue signs and symptoms that developed 3 months after treatment for hyperthyroidism in this 70-year-old man.

symptoms at the beginning of orbital radiotherapy; this is usually resolved by the end of the second week, and can be modified by a very short course of steroids during treatment. Soft tissue changes respond in two to four weeks. Proptosis and ophthalmoplegia have little response to any form of conservative medical therapy. In our treatment center, the technique has been modified to use supervoltage irradiation (2000 cGy in ten fractions over 12 days using a 4-MeV linear accelerator) delivered only to the posterior two thirds of the orbit, avoiding the globe itself. We found that the extraocular muscle and orbital CT changes tend to parallel the response after radiotherapy. Only 14% of our patients had recurrence of symptoms following radiotherapy. An added benefit is

that this appears to be a single-course treatment modality.

There are a number of questions about the use of radiotherapy in Graves' orbitopathy; "Why does it work?" is not the least of them. Local immunosuppression is an attractive theory and was the initial impetus for using this modality. If an abnormal systemic immune response is the basis of the disease process, it is surprising that symptomatic local recurrences are not more common. Possibly, orbital radiotherapy interferes with a target other than just the inflammatory cells, such as the muscle membrane or fibroblastic component, to prevent the development of progressive infiltrative changes. We believe that orbital radiotherapy is indicated for rapidly progressive severe orbitopathy, for troublesome soft tissue signs and symptoms, for patients in whom steroids are contraindicated, or for those not controlled by or who develop side-effects on modest doses of steroids. The effect of radiotherapy as a primary modality in very early disease is not known, and potentially may lead to permanent arrest of disease progression and prevent disabling and disfiguring problems. The role of early radiotherapy is currently being investigated. Generally speaking, we have tended to avoid the use of radiotherapy in young patients because the disease tends to be much milder and the long-term effects of radiotherapy are not known. An additional important contraindication to radiotherapy is known diabetes or vascular disease, because radiotherapy may significantly accelerate the course of vascular retinopathy.

Surgical decompression for the acute infiltrative situation should be limited to sight-threatening manifestations because the large majority of the remaining patients can be treated early by nonsurgical means. We believe (and McCord's review of the literature suggests) that the apical syndrome is best treated by a mechanical decompression that addresses the location of the compressive component. In effect, in our experience the most direct and effective method of dealing with optic neuropathy has been decompression with a short-term (1 to 2 weeks) and moderate dose (30 to 40 mg/day) of prednisone. It is exceedingly important to ensure that, whatever technique is used, the apical portion of the orbit is decompressed (Fig. 11-26; see also Fig. 11-19). There are a number of relatively safe surgical procedures for decompression, and the choice is governed by the experience of the particular center doing it. It is necessary to emphasize that proper decompression requires breaching or removing the periorbita. We prefer anterior orbital decompressive routes because of the ease of visualizing the orbital anatomy, but many advocate antral or combined orbital–antral decompression. Regardless of the surgical approach, the key element to decompression for optic neuropathy is removal of the apical portion of the orbital walls.

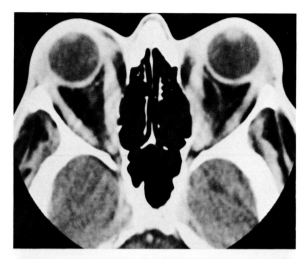

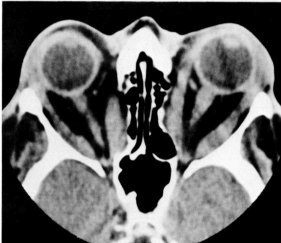

FIGURE 11-26. Axial CT scans taken before *(top)* and after *(bottom)* ethmoid decompression demonstrate relief of apical compression.

Decompression for optic neuropathy is followed by a rapid resolution of visual symptoms in the large majority of instances, and failure to observe rapid resolution may infer that the decompression was not apical enough. In addition, there is a dramatic resolution of the congestive component of this disease due to the release of orbital pressure. We have been impressed with the abatement of soft tissue signs, the improvement in motor excursion, and the appearance of lid retraction following decompression for the apical orbital compressive syndrome of thyroid orbitopathy (Fig. 11-27). Because these patients generally have a significant motor component to their disease, they should be warned that diplopia may become more troublesome due to increased scarring postoperatively in about one third of instances.

Exposure

Exposure can be managed by conservative measures consisting of elevation of the head, ocular lubricants, moisture chambers, humidifiers, and night-time taping of the lids. Moisture chambers are very effective in abating acute symptoms. One can simply obtain swimming or ski goggles, occlude the vents, and place a small pledget of moist cotton gauze in the goggles to develop a misted chamber. Alternatively, some of the commercially available bubble-shaped ocular bandages can be used in the same way. We have rarely found it necessary, and eschew the philosophy of tarsorrhaphy for exposure because tarsorrhaphy tightens rather than loosens the orbital lid septal complex. We prefer, when necessary, to treat a widened interpalpebral fissure with lid-lengthening procedures. Another factor that increases corneal exposure is inferior rectus tethering, which interferes with Bell's phenomena, thus contributing to nocturnal exposure. In these circumstances, recession of the inferior recti to improve mobility may become necessary as a factor in treatment of exposure. In addition, severe proptosis may have to be dealt with surgically for similar reasons.

Surgery for Thyroid Orbitopathy

Surgery for the oculomotor abnormalities, lid malposition, and cosmetic deformity of thyroid orbitopathy or for non-sight-threatening reasons should be done only when the disorder becomes quiescent for at least 6 months. The order of the procedures must be designed within the context of the specific disease process, its effect on the patient, and expectations of the patient. There are five categories of procedures for thyroid orbitopathy, and the order in which they should be done *when indicated* is as follows:

1. Decompression
2. Ocular muscle surgery
3. Upper lid-lengthening procedures
4. Lower lid procedures
5. Blepharoplasty

One can achieve very satisfying cosmetic results in the majority of patients by lid surgery alone. It is the lid retraction and the orbital fat prolapse that give these patients a much more proptotic appearance. Generally speaking, unless it is a sight-threatening situation, we do not consider orbital decompression with less than 23 mm to 24 mm of proptosis. The three lid procedures available are upper lid lengthening, lower lid elevation, and blepharoplasty. To reiterate, the major principles in elective surgery are treatment when the disease is quiescent, choice of the least potentially damaging procedure that will

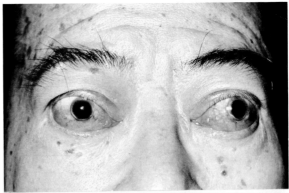

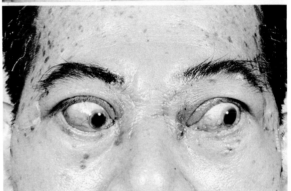

FIGURE 11-27. This 75-year-old man presented with a severe congestive orbitopathy and optic neuropathy that developed over a 6-month period 8 years after he first noted prominence of his eyes and 5 years after treatment for hyperthyroidism. He had left macular degeneration with hand movements vision and a right visual acuity of 20/100, proptosis of 22 left and 21 right, severe chemosis, and marked limitation of extraocular movements *(top, attempted left gaze)*. Postoperatively *(bottom, attempted left gaze)*, note improvement in soft tissue signs, reduction of proptosis, increased lid retraction, and increased extraocular movements. VEP returned to normal postoperatively and vision improved to 20/70 due to the presence of a cataract. Following cataract extraction, vision on the right side was 20/25. Such dramatic resolution of soft tissue features is often seen due to relief of venous congestion.

achieve good results, and an order of procedures within the context of the disease process and patient expectation.

DECOMPRESSION

Decompression is discussed technically elsewhere in this book. We generally will choose this as an elective procedure in non-sight-threatening situations only in patients who have more than 23 mm of proptosis and who are well motivated. Many patients are severely disturbed by the cosmetic changes and may be willing to undergo the risks of orbital decompression for the sake of the severe cosmetic abnormality. It should be noted that the smaller the muscle involvement on CT scan, the better the degree of decompression achieved. Technically, there are many different approaches to orbital decompression, including anterior ethmoidal (Sewall), transantral (Ogura), lateral (Kronlein), transfrontal (Naffziger), and maxillary (Hirsch) (Fig. 11-28). Our modification of the ethmoidal approach allows for removal of the medial two thirds of the floor of the orbit (Fig. 11-29). Decompression by means of an anterior cul-de-sac or skin incisions may be augmented by blepharoplasty. Overall, the best philosophy for elective decompression is to tailor it to the specific needs of the individual patient, and to choose a

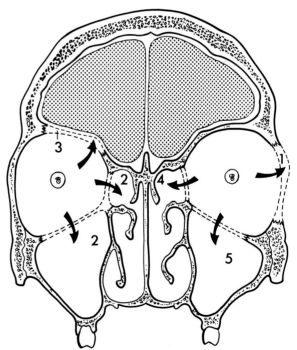

FIGURE 11-28. Schematic diagram demonstrates various sites of orbital decompression: *(1)* lateral (Kronlein); *(2)* transantral (Ogura); *(3)* transfrontal (Naffziger); *(4)* ethmoidal (Sewall); and *(5)* maxillary (Hirsch).

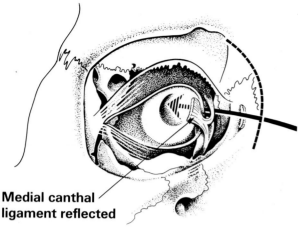

Medial canthal ligament reflected

FIGURE 11-29. Schematic drawing demonstrates the potential site of bony removal possible with a medial orbital decompression *(absent bone stippled black)*. This procedure is accomplished through an ethmoidal incision with reflection of the lacrimal sac and medial canthal ligament. The medial canthal ligament is resutured along with the periosteum postoperatively.

single to three-wall decompression depending on the degree of proptosis and patient expectation (Fig. 11-30). Generally speaking, the degree of success in alleviating proptosis correlates well with the degree of myopathy, and to some extent with adjacent changes in orbital fat. In effect, patients who have more severe orbitopathy and as such more scarring tend to have poorer decompressive results than patients with lesser degrees of fibrosis. To some extent the risks of orbital decompression have been overemphasized, and this procedure has probably been withheld in many circumstances when it might have

helped the patient. A well-controlled, experienced surgical approach to the orbit for decompression carries relatively few complications. Although one would not encourage a cavalier attitude towards this procedure, it has almost certainly been underutilized. The most important factors contributing to success are experience in evaluating the patients and with the procedure itself.

LID RETRACTION

Lid retraction may be treated medically by adrenergic blocking agents; however, the results are inconsistent and often locally irritating. About 10% to 15% of the patients we have treated with guanethidine (Ismelin) have had a positive response. Some of them require the addition of weak topical steroids to deal with the injection associated with guanethidine.

The surgical management of lid retraction may be most gratifying. The procedure that we prefer for upper lid retraction is graded Müllers' and aponeurosis weakening (Fig. 11-31). The surgery is best performed under local anesthesia to permit intraoperative evaluation of lid position and function. This can be achieved with local subconjunctival injection along the upper tarsal border and fornix after everting the lid over a pediatric Desmarres retractor (Fig. 11-31B). A buttonhole incision is made in the conjunctiva about 1 mm above the border of the tarsus (Fig. 11-31C). Conjunctiva is then carefully dissected free of the underlying Müllers' muscle (Fig. 11-31D). This dissection is aided by the subconjunctival injection and hydrodissection produced by the local anesthetic. The dissection is carried laterally and medially along the edge of the upper tarsal border and superiorly

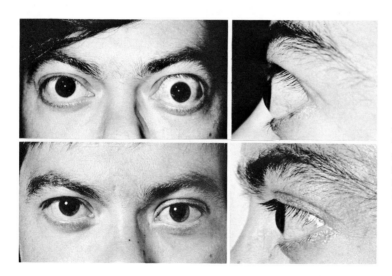

FIGURE 11-30. These photographs demonstrate the preoperative *(top)* and postoperative *(bottom)* appearance of a 30-year-old man who developed proptosis with hyperthyroidism 3 years prior to presentation. He underwent bilateral, medial, and floor decompression through an ethmoidal incision and a left müllerectomy for a cosmetic and functional disorder that troubled him greatly in his job as a schoolteacher.

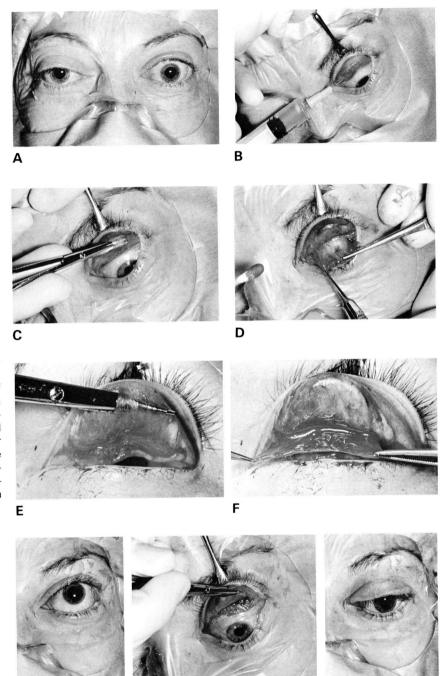

FIGURE 11-31. These photographs demonstrate a graded müllerectomy for left upper lid retraction (A). The lid is everted over a pediatric Desmarres retractor and a local anesthetic with epinephrine is injected subconjunctivally (B). A buttonhole incision is then made in the conjunctiva at the tarsal margin, and the conjunctiva is elevated (C), detached, and dissected free of the underlying Müller's muscle (D). Müller's muscle is then buttonholed and detached from the tarsal plate (E), and is dissected free of the underlying levator aponeurosis (F). The patient's lid position is assessed (G). Note persistent lateral arching. The lid is then everted over the Desmarres retractor, and the lateral half to two-thirds of the levator aponeurosis is incised and allowed to retract (H) to achieve a normal lateral curvature (I).

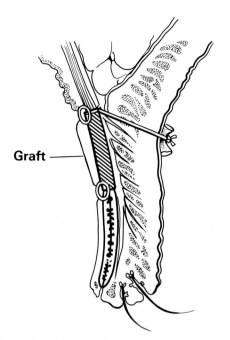

Graft

FIGURE 11-32. Schematic diagram of sagittal section of the lid demonstrates the position of a spacer graft between the levator aponeurosis and the tarsal plate. Note the placement of a suture through the lid to a bolster to create an upper lid fold.

anterior incision and myotomy or by placing a scleral graft laterally.

We have found this a useful approach for most patients, but several additional or alternative procedures may be chosen, including percutaneous levator aponeurotic and Müllers' muscle recession with and without scleral grafts or marginal myotomies of the levator (Fig. 11-32). These alternative methods include Grove's levator aponeurotic marginal myotomies for mild retraction; scleral extension techniques (Doxanas and Dryden and Iliff's modifications); posterior müllerectomy described by Putterman; anterior levator recession and müllerectomy as outlined by Harvey and Anderson; and Sisler's recession of Müller's superior tarsal muscle.

As a general guideline for the surgical management of lid retraction, if the upper lid is at the limbus or is retracted up to 3 mm, a müllerectomy with lateral tenotomy as described is usually adequate. In addition, marginal myotomy from an anterior route may correct relatively small degrees of lid retraction. Lid retraction of 3 mm to 4 mm requires a recession of either the levator muscle or the aponeurosis along with the müllerectomy. Lid retraction of 4 mm or greater requires a recession, müllerectomy, and a scleral graft.

SURGICAL MANAGEMENT OF THYROID OCULOMYOPATHY

Jack Rootman, Larry Allen, and John Pratt-Johnson

In a retrospective study of our experience with thyroid orbitopathy, we found that 9% of the patients required muscle surgery, which was performed on average about 20 months after onset of diplopia. The majority of these patients (63.5%) have combined vertical and horizontal deviations, with a smaller percentage demonstrating pure vertical (27%) or pure horizontal (9.7% esotropia) deviations. We found that about equal numbers had an increase or decrease in their esodeviation in downgaze (V and A pattern). In addition, the degree of deviation, nature of muscle involvement, clinical indices of proptosis, and degree of forced duction abnormality correlated well with CT findings. (That is, the larger the muscle and the more muscles involved, the greater the deviation, proptosis, and forced duction abnormality.) In some instances of severe apical disease, the proptosis and deviation may not be great because of symmetry of involvement, but the severity of myopathy will be evident on vergence and ductions. Our study reconfirmed that the typical thyroid eye patient with disabling diplopia was a woman (female:male, 4:1) in her middle years (average age 53.8 years).

The goal in the surgical management of thyroid myopathy is the restoration of as large an area of fused single

into the fornix. One should be careful not to dissect the superolateral fornix in order to avoid the lacrimal ducts. The upper limit of dissection is usually identified by the appearance of the white aponeurosis of the levator. Following dissection and retraction of the conjunctiva, Müllers' muscle is detached at the very border of the tarsus. It is then freed from the underlying levator aponeurosis, which can be identified by its smooth white surface (Fig. 11-31F). Generally, this dissection is carried 8 mm to 10 mm to the upper fornix, where a small fat pad is noted. The patient then sits up or looks up and the level of the lid evaluated (Fig. 11-31G). If an appropriate degree of ptosis is achieved, Müllers' muscle is allowed to retract or is resected and the conjunctiva is sutured to the upper tarsal border. Because residual retraction is almost universally present laterally, lysis of the outer one half to one third of the levator aponeurosis is routinely performed (Fig. 11-31H and I). This can be safely achieved by everting the tarsus and incising the levator aponeurosis at the very tarsal margin, avoiding the lacrimal ducts. If retraction is severe and persistent, a graded recession of the levator aponeurosis is then performed. In severe instances, this may be aided by scleral graft and conjunctival recession. In the event that a routine müllerectomy fails to rid the patient of significant lateral arching, the lateral portion of the muscle can be dealt with from an binocular vision as possible. Particular emphasis should be placed on obtaining stable fusion in the primary position and on looking down in the position normally used for reading and negotiating stairs. The patient should not undergo surgery unless stable in terms of the thyroid disease and off steroids for at least 6 months. A useful but not totally accurate method for assessing stability of the oculomotor deviation is persistent flattening of the base of the Hess screen, which usually infers a stable end to the cicatricial process (Fig. 11-33). Where possible, correction of the muscle imbalance should utilize adjustable recessions of muscles in either eye rather than resection because of the inherent scarring and contractures produced by the myopathy. Adjustable sutures should be used routinely and an attempt made to do all of the surgery as a primary procedure, because secondary surgery is technically more difficult. Preoperative and intraoperative forced duction testing must be employed and one must be ready to change the operative plan depending upon the results of forced duction.

The following outlines the surgical technique that we prefer. The adjustable suture method is carefully explained to the patient to assure postoperative cooperation. We inform the anesthetist preoperatively so that minimal narcotic, sedative, and anesthetic agents are used to avoid excessive postoperative emesis and drowsiness. Droperidol, which is frequently used in routine strabismus surgery as an antinauseant, is to be totally avoided in the adjustable suture patient because of the disassociating effect on eye muscle coordination that sometimes occurs. Forced duction testing is done at the start of the procedure and the results are recorded. The plan of surgery is adjusted according to the forced duction findings. We make a conjunctival incision 2 mm to 4 mm posterior to the limbus, isolate the muscle on a muscle hook, and proceed with deep orbital dissection of all the cheek ligaments and fibrous bands attached to the peripheral aspect of the muscles. Dissection often goes far enough to expose the vortex veins adjacent to the grossly enlarged muscles, where direct trauma should be avoided. Meticulous attention is warranted in freeing all adhesions and connections between the lower lid retractors and the inferior rectus muscle if it is to be recessed. A 6-0 double-armed Vicryl suture on a spatula needle is threaded through the muscle 1 mm to 2 mm from the insertion and is locked at either side. The muscle is cut from the sclera with scissors between the suture and the insertion to sclera. In some cases, such as severely tethered inferior rectus with the affected eye held 30 D or more below the horizontal position, it may not be possible to pull the eye up to a position where the tendon can be safely cut from the sclera with scissors without the danger of inadvertent cutting of the sclera. In such instances, it is safer to cut the muscle from the sclera using a 15 Bard Parker blade to cut through the tendon onto the muscle hook (Fig.

11-34). Once cut, forced duction testing is repeated to identify any persistent tethering and further dissection of any remaining bands is done. The muscle is secured by inserting each needle of the double-armed suture through the insertion site obliquely to spread the muscle as wide as possible and yet bring the suture ends to approximately 3 mm apart. A double throw followed by a half bow secures the muscle, allowing it to hang back against the sclera the measured or desired amount. The muscle is recessed 1 mm to 2 mm more than predicted on the basis of the preoperative evaluation.

The suture in the muscle is tied with a slip knot, the conjunctiva closed temporarily, and *repeat forced duction* performed to rule out conjunctival tethering. If after suturing the conjunctiva, the forced duction test demonstrates more tethering than before closure, we may recess the conjunctiva as needed. About 4 hours later, using topical 4% cocaine as anesthesia, a final adjustment is made. Because it is technically easier to tighten the muscle (*i.e.* reduce a recession), we would emphasize the concept of slight over-recession at the time of surgery. Using the above principles and adjustable sutures, we were able to obtain fusion in the primary and downgaze positions in a single surgical procedure in 75% of our cases, and fusion in primary gaze alone in 85% of cases.

Generally, we have found with multiple muscle involvement one can predict about 2.5 D to 3 D achieved per millimeter of recession, whereas with single muscle involvement 3 D and even 4 D can be achieved with 1 mm of recession. Usually, more effect is obtained the more the recessed muscle was tethered. From our study, we noted that when adjustable inferior rectus recession surgery alone was performed, an average correction of 3.4 D per millimeter of surgery could be expected. If bimedial recessions were done, values of 2.5 D per millimeter of surgery were obtained. When operating on combined deviations, horizontal changes of 3.3 D per millimeter and vertical changes of 2.7 D per millimeter of surgery were obtained. Recession of the inferior rectus alters its adducting influence and promotes exodeviation, thus accounting for this greater horizontal measurement. Generally speaking, the maximum recessions done are 8 mm to 10 mm on the inferior rectus, 8 mm on the medial rectus, and 5 mm on the superior rectus. Over-recessions may lead to problems, particularly in downgaze, and should be avoided. These figures can be used as preoperative guidelines to help predict the amount of surgery necessary.

The major complication of strabismus surgery in our experience has been lower lid retraction despite meticulous dissection of the lower lid retractors. If this is cosmetically noticeable and disturbing, further corrective procedures as outlined can be done at a later stage under local or general anesthetic (Figs. 11-35, 11-36). Some au-

(Text continues on p. 274.)

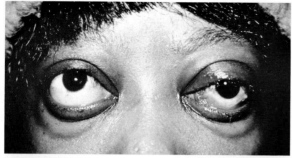
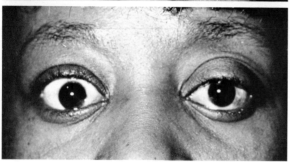

FIGURE 11-33. *(A)* This patient demonstrates the various stages of management of severe thyroid orbital disease. *(Top)* She presented with severe congestive orbitopathy; corneal exposure; optic neuropathy with a vision of 20/200 right and 20/30 left; exophthalmometry of 25 mm right and 20 mm left; and a marked vertical deviation. She was treated with a short course of corticosteroids and underwent bilateral transantral orbital decompression (procedure preferred in dark-skinned persons to avoid keloid formation) with recovery of vision. She subsequently underwent left inferior rectus recession and right superior rectus recession on adjustable suture for tethering of the inferior and superior recti. She was orthophoric in primary position and downgaze, and had 18 mm of proptosis on the right and 16 mm on the left postoperatively. *(B)* The preoperative and postoperative Hess screens show flattening of the base preoperatively and recovery of binocularity following surgery. *(C)* The preoperative and postoperative field of binocular single vision (FBSV).

A

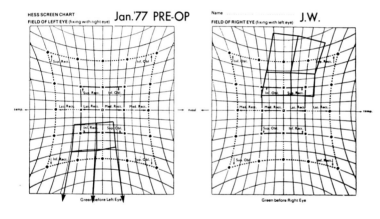

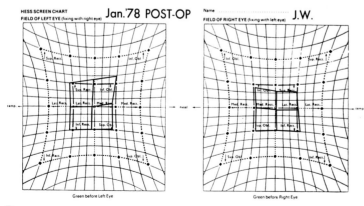

B

272

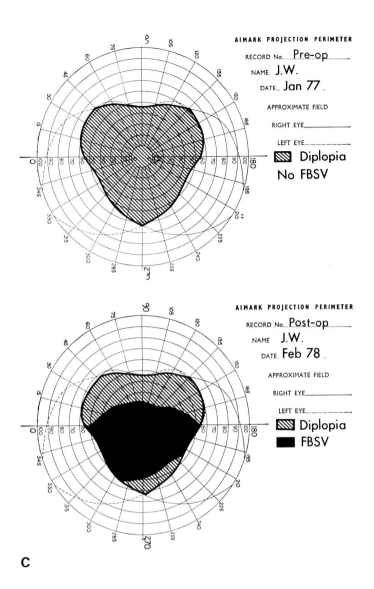

AIMARK PROJECTION PERIMETER

RECORD No. Pre-op

NAME J.W.

DATE Jan 77

APPROXIMATE FIELD

RIGHT EYE_____

LEFT EYE_____

▨ Diplopia

No FBSV

AIMARK PROJECTION PERIMETER

RECORD No. Post-op

NAME J.W.

DATE Feb 78

APPROXIMATE FIELD

RIGHT EYE_____

LEFT EYE_____

▨ Diplopia

■ FBSV

C

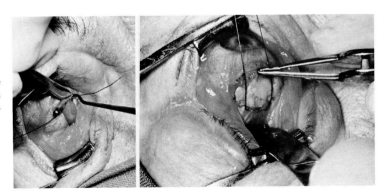

FIGURE 11-34. Photographs demonstrate the disinsertion of a muscle at the time of strabismus surgery *(left)*, and placement of an adjustable suture *(right)* for thyroid myopathy.

273

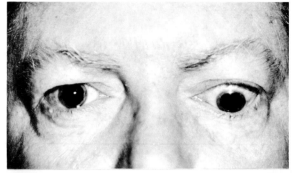

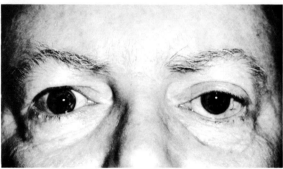

FIGURE 11-35. *(Top)* This 54-year-old woman presented with a 2-year history of intermittent and subsequently permanent diplopia due to a euthyroid orbitopathy. She had a 40-D right hypotropia due to tethering of the inferior rectus. She underwent a maximal recession of the inferior rectus on the right side using an adjustable suture technique. *(Bottom)* Postoperatively she achieved orthophoria in the primary position and had 2 mm of lower lid retraction on the right side, which was subsequently treated by a lower lid elevation and scleral graft. This patient demonstrates the correction of a large deviation in single muscle involvement where the amount achieved per millimeter is frequently greater than in patients with multiple muscle involvement.

thors have advocated release of the lower lid retractors at the time of inferior rectus surgery, but because this is an unpredictable complication, we advocate waiting and then correcting.

There are two special aspects of strabismus surgery for thyroid oculomyopathy that should be reemphasized. The first is awareness of the importance of the forced duction test. There are a small percentage of patients (roughly 8% of those operated upon in our series) that have superior rectus involvement accounting for a hyperdeviation rather than the usual contralateral inferior rectus tethering. One should be on guard to recognize these patients so that appropriate superior rectus recession is done in these circumstances. The other important caveat in strabismus surgery is that one should aim for single binocular vision in the primary position and 20 to 30 degrees of downgaze. Patients who do not achieve single binocular vision in downgaze may be particularly upset, because this makes it difficult to read and to negotiate stairs.

Fusion is usually achieved immediately and is sustained in almost all cases. Rare instances of redevelopment of diplopia due either to progressive disease or loss of fusion are noted. We found that about 49% of our cases required medial rectus surgery, 41% inferior rectus surgery, 8% superior rectus surgery, and 1% lateral rectus surgery. About half of the patients had single muscle involvement, 27% required surgery on two muscles, and the remainder had surgery on three or more muscles. No more than two muscles per eye were operated on.

As to complications, about 40% of our patients having inferior rectus surgery had increased lower lid retraction; 80% of these patients needed lower lid elevations. Another rare complication of muscle surgery, which we have not encountered, is anterior segment ischemia, which is believed to be more common in thyroid eye disease patients. For this reason, operations on more than two muscles per eye should be avoided.

In summary, we suggest that strabismus surgery in thyroid myopathy should aim for cure in the primary position and downgaze, should be done on a patient who does not have active thyroid disease, and should involve release of a tethered muscle by recession rather than any resections. Furthermore, the amount of and the muscle to recess should be predicted on the basis of degree of involvement (clinical deviation and versions), symmetry, forced duction (prior to and repeated during surgery), and amount of scarring noted intraoperatively. The use of adjustable sutures is strongly advocated.

LOWER LID ELEVATION

Lower lid retraction contributes to the appearance of proptosis and degree of exposure, and may be a complication of operations on the inferior rectus muscle. In

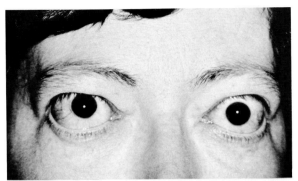

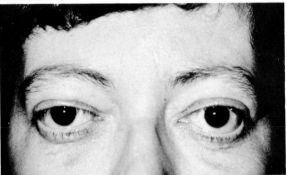

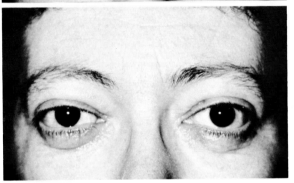

FIGURE 11-36. *(Top)* This 36-year-old woman presented 1 year after treatment of hyperthyroidism with radioactive iodine. She had a 16-D left hypotropia and a 10-D esotropia. Exophthalmometry measurements were 23 mm right and 24 mm left, with marked upper lid retraction. She underwent an adjustable left inferior rectus recession and right medial rectus recession, followed by a müllerectomy *(center)* and bilateral lower lid elevation *(bottom)*.

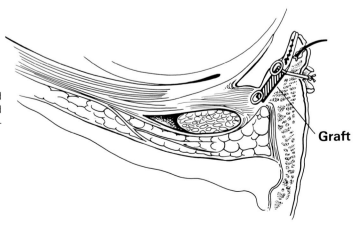

FIGURE 11-37. A schematic drawing of the lower lid shows placement of a graft between the tarsus and lower lid retractors. Note that the upper border is attached to a bolster on the anterior lid surface.

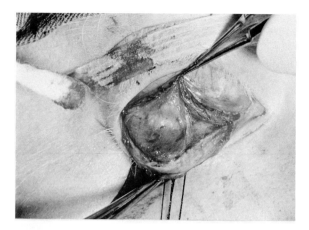

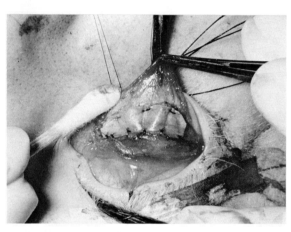

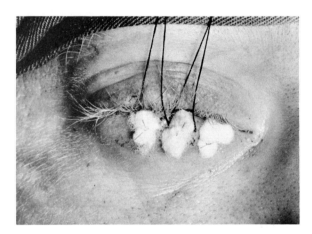

FIGURE 11-38. Surgery for lower lid retraction. *(Top)* The lower lid retractors are detached from the border of the tarsus. *(Bottom left)* Placement of the scleral graft. Note that the graft is wider laterally than medially. *(Bottom right)* The anterior lid bolsters are shown.

essence, all of the procedures on the lower lid achieve their results by disinsertion of the capsulopalpebral fascia from the lower tarsus with placement of a spacer using sclera, cartilage, or fascia (Fig. 11-37).

The method we prefer can be done under local or general anesthesia (Fig. 11-38). A suture is placed in the lid, which is everted over a Desmarres retractor. A conjunctival incision is made at the lower tarsal border. The capsulopalpebral fascia is exposed by dissection of the conjunctiva into the fornix. The retractors are then disinserted from the tarsus, gently swept inferiorly, and separated from the orbicularis with cotton-tipped applicators or dissectors. A scleral graft of a width two to three times the amount of retraction is then prepared and sutured to the capsulopalpebral fascia. The other margin of the graft is then attached at the lower edge of the tarsus by passing a suture through the tarsal margin onto the skin of the lid to produce a mild lash eversion. The conjunctiva is then

TABLE 11-5.
AGE OF ONSET AND SEX DISTRIBUTION OF THYROID ORBITOPATHY, UNIVERSITY OF BRITISH COLUMBIA ORBITAL CLINIC, 1976–1986

	Decade								**Total**
	2nd	3rd	4th	5th	6th	7th	8th	9th	
Female	18	73	105	117	119	54	16	1	503
Male	6	16	26	42	39	25	7	0	161
Total	24	89	131	159	158	79	23	1	664
Ratio F:M	3:1	4.6:1	4:1	2.8:1	3.1:1	2.2:1	2.3:1		3.2:1

TABLE 11-6.
AGE AND NATURE OF ONSET OF THYROID ORBITOPATHY, UNIVERSITY OF BRITISH COLUMBIA ORBITAL CLINIC, 1976–1986

	2nd			3rd			4th			5th			6th			7th			8th			9th		
	M	F	T	M	F	T	M	F	T	M	F	T	M	F	T	M	F	T	M	F	T	M	F	T
Acute or subacute	3	0	3	0	25	25	10	35	45	15	51	66	15	52	67	11	27	38	6	10	16	0	1	1
Ratio F:M								3.5:1			3.4:1			3.7:1			2.5:1			1.7:1				
Chronic	M	F	T	M	F	T	M	F	T	M	F	T	M	F	T	M	F	T	M	F	T			
	6	15	21	16	48	64	15	70	85	27	66	93	24	67	91	14	27	41	1	7	8			
Ratio F:M		2.5:1			3:1			4.7:1			2.4:1			2.8:1			1.9:1							
% Chronic		87.5			71.9			65.3			58.5			57.6			51.9			33.3				

M = male; F = female; T = total

closed or, rarely, may be recessed. The lid is taped to the brow with Frost sutures for the first 24 hours to hold the graft in position.

BLEPHAROPLASTY

Blepharoplasty is another procedure that should attend to the nature of the abnormality produced by the disease. In addition, one should assiduously avoid blepharoplasty on patients who have severe preseptal edema, that is, one should await resolution or manage the medical aspects of the disease prior to surgery. By and large, these patients do not have the kind of fat prolapse or, for that matter, the kind of skin that you see in senile patients, and they require more radical excision of anterior orbital fat and lesser excision of their often thickened skin. Thus, blepharoplasty should include blunt dissection through the orbicularis and orbital septum with more radical removal of anterior orbital fat. A special note of caution: Avoid excessive skin resection because complications of lagophthalmos can result. This is best avoided by doing it under local anesthesia and maintaining a conservative attitude towards vertical skin resection. Rather, the con-

tour of the lid should be altered by the fat resection and lateral tension rather than by vertical shortening.

■ EPIDEMIOLOGIC CONSIDERATIONS

We have had an opportunity to review our cases of thyroid orbitopathy in an attempt to assess three specific factors: age of onset, nature of onset, and thyroid status. Not all of the information was available in each instance; however, it could be obtained in the majority of patients, and certain useful clinical information can be gleaned from this analysis. Although the overall female:male ratio is about 3.2:1, it can be noted that the female:male ratio tends to decrease with age, suggesting that a larger proportion of males develop this disease later in life (Table 11-5). The inquiry into nature of onset suggests that the number of patients presenting with relatively mild or insidious onset of disease tends to diminish with age (Table 11-6). In effect, the corollary suggests that disease in the elderly is more often of an acute and more fulminant nature, a feature we have noted clinically. Finally, where possible, we have tried to determine the thyroid status of patients who develop orbitopathy (Table 11-7). These have been divided into patients who

TABLE 11-7.
THYROID STATUS OF PATIENTS WITH THYROID ORBITOPATHY, UNIVERSITY OF BRITISH COLUMBIA ORBITAL CLINIC, 1976–1986

	Total	Male	Female	Ratio
Hyperthyroid	532	121	411	3.4:1
Hypothyroid	11	0	11	
Euthyroid (nonsuppressible autonomous gland)	37	15	22	1.5:1
Euthyroid (suppressible)	17	8	9	1.1:1
Euthyroid (unknown)	36	15	21	1.4:1
Total euthyroid	90	38	52	1.4:1
Thyroiditis	7	0	7	

have had or experienced hyperthyroidism and hypothyroidism, who were euthyroid, or who had thyroiditis. In each instance, the specific thyroid status was established by history or medical consultation. The 90 patients with euthyroid status were divided into those who had proven glandular autonomy; those with thyroid orbitopathy and completely normal or suppressible gland function; and those who had normal thyroid function clinically and chemically but who were not assessed for glandular autonomy. The female : male ratio of patients with a history of hyperthyroidism was roughly that seen in the general population of thyroid orbitopathy. Hypothyroidism and thyroiditis was dominated by women; there were no men in either instance. Among those patients who were euthyroid, the female : male ratio was much more nearly equal when compared to the overall ratio.

The above analysis provides some useful generalizations about thyroid orbitopathy. This is a disease that peaks in middle life and is dominated by female occurrence, but this dominance decreases with age. It is usually insidious in onset, but is more frequently acute in the elderly. The majority of patients have had hyperthyroidism. The female : male ratio in the euthyroid patient is much more nearly equal.

Conclusion

Graves' orbitopathy can be an exceedingly disabling disease. The road to recovery is paved with a number of different kinds of treatment that require careful analysis and individualization. These patients require prolonged, multidisciplinary, and sensitive care. Proper timing and careful study of the patient is of paramount importance in the management of this disorder.

Bibliography

GENERAL

Bouzas AG: Endocrine ophthalmopathy. Trans Ophthalmol Soc UK 100:511, 1980
Char DH: Thyroid Eye Disease. Baltimore, Williams & Wilkins, 1985
Gamblin GT, Harper DG, Galentine P et al: Prevalence of increased intraocular pressure in Graves' disease — evidence of frequent subclinical ophthalmopathy. N Engl J Med 308:420, 1983
Gorman CA, Waller RR, Dyer JA: The Eye and Orbit in Thyroid Disease. New York, Raven Press, 1984
Sergott RC: Oculocutaneous manifestations of thyroid disease. In Callen JP, Eiferman RA (eds): Ocultaneous Diseases p 117. Boston, Little, Brown & Co, 1985
Sisler HA, Jakobiec FA, Trokel SL: Ocular abnormalities and orbital changes of Graves' disease. In Duane TD, Jaeger EA (eds): Clinical Ophthalmology, Vol 2, Chap 36. Philadelphia, Harper & Row, 1986

Solomon DH, Chopra IJ: Graves' disease — 1972. Mayo Clin Proc 47:803, 1972
Uretsky SH, Kennerdell JS, Gutai JP: Graves' ophthalmopathy in childhood and adolescence. Arch Ophthalmol 98:1963, 1980
Walfish PG, Wall JR, Volpe R: Autoimmunity and the Thyroid. Orlando, Academic Press, 1985
Weetman AP, McGregor AM, Hall R: Ocular manifestations of Graves' disease: A review. J R Soc Med 77:936, 1984
Werner SC: The eye changes of Graves' disease. Mayo Clin Proc 47:969, 1972

PATHOGENESIS

Anderson DR: Mechanisms of Graves' disease and endocrine exophthalmos. Am J Ophthalmol 68:46, 1969
Atkinson S, Holcombe M, Kendall-Taylor P: Ophthalmopathic immunoglobulin in patients with Graves' ophthalmopathy. Lancet August 18:374, 1984
Doniach D: The pathogenesis of endocrine exopthalmos: A short review. Proc R Soc Med 70:695, 1977
Doniach D, Florin-Christensen A: Autoimmunity in the pathogenesis of endocrine exophthalmos. Clin Endocrinol Metab 4:341, 1975
Frueh BR, Musch DC, Grill R et al: Orbital compliance in Graves' eye disease. Ophthalmology 92:657, 1985
Hufnagel TJ, Hickey WF, Cobbs WH et al: Immunohistochemical and ultrastructural studies on the exenterated orbital tissues of a patient with Graves' disease. Ophthalmology 91:1411, 1984
Kennerdell JS, Rosenbaum AE, El-Hoshy MH: Apical optic nerve compression of dysthyroid optic neuropathy on computed tomography. Arch Ophthalmol 99:807, 1981
Kriss JP: Graves' ophthalmopathy: Etiology and treatment. Hosp Pract, March:125, 1975
McKenzie JM: Thyroid-stimulating antibody (TSAb) in Graves' disease. Thyroid Today 3:1, 1980
Sergott RC, Felberg NT, Savino PJ et al: E-rosette formation in Graves' ophthalmopathy. Invest Ophthalmol Vis Sci 18:1245, 1979
Sergott RC, Felberg NT, Savino PJ et al: Association of HLA antigen Bw35 with severe Graves' ophthalmopathy. Invest Ophthalmol Vis Sci 24:124, 1983
Sergott RC, Glaser JS: Graves' ophthalmopathy: A clinical and immunologic review. Surv Ophthalmol 26:1, 1981
Strakosch CR, Wall JR: Pathogenesis of autoimmune thyroid disease: Some facts and some speculation. Can Med Assoc J 126:10, 1982
Volpe R: The pathogenesis of Graves' disease. Comp Ther 2:43, 1976
Volpe R, Lamki L, Clarke PV et al: The pathogenesis of Graves' disease: A disorder of delayed hypersensitivity. Mayo Clin Proc 47:824, 1972
Wall JR: Humoral mechanisms in relationship to Graves' ophthalmopathy. In Walfish PG, Wall JR, Volpe R (eds): Autoimmunity and the Thyroid, p 125. Orlando, Academic Press, 1985
Wall JR, Henderson J, Strakosch CR et al: Graves' ophthalmopathy. Can Med Assoc J 124:855, 1981
Wall JR, Odgers R, Metzel BS: Immunological studies of the eye changes of thyrotoxicosis. Aust NZ J Med 3:162, 1973

CLINICAL CONSTELLATION

Berta A, Kalman K, Patvaros I et al: Changes in tear protein composition in Graves' ophthalmopathy. Orbit 5:97, 1986

Feldon SE, Muramatsu S, Weiner JM: Clinical classification of Graves' ophthalmopathy: Identification of risk factors for optic neuropathy. Arch Opthalmol 102:1469, 1984

Kennerdell JS, Rosenbaum AE, El-Hoshy MH: Apical optic nerve compression of dysthyroid optic neuropathy on computed tomography. Arch Ophthalmol 99:807, 1981

Neigel JM, Rootman J, Belkin RI et al: Dysthyroid optic neuropathy in the crowded orbital apex syndrome. (Accepted for publication, Ophthalmology)

Panzo GJ, Tomsak RL: A retrospective review of 26 cases of dysthyroid optic neuropathy. Am J Ophthalmol 96:190, 1983

Rootman J, Patel S, Berry K et al: Pathological and clinical study of Muller's muscle in Graves' ophthalmopathy. Can J Ophthalmol 22:32, 1987

Trobe JD, Glaser JS, Laflamme P: Dysthyroid optic neuropathy: Clinical profile and rationale for management. Arch Ophthalmol 96:1199, 1978

Van Dyk JHL: Orbital Graves' disease: A modification of the "NO SPECS" classification. Ophthalmology 88:479, 1981

DIAGNOSIS

Bassett F, Eastman CJ et al: Diagnostic value of thyrotropin concentrations in serum as measured by a sensitive immunoradiometric assay. Clin Chem 32:461, 1986

Belkin RI, Neigel JM, Rootman J et al: Clinical-computed tomographic correlations in thyroid orbitopathy. (submitted)

Calissendorff BM, Soderstrom M, Alveryd A: Ophthalmology and hyperthyroidism: A comparison between patients receiving different antithyroid treatments. Acta Ophthalmol 64:698, 1986

Clague R, Mukhtar ED, Pyle GA et al: Thyroid-stimulating immunoglobulins and the control of thyroid function. J Clin Endocrinol Metab 43:550, 1976

Coleman DJ, Jack RL, Franzen LA et al: High resolution B-scan ultrasonography of the orbit. V: Eye changes of Graves' disease. Arch Ophthalmol 88:465, 1972

Dal Pozzo G, Boschi MC: Extraocular muscle enlargement in acromegaly. Comput Assist Tomogr 6:706, 1982

Dresner SC, Rothfus WE, Slamovits TL et al: Computed tomography of orbital myositis. AJR 143:671, 1984

Enzmann DR, Donaldson SS, Kriss JP: Appearance of Graves' disease on orbital computed tomography. J Comput Assist Tomogr 4:815, 1979

Feldon SE, Lee CP. Muramatsu SK et al: Quantitative computed tomography of Graves' ophthalmopathy: Extraocular muscle and orbital fat in development of optic neuropathy. Arch Ophthalmol 103:213, 1985

Feldon SE, Weiner JM: Clinical significance of extraocular muscle volumes in Graves' ophthalmopathy. Arch Ophthalmol 100:1266, 1982

Forbes G, Gehring DG, Gorman CA et al. Volume measurements of normal orbital structures by computed tomographic analysis. AJNR 6:419, 1985

Forbes G, Gorman CA, Gehring D et al: Computer analysis of orbital fat and muscle volumes in Graves' ophthalmopathy. AJNR 4:737, 1983

Franco PS, Hershman JM, Haigler ED Jr et al: Response to thyrotropin-releasing hormone compared with thyroid suppression tests in euthyroid Graves' disease. Metabolism 22:1357, 1973

Haiback H. Avioli LV: Hyperthyroidism in Graves' disease: Current trends in management and diagnosis. Arch Intern Med 136:725, 1976

Harris GJ, Syvertsen A: Multiple projection computed tomography in orbital disorders. Ann Ophthalmol, February, p 183, 1981

Hart I: Testing thyroid function. Ann R Coll Physic Surg Can 17:399, 1984

Healy JF, Metcalf JH, Brahme FJ: Thyroid ophthalmopathy: Bony erosion on CT and increased vascularity on angiography. AJNR 2:472, 1981

Healy JF, Rosenkrantz H: Enlargement of the optic nerve sheath complex in thyroid ophthalmopathy. CT 5:8, 1981

Hershman JM: Clinical application of thyrotropin-releasing hormone. N Engl J Med 290:886, 1974

Hopton MR, Harrop JS: Immunoradiometric assay of thyrotropin as a "first-line" thyroid function test in the routine laboratory. Clin Chem 32:691, 1986

Hyman BN, Johnson PC: Thyrotropin-releasing hormone (a test to diagnose Graves' ophthalmopathy). Trans Am Acad Ophthalmol Otolaryngol 79:OP524, 1975

Laibovitz RA, Karsell P: Thyroid eye disease and normal computerized tomography. Tex Med 76:58, 1980

Merlis AL, Schaiberger CL, Adler R: External carotid-cavernous sinus fistula simulating unilateral Graves' ophthalmopathy. J Comput Assist Tomogr 6:1006, 1982

Perrild H, Feldt-Rasmussen U, Bech K et al: The differential diagnostic problems in unilateral euthyroid Graves' ophthalmopathy. Acta Endocrinol 106:471, 1984

Rosenberg IN: Euthyroid Graves's disease. N Engl J Med 296:223, 1977

Rothfus WE, Curtin HD: Extraocular muscle enlargement: A CT review. Radiology 151:677, 1983

Schrooyen M, Winand R, Glinoer D: Plasma exchange therapy for severe Graves' ophthalmopathy. Orbit 5:105, 1986

Shammas HJF, Minckler DS, Ogden C: Ultrasound in early thyroid orbitopathy. Arch Ophthalmol 98:277, 1980

Solomon DH, Chopra IJ, Chopra U et al: Identification of subgroups of euthyroid Graves' ophthalmopathy. N Engl J Med 296:181, 1977

Surks MI: Assessment of thyroid function. Ophthalmology 88:476, 1981

Trokel SL, Hilai SK: Recognition and differential diagnosis of enlarged extraocular muscles in computed tomography. Am J Ophthalmol 87:503, 1979

Trokel SL, Jakobiec FA: Correlation of CT scanning and pathologic features of ophthalmic Graves' disease. Ophthalmology 88:553, 1981

Walfish PG, Gottesman IS, Baxter JL: Graves' ophthalmopathy and subclinical hypothyroidism: Diagnostic value of the thyrotropin releasing hormone test. Can Med Assoc J 127:291, 1982

Weetman AP, Ludgate M, Mills PV et al: Cyclosporin improves Graves' ophthalmopathy. Lancet 27:486, 1983

MANAGEMENT

Anderson RL, Linberg JW: Transorbital approach to decompression in Graves' disease. Arch Ophthalmol 99:120, 1981

Baylis HI, Call NB, Shibata CS: The transantral orbital decompression (Ogura technique) as performed by the ophthalmologist: A series of 24 patients. Ophthalmology 87:1005, 1980

Bigos ST, Nisula BC, Daniels GH et al: Cyclophosphamide in the management of advanced Graves' ophthalmopathy. Ann Intern Med 90:921, 1979

Blahut RJ, Beierwaltes WH, Lampe I: Exophthalmos response during roentgen therapy. Am J Roentgenol 90:261, 1963

Bowden AN, Rose FC: Investigation of endocrine exophthalmos. Proc R Soc Med 62:13, 1969

Brennan MW, Leone CR Jr, Janaki L: Radiation therapy for Graves' disease. Am J Ophthalmol 96:195, 1983

Brown J, Coburn JW, Wigod RA et al: Adrenal steroid therapy of severe infiltrative ophthalmopathy of Graves' disease. Am J Med 34:786, 1963

Buffam FV, Rootman J: Lid retraction — its diagnosis and treatment. Ocular Plastic Surg 18:75, 1978

Burrow GN, Mitchell MS, Howard RO et al: Immunosuppressive therapy for the eye changes of Graves' disease. J Clin Endocrinol 31:307, 1970

Calcaterra TC, Thompson JW: Antral-ethmoidal decompression of the orbit in Graves' disease: Ten-year experience. Laryngoscope 90:1941, 1980

Cooper WC: The surgical management of the lid changes in Graves' disease. Ophthalmology 86:2071, 1979

Dandona P, Marshall NJ, Bidey SP et al: Successful treatment of exophthalmos and pretibial myxoedema with plasmapheresis. Br Med J 10:374, 1979

Day RM, Carrol FD: Corticosteroids in the treatment of optic nerve involvement. Arch Ophthalmol 79:279, 1968

Dixon R: The surgical management of thyroid-related upper eyelid retraction. Ophthalmology 89:52, 1982

Donaldson SS, Bagshaw MA, Kriss JP: Supervoltage orbital radiotherapy for Graves' ophthalmopathy. J Clin Endocrinol Metab 37:276, 1973

Doxanas MT, Dryden RM: The use of sclera in the treatment of dysthyroid eyelid retraction. Ophthalmology 88:887, 1981

Dyer TA: The oculorotary muscle in Graves' disease. Trans Am Ophthalmol Soc 74:425, 1976

Ellis FO: Strabismus surgery for endocrine ophthalmopathy. Ophthalmology 86:2059, 1979

Evans D, Kennerdell JS: Extraocular muscle surgery for dysthyroid myopathy. Am J Ophthalmol 95:767, 1983

Feldon SE: Management of thyroid-eye disease. Am Acad Ophthalmol, Member Benefit Module 2, 1984

Garber MI: Methylprednisolone in the treatment of exophthalmos. Lancet 30 April:958, 1966

Gorman CA, DeSanto LW, MacCarty CS et al: Optic neuropathy of Graves' disease: Treatment of transantral or transfrontal orbital decompression. N Engl J Med 290:70, 1974

Grove AS: Upper eyelid retraction and Graves' disease. Ophthalmology 88:499, 1981

Gwinup G, Elias AN, Ascher MS: Effect on exophthalmos of various methods of treatment of Graves' disease. JAMA 247:2135, 1982

Harvey JT, Anderson RL: The aponeurotic approach to eyelid retraction. Ophthalmology 88:513, 1981

Ivy HK, Medical approach to ophthalmopathy of Graves' disease. Mayo Clin Proc 47:980, 1972

Jones A: Orbital x-ray therapy of progressive exophthalmos. Br J Radiol 24:637, 1951

Kramar P: Management of eye changes of Graves' disease. Surv Ophthalmol 18:369, 1974

Lanier VC Jr: The surgical treatment of exophthalmos. Plas Reconstri Surg 55:56, 1975

Leone CR: The management of ophthalmic Graves' disease. Ophthalmology 91:770, 1984

Leone CR Jr, Bajandas FJ: Inferior orbital decompression for dysthyroid optic neuropathy. Ophthalmology 88:525, 1981

McCord CD Jr: Orbital decompression for Graves' disease: Exposure through lateral canthal and inferior fornix incision. Ophthalmology 88:533, 1981

Ogura J, Wessler S, Avioli LV: Surgical approach to the ophthalmopathy of Graves' disease. JAMA 216:1627, 1971

Olivotto IA, Ludgate CM, Allen LH et al: Supervoltage radiotherapy for Graves' ophthalmopathy: CCABC technique and results. Int J Radiat Oncol Biol Phys 11:2085, 1985

Putterman AM: Surgical treatment of dysthyroid eyelid retraction and orbital fat hernia. Otolaryngol Clin North Am 13:39, 1980

Putterman AM: Surgical treatment of thyroid-related upper eyelid retraction. Ophthalmology 88:507, 1981

Ravin JG, Sisson JC, Knapp WT: Orbital radiation for the ocular changes of Graves' disease. Am J Ophthalmol 79:285, 1975

Schimek RA: Surgical management of ocular complications of Graves' disease. Arch Ophthalmol 87:655, 1972

Scott WE, Thalacker JA: Diagnosis and treatment of thyroid myopathy. Ophthalmology 88:493, 1981

Sergott RC, Felberg NT, Savino PJ et al: Graves' ophthalmopathy — immunologic parameters related to corticosteroid therapy. Invest Ophthalmol Vis Sci 20:173, 1981

Shorr N, Neuhaus RW, Baylis HI: Ocular motility problems after orbital decompression for dysthyroid ophthalmopathy. Ophthalmology 89:323, 1982

Sisler HA: Preserving and maximizing the effect of Muller's superior tarsal muscle in levator surgery for blepharoptosis. Orbit 1:113, 1982

Small RG, Meiring NL: A combined orbital and antral approach to surgical decompression of the orbit. Ophthalmology 88:542, 1981

Teng CS, Crombie AL, Hall R et al: An evaluation of supervoltage orbital irradiation for Graves' ophthalmopathy. Clin Endocrinol 13:545, 1980

Trokel SL, Cooper WC: Orbital decompression: Effect on motility and globe position. Ophthalmology 86:2064, 1979

Walsh TE, Ogura JH: Transantral orbital decompression for malignant exopthalmos. Laryngoscope 67:544, 1957

Werner SC: Prednisone in emergency treatment of malignant exophthalmos. Lancet 7 May:1004, 1966

White IL: Total thyroid ablation: A prerequisite to orbital decompression for Graves' disease ophthalmopathy. Laryngoscope 84:1869, 1974

CHAPTER 12

Tumors

■ NEUROGENIC TUMORS

Jack Rootman and William D. Robertson

Neurogenic tumors constitute an apparently disparate group of lesions originating from the neuroectoderm and from nonmesenchymal support cells that are, in turn, derived from the neural crest. The four cell lines included in this category are schwannian, melanocytic, ganglion, and leptomeningeal. The classification and nomenclature within these groups are confusing, but logic compels us to include them all as neurogenic tumors. For purposes of discussion and description, we have tried to emphasize our clinical experience.

Optic Nerve Glioma

PILOCYTIC (JUVENILE) ASTROCYTOMA

Optic nerve gliomas are best understood within the context of histogenesis, site, biologic behavior, and systemic associations. They have been described since the nineteenth century, and have been the subject of controversy in numerous retrospective surveys. Gliomas are of glial origin and the overwhelming majority are of low biologic growth potential. In 1969, Hoyt and Baghdassarian suggested that childhood chiasmal gliomas had a good prognosis for survival and behaved more like hamartomatous than neoplastic lesions, based on an apparent tendency for early growth followed by long-term quiescence. A recent update by Imes and Hoyt reviewed the same population of patients and concluded that the prognosis was less favorable, because 57% (16/28) of their patients are dead. However, they note that only five of the patients died directly from the chiasmal glioma, and the deaths occurred largely during the first decade of follow-up. They also noted that of the 16 patients (57%) with neurofibromatosis, 9 (56%) died, a comparable figure to the patients without neurofibromatosis. Further, two thirds of those who died and who had neurofibromatosis died from nonchiasmal sarcomas and gliomas. The 12 patients

who survived have had stable vision and a good quality of life.

Optic nerve gliomas, therefore, are low-grade pilocytic (juvenile) astrocytomas that parallel the biology and behavior of similar tumors seen elsewhere in the central nervous system. The majority are isolated lesions, but a significant proportion arise within the context of neurofibromatosis (10% to 57% overall have been noted in different series, with an average of one third of patients) wherein the biologic behavior and associations appears to be different. Bilaterality is pathognomonic for von Recklinghausen's disease. From another perspective, optic nerve gliomas are actually the least common cranial nerve neoplasm in neurofibromatosis as pointed out by Reese in his text and by Lewis, who noted that 12% of their patient populations with neurofibromatosis had optic nerve glioma.

There is a female predominance, with 75% occurring during the first decade of life. Defining the location and extent of these tumors is difficult; however, based on a review of our experience and 15 series in the literature about 22% are unilateral and limited to the orbital portion of the optic nerve, 11% involve the optic nerve up to but not including the chiasm, 8% are diffuse but limited to the optic nerve, 43% are chiasmal, and about 16% are diffuse with extra chiasmal involvement. The important factors to establish in optic nerve gliomas (for that matter, in any case of visual deterioration due to an optic nerve tumor) are a correct and specific diagnosis; the extent of the lesion; the functional deficits caused by the tumor; and the predictable biologic behavior. The major controversy with these tumors concerns their biologic behavior or growth potential. Most authors agree they are biologically slow growing. Clinical criteria based on their location, extent, and behavior (assessed with accurate imaging) can provide management guidelines. The general principle of management, governed by their low biologic potential, is essentially conservative treatment. When limited to the orbit or the optic nerve and when either large or rapidly progressing, excision is recommended. When there is significant chiasmal or parachiasmal involvement with stability, they can be observed, but

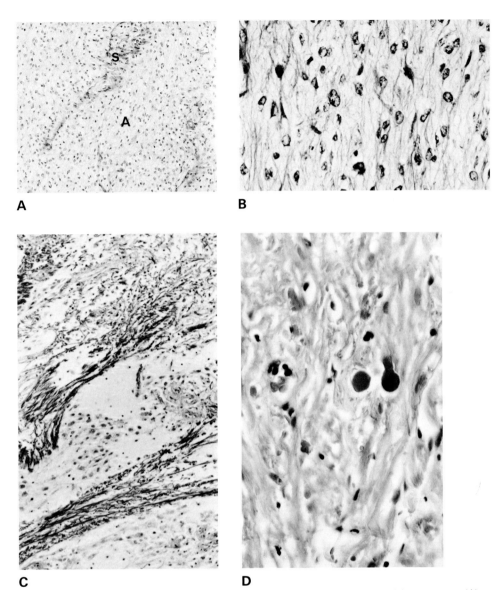

FIGURE 12-1. Histologic features of optic nerve gliomas. *(A)* Diffuse proliferation of the astrocytes (A) and expansion of the compartments. In addition, there is thickening of the septae (S) with loss of the normal architecture (hematoxylin-eosin, original magnification × 10). *(B)* Fibrillary astrocytes that are minimally pleomorphic and hyperchromatic (Bodian, original magnification × 25). *(C)* Cysts formed by pools of mucopolysaccharide containing bloated macrophages (phosphotungstic acid–hematoxylin, original magnification × 10). *(D)* Dilated processes of the glial cells (Rosenthal fibers) in an ancient glioma surrounded by hyalinized connective tissue. The presence of these Rosenthal fibers helps to distinguish this tumor from meningioma or peripheral nerve sheath tumors.

if they progress, either radiotherapy or shunting procedures, or both, should be employed.

Histopathology

Optic nerve gliomas are well-differentiated (low-grade) pilocytic astrocytomas. Two growth patterns have been described. The majority arise intrinsically, expanding the individual fascicles and the overall dimension of the nerve. The second pattern is extraneural extension of glioma in the arachnoid space, and is believed to be more common in neurofibromatosis. Not infrequently there is hyperplasia of the surrounding arachnoidal cells, which may lead to an incorrect diagnosis of meningioma in small biopsy specimens. However, gliomas characteristically do not invade the dura, which remains intact (see Fig. 12-5C). They are composed of fibrillary astrocytes, which may develop many brightly eosinophilic nodes (called Rosenthal fibers) in their processes (Fig. 12-1). Optic nerve gliomas rarely show malignant degenerative changes or mitoses; however, cystic and mucinous changes are frequently noted. Histologically, there may be considerable sparing of the axonal component of the nerve (see Fig. 12-5C, D). Vascular proliferation and atypia are common in piloid astrocytomas and do not indicate malignancy. However, mitotic figures and necrosis are frequently associated with malignant degeneration. Therefore, factors that may account for expansion or growth of gliomas include deposition of mucin; astrocytic proliferation; and to lesser degrees necrosis, hemorrhage, and arachnoidal hyperplasia.

As noted previously, a small or peripheral biopsy specimen may only include an area of arachnoidal hyperplasia, which can be difficult to distinguish from a meningioma. Occasionally, gliomas within the subarachnoid space may be confused with a peripheral nerve sheath spindle cell tumor. They may be distinguished by histochemical stains for glial fibrillary acidic protein (GFAP) and phosphotungstic acid-hematoxylin (PTAH) to identify glial filaments. Electron-microscopically, astrocytomas usually have a very loose lacey appearance and only rarely demonstrate basement membranes. Rosenthal fibers are electron-dense condensations of glial filaments that are unique to astrocytes and help to distinguish them from peripheral sheath tumors.

The clinical character and management of optic nerve gliomas can be best understood by dividing them into orbital, orbital-cranial, chiasmal, and diffuse types.

Orbital Pilocytic Astrocytoma

Approximately 20% to 23% of orbital pilocytic astrocytomas (Fig. 12-2) arise within the orbit where they are characterized by proptosis (frequently nonaxial and temporal), visual loss, optic atrophy, and unilateral papil-

ledema. The degree of visual loss tends to be profound at initial diagnosis (Fig. 12-3), but may be minimal (Fig. 12-5). Proptosis is usually insidious in onset but may occur rapidly as a result of increased mucosubstance, necrosis, or hemorrhage.

Examination reveals pupillary abnormalities, visual deficit, visual field changes (including irregular defects, increased blind spot, and peripheral contraction), and (in some younger patients) strabismus. On CT scan, gliomas present as enlarged fusiform optic nerves with smooth, well-defined, intact dural margins (Fig. 12-3A, B). Involvement of the entire optic nerve within the orbit is common. Anterior kinks adjacent to the globe and low-density cystic areas are frequent and characteristic, reflecting pliability of the nerve and focal areas of degeneration within the tumor. Calcification visible on CT scan does not occur. The density of these lesions is similar to normal optic nerve and shows uniform intense enhancement after contrast infusion. A central linear lucency within the optic nerve sheath, as seen with meningiomas after contrast infusion, is never seen in optic nerve gliomas. Angiographically, these lesions do not demonstrate a tumor blush, in contradistinction to optic nerve meningiomas. Ultrasonographic examination demon-

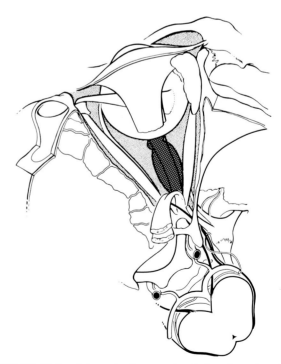

FIGURE 12-2. Schematic diagram of typical configuration of intraorbital optic nerve glioma showing smooth fusiform expansion of the nerve with kinking at the distal end (see Figure 12-7).

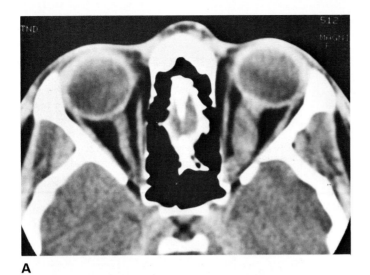

A

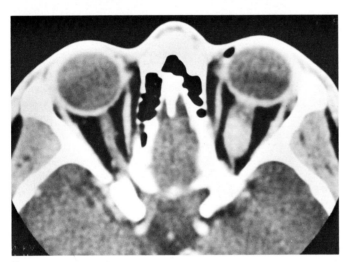

B

FIGURE 12-3.   *(A, B)* Axial CT scans show a fusiform dilatation of the optic nerve with slight kinking of the anterior portion of the nerve due to a glioma. The patient, a 22-year-old woman, had noted left visual problems for 4 years. *(C)* Axial scan using bone settings demonstrates a normal-sized optic canal on the affected side.

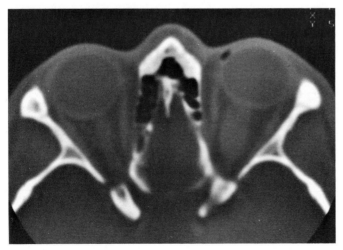

C

strates relatively homogeneous enlargements of the optic nerve (Fig. 12-4).

Clinical progression is characterized by increasing visual loss, visual field defects, optic atrophy, proptosis, papilledema, and, rarely, the development of optociliary shunts (Fig. 12-5B).

Management. Many series have noted that isolated intraorbital gliomas have an excellent prognosis for life but a poor one for vision. Their slowly progressive nature and tendency to a declining growth pattern with time imply that the clinician's responsibilities are to establish their isolated nature and to observe them unless there is disfiguring proptosis or significant progression. In case of either circumstances, adequate resection of the tumor is indicated. Resection may be achieved through a lateral orbital approach; however, we believe a temporofrontal panoramic orbitotomy is the method of choice, since the onus on the surgeon at the time of extirpation is to achieve a complete removal. The reason for this preferred route is based on intervention only for tumors that are of significant size, extend to the apex, or have shown evidence of rapid progression. The tumor should be excised within the dura of the optic nerve distally at the globe, and the proximal extent should be identified grossly, resected, and defined histologically as clear. Several reports have suggested that even incompletely excised gliomas may not progress.

Orbital-Cranial Gliomas

The second group of optic nerve gliomas are those with both orbital and intracranial involvement (Fig. 12-6). They fall into three subgroups: anterior to the chiasm; with chiasmal involvement; and with adjacent parachiasmal involvement. The first subgroup consists of tumors that extend from the orbit up to, but not involving, the chiasm. These patients generally require more prompt surgical action, because once tumors involve the chiasm, excision is impossible. The patient may have evidence of tumor involving the nerve but not the chiasm on the basis of absence of contralateral visual field defect and careful radiologic and CT evaluation of the optic canal and chiasmal region (Fig. 12-7). High-resolution axial and coronal CT scans with thin cuts are mandatory to evaluate the parachiasmal region and define the extent of the lesions, which demonstrate a dense oval to round enhancing chiasmal mass. The tumor is isodense on noncontrast CT and may be missed if contrast infusion is not used. Loss of the normal suprasellar cisterns is an indirect sign of a chiasmal lesion. CT scans may demonstrate expansion of the optic canal (Figs. 12-7 and 12-8). Magnetic resonance imaging appears useful for the differential diagnosis of optic nerve lesions with the optic canal, and may play a role in defining the degree of involvement. This subgroup of optic nerve astrocytomas can be man-

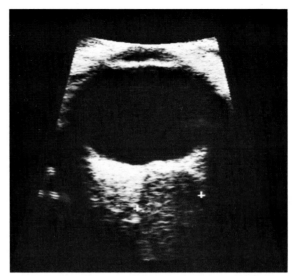

FIGURE 12-4. B-scan ultrasound demonstrates enlargement of the optic nerve by the solid glioma shown in Figure 12-7.

aged by surgical excision of the involved nerve up to the chiasm with confirmation of clear margins.

Chiasmal Gliomas

From looking at combined series, it appears that about two thirds of optic nerve astrocytomas involve the chiasm in one way or another (Fig. 12-9). They may either be restricted to the chiasm or involve the parachiasmal structures including the optic nerve, third ventricle, and adjacent brain. Patients with chiasmal involvement represent the most distressing group, because there is no reliable, agreed-upon, and definitive therapy. Operative intervention is of no benefit other than to establish diagnosis when unsure. Intervention may even ablate residual vision. In addition, several authors have noted intraoperative and perioperative deaths during and following biopsy. Furthermore, a significant number of patients in this group have involvement of the adjacent central nervous system structures, and may develop symptoms and signs of precocious puberty and obstructive hydrocephalus that reflect hypothalamic and ventricular system invasion. Miller has divided the chiasmal groups into anterior and posterior types based on dominant location, with the posterior type having a much more serious prognosis. Shunting may be required to relieve obstructive hydrocephalus. Nonsurgical treatment, such as radiotherapy and chemotherapy, remains controversial; some authors have found clinical improvement in vision and diminution in growth, whereas others fail to confirm this. Still others have noted that surviving patients tend to have stable vision regardless of the mode of therapy. In

(Text continues on p. 290.)

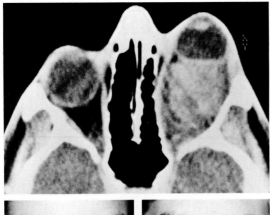

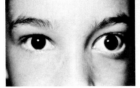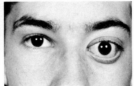

A

FIGURE 12-5. *(A)* The lower figure demonstrates the clinical features of a developing optic nerve glioma. This boy presented at age 11 years *(left)* with a history of proptosis first noted at age 6 years and documented progressive anisometropic hyperopia. At this stage his vision was 20/70 with a +3.50 sphere; in addition, he had 7 mm of proptosis, an afferent pupillary defect, and a raised gliotic disc. Over the next 5 years he showed documented fluctuations of vision between 20/40 and 20/80 with progressive proptosis and increasing hyperopia. At age 16 years *(right)* he had 11 mm of proptosis, 7 D of hyperopia, increased optic nerve atrophy, and an unsightly globe. Axial CT scan done at that time shows a massive inhomogeneous lesion that has led to flattening of the posterior aspect of the globe and expansion of the orbit. The tumor and optic nerve were removed, and histologically there were multiple cystic areas (shown in *C*). *(B)* The raised gliotic disc and optociliary shunt of the patient's left nerve head.

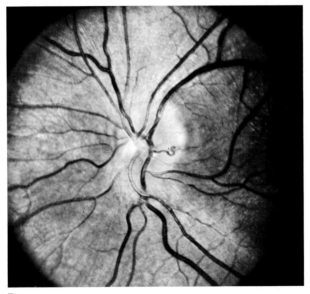

B

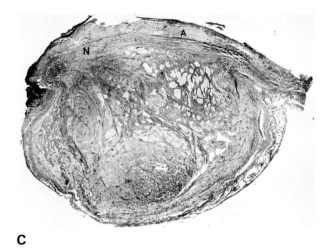

C

FIGURE 12-5. *(Continued).*   *(C)* This massive glioma had multiple cystic areas and hyperplasia of the arachnoid (A) with considerable preservation of the axonal elements (N) (luxol fast blue hematoxylin, original magnification × 4). *(D)* The cross section of the cut end of the optic nerve at the orbital apex. Note the arachnoidal hyperplasia (A) and preserved optic nerve (hematoxylin-eosin, original magnification × 10, inset × 2.5). *(E)* Electronmicroscopic features of the above astrocytoma. The tumor cells have delicate cytoplasmic processes, some filled with bundles of intermediate filaments (original magnification, × 9828). *(Inset)* The black condensation of the glial filaments in an astrocytic process is a Rosenthal fiber (original magnification, × 6725). (Electron micrograph courtesy C. Dolman.)

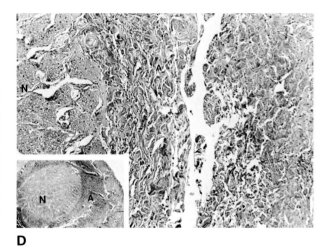

D

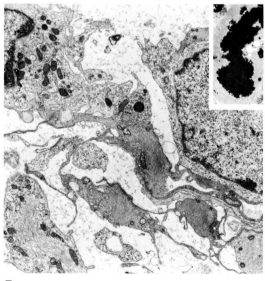

E

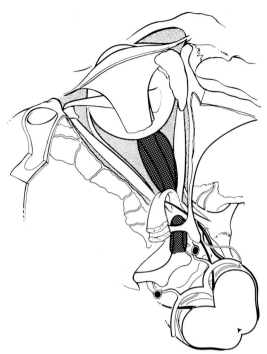

FIGURE 12-6. Schematic diagram of orbitocranial glioma extending to the chiasmal region.

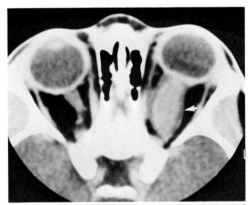

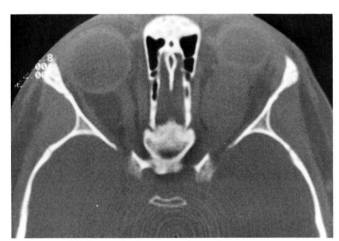

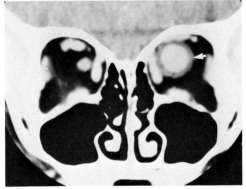

FIGURE 12-7. *(A)* Axial and coronal contrast-enhanced CT scan of a 5-year-old child with a fusiform optic nerve lesion causing flattening of the posterior margin of the globe. Note the low-density expansion of the left optic nerve sheath that corresponded histologically to arachnoidal meningeal hyperplasia *(arrow)*. Clinically, the patient had slight proptosis and mere light perception. *(B)* Axial CT scan of the same patient with bone settings demonstrates widening of the left optic canal due to involvement of the intracanalicular portion of the nerve.

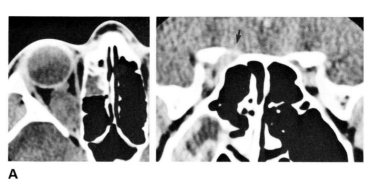

FIGURE 12-8. *(A, left)* Axial CT scan of a glioma shows a typical fusiform expansion of the right optic nerve with distal kinking adjacent to the globe. Coronal scan *(right)* shows erosion of the roof of the optic canal in the lesser sphenoid wing *(arrow)*. Clinically, this was associated with an 8-month history of decreased vision in a 14-year-old girl. On examination, she had counting fingers vision, a dense temporal pallor, and a central scotoma. *(B, top)* Coronal scan of the same lesion more posteriorly shows glioma expanding the intracranial portion of the optic nerve *(arrow)*. *(Bottom)* A reformatted sagittal scan of the same lesion. This glioma was resected with clear margins just anterior to the chiasm by temporal frontal craniotomy.

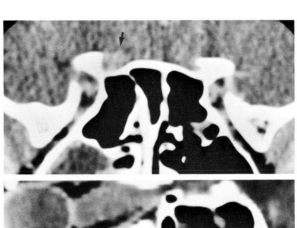

A

B

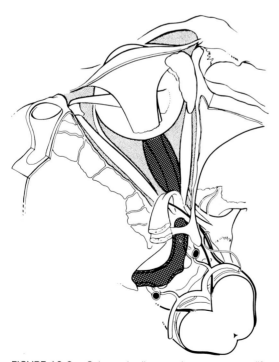

FIGURE 12-9. Schematic diagram demonstrates a diffuse glioma of the optic nerve, tract, and chiasm.

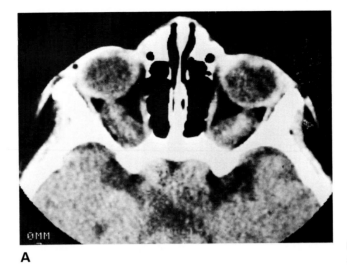

A

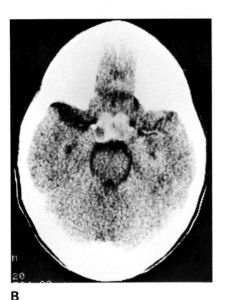

B

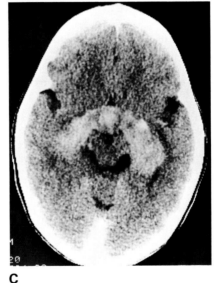

C

FIGURE 12-10. Axial CT scans show a diffuse glioma involving both optic nerves *(A)*, the chiasm *(B)*, and optic tracts *(C)*. The patient was a 5-year-old boy with neurofibromatosis; he had bilateral blindness and optic pallor.

the absence of randomized prospective studies, it is difficult to derive a clear conclusion. Nevertheless, the majority of authors still favor radiotherapeutic intervention if there is evidence of deterioration of vision, and in many patients, improvement in vision has occurred following treatment.

Diffuse Pilocytic Astrocytoma

The final type is the multifocal or diffuse optic nerve glioma (Fig. 12-10). They occur in patients with von Recklinghausen's disease, and some believe their histology and biologic behavior are different. Several reports have indicated a good visual prognosis in these patients even without intervention. Jakobiec has suggested that

diffuse gliomas tend to extend and grow as pilocytic masses in the subarachnoid space about the pia without breaching the dura. In practical terms, patients with neurofibromatosis and evidence of an optic nerve glioma of a multifocal or diffuse nature are probably best left alone and simply observed unless documented progression is noted. It is worth emphasizing that patients with neurofibromatosis are prone to sarcomas and malignant gliomas in other sites and bear close follow-up.

Although limited, our own experience (Table 12-1) with pilocytic astrocytomas of the optic nerve reflects the clinical gamut of these lesions. We have seen a total of 12 cases, three of which have occurred in patients with von Recklinghausen's disease. The patients with neurofibromatosis have shown considerable fluctuations in vision, with spontaneous improvement and deterioration occurring over very short periods of time. All three had chiasmal involvement; two were bilateral and diffuse, and one had associated precocious puberty. Two have simply been observed, and one was treated with radiotherapy with improvement of deteriorating vision. Two of our patients have had chiasmal involvement without evidence of orbital disease. Both were treated with radiotherapy, leading to improvement in vision. The remaining seven patients have had gliomas without apparent involvement of the chiasm. Three were clearly intraorbital; one was of enormous size, yet was not associated with as profound a loss of vision as one would expect given the size of the lesion (see Fig. 12-5). The large orbital glioma was resected, and the other two patients are under observation. The remaining four patients had lesions that extended from the orbit to the optic tract anterior to the chiasm on CT scanning and no involvement of the opposite optic nerve from a functional point of view. Two of these underwent temporal frontal craniotomy and surgical excision, whereas the others were observed and have not progressed to date.

The major lesion to differentiate from optic nerve gliomas remains optic nerve meningioma. The numerous epidemiologic, clinical, orbital imaging, and histopathologic differences between these two lesions are summarized in Table 12-2.

MALIGNANT OPTIC GLIOMA (GLIOBLASTOMA) OF ADULTHOOD

In 1973 Hoyt and co-workers described a malignant optic nerve glioma of adulthood (Fig. 12-11). It appeared to constitute a distinct syndrome occurring in middle-aged males, causing rapid deterioration of vision mimicking optic neuritis with relentless progression to blindness and fatality. The early symptoms consisted of monocular visual blurring, retrobulbar pain, features of increased venous congestion, edema, and infarction of the nerve at the disc. The tumor progresses to cause blindness, hemiparesis, and hypothalamic abnormalities. Pathologically, it is an aggressive glioblastoma that invades the surrounding tissues, leading to a rapid downhill course and death. Most patients were not diagnosed before craniotomy or autopsy.

TABLE 12-1.
OPTIC NERVE GLIOMAS, UNIVERSITY OF BRITISH COLUMBIA ORBITAL CLINIC, 1976–1986

Site	Age When Seen (Years)	Sex*	Neurofibromatosis*	Presentation*	Site*	Management	Follow Up*
Orbital							
TH	11	M	—	Changing refraction by 1 year, increasing hyperopia, VA 20/25, 7 mm proptosis, disc pallor	L orbit	Observed for 7 years, VA 20/80; marked proptosis (11 mm); optociliary shunt, resected	No recurrence at 5 years
RF	22	F	—	4 years decreased vision OS; 2 mm proptosis, optic atrophy	L orbit	Observed for 1 year	No growth
DK	13	M	—	OD reduced vision 20/25	R optic nerve enlarged	Observed since 1981	No change at 5 years
Orbital-Cranial							
JD	16	M	3 café au lait spots	7-year history of progressive visual loss OD; now NLP	R optic nerve	Observation	No progression at 2 years
HD	14	F	—	8 months progressive VA OD (counting fingers 40 cm), elevated optic nerve head	R optic nerve anterior to chiasm	Resection	No recurrence at 2 years

(Continued)

TABLE 12-1. (Continued)

Site	Age When Seen (Years)	Sex*	Neurofibro-matosis*	Presentation*	Site*	Management	Follow Up*
KL	30	F	−	Decreased VA OD for 5 years, diagnosis astrocytoma grade II; treated with radiotherapy 5600 rad, resected (elsewhere)	R optic nerve to chiasm	Observation	Enucleation following radiation keratopathy and painful eye
AQ	6	F	1 café au lait spot	OS strabismus since age 9 months, proptosis age 4 years, LPP only OS	L optic nerve to chiasm	Resected; gross complete, microscopic residual	No recurrence at 1 year
Chiasmal and Parachiasmal							
KC	9	M	+	Decreased VA OU, 6/200 OD, 6/40 OS, bilateral optic atrophy OD greater than OS, precocious puberty	Chiasmal	Observed for 2 years, decreased VA to 20/400 and 20/60, led to radiotherapy 5000 rad	Vision improved to 20/100 OD, 20/40 OS at 2 years; second cerebral glioma at 3 years
DA	7	M	−	Visual loss, left eye	Left optic nerve to chiasm	Biopsied and irradiated prior to referral	7 years—NLP left with optic atrophy and right nasal field defect
Diffuse							
DC	2	F	+	Right pupil noted to be larger than left, 4 months of progressive right proptosis (OD 14 mm, OS 8 mm)	Diffuse optic nerve and chiasm	Under observation	8 months
JC	4	F	+	OS prominent for several months, VA 20/40 OD 20/200 OS	Diffuse optic nerve and chiasm	Observed, variable vision, fluctuates to levels of 20/40 OD 20/50 OS	Follow up at 7 years
JH	4	M	+	Bilateral blindness progressive since age 1 year, nystagmus, optic atrophy	Optic nerves, chiasm, and radiations	Observed	Follow up at 1 year
Malignant							
WM	54	M	−	Blurred vision OS, VA 20/20 OD counting fingers 2 m OS, bilateral temporal field defect	Chiasm, hypothalamus	Biopsy; glioblastoma; radiotherapy	Dead in 6 months

* M, male; F, female; VA, visual acuity; LPP, light perception and projection; +, neurofibromatosis present; −, neurofibromatosis absent; L, left; R, right; NLP, no light perception.

TABLE 12-2.
MAJOR FEATURES OF OPTIC NERVE GLIOMA AND OPTIC NERVE MENINGIOMA

Optic Nerve Glioma	Optic Nerve Meningioma
Epidemiology	
Age	
Median 5 years (may be first symptomatic after age 20 years)	Mean 42 years (4% under 20)
Associations	
Up to 50% have von Recklinghausen's	Rare association with von Recklinghausen's
Bilateral involvement is pathognomonic of von Recklinghausen's	Bilateral involvement is not associated with von Recklinghausen's
Sex	
Slight female dominance	Significant female dominance
Clinical Features: Visual	
Disproportionate visual loss with minimal proptosis	Disproportionate visual loss to degree of proptosis
Generally worse vision than meningioma	Vision may be better preserved than glioma
Optociliary shunt rare	Optociliary shunt a characteristic feature
Optic nerve head invasion rare	Optic nerve head may be invaded
CT Features	
Intact dura, smooth margins	Dura invaded; irregular margins; orbital invasion
Most are fusiform	Diffuse with apical bulbous enlargement
May have central remnant of optic nerve	Railroad tracking
Kinking and cystic degeneration	Straight or splinted
Rare calcification	Calcification a typical feature
Rare bone change	Bone change at the apex
Histologic Features	
Astrocytic filaments (PTAH and GFAP)	Intranuclear vacuoles
Rosenthal fibers	Clusters and whorls
Arachnoidal hyperplasia frequent	All are meningothelial or transitional PAS-positive glycoprotein in cytoplasm
Electron-microscopic Features	
Elongated and spindle-shaped	Intertwining cell processes with many desmosomes
Abundant cytoplasmic glial filaments	Little extracellular space or matrix
Focal degeneration	Cytoplasm numerous filaments
Rosenthal fibers; electron-dense condensations of glial filaments	Few organelles

(After Jakobiec FA, Depot MJ, Kennerdell JS et al: Combined clinical and computed tomographic diagnosis of orbital glioma and meningioma. Ophthalmology 91:137, 1984; and Jakobiec FA, Font RL: Tumors of the optic nerve. In Spencer WH (ed): Ophthalmic Pathology: An Atlas and Textbook, 3rd ed, Vol 3, p 2632. Philadelphia, WB Saunders, 1986)

More recently, the syndrome has been broadened to include middle-aged persons of both sexes (roughly in equal proportion) with binocular visual symptoms also occurring in equal numbers. In spite of visual and retrobulbar symptoms, 25% of cases show normal ophthalmologic and neuroradiologic findings. Roughly 50% have or develop disc edema and may go on to hemorrhagic glaucoma and orbital involvement (proptosis and ophthalmoplegia) as a result of growth and extension. The ocular symptoms occur early, and as the tumor rapidly extends into the nervous system neurologic symptoms develop. CT scanning will demonstrate enlargement of the optic nerve or chiasm in 75% of patients. Diagnosis is by open biopsy. Kennerdell has described one case in which the biopsy was made by fine needle aspiration. The fulminant and relentless course of this disease is unaffected by any therapeutic modality. Histologically, the majority of cases have been pleomorphic astrocytomas with many mitoses and vascular endothelial proliferation, characteristic of a glioblastoma multiforme. A few cases have been described with histologically more well-differentiated astrocytomas.

Meningiomas

Meningiomas may affect the orbit and its contents as tumors arising from the intracranial cavity, optic nerve, or rarely the orbital soft tissues. They are usually slow-growing neoplasias that declare themselves clinically by compression or encasement, or both, of normal anatomic structures. Meningiomas frequently lead to visual loss;

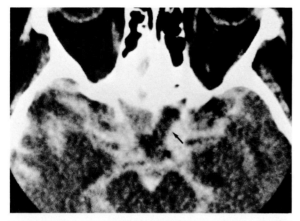

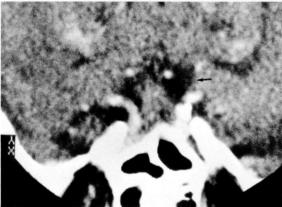

FIGURE 12-11.   Axial *(top)* and coronal *(bottom)* CT scans of the chiasmatic region obtained with metrizamide in the basal cisterns shows expansion of the optic chiasm *(arrows)* due to a malignant optic nerve glioma (glioblastoma multiforme). This 54-year-old man presented with a 3-week history of left blurred vision (counting fingers at 2 feet), bilateral temporal field loss, a left afferent pupillary defect, and normal discs. In spite of radiotherapy, this patient succumbed to the tumor within 5 months.

those confined to and arising from the optic nerve sheath cause unilateral deterioration, whereas those arising intracranially often ultimately affect vision bilaterally. The more confined the space and the closer to the optic nerve they arise, the earlier their effect on vision; thus, even small tumors of the optic canal cause early visual disturbances, whereas more remote lesions lead to structural displacement and disfigurement first, with functional deficits appearing later. At the time of writing this chapter, we have seen 23 meningiomas, of which 7 were of primary optic nerve sheath origin and the remaining 16 arose extrinsic to the optic nerve involving either the sphenoid wing (8), parasellar region (1), or both (7). One appeared to arise as a primary tumor of the soft tissues of the orbit. Most intracranial meningiomas that affect the orbital or visual structures arise from the dura of the sphenoid bone (ridge, planum, parasellar region, or optic canal).

Histogenesis and Growth

The meningothelial cap cells of the arachnoid villi (pacchionian granulations) are considered the stem cell of meningiomas. They arise from and incorporate the middle meningeal layer adjacent to the pia-arachnoid. Growth is slow and tends to be in cohesive clusters with or without evidence of encapsulation. When infiltrating soft tissues the tumors frequently cause reactive desmoplasia. Infiltration of bone can cause hyperostosis, which may make meningiomas difficult to distinguish clinically from primary bone tumors. These tumors tend either to displace structures; extend along paths of least resistance through foramina and adventitial spaces; encase structures in dense connective tissue; or cause compression due to hyperostosis and expansion of bone.

There are a number of histologic patterns of meningioma. The fundamental cell is usually round or polygonal, but may be more spindle shaped. Varying admixtures of blood vessels, fibroblasts, and psammoma bodies account for the differing patterns. Although they usually arise as a cohesive mass that develops in continuity, concurrent multiple sites of occurrence and seeding have been described.

Two thirds of meningiomas are meningotheliomatous (syncytial), consisting of sheets of polygonal cells, or transitional (mixed—psammomatous) where they are composed of eddies or whorls of spindle cells that frequently surround a central psammoma body. Dense, randomly woven bundles of spindle-shaped meningothelial cells and fibroblasts constitute the fibrous pattern (Fig. 12-12). Meningiomas may be quite vascular, as demonstrated in the histopathology of the lesion shown in Fig. 12-13*B*.

Two aggressive patterns exist: the angioblastic (capillary hemangioblastoma) and sarcomatous. Angioblastic meningiomas are exceedingly rare, constituting 3% of meningeal tumors, and have also been called *hemangiopericytoma* of the meninges because of a similar histologic pattern to soft tissue hemangiopericytoma. Angioblastic meningiomas have a tendency to recur, and up to one third are reported to metastasize eventually. Spread of angioblastic meningiomas is not predictable histologically. At the University of British Columbia, Holden, Dolman, and Churg have provided recent immunohistochemical evidence of meningothelial origin, and they included in this series a case of ours that arose from the optic nerve sheath. (The case was included in Chapter 14.) The patient returned recently with a recurrence and optic atrophy due to his apical tumor (Fig. 12-14). At

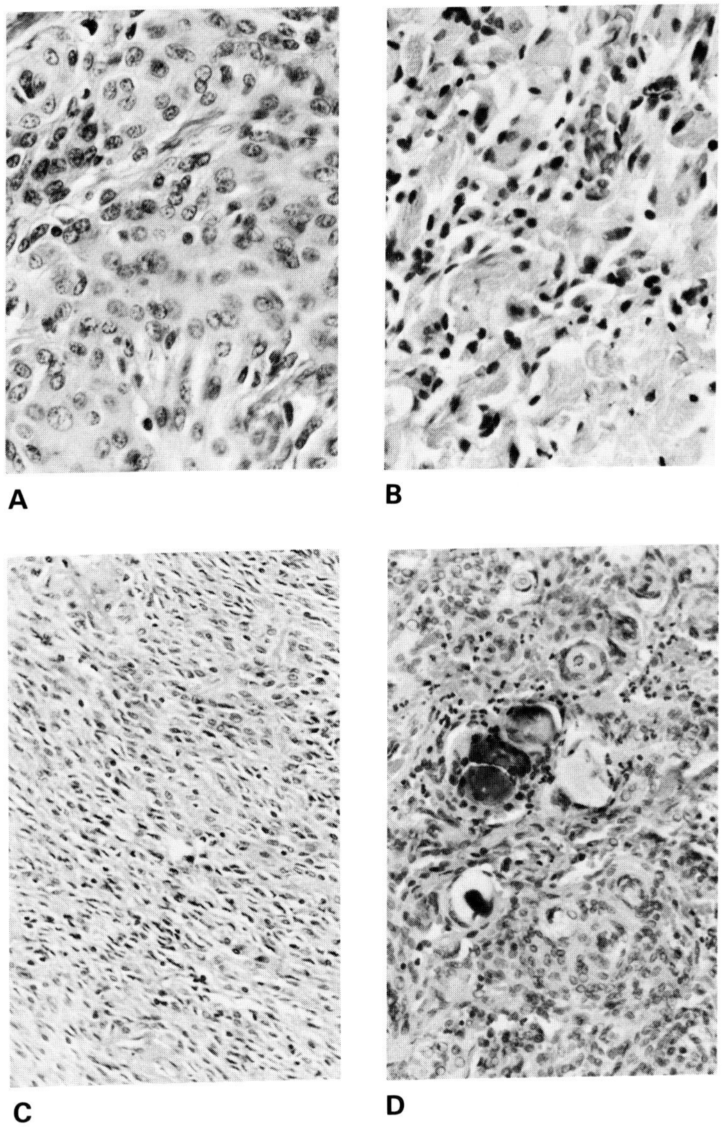

FIGURE 12-12. Histopathology of meningioma, showing varying patterns of meningothelial growth. (A) A dense syncytial pattern of whorling, plump, polygonal cells of a meningotheliomatous type. The nuclei are oval, lightly stained, and show slight indentation. (B) The mixture of fibroblasts, connective tissue, and meningothelial cells of the fibroblastic pattern. (C) A transitional pattern with a mixture of meningothelial and slender, elongated spindle-shaped cells. (D) An example of a psammomatous meningothelial meningioma (H&E, original magnifications: A, × 40; B, × 25; C, × 10; D, × 25).

combined orbitotomy the largely exophytic lesion and adjacent optic nerve were removed. Histochemically this hemangiopericytoma was positive for Vimentin and variably positive for keratin, as were meningiomas and arachnoidal granulations. In contrast, soft tissue hemangiopericytomas and normal pericytes were negative for both. Angioblastic meningiomas ultrastructurally show much basement membrane material and usually have more primitive junctions than meningiomas. This study suggests they are meningiomas. Boniak and co-workers have reported a hemangiopericytoma of the optic nerve that was intrasheath, whereas our case was mainly exophytic with an intrasheath component.

Sarcomatous intracranial meningiomas occur in a younger age group (second decade), are more pleomorphic and invasive, and may metastasize outside the central nervous system.

Clinical Presentation and Topography

In spite of the varying histologic patterns, growth is generally measured in years and clinical manifestations are largely governed by location. The less confined and the more remote, the longer the tumor will be present prior to clinical manifestation. Thus, tumors in the optic canal cause profound early visual symptoms, in contrast to

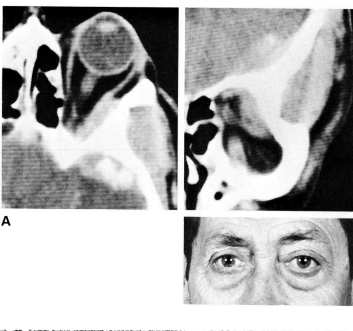

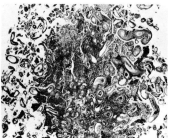

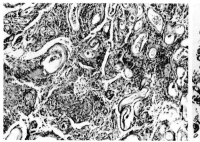

FIGURE 12-13. *(A)* This meningioma of the outer two-thirds of the sphenoid wing is causing hyperostosis with an associated soft tissue mass involving the adjacent lateral orbit, middle cranial, and temporalis fossa (axial and coronal contrast-enhanced scans). Note fullness of the left temporalis fossa in clinical photograph of this 67-year-old man, who had become aware of a decrease in his vision. Clinically, there was medial displacement (2 mm), proptosis (7 mm), and decreased visual field. He underwent resection of the tumor and bone, with recovery of field and vision. *(B)* Histopathology of the lesion shown in *A*. Note rich vascular pattern with islands of meningothelial cells (hematoxylin-eosin, original magnification: *left*, ✕ 10; *right*, ✕ 2.5).

large meningiomas of the outer third of the sphenoid ridge, which lead to mass effect early and dysfunction late.

INTRACRANIAL MENINGIOMAS

Intracranial meningiomas constitute 15% of adult and 2% of childhood intracranial tumors. The major sites affecting the orbital and visual structures are the sphenoid ridge, suprasellar area (tuberculum sellae, presellar), and olfactory groove. Overall, 18% of all intracranial meningiomas occur in the sphenoid wing, 8% suprasellar, and 8% along the olfactory groove. Tumors of the middle portion of the sphenoid ridge arise from the posterior margins of the lesser wing (Fig. 12-15, 2). The deep inner or clinoidal portion and the middle third of the sphenoid

ridge make up the medial portion and by contiguity affect neural and vascular structures coursing through the optic canal and superior orbital fissure early in the course of their development (Fig. 12-15, *1* and *2*). Similarly, parasellar meningiomas affect adjacent vessels and structures of the cavernous sinus early, leading to motor and sensory deficits followed by optic nerve compression (Fig. 12-15, *5*). In contrast, tumors of the olfactory groove (Fig. 12-15, *4*) and lateral third of the sphenoid ridge (greater wing; Fig. 12-15, *3*) tend to be large and globular before causing symptoms as a result of raised intracranial pressure or displacement. En plaque meningiomas have a propensity to occur along the greater wing of the sphenoid and are frequently desmoplastic, infiltrative, and hyperostotic, making effective removal extremely difficult and recurrence frequent.

The orbital and visual manifestations reflect the location of the mass with the more medial tumors causing cranial nerve palsies, visual deficits, and venous obstructive signs and symptoms (edema and chemosis). More remote tumors exert their effect by virtue of raised intracranial pressure or mass effect, with those of the greater wing of the sphenoid presenting as enlargement of the temporalis fossa with late intracranial symptoms and those of the olfactory groove with both intracranial and visual symptoms. Physical distortion of the orbit is the result of expanded bone or tumor encroaching on the soft tissues. Enlargement of the temporalis fossa may be easily noted in patients wearing glasses wherein the gap between the temporalis and the temple of the glasses shows marked narrowing compared to the other side. In addition, retrospective review of photographs can often be useful in assessing expansion of the temporalis fossa or orbital displacement (Figs. 12-13, 12-16, 12-17). By the time tumors of the olfactory groove manifest clinically with visual loss, they have often affected both optic nerves.

Intracranial meningiomas occur three times more frequently in women than in men and are seen generally in the fifth decade. In contrast, Wright has noted that optic nerve and orbital meningiomas may have a bimodal peak in the second and fifth decades. Those in the young are said to be more aggressive. Multifocal simultaneous meningiomas may occur, and there is an increased frequency of intracranial and orbital meningiomas in neurofibromatosis.

The visual and other functional deficits due to intracranial meningiomas reflect their direct early or late compressive effects based on location. Wilson, in a summary of data from prospective studies, has noted that the characteristic visual loss of intracranial meningiomas is slowly progressive in 90% and acute in 8% to 12%. In addition, the visual progression may be slow but intermittent in character in about 12% of instances. Fifty percent have initial unilateral loss with bilateral visual loss occurring in the other 50%, except for olfactory groove meningiomas, which have a higher incidence of bilateral visual acuity loss. Deterioration of color vision is an earlier and more sensitive index of compression of the optic nerve.

Investigations

The most useful imaging modality for meningiomas is CT scan. Bony change, hyperostosis (see Fig. 12-17) and lysis, and the soft tissue component of the tumor are easily visible (Fig. 12-18). The lesion is well defined, homogeneous, and characteristically of increased density with uniform enhancement postcontrast infusion. In addition, the tumor may show encasement of adjacent structures (Fig. 12-19). Smaller intracranial meningiomas may be identified with CT scanning (Fig. 12-20). Contrast angiography may be useful primarily in demonstrating preoperative relationship to blood vessels or to identify tumor blush, a frequent feature of meningioma. Fine calcification may be evident in highly psammomatous lesions.

Management

The management of intracranial meningiomas is mainly surgical. Providing the tumor is well defined and encapsulated, microsurgical excision is extremely effective. However, invasion of bone and soft tissues or encasement of vital structures may obviate complete excision. Major debulking may be effective in improving cosmesis and alleviating compressive symptoms with reversal or postponement of visual loss. The introduction of surgical lasers, high-speed drills, and ultrasonic fragmentizers has aided considerably in the surgical management of these lesions. We have recently introduced a combined panoramic orbitotomy approach to the removal of sphenoid wing meningiomas. The orbitotomy craniotomy allows complete removal of the bone surrounding the superior orbital fissure as well as affected dura and soft tissues. The role of radiotherapy, often suggested after incomplete excision, remains somewhat controversial, and chemotherapy is ineffective.

OPTIC CANAL MENINGIOMAS

Canal meningiomas typically present with visual loss due to early compression of the optic nerve. Even with the use of thin section axial and coronal CT scans, it may be very difficult to identify small tumors of the canal. Subtle, round expansion of the orbital end of the optic canal should be sought. Magnetic resonance imaging will aid in the study of the intracanalicular portion of the optic nerve and the identification of these lesions. These tumors have a tendency to spread posteriorly and extend over the planum to affect the opposite optic nerve even 10 to 20 years after initial diagnosis. Because of their intimate relationship to the vascular supply in the optic canal, excision without damage to the nerve is highly unlikely and therapeutic intervention should aim for complete excision based on the risk of spread to the chiasm and opposite optic nerve. It has been suggested that bilateral optic nerve meningiomas may represent multicentric origin. On the other hand, intracranial continuity may not be detectable radiologically yet may be evident on histologic or operative inspection (Fig. 12-21). Bilaterality is also a feature of basofrontal or sphenoid meningiomas, particularly if they are of the en plaque variety.

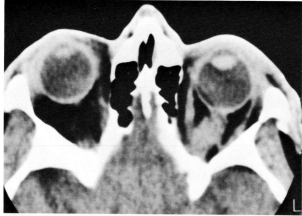
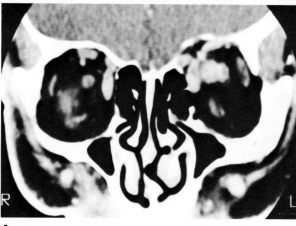

A

FIGURE 12-14. *(A)* An axial (unenhanced) and coronal (enhanced) CT scan of a recurrent angioblastic meningioma. The original tumor is shown in Figure 14-18*B*. The electronmicroscopy was characteristic for hemangiopericytoma. However, immunohistochemistry was positive for vimentin and keratin, a feature of meningiomas and arachnoidal granulations that was not noted with soft tissue hemangiopericytomas. The bulk of the mass was exophytic, but it also clearly involved the subarachnoid space, as shown in *B* and *C* (H&E, original magnifications: *B*, × 2.5; *C, left,* × 10; *C, right,* × 25).

OPTIC NERVE MENINGIOMAS

Histogenesis

The pathology of optic nerve meningiomas is essentially the same as described for meningiomas in general. However, they are almost always meningotheliomatous or transitional in pattern and characterized by slow growth, local extension, and invasion as cohesive masses along the lines of least resistance. A subgroup of optic nerve meningiomas is densely psammomatous and calcified. They may be multicentric (as noted previously) but are largely tumors that grow in continuity. Three basic gross patterns occur within the optic nerve: extradural, subdural, or combined extradural and subdural. Meningiomas of the nerve sheath have a propensity to breach the dural sheath and grow as nodular cohesive extradural masses (Fig. 12-22).

Clinical Manifestations

The majority of optic nerve meningiomas occur between the third and sixth decades with about two thirds of cases affecting females. They have been described in childhood wherein they are believed to be more invasive and frequently associated with neurofibromatosis.

The essential clinical features are a slowly developing compressive optic neuropathy with several types of onset and progression. Optic nerve meningiomas present with transient visual obscurations similar in character to those in papilledema. Obscurations may be duction-induced in extremes of gaze. These early symptoms correlate with minimal visual impairment, mild dyschromatopsia, enlargement of the blind spot, and contraction of the visual field. On physical examination the optic nerve head may be mildly edematous in spite of apparently normal visual acuities. The patient's subjective complaint of visual dif-

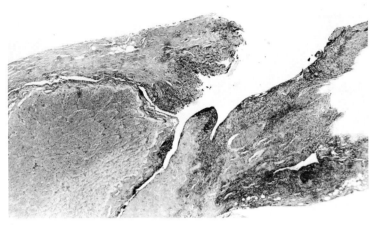

B

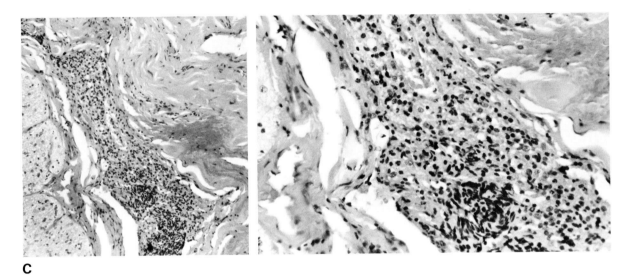

C

ficulty may be substantiated by more sensitive psychophysical testing, such as contrast sensitivity and accurate color vision studies. The early development may be difficult to differentiate from other entities with similar clinical presentations such as diabetic papillopathy, thyroid optic neuropathy, congenital pseudopapilledema, perineuritis, asymmetric or unilateral papilledema, cavernous hemangiomas, papillophlebitis, disc drusen, and some infective lesions of the optic nerve.

As the tumor grows, greater degrees of impairment of vision and psychophysical function become evident. Proptosis may increase, but in all instances is usually mild and between 2 mm and 6 mm. There is progressive constriction of the visual fields, leading to residual visual islands. Increasing disc edema is associated with dilatation of papillary and peripapillary vessels, increasing

gliosis, and the appearance of refractile bodies (Fig. 12-23). Vascular compromise may be associated with the appearance of optociliary shunt vessels (see Fig. 12-21) and choroidal folds. Ultimately, the nerve becomes increasingly gliotic, the refractile bodies disappear, and atrophy supervenes. Progression usually is exceedingly slow, providing a safe temporal framework for evaluation and follow up of these patients.

Orbital Imaging

High-resolution CT scans are the mainstay of investigation. They allow accurate definition of size and extension of the tumor. Careful axial cuts in the plane of the optic nerve and coronal scans will define these lesions. Subtle
(Text continues on p. 304.)

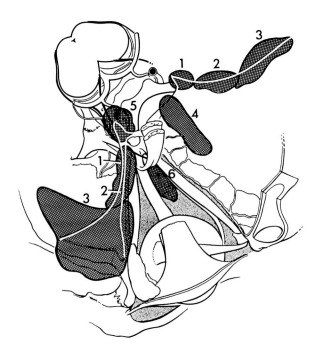

FIGURE 12-15. Schematic diagram demonstrates the sites of nonoptic nerve meningiomas that may affect vision and the orbit: *(1)* inner, *(2)* middle, and *(3)* outer thirds of the sphenoid; *(4)* olfactory groove, *(5)* parasellar, and *(6)* intraorbital.

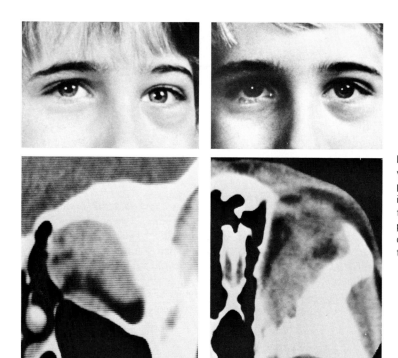

FIGURE 12-16. Clinical photograph of an 11-year-old boy *(top, left)* who presented with a left proptosis (8 mm), and downward (3 mm) and inward (2 mm) displacement. A photograph taken 2 years earlier *(top, right)* demonstrates prior "swollen lids." Axial and coronal CT scans of the meningioma demonstrate hyperostosis of the orbital roof and lateral wall.

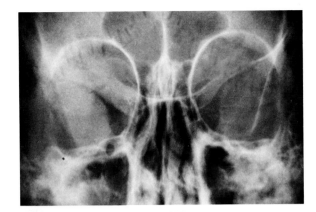

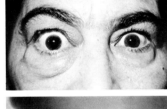

FIGURE 12-17. Plain film and tomographic features of hyper-ostosis associated with a right sphenoid wing meningioma. Note narrow right superior orbital fissure. Clinical features consisted of temporal and supraorbital pain with proptosis for a 5-year period. The patient had slight decreased vision (20/25) with minimal temporal pallor. Clinical photograph demonstrates swelling of lids and chemosis due to venous obstruction, a common feature of apically located meningiomas. She had lid retraction, making the differential diagnosis one of thyroid orbitopathy.

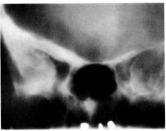

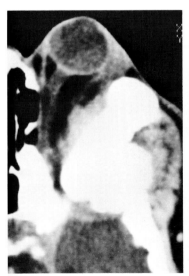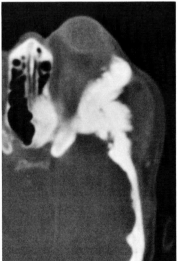

FIGURE 12-18. Axial CT scans with bone *(right)* and soft tissue *(left)* settings demonstrate the bony and soft tissue components of an exten-sive meningioma affecting the orbit and adjacent structures. Note the marked proptosis.

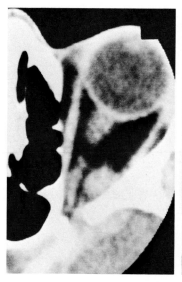
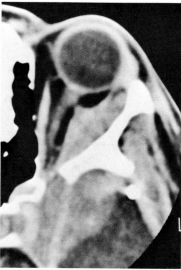

FIGURE 12-19. Axial CT features of two different meningiomas of the sphenoid wing showing variation in patterns of growth and biologic character. The lesion shown on the left was seen in a 57-year-old woman with visual deterioration for 1 year, lid swelling, and proptosis for 7 years. She had 2 mm downward and 2 mm inward displacement and 6 mm of proptosis with a minimal afferent pupillary defect and decreased color vision. Note small *en plaque* meningioma of both sides of the inner sphenoid wing. In contrast, the patient shown on the right was a 21-year-old woman with a 2-months' history of progressive proptosis (6 mm), slight decreased color vision, and reduction of extraocular movements in left abduction. A large meningioma involves the orbit, middle fossa, cavernous sinus, and temporal fossa.

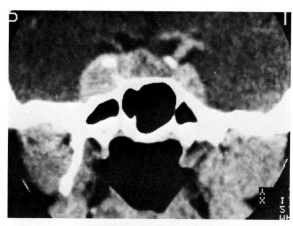

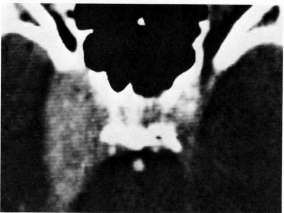

FIGURE 12-20. Axial *(bottom)* and coronal *(top)* enhanced CT scans of a right cavernous sinus meningioma in a 48-year-old woman who had minimal third nerve palsy and 2 mm of proptosis.

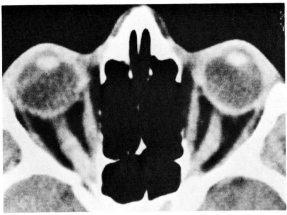

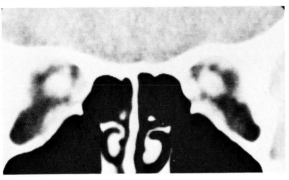

FIGURE 12-21. *(A)* Axial and coronal CT scans show diffuse bilateral optic nerve meningioma in a 33-year-old woman who presented with an 8-year history of intermittent reduction of vision. She had no perception of light on the right, and a right afferent pupillary defect and 20/30 vision on the left. She had concurrent basilar aneurysms. The meningioma was proven on biopsy, and continuity was noted over the planum sphenoidale at the time of aneurysm surgery following an intracranial hemorrhage. *(B)* Photographs of the fundi of the patient shown in *A* demonstrate chalky white pallor and optociliary shunts (on the right) with left superior temporal pallor.

A

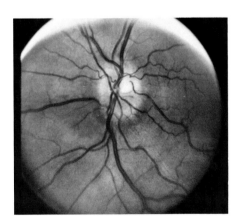

B

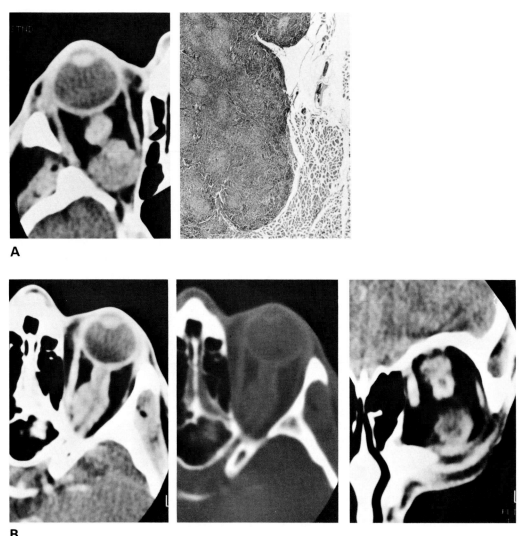

FIGURE 12-22. *(A)* Axial CT scan and histologic features of a nodular extradural sheath meningioma. It had recurred after previous sheath and tumor resection (H&E, original magnification ✕ 2.5). *(B)* Contrast-enhanced axial and coronal CT scans of a nodular extradural meningioma in a 32-year-old woman with normal visual acuity and optic nerve function. She had a 6-month history of intermittent diplopia, particularly in lateral gaze, and progressive proptosis. The optic canal is of normal dimension, and there is a central lucent zone representing the optic nerve (''railroad track'').

expansion of the optic canal may be seen. Optic nerve meningiomas generally demonstrate one of three radiologic patterns: diffuse thickening, fusiform swelling, and either anterior or (more frequently) posterior globular enlargement (Fig. 12-24). Often the border of optic nerve meningioma has a slightly nodular or irregular surface pattern (see Figs. 12-22, 12-24B). Central lucent areas after contrast infusion are characteristic and may identify the residual optic nerve. Dense uniform enhancement of

the lesion occurs, and, in contrast to optic nerve gliomas, buckling or kinking of the optic nerve is not seen. There is a pathognomonic subgroup characterized by calcification that may have areas of negative optic nerve shadow (Figs. 12-25, 12-26) and railroad tracking, which has also been noted in some of the noncalcified meningiomas (see Fig. 12-22B). Intracranial extension of meningiomas may be noted as small tumors in the region of the anterior clinoids without evidence of optic canal involvement, so it is important to evaluate this area (see Fig. 12-26). A significant feature on CT imaging is evidence of a finely nodular surface reflecting the typical extradural growth pattern. This particular appearance is in contrast to gliomas, which retain a smooth, well-defined margin. Other radiologic studies are less useful and are essentially supplementary to CT scans. Ultrasonography may help to define the nodular margins and the presence of calcification (Fig. 12-27) as well as the absence of cystic change (a feature more characteristic of glioma). The clinical syndromes of optic nerve glioma and meningioma rarely overlap because of the large difference in age. However, on CT evaluation there is an overlapping pattern noted in both optic nerve glioma and meningioma, consisting of a fusiform diffuse expansion of the nerve (Fig. 12-28). In this instance, angiography may display a blush in meningioma as opposed to optic nerve glioma, which does not blush.

Meningioma and optic nerve glioma are not the only lesions to enlarge the optic nerve. Expansion of the optic nerve may be seen in the perineuritis of multiple sclerosis, wherein the optic nerve sheath may enhance. Perineural hemorrhage may be seen as a high-density sleeve on noncontrast CT scan surrounding the optic nerve. Tubular enlargement of the optic nerve may be noted with leukemic infiltration, papilledema, optic neuritis, idiopathic orbital inflammatory disease (apical type), thyroid orbitopathy, and patulous subarachnoid space. The last condition can be diagnosed with metrizamide cisternography; metrizamide will extend along the subarachnoid space of the optic nerve from the basal cistern. In addition, a lucent zone between the nerve and dural sheath may be noted on high-resolution CT scan. The differential diagnostic features of optic nerve meningiomas and gliomas have been described in the section on optic nerve glioma (see Table 12-2).

Management

Management of optic nerve meningioma should be governed by its slow growth and confined location. The major reasons for therapeutic intervention are evidence or risk of spread to the central nervous system, progressive or aggressive growth, and visual deterioration. Although numerous reports of microsurgical excision with return of vision have been documented, the majority of these have subsequently recurred with more locally infiltrative features. However, this may be a temporizing method in selected cases.

Patients can be safely and reasonably observed for long periods of time as long as there is little progression or evidence of intracranial involvement. If there is evidence of visual deterioration or if the diagnosis is insecure, fine needle aspiration biopsy under CT scan control

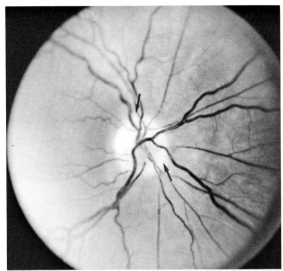

FIGURE 12-23.   Mild optic nerve pallor with a few refractile bodies *(arrows)* in an optic nerve meningioma.

may be a useful adjunct to planned further therapy. Surgical intervention ought to be designed to achieve complete excision of the tumor with the nerve, except in the rare circumstances where the growth is primarily exophytic and anterior and successful microsurgical excision might be anticipated without resection of the adjacent optic nerve. When confined to the anterior two thirds of the optic nerve in the orbit, the optic nerve and meningioma may be excised by lateral orbitotomy. If there is apical or intracranial involvement, a more appropriate approach is a combined neurosurgical ophthalmic panoramic orbitotomy. The object here would be complete excision of the optic nerve and surrounding meningioma. Radiotherapy in instances of progressive visual loss has been described as useful and may have particular application in progressive apical lesions.

Surgery, when indicated, should consist of total excision with the optic nerve when there is progression and the patient is blind; tumor excision alone when there is progression of an anterior exophytic tumor; and decompression (or radiotherapy) when the vision of the fellow eye is lost and the optic canal is involved.

Other Optic Nerve Tumors

The majority of clinically relevant other optic nerve tumors are either secondary by contiguity or metastatic in origin. There are also a large number of pseudoneoplastic causes of optic nerve enlargement including inflammatory, structural, and choristomatous lesions.

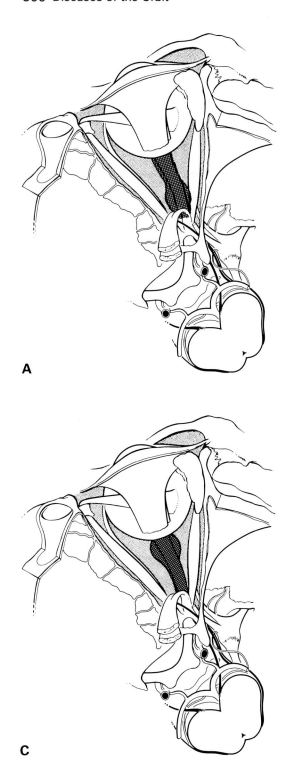

A

B

C

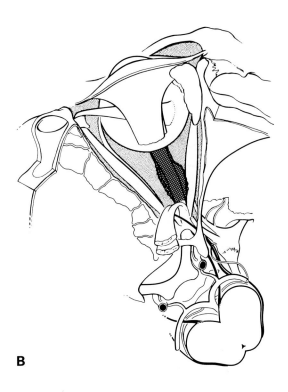

FIGURE 12-24. (A) Schematic drawing of a fusiform pattern of meningioma causing posterior expansion of the optic nerve. (B) Schematic drawing of a meningioma showing slight posterior nodularity of the optic nerve. (C) Schematic drawing of an anterior meningioma of the optic nerve.

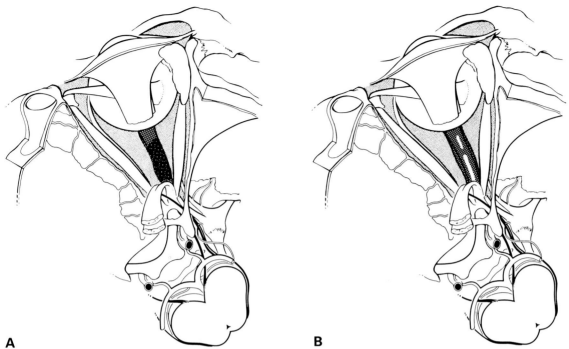

A **B**

FIGURE 12-25. *(A)* Schematic drawing of a calcified meningioma of the optic nerve. *(B)* Schematic drawing of a calcified meningioma of the optic nerve with railroad tracking.

MEDULLOEPITHELIOMAS (NEUROEPITHELIOMAS)

Medulloepithelioma of the optic nerve is a clinical curiosity usually seen in children. It affects the nerve head and extends into the substance of the optic nerve. The tumors arise from the medullary epithelium of the optic vesicle and are more common in the ciliary body region. Several cases of benign and malignant medulloepitheliomas of the optic nerve have been described. The obvious important differential diagnosis is optic nerve glioma.

SECONDARY AND METASTATIC TUMORS

Tumors arising from the globe and surrounding tissues may invade and extend down the optic nerve. The clinical context is usually obvious in the case of retinoblastoma and melanoma, unless the lesion arises within a phthisical eye. Retinoblastoma has a greater propensity to involve the optic nerve, a feature readily detectable with the new imaging modalities.

An increasingly more significant source of optic nerve tumors is metastatic and primary central nervous system neoplasia. In particular, leukemia can affect the central nervous system, and hence the optic nerve and eye, usually in the late and aggressive stages because of the relative pharmacologic isolation of these sites. Leukemia frequently affects the optic nerve head but may independently deposit in the arachnoid of the sheath as part of a widespread meningial process. Generalized carcinomatous meningiomatosis may also infiltrate the optic nerve. Usually in this instance the patient presents with papilledema, a known history of carcinoma, and negative CT findings because of widespread superficial involvement of the meninges without significant mass effect. The diagnosis can be secured by cytologic examination of cerebrospinal fluid. We have encountered three cases of meningiomatosis due to metastatic tumors; two were in patients with breast carcinoma and the other was in a patient with a metastatic melanoma of the skin. In all instances the diagnosis was made on CSF tap in the presence of normal CT findings. Direct metastases to the substance of the optic nerve have also been described as a cause of optic nerve enlargement.

Primary neoplasia in the central nervous system may also extend into the optic nerve. We have experienced just such a circumstance in two instances, one a medulloblastoma and the other a dural melanoma. Both were diagnosed by aspiration needle biopsy of the affected nerve sheath and are described later in this chapter in the section on Secondary Tumors of the Orbit. The primary

(Text continues on p. 310.)

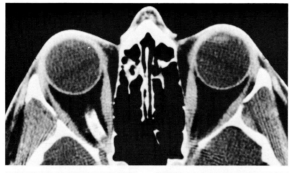

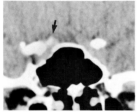

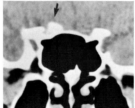

A

FIGURE 12-26. *(A)* Axial CT scans of a calcified meningioma of the optic nerve that occurred in a 41-year-old woman with progressive reduction in vision. Note slight central lucency in the nerve. The coronal scan *(bottom)* demonstrates an intracranial component *(arrow)*. The lesion was successfully resected by combined panoramic orbitotomy. *(B)* Histopathology of the meningioma shown in A. Note islands of invasion by the psammomatous meningioma into the optic nerve and dural sheath (H&E, original magnifications: *left* × 2.5, *right* × 10).

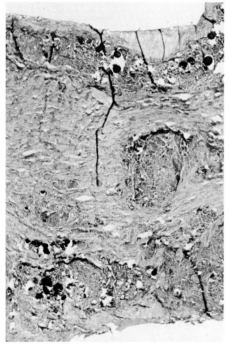

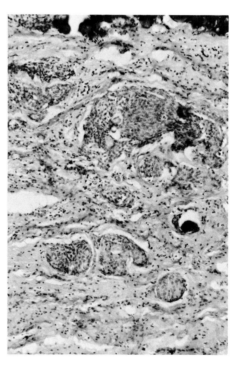

B

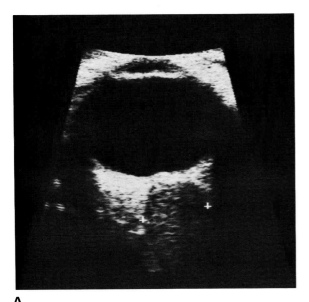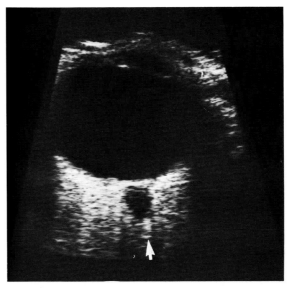

A   **B**

FIGURE 12-27. *(A)* B-scan ultrasonography demonstrates enlargement of the optic nerve due to a solid glioma. *(B)* In contrast, B-scan ultrasonography also shows a lesion of the optic nerve with increased irregular high reflectivity due to the presence of calcium. This lesion was an optic nerve meningioma.

FIGURE 12-28. Clinical and CT features of fusiform meningioma in a 46-year-old woman with progressive loss of vision (for 6 years), optic atrophy, and optociliary shunts.

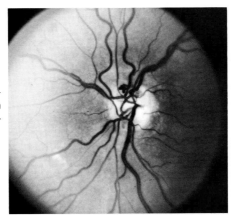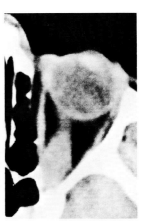

reticuloendothelial sarcoma (lymphoma) of the brain has a specific propensity for ocular involvement, usually as a cryptogenic chronic uveitis and vitritis.

PSEUDONEOPLASMS

There are a number of inflammatory processes affecting the orbit or the optic nerve that may lead to swelling of the nerve. We have encountered this in one case of orbital cellulitis and another of Wegener's granulomatosis with optic neuropathy.

Arachnoidal cysts of the optic nerve may simulate a neoplasm and can be effectively treated by a surgical window in the optic nerve sheath. However, it is important to rule out the possibility of an undetected small tumor of the optic canal, which may obstruct the CSF and distend the subarachnoid space. Nevertheless, true arachnoid cysts have been repeatedly described. The subarachnoid space may become patulous in any instance of raised intracranial pressure, particularly pseudotumor cerebri. In such instances, a dural window may relieve chronic papilledema.

The non-neoplastic causes of optic nerve swelling that we have encountered over the last 10 years include Wegner's granulomatosis (2), postcellulitis (1), optic nerve lymphoma and leukemia (3), carcinomatous meningitis (2), sarcomatous meningitis (metastatic melanoma) (1), medullobastoma (1), dural melanoma (1), arachnoid cyst (1), ischemic optic neuropathy (1), and chronic papilledema (2).

Peripheral Nerve Sheath Tumors

Tumors of nerve sheath origin include a large number of entities, but in the clinical setting only two—neurofibromas and schwannomas—are of importance in the orbit. These tumors share schwannian origin but have differing associations, histopathology, and prognosis. In brief, neurilemmomas are composed of Schwann cells and are localized, slow-growing, benign tumors of the adult. On the other hand, neurofibromas are made up of a mixture of Schwann cells, perineural cells, and fibroblastoid cells and often contain residual axons. They are plexiform, fusiform, or diffuse and are less well contained. When not isolated, they have a classic and frequent association with multiple neurofibromatosis (implying an underlying tendency to widespread involvement, progression, mesodermal defects, and potential malignant transformation). Most series suggest an overall 2 : 1 occurrence of neurofibroma versus schwannoma. Overall, peripheral nerve tumors constitute 4% of all orbital neoplasia, 2% occurring as plexiform neurofibromas, 1% as isolated neurofibromas, and 1% as schwannomas.

NEUROFIBROMAS

Throughout the body, neurofibromas occur in three different settings: as isolated (generally dermal) tumors; as diffuse infiltrations; and as plexiform lesions. All three types can be seen as part of the protean manifestations of neurofibromatosis. Isolated, solitary neurofibromas (versus multiple) are in 90% of instances unassociated with neurofibromatosis. It should be noted, however, that neurofibromatosis has low penetrance. Therefore, persons with a single neurofibroma may carry the gene but not show the disease. Diffuse neurofibromas are part of the syndrome in about 10% of occurrences, according to Enzinger. In contrast, many believe that clinically apparent (versus small histologically diagnosed) plexiform lesions are virtually pathognomonic of von Recklinghausen's disease. The fundamental pathologic abnormality in each consists of a proliferation of schwannian and endoneurial elements with separation of the component axons of the nerve of origin.

We have seen 14 cases of neurofibromas of the orbit (5% of our neoplasia) and periorbital tissues (11 plexiform, 1 multiple neurofibroma, and 2 solitary lesions).

Neurofibromatosis

Neurofibromatosis is an autosomal dominant disease with an incidence of 1 in 2500 to 3300 live births. It may arise from more than one neurogenic cell line and could be associated with a nerve growth factor that accounts for its relentless and progressive course. Although heritable, the character and degree of involvement varies so much even within a single family that a consistent and uniform constellation of findings does not exist. The diagnostic criteria and severity grading for neurofibromatosis are listed in Table 12-3. Generally, there are two forms, central and peripheral, that occur and they rarely overlap.

Peripheral neurofibromatosis is usually heralded by the development and progression of café-au-lait spots within the first few years of life. By definition these must be over 1.5 cm in size and occur in six or more sites (characteristically in unexposed areas such as the axilla; Fig. 12-29) in order to diagnose von Recklinghausen's disease. Even fewer carry a risk of the disease, and number of spots roughly correlates with severity. The neurofibromas generally appear during late childhood and adolescence, but may be noted at any time (even at birth) or any site. Visceral neurofibromas may also develop in the gastrointestinal tract, larynx, heart, and blood vessels. Diverse skeletal abnormalities (both primary mesodermal and due to pressure expansion) are seen in 40% of patients. In the orbital region, associated absence of the sphenoid wing may cause pulsating exophthalmos (see Fig. 12-35). In addition, other anomalies including

TABLE 12-3.
CRITERIA AND GRADING FOR NEUROFIBROMATOSIS

Diagnostic Criteria for Neurofibromatosis
Six or more café-au-lait spots, at least 15 mm in diameter
Axillary freckling
Cutaneous neurofibromas
Positive family history of neurofibromatosis

Severity Grading for Neurofibromatosis
Grade I: Minimal (dermal manifestations, café-au-lait spots, uncomplicated neurofibromas)
Grade II: Mild complications (mild scoliosis, precocious puberty, behavior disorder)
Grade III: Moderate complications (requiring palliative medical attention: hemihypertrophy, controlled seizures, gastrointestinal involvement)
Grade IV: Major sensory or motor impairment (intracranial masses, severe mental retardation, severe scoliosis, uncontrolled seizures)

(After Lewis RA, Riccardi VM: Von Recklinghausen neurofibromatosis: Incidence of iris hamartomata. Ophthalmology 88:348, 1981)

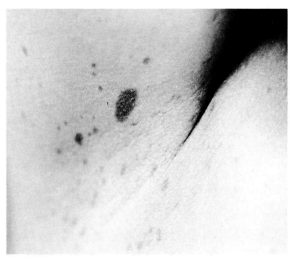

FIGURE 12-29. Typical site and appearance of café-au-lait spots in the axilla of a 9-year-old child with neurofibromatosis.

growth and mental disorders and tumors (pheochromocytoma, neurilemmoma) may be seen. Malignant degeneration is believed to occur in about 10% to 15% of neurofibromas in the context of neurofibromatosis.

Central neurofibromatosis is characterized by the development of a variety of tumors including astrocytomas, meningiomas, schwannomas (especially eighth and fifth nerves), and ependymomas in the central nervous system with few peripheral manifestations. Most of the astrocytomas are in the cerebrum, but some occur in the third ventricle and the optic nerves.

Overall, the orbital manifestations of neurofibromatosis can include optic gliomas, perioptic meningiomas, neurofibromas, schwannomas, osseous dysplasia, and buphthalmos. Table 12-4 summarizes the ocular and orbital manifestations of von Recklinghausen's disease and ascribes relative incidence.

Plexiform Neurofibromas

Plexiform neurofibromas are the most common and complex peripheral nerve tumors of the orbit. Because of the association with neurofibromatosis, they are of early onset (first decade) and of protean manifestation. Pathologically, they consist of diffuse intertwining bundles of Schwann cells, axons, and endoneural fibroblasts surrounded by a cellular perineural sheath (Fig. 12-30). The lesions are not encapsulated, grow along the nerves of origin in a centripetal manner, and insinuate throughout the orbital tissues. Virtually any of the cranial, sympathetic, and parasympathetic nerves may be involved with a propensity to affect sensory nerves in the orbit. With Bodian stains the axons are demonstrable throughout the fascicles of these grotesquely distorted nerves (Fig.

12-30B). The overlying skin may be thickened (elephantiasis neuromatosa; Fig. 12-31). The tortuous, ropey, tangled nerves produce a characteristic palpable "bag of worms" (Fig. 12-32). Plexiform neurofibromas are highly vascular and so diffusely intertwined with the normal tissues that removal is fraught with hemorrhage and is extremely difficult, if not impossible. Combined with a tendency to continued growth, these make it a surgical frustration. Malignant transformation of plexiform neurofibromas of the orbit is exceedingly rare.

The clinical and investigative findings of plexiform neurofibromatosis consist of soft tissue, bony, and ocular abnormalities. The soft tissues of the lid, periorbita, and face are thickened, hypertropied, or even pendulous producing varying degrees of proptosis or facial disfigurement or both (see Figs. 12-31, 12-32; Figs. 12-33 to 12-37). Thirty-one percent of plexiform neurofibromas occur in the lid and periorbital region. CT scanning demonstrates the changes as contrast-enhancing irregular soft tissue infiltration involving these structures. Frequently, the extraocular muscles are enlarged due to nerve involvement (see Fig. 12-34). In addition, the retrobulbar fat may show increased density, and when the nerves in the cavernous sinus are involved it is enlarged (see Fig. 12-34).

Bony changes may be compensatory with expansion due to mass effect or primary mesodermal defects. They consist of enlargement of the orbit, widening of the superior and inferior orbital fissures (see Figs. 12-34, 12-37; Fig. 12-38), hypoplasia of the ethmoid and maxillary sinus (see Fig. 12-33), abnormalities of the sphenoid (defects in the greater wing, elevation of the lesser wing), and enlargement and distortion of the middle cranial fossa (see Fig. 12-35).

TABLE 12-4.
OCULAR AND ORBITAL MANIFESTATIONS IN 77 PATIENTS WITH NEUROFIBROMATOSIS

Location	Number of Patients (Eyes)	Percent
Uveal		
Iris nodules	59	77%
Patients over 6 years old	59/61	92%
Choroidal hamartomas	30/59 (Caucasian)	51%
Eyelid		25%
Punctate neurofibromat a of lid or lid border	14 (26)	
Plexiform neurofibromata	4 (4)	
Café-au-lait spots	2 (2)	
Cornea		25%
Prominent nerve fibers	17 (34)	
Posterior embryotoxon	2 (4)	
Optic nerve glioma (suspected or proven)	9 (13)	12%
Strabismus		10%
Congenital esotropia	3	
Partially accommodative esotropia	2	
Alternating extropia	1	
Overacting inferior oblique muscles	1	
Rotatory nystagmus (congenital)	1	
Retina		9%
Sectoral chorioretinal scar, cause unknown	1 (1)	
Optic disc drusen	1 (2)	
Myelinated nerve fibers	1 (1)	
Typical peripheral retinoschisis	1 (2)	
Congenital hypertrophy of retinal pigment epithelium	3 (3)	
Conjunctiva		5%
Presumptive neurofibromata	4 (5)	

(After Lewis RA, Riccardi VM: Von Recklinghausen neurofibromatosis: Incidence of iris hamartomata. Ophthalmology 88:348, 1981)

The ocular features of neurofibromatosis are as protean as the general condition and reflect involvement of the uveal tract and emissarial nerves. Patients may have uveal neurofibromas varying from a few characteristic round, dome-shaped, avascular nodules that are clear or orange-brown (burnt sienna) in coloration (Lisch nodules; see Fig. 12-36) to diffuse infiltrations of the uveal tract. The choroidal lesions appear as flat, ill-defined, yellow-white to brown areas noted in whites. When carefully looked for, Lisch nodules are present in 77% of patients with neurofibromatosis and 90% of those over 6 years of age. In our experience the most severe ocular involvement correlated with childhood glaucoma, diffuse uveal neurofibroma (enlarged and thickened globes), and marked orbital anomalies including irregular nodular thickening of the optic nerve sheath outline with central lucency reflecting plexiform neurofibromas of the perineural and ocular emmissaria (see Figs. 12-34, 12-38). Involvement of single or multiple nerve bundles may produce dramatic enlargement (Fig. 12-39).

The management of plexiform neurofibromas is difficult, treacherous, and frustrating, and usually produces cosmetically inadequate and temporary results. Therefore, some authors have suggested that in the case of significant involvement only exenteration will produce an effective result. The usual surgical management is cosmetic surgery, consisting of repeated debulking or orbital bony enlargement or both by combined cranial–facial teams; it produces less than gratifying results in most instances.

Solitary (Isolated) Neurofibromas

An exact incidence of localized neurofibromas in the orbit is hard to obtain because statistics may be marred by the inclusion of cases that may be the early manifestation of neurofibromatosis. This lesion (when compared to occurrence elsewhere in the body) is infrequent in the orbit; Henderson reported that 5 of 18 neurofibromas

(Text continues on p. 319.)

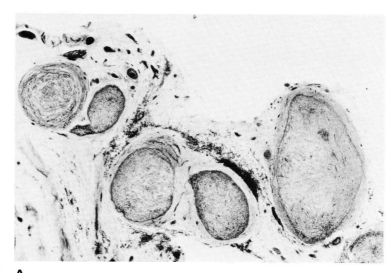

A

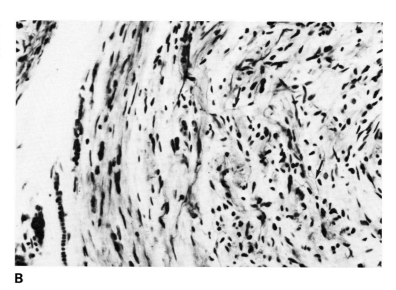

B

FIGURE 12-30. *(A)* Low-power photomicrograph of a plexiform neurofibroma that was associated with von Recklinghausen's disease. Each nerve bundle is surrounded by a thickened perineurium (H&E, original magnification × 2.5). *(B)* Higher-power view of the lesion shown in *A* shows the thickened perineurium and randomly distributed axons *(arrow)* in the loose matrix of Schwann cells, and endoneural fibroblasts (Bodian, original magnification × 25).

FIGURE 12-31. This 19-year-old woman presented with a left periorbital lesion that had been increasing over a 3-year period. It had a chordlike consistency with thickening of the overlying skin (elephantiasis neuromatosa) and was associated with an isolated neurofibroma of the left iris (Lisch nodule). The axial CT scan demonstrates thickening of the lateral portion of the lid and the skin in subcuticular tissue overlying the temporalis fossa.

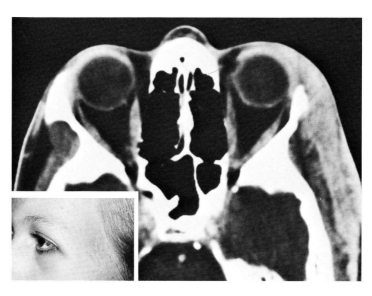

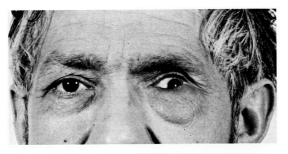
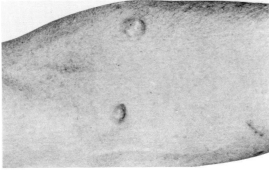

A

FIGURE 12-32. *(A)* This 50-year-old man has a plexiform neurofibroma of the lower lid *(top)*, which was associated with multiple neurofibromas throughout the body *(bottom)*. In addition, he had diffuse neurofibromatosis of the uveal tract and iris, which led to glaucoma and phthisis of the left globe. *(B)* Histopathology of this patient's plexiform neurofibroma. Note loosely arranged swollen nerve bundles surrounded by fibroblasts and collagen (H&E, original magnification × 10). *(C)* Electron micrograph of this plexiform neurofibroma shows Schwann cells and occasional fibroblasts separated by abundant extracellular matrix. *(Inset)* The basement membrane invests the cytoplasmic processes, indicating that this cell is of Schwannian origin (original magnifications × 9828, *inset* × 4050). (Electron micrograph courtesy C. Dolman.)

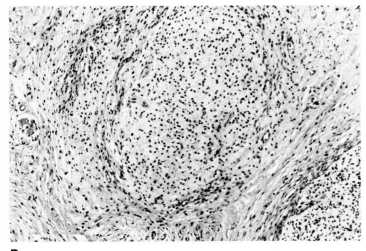

B

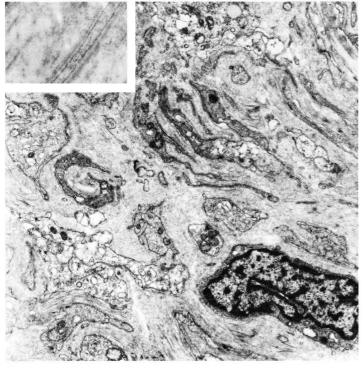

C

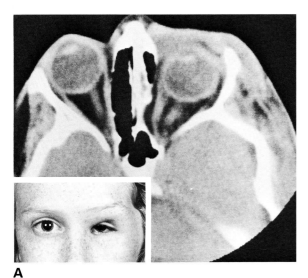

A

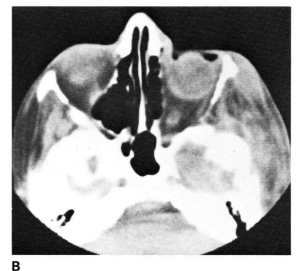

B

FIGURE 12-33. *(A)* A 15-year-old boy presented with a progressive enophthalmic appearance noted since age 2 years. It was associated with thickening of the skin of the upper lid and over the temporalis fossa. In addition, he had a light pigmentary patch in the temporal region of his forehead. On physical examination, he had 11 mm of enophthalmos with spongy thickening of the superior lid, infraorbital region, and the zygomatic arch. The enhanced axial CT scan shows marked thickening of the upper eyelid and periorbital soft tissues on the left. The globe is enophthalmic because of enlargement of the orbit, reduction in the size of the ethmoid sinus, and decrease in the volume of intraconal fat. The intraconal fat also shows increased density compared to the normal side. *(B)* The patient also had absence of a portion of the sphenoid wing and lateral orbital wall, which was associated with an unusual feature of ocular bobbing on mastication due to the intimacy of the periorbita and temporalis muscle.

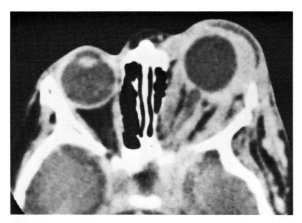

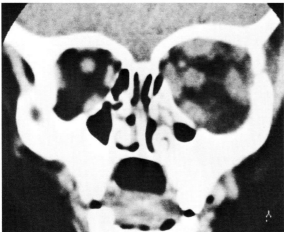

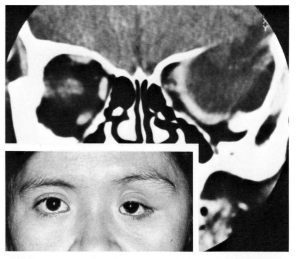

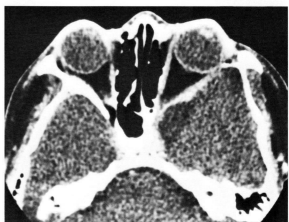

FIGURE 12-34. Axial and coronal CT scans of a 1-year-old child who presented at birth with an enlarged left eyeball and glaucoma due to uveal neurofibromatosis. On clinical examination he had left proptosis, a thickened doughy lid with megaloglobus, a thickened iris, and pale choroid. The axial CT scan demonstrates extensive orbital plexiform neurofibroma with the full constellation of findings. The left orbit is enlarged. The left ethmoid and maxillary sinuses are small. The upper eyelid and periorbital soft tissues, both medially and laterally, are thickened as are the four rectus muscles. There is increased density of intraconal fat with several linear densities, and a thickened irregular optic nerve sheath complex due to posterior ciliary involvement. The left globe is buphthalmic and proptotic. The contrast-enhanced axial scan shows marked thickening and enhancement of the uveal–scleral layer. The optic nerve is a central low-density area surrounded by the irregular enhancing plexiform neurofibroma. The cavernous sinus is enlarged on the left side.

FIGURE 12-35. A 28-year-old woman presented with a throbbing, rhythmic pulsation of the left eye associated with drooping of the lid; the condition had been present for many years. On physical examination she had 4 mm of downward displacement of the eye, a deepened superior sulcus, and 3 mm of enophthalmos. A rhythmic pulsation of the left orbit was noted, and she had multiple café-au-lait spots as well as Lisch nodules of the iris. Axial and coronal CT scans demonstrate absence of the greater sphenoid wing with herniation of the contents of the temporal fossa.

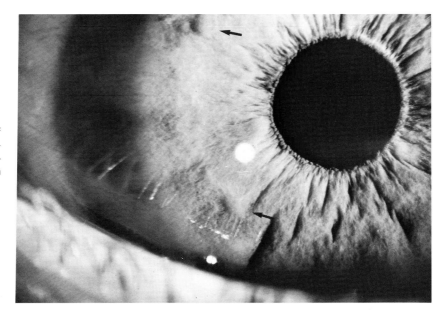

FIGURE 12-36. A photograph of the iris of a patient with neurofibromatosis demonstrates the characteristic round, dome-shaped, Lisch nodules of the iris.

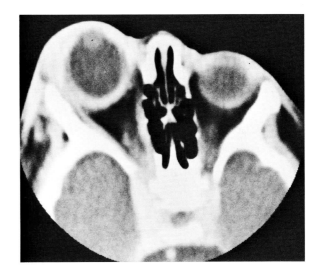

FIGURE 12-37. Enhanced axial CT scan of a 1-year-old child who presented with gross enlargement of the right eye and thickening of the eyelid, which was associated with congenital glaucoma due to diffuse uveal neurofibromatosis. The child's mother also suffered from neurofibromatosis. The CT scan demonstrates thickening of the uveal-scleral envelope and widening of the superior oribtal fissure as well as slight enlargement of the cavernous sinus. The globe is enlarged due to a combination of buphthalmos and thickened uveal-scleral envelope.

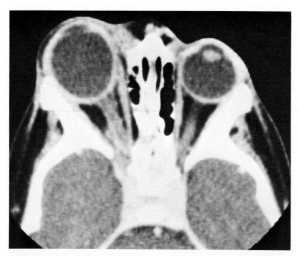

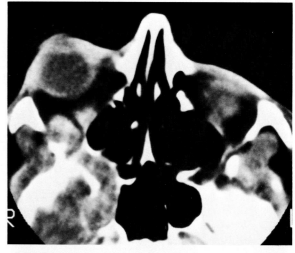

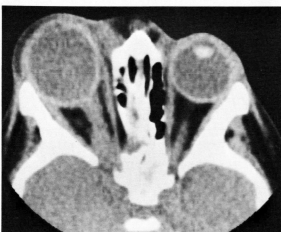

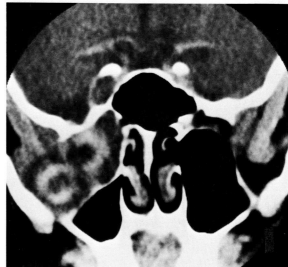

FIGURE 12-38. Enhanced *(top)* and unenhanced *(bottom)* axial CT scans demonstrate a buphthalmic right globe with slight thickening and enhancement of the uvea and sclera. The optic nerve outline is thick and irregular, and there is a central low-density apparent after-contrast enhancement that represents the normal optic nerve. Linear densities due to plexiform neurofibroma involving the small nerves are seen in the intraconal fat, and the superior orbital fissure appears slightly enlarged.

FIGURE 12-39. Axial and coronal contrast-enhanced CT scans demonstrate a neurofibroma that appears to involve primarily the second division of the fifth nerve with a small first division component. Note enlargement of the cavernous sinus, infraorbital fissure, pterygopalatine fossa, and apical orbit. Two areas of ring enhancement surround the lesion. The patient was 34 years old and had known neurofibromatosis.

were solitary, and Kuo reported a 0.6% occurrence in a large series of orbital tumors. We have encountered only two cases of solitary neurofibromas (Fig. 12-40). Krohel has reported on nine cases of isolated neurofibromas in the orbit.

These lesions tend to be seen in middle-aged persons, and manifest as solitary masses with a preponderance of occurrence in the upper quadrants (see Fig. 12-40A). Clinically they are solid, isolated, circumscribed, slow-growing mass lesions. Thus, the major findings reflect mass effect leading to localized expansion of the orbit. When in the lacrimal fossa they may be virtually indistinguishable preoperatively from a benign mixed tumor. Because they chiefly affect sensory nerves, anesthesia, paresthesia, and hypesthesia have been frequently noted.

Grossly, at the time of surgery they are noted to arise from a major nerve and appear as well-defined, firm, circumscribed, rubbery, gray masses with little vascularity. Histologically, they may not be well encapsulated (rather, they show condensation of adjacent tissues) and contain loosely arranged interlacing bundles of spindle cells (two to three cells thick) and collagen fibrils within a mucoid matrix (see Fig. 12-40, B and C). Small, frequently varicose axons may be demonstrated throughout the tumor with special stains. The common histologic variants include a cellular type with dense Schwann cell populations and myxoid neurofibromas with a striking mucoid component (Fig.12-40B). In addition there are several of interest only to the pathologist, including paccionian, epitheliod, pigmented, and granular neurofibromas. Malignant transformation is exceedingly rare, but is believed to be more common than in the case of schwannomas.

On CT scan they appear as well-circumscribed, usually homogeneous masses and on ultrasonography they display low reflectivity. Although multiple tumors may be evident at the time of surgery, these are rarely detected preoperatively.

Management of solitary neurofibromas does not imply the same risks noted in the hereditary forms, and they can be removed even partially with impunity. At surgery they appear as isolated tumors but require careful dissection of the capsule, which can be adherent in areas. Recurrences may represent undetected multiple lesions. Resection implies transecting the nerve of origin, and extreme care should be taken to identify it as a sensory rather than motor nerve before resecting it.

Diffuse Neurofibroma

Diffuse neurofibroma is a rare dermal form characterized by infiltration and envelopment of normal structures. It is histologically ill-defined and made up of cells with ovoid nuclei mainly growing diffusely, but in some areas showing an arrangement reminiscent of Wagner-Meissner corpuscles. A variable amount of collagen is present. About 10% of diffuse neurofibromas occur in the context of neurofibromatosis. The majority of these lesions do not imply a high risk of malignant change. Their rare occurrence in the orbit is characterized by a diffuse infiltration of fat, muscles, and soft tissues. Resection implies the same hazards and frustrations as plexiform neurofibromas.

Amputation Neuromas

In spite of frequent nerve transection in the orbit, amputation neuromas rarely occur and have been reported in only seven cases. We have encountered a single case of amputation neuroma. They represent a regenerative overgrowth of transsected peripheral nerves. Clinically, they may be associated with pain that is curable by excision. It is believed that mechanical factors such as movement, pressure, and scar tissue contribute to and increase irritation, and this may explain the relative infrequency of these lesions in the orbit. Grossly, they are circumscribed and continuous with the transected nerve. Histologically, they consist of a disorganized proliferation of nerve fascicles with a background of collagen.

SCHWANNOMA (NEURILEMMOMA)

Schwannomas are well-defined, encapsulated, slowly progressive tumors that arise as eccentric growths from peripheral nerves. They are usually solitary, occur between the ages of 20 and 50 years, and have a predilection for the head and neck region. In general series they may be noted in association with von Recklinghausen's disease (18% of schwannomas and 1.5% of patients with neurofibromatosis). In the orbit they represent 1% to 2% of tumors, and in our series they were 1.5% of nonthyroid orbital lesions and about 3% of neoplasia. They are rarely multiple and malignant transformation is rare.

They consist of proliferations of Schwann cells within a perineural capsule that displace and may compress the nerve of origin. The characteristic pathology is an admixture of tightly ordered cellular Schwann cells (Antoni A area) and a loosely arranged component (Antoni B area) within the capsule (Fig. 12-41). When studied with special stains, axons are not noted within the substance of the tumor, but rather are seen as eccentric nerve bundles in the capsule. They contain less acid mucopolysaccharide than neurofibromas, have many reticulin fibers, and are S-100 protein positive. On electron-microscopy, in contrast to neurofibromas, schwannomas are made up almost exclusively of Schwann cells and their processes. In the Antoni A areas, stacks of processes are surrounded by a well-marked basal lamina (500 nm). In the Antoni B areas, the processes are less densely arranged. Long spacing collagen is often seen in schwannomas (Luse bodies;

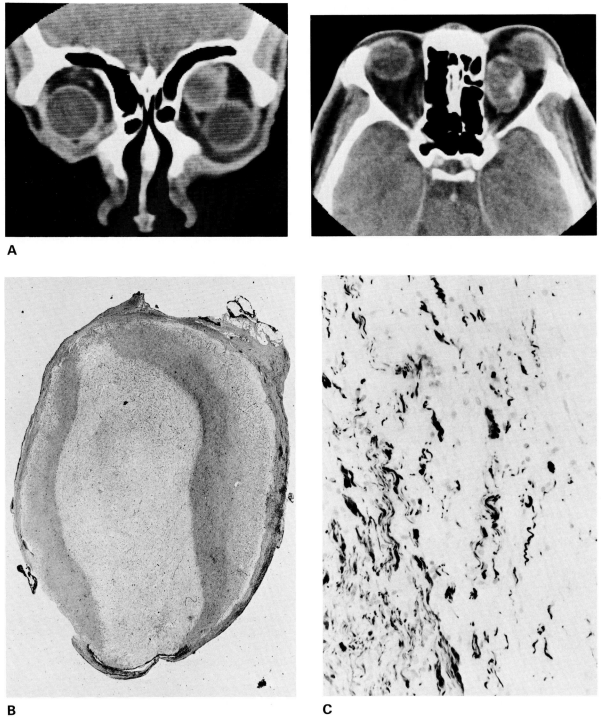

FIGURE 12-40. *(A)* Coronal and axial CT scans demonstrate a well-defined isolated superior medial orbital mass. The downward displacement of the globe, and capsular and focal density reflect a largely myxomatous lesion shown in *B* under low power. *(C)* Immunoperoxidase stain for S-100 demonstrates the dispersed fibrillary component of this isolated neurofibroma.

Fig. 12-42). The cytoplasm contains few mitochondria, microfibrils, occasional lysosomes, and rarely cilia (Fig. 12-43B), and the nucleus is usually flat.

Aside from these typical areas there is a gamut of findings that reflects the varying organization and maturational features of these tumors. This includes characteristic organoid cellular patterns (Verocay bodies; see Fig. 12-41B), palisading, lymphocytoid cells, and hyalinized vessels (see Fig. 12-41B) (with PAS-positive basement membrane). Because they are slow growing and late in presentation, features of degeneration may dominate the larger masses. These include cyst formation, hemorrhage (Fig. 12-44), calcification (see Fig. 12-41C), collagen deposition, and hyalinization with infiltration of siderophages and lipid-laden Schwann cells. In addition, ancient lesions may display distressing nuclear atypia with large hyperchromatic, frequently multilobed nuclei without mitoses, yet usually they behave as benign lesions. Ten percent of schwannomas occur in neurofibromatosis and 50% of malignant schwannomas occur within this group. The clinical development, investigational features, and management of schwannomas reflect the underlying pathology.

No single feature is pathognomonic, but a multiplicity of clinical, radiographic, and surgical features point to the diagnosis of schwannoma. It is a tumor of adults (average 31 in our series with a range from the third to the seventh decade), has an insidious onset, is slow growing and noninvasive with findings governed by the position and size of the lesion (mass effect). In our experience, when intraconal (7 of 10) the major findings were proptosis (6), lid swelling (3), posterior indentation of the globe (2), diplopia in extremes of gaze (3), and in an apically located tumor a central scotoma with marked fluctuation of vision on lateral movement (see Fig. 12-43). Extraconal schwannomas may occur virtually anywhere in and about the orbit including the sinuses, the gassarian ganglion, and the lacrimal sac. We have seen tumors in the ethmoid (one of which presented with sinusitis; Fig. 12-45), lid, and in the roof of the orbit (see Fig. 12-42). All were localized except for one multinodular tumor that affected the entire orbital portion of the frontal nerve in a patient suspicious for form fruste of neurofibromatosis (two large café-au-lait spots and similar spots in two of her children; see Fig. 12-42). Most series suggest that sensory nerves are more commonly involved in the orbit. However, we have experienced two affecting motor nerves (sixth and superior division of the third).

On routine radiologic investigation, features of longstanding pressure effect with expansion may be noted when the tumor is next to bone (Fig. 12-46), and rarely focal intratumoral calcification may be seen (see Fig. 12-41). CT scanning demonstrates well-defined, smooth, rounded contours (both anterior and posterior), with variation in density based on cyst formation, degeneration, and lipid deposition in some tumors (see Fig. 12-44).

With contrast injection, mild enhancement may be noted and arteriography is generally negative showing displacement, except in one of our cases where a blush was observed. Ultrasonography will confirm discrete, generally solid tumor masses with occasional cysts in some. Overall, the investigative features parallel those of solitary neurofibromas.

Management

Large or symptomatic tumors can be managed definitively by surgery, the approach being governed by location. At surgery they are characteristically yellow-tan, solid, encapsulated, and have typical varicose, violaceous tumor vessels on the surface (see Fig. 12-42B). Because they arise as outpouchings, they may be stripped off the nerve of origin by microsurgical technique. Removal may be total or subtotal, in piecemeal fashion or by evacuation of the tumor within its capsule. Evacuation of these tumors may be wise when critically located and can be aided by using ultrasonic fragmentation suction devices (Cavitron Ultrasonic Aspiration, CUSA). Overall, recurrence is extremely rare even when the tumor is only partially removed. We saw a single recurrence of a schwannoma, which was removed from the ethmoid sinus.

In summary, schwannomas are rare periorbital and orbital tumors with variable anatomic and pathologic features. They are slow growing, solitary, noninfiltrative, and almost universally benign. A constellation of investigative features points to this diagnosis and surgical intervention, when indicated, is successful.

MALIGNANT PERIPHERAL NERVE SHEATH TUMORS

The principal malignancy among nerve sheath tumors appears to be the malignant schwannoma, but not all tumors in this group arise exclusively from Schwann cells, and they may have diverse histologic manifestations reflecting a pluripotential neural crest origin. Thus, some may arise principally from neural fibroblasts or perineural cells. In the past, these tumors have been described as neurofibrosarcoma, neurogenic sarcoma, and malignant schwannoma. Despite the fact that close to 50% of those described throughout the body are associated with von Recklinghausen's disease or with antecedent neurofibroma, many authors prefer the designation *malignant schwannoma* for this group. The term *malignant peripheral nerve sheath tumor* is a broader umbrella for lesions we have included in this category.

In general, these tumors represent 10% of all soft tissue sarcomas throughout the body with approximately half occurring within the context of neurofibromatosis. Three percent to 13% of patients with neurofibromatosis

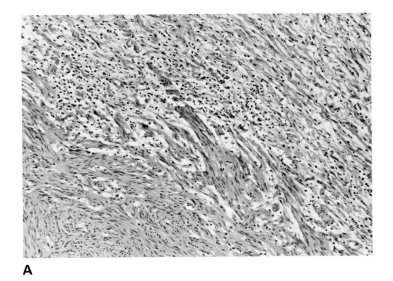

A

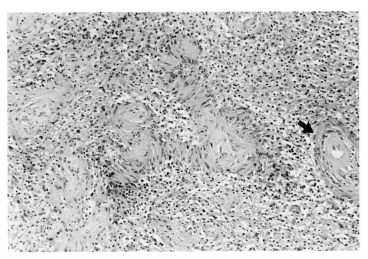

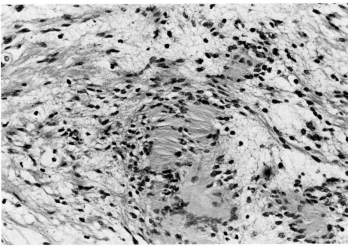

B

FIGURE 12-41. *(A)* Histopathology of an intraconal schwannoma demonstrates an admixture of compactly arranged interlacing fascicles (Antoni A pattern, *lower left*) and more loosely arranged cells separated by a clear matrix (Antoni B pattern) with a background of lymphocytoid cells (H&E, original magnification × 10). *(B, top)* Histopathology of another area of the same tumor shows a hyalinized vessel *(arrow)* with an organoid cellular pattern centrally (Verocay body). Background pattern is essentially Antoni B with lymphocytoid and lipid-laden foam cells. *(Bottom)* A higher-power view of a Verocay body (H&E, original magnifications *top* × 10, *bottom* × 25).

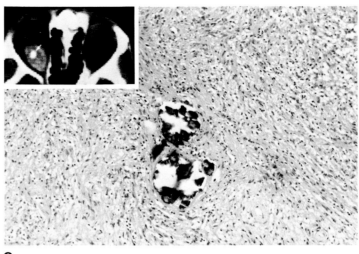

FIGURE 12-41 *(Continued)*. *(C)* Light microscopy of the intraconal schwannoma shown in axial CT scan *(inset)*. Note the smooth, well-defined, oval intraconal mass with central calcification *(arrow)*. Histopathology shows a basically Antoni B pattern with a central area of calcification (H&E, original magnification × 10). (Rootman J, Goldberg C, Robertson W: Primary orbital schwannomas. Br J Ophthalmol 66:194–204, 1981)

C

will develop a malignant peripheral nerve sheath tumor with a latent period of 10 to 20 years. They largely occur between the second and fifth decades. In the context of neurofibromatosis, they are noted earlier, and males dominate females. Most arise from major nerves and are associated with mass effect and variable sensory and motor symptoms. They usually arise from deeper nerves, and few are seen in the head and neck. There is a high incidence of local recurrence and metastases and a poor prognosis, in part based on their large size at diagnosis. They generally have a much poorer prognosis when associated with von Recklinghausen's disease.

In the orbit, the malignant peripheral nerve sheath tumors are exceedingly rare; Schatz has documented 14, Henderson 2, and Jakobiec and colleagues 8 cases. The age occurrence in this site is wide (2–75 years). About one quarter of the patients described have had lesions arising within the context of long-standing neurofibromatosis.

Biologically, these are usually locally aggressive tumors. Thus, the onset when *de novo* or due to transformation in the context of neurofibromatosis is usually over several months. More indolent and slowly recurrent tumors have been described. A higher incidence of superior nasal lesions has been noted and affectation of the frontal or supraorbital nerve may be associated with pain, paresthesia, and tenderness in its distribution. Patients with known neurofibromatosis may have a more indolent course or sudden explosive onset of mass and infiltrative effect. Because of frequent incomplete excision or simple biopsy as the initial procedure, rapid recurrence within 3 to 6 months is common. In addition, a propensity for extension along the nerve sheath and systemic or regional spread make these a prognostically poor neoplasm.

Microscopically, the majority of these tumors resemble fibrosarcomas. However, the cells are arranged in a more irregular pattern with wavy, often buckled or comma-shaped nuclei (Fig. 12-47B). In addition, myxoid areas may be noted, particularly in the context of neurofibromatosis. More common features of Schwann cell character may be seen, including palisading. Heterotopic elements such as bone, skeletal muscle, glandular tissue, and cartilage may be noted. Many of these tumors contain an epithelioid cell component in addition to the spindle-cell proliferation (biphasic). Rhabdomyosarcomatous differentiation and glandular formation have been noted elsewhere but not in the orbital cases. Electron-microscopy and immunohistochemistry (S-100 protein) may help to differentiate these tumors from other spindle-cell and epithelioid neoplasias.

Management of malignant peripheral nerve tumors implies radical and complete excision, which in the orbital context infers exenteration. Because of a propensity to spread along the nerves, combined craniotomy with frozen section may be required. Although recommended, radiotherapy and chemotherapy are not of proven value. Overall, the prognosis for survival is poor, but some tumors may display low-grade behavior with multiple recurrences before succumbing to the malignancy. The introduction of more radical craniofacial techniques may improve the prognosis from an overall 60% to 75% mortality.

We have encountered two cases of malignant schwannoma, both of which appeared to have arisen from the ethmoid sinus and secondarily involved the orbit. One was a low-grade recurrence (see Fig. 12-45) and the other was a primary tumor (see Fig. 12-47). Both patients underwent radical combined surgery for excision of the masses, and are alive and well 1 year and 4 years postoperatively.

(Text continues on p. 326.)

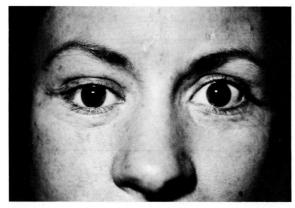

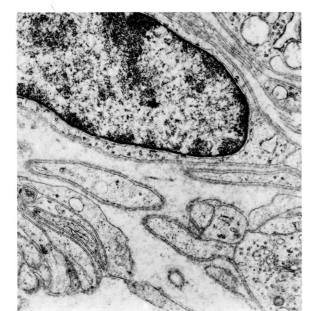

A

B

FIGURE 12-42. *(A)* This 32-year-old woman had 4 mm downward displacement of the right globe and slight facial asymmetry. *(B)* Intraoperative photograph of the superior orbital schwannoma removed from this patient. There is a multilobular solid tumor mass with slightly varicose surface vessels. *(C)* Electron micrograph of tissue taken from this patient shows Schwann cells with interdigitating and convoluted cell membranes with few subcellular organelles and a prominent extracellular basement membrane (original magnification × 18,110). *(D)* Electron micrograph from this schwannoma demonstrates "long spacing" collagen adjacent to a cell membrane (Luse body) (original magnification × 50,700). (Rootman J, Goldberg C, Robertson W: Primary orbital schwannomas. Br J Ophthalmol 66:194–204, 1981)

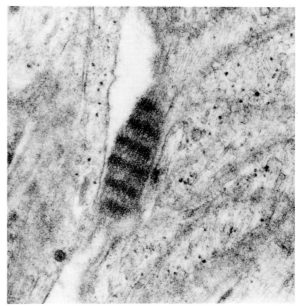

C

D

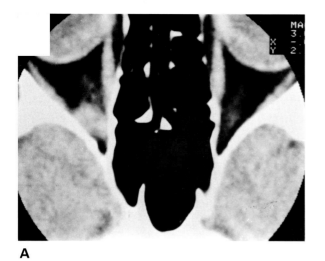

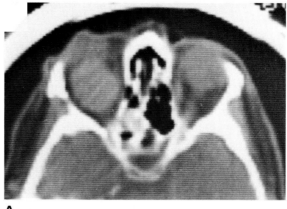

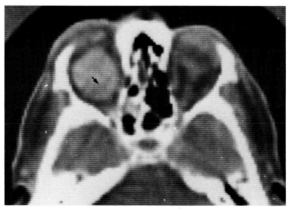

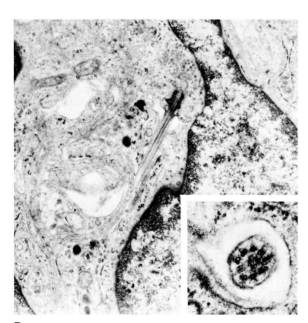

B

FIGURE 12-43. *(A)* Axial CT scan demonstrates an apical intraconal lesion in a 54-year-old woman. She had a history of a right central scotoma and vision that fluctuated between finger counting and 20/25. Her vision diminished on right lateral gaze. The intraconal lesion displaced the optic nerve and had a well-defined posterior margin that spared the apex. *(B)* Electron micrograph from the lesion described in *A*. It was histologically a schwannoma. The micrograph demonstrates a longitudinal section of a cilia adjacent to the nuclear membrane. *Inset* shows a cilium in cross section (original magnification, × 8500, *inset* × 66,000). (Rootman J, Goldberg C, Robertson W: Primary orbital schwannomas. Br J Ophthalmol 66:194–204, 1981)

A

B

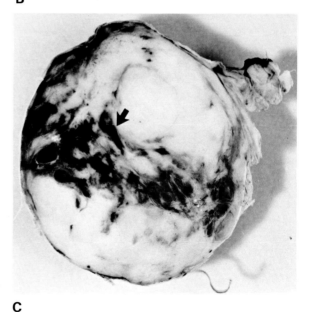

C

FIGURE 12-44. *(A)* Axial CT scan demonstrates a well-defined intraconal schwannoma, which was mildly enhancing following contrast injection *(B)*. *(C)* Gross photograph of the excised schwannoma demonstrates focal necrosis and hemorrhage in the center of the lesion, which reflected the low-density nonenhancing areas noted on axial CT scan *(arrows)*. (Rootman J, Goldberg C, Robertson W: Primary orbital schwannomas. Br J Ophthalmol 66:194–204, 1981)

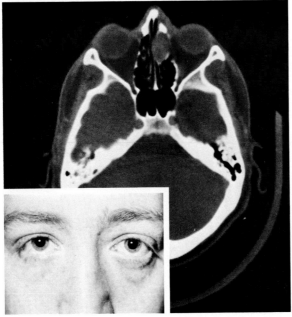

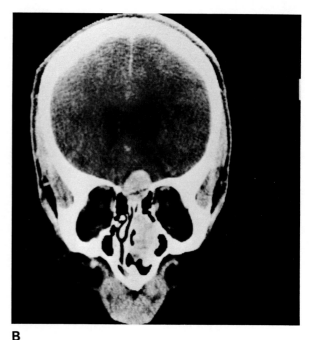

A **B**

FIGURE 12-45. *(A)* This 23-year-old man had mild periorbital swelling, proptosis, and displacement of the left eye as a result of the presence of a mass in the anterior ethmoid portion of the sinus shown on CT scan. Surgically, it was associated with an accumulation of mucopurulent material and an underlying tumor mass, which proved to be a schwannoma with slight cellular atypia. *(B)* Coronal CT scan of the same patient taken 3 years later shows extension and growth of a residual tumor into the anterior cranial fossa and nasopharynx. He underwent a combined craniotomy-ENT resection, and is alive and well 4 years later. (Rootman J, Goldberg C, Robertson W: Primary orbital schwannomas. Br J Ophthalmol 66:194–204, 1981)

Rare Tumors of Neuroectodermal Origin

ALVEOLAR SOFT PART SARCOMA

Alveolar soft part sarcoma constitutes 0.5% to 1% of all soft tissue sarcomas. It most frequently occurs on the extremities, particularly the lower and on the right side. Overall, it tends to occur in adolescents and young adults with a 3:1 female predominance. In children, it is believed to affect the head and neck more often, where the orbit is a preferential site. In Enzinger's series, 11% of alveolar soft part sarcomas were in the orbit.

In the orbit, it is characteristically a slow-growing noninvasive mass that leads to proptosis, generally over a 4-month period. The overall 5-year survival rate is 59% and the 20-year rate is 47%. In contrast, when it occurs in the orbit the survival rate is 77%. It is a locally aggressive tumor with a protracted course when it recurs locally. In contrast to rhabdomyosarcoma, it occurs in a slightly older age group and is associated more frequently with decreased vision and proptosis.

Grossly, it is a relatively circumscribed, tan-to-red, vascularized tumor. The characteristic histologic pattern is one of an organoid arrangement of plump, rounded to polygonal cells. The reticulin pattern emphasizes the organoid or nestlike arrangement and the presence of dilated vascular channels. The cells have a rich eosinophilic, occasionally vacuolated cytoplasm with vesicular nuclei. The cytoplasm in 80% of these tumors contains a characteristic PAS-positive, diastase-resistant crystalline material. The electron-microscopic picture identifies within the abundant cytoplasm numerous mitochondria, a prominent smooth endoplasmic reticulum and Golgi apparatus, and rod-shaped crystalloid bodies with occasional electron-dense secretory granules. The crystals and dense granules are characteristically membrane bound and have a lattice pattern with 100-nm periodicity. These diastase resistant crystals characteristically occur in the paranuclear region.

Several theories of histogenesis have been proffered. There have been numerous suggestions that this tumor may be of neural origin, and more recently it has been noted that they may originate from a modified mural cell that stains positively for renin. Thus, an alternative name of *malignant angioreninoma* has been suggested but not confirmed.

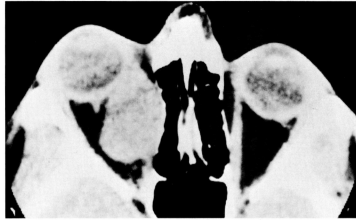

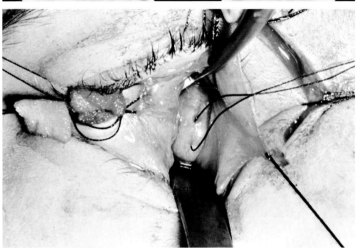

FIGURE 12-46. *(Top)* An axial CT scan of a medial orbital schwannoma in a 23-year-old woman who presented with cephalgia of 8 weeks' duration and a history (on retrospective photographic analysis) of gradual right proptosis. She had 4 mm proptosis and 1 mm lateral displacement. Note the well-defined intraorbital mass with bowing of the medial wall. *(Bottom)* The schwannoma was removed by medial orbitotomy, when it was found to be medial to the medial rectus muscle.

Wide local excision accompanied by radiotherapy is the recommended form of treatment. Exenteration is advised in lesions that cannot be completely excised or for local recurrence. Survival following successful excision of the primary tumor and its metastatic lesions has been reported.

GRANULAR CELL TUMOR

Of 500 cases of granular cell tumor reported in the literature, 16 have been described in the orbit. In addition, cases in or near the eye have been noted arising in uvea, conjunctiva, caruncle, lacrimal sac, eyebrows, and eyelids.

The tumor may occur at any age, most commonly between 40 and 70 years. There is a female predominance. The typical presentation is a solitary, nontender, firm nodule less than 6 cm in diameter that has been present for less than 1 year. It may be well circumscribed

or may infiltrate into surrounding tissues (Fig. 12-48). Overall, 10% to 15% are multicentric and 1% to 3% are malignant. In the orbit, they may occur as discrete or infiltrating, indolently growing tumors of soft tissue or extraocular muscle.

The tumor consists of nests and ribbons of large, round, and polygonal cells. The cells have paracentral, vesicular nuclei with prominent nucleoli and abundant cytoplasm replete with striking coarse eosinophilic granules. The cells lie close to peripheral nerve bundles and normal striated muscle (see Fig. 12-48, *B* and *C*). They are well differentiated and no mitotic activity is noted.

The cytoplasmic granules are periodic acid–Shiff (PAS) positive and diastase resistant. The characteristic ultrastructural features demonstrate clusters of cells with short interdigitating processes and rare primitive intercellular junctions. The nuclei are irregularly oval or round with dispersed chromatin and medium-sized nucleoli. Within the cytoplasm are numerous pleomorphic lysosomal-like round bodies lined by single and occasionally

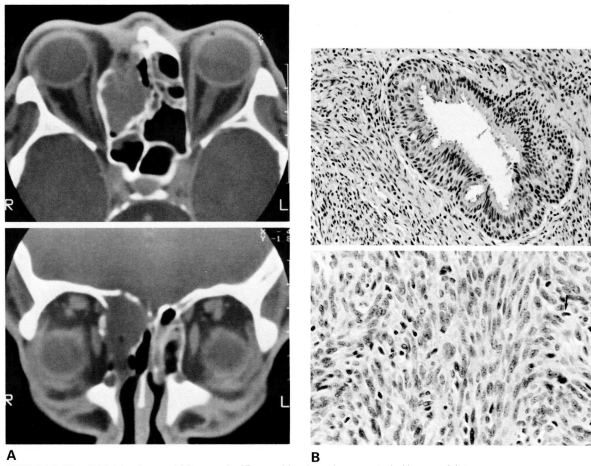

FIGURE 12-47. *(A)* Axial and coronal CT scans of a 45-year-old patient who presented with a complaint of tearing present over the previous 2 years. Investigations revealed an ethmoid mass that was believed to be a nasopharyngeal carcinoma. However, biopsy revealed a spindle cell tumor diagnosed as a low grade malignant schwannoma. The lesion has destroyed the cribriform plate and medial orbital wall. The patient underwent a combined craniofacial excision of the mass, and is alive and well 1 year later. *(B)* Histologically the mass was a low grade malignant schwannoma infiltrating beneath the sinus mucosa. The pattern is one of a spindle cell neoplasm with plump, ovoid, slightly irregular nuclei and occasional comma shapes *(arrow)* arranged in fascicles (H&E, original magnification *top* × 10, *bottom* × 40).

double limiting membranes and filled with granular dense material, numerous small vesicles and concentric laminated bodies. A second, usually more sparse population of spindled mesenchymal cells is frequently noted. They often contain oblong, filamentous, angulate bodies surrounded by a unit membrane (see Fig. 12-48D). The histogenesis of granular cell tumor remains controversial, but most recent evidence supports a neural origin.

The treatment of granular cell tumor is wide surgical excision. The reported local recurrence rate is less than 7%. Malignant granular cell tumor of the orbit is unknown.

CHEMODECTOMA (PARAGANGLIOMA)

Chemodectomas are said to arise from the chemoreceptor system, particularly the carotid and jugulotympanic bodies. They are also called *paragangliomas* and are part of a more widely dispersed collection of chemoreceptor cells that arise from neural crest cells throughout the body. The paraganglion system can be divided into three anatomical groups: branchiomeric, which essentially arises from the head and neck; intravagal, arising from the perineurium of the vagus nerve; and aorticosympathetic, which arises from the sympathetic nervous system. Paraganglioma may occur in any of these sites; it occurs most commonly in the carotid body. Overall, there is no sex dominance and they occur between 30 and 60 years of age. In addition, they may be sporadic, familial, or multiple. They have a tendency to recur following resection and may metastasize.

In the orbit they are exceedingly rare; about 16 cases have been reported, all of which have been benign. Ten of these were collected from 1951 through 1980 from all of China. The previously reported malignant cases have been believed to be alveolar soft part sarcomas. Clinically, they have been associated with slowly developing (years) proptosis, visual loss, diplopia, and occasionally a throbbing orbital pain. Some tumors reported were attached to extraocular muscles. These tumors may be locally infiltrative, but are usually well defined at the time of surgery.

Pathologically, these firm or rubbery reddish-to-tan lesions appear circumscribed and vascular. The component cells are arranged in an organoid or nestlike (Zellballen) pattern and the individual tumor cells are polygonal or ovoid with abundant pale or eosinophilic granular or slightly vacuolated cytoplasm. These nests are surrounded by reticulin. The cell nuclei have finely clumped chromatin (Fig. 12-49). The cytoplasmic granules may be argentaffin- or argyrophil-positive, reflecting small amounts of catecholamines that may be more reliably identified using a formaldehyde-induced fluorescence.

Chemodectomas are best treated surgically with wide excision to avoid recurrence and are not believed to be significantly radiosensitive.

PRIMARY ORBITAL CARCINOID

A single case of primary orbital carcinoid has been described by Zimmerman and colleagues in a series that had seven in this site (remainder metastatic) and eight in the uveal tract. Carcinoids characteristically occur as slow-growing neoplasia of the gut, arising from the Kulchitsky's cells. They belong to a larger group of tumors arising from amine precursor uptake and decarboxylation (APUD) cells, which may arise in the pituitary, hypothalamus, adrenal medulla, thyroid, pancreas, and lung. These cells and tumors derived from them are distinguished by their ability to synthesize bioactive amines or polypeptide hormones. Of tumors arising from this system, 81% are in the upper and lower GI tract, 14% occur in the lungs and bronchi, and 5% occur in all other sites. About 5% to 10% of patients with GI carcinoid develop the carcinoid syndrome due to a significant hepatic metastatic load producing serotonin and other secretory products. Degredation to 5-hydroxyindoleacetic (5-HIAA), which can be detected in the urine, is a marker for

this syndrome. All but one of the patients in Zimmerman's series had either clinical or chemical evidence of nonocular or orbital primaries (12 before and 3 after orbital and ocular occurrence).

The case described in the orbit was marked by an 11.5-year history of progressive proptosis, which led to exenteration. The orbit contained a tumor made of two cell types arranged in basaloid, tubular, trabecular, and rosette patterns. The tumor cells had either a clear cytoplasm with faint eosinophilic granules and a light basophilic central nucleus with stippled chromatin, or an eosinophilic cytoplasm and densely basophilic nucleas. It had an intense argentaffic reaction (Gremelius) and a light argyrophilic reaction. The patient had no primary lesion detected and was alive and well without recurrence 3 years after exenteration.

NEUROEPITHELIAL TUMORS

The neuroepithelial tumors are a family of neoplasia thought to arise from the primitive neuroectoderm. They bear close histologic resemblance and differences are based on sites of origin; the neuroblastoma and ganglioneuroma arise from the sympathetic system, the neuroepithelioma arises from the nonautonomic nerve, and the olfactory neuroepithelioma arises from the olfactory placode.

Neuroepithelioma

Neuroepithelioma is an exceedingly rare tumor that occurs at any age (most patients are over 20 years) and is thought to arise from peripheral nerves. A single case has been reported in the orbit. Histologically, it was composed of sheets or lobules of rounded cells with indistinct cytoplasm. Some of these groups of cells formed neurotubular units. Lesions decribed elsewhere in the body may form rosettes with a core of neurofibrillary material. The single case in the orbit was locally aggressive and ultimately rapidly metastasized despite surgery and radiotherapy.

Olfactory Neuroblastoma (Esthesioneuroblastoma)

Olfactory neuroblastoma is a tumor that arises from the olfactory epithelium in the upper nasal cavity and may extend into the orbit secondarily. Histologically, it is similar to neuroblastoma except for site and age of occurrence. In contrast to neuroblastoma, these characteristically occur in a bimodal peak in the second and fifth decades.

(Text continues on p. 333.)

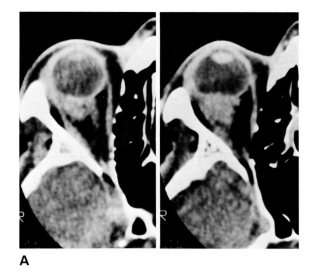

A

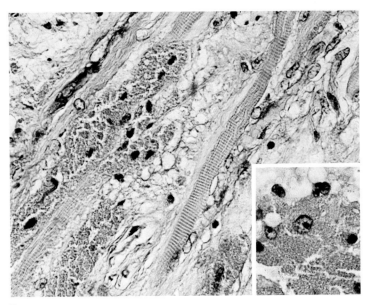

B

FIGURE 12-48. *(A)* Axial CT scan shows an irregular right retrobulbar mass displacing the optic nerve medially and indenting the globe. *(Left)* Superior cut; *(right)* inferior cut. The mass was seen in a 44-year-old man who presented with horizontal diplopia and restricted extraocular movements of 10 months' duration. Vision was 20/60, and the globe was elevated 2 mm and proptosed 3 mm. He had posterior choroidal folds. *(B)* Tumor from the orbit shows plump granular cells invading striated muscle; *inset* shows individual cells with prominent nucleoli and cytoplasmic granules (H&E, original magnification × 10, *inset* × 40). *(C)* Granular tumor cell positive for S-100 lies among nonstaining striated muscle cells (H&E, original magnification × 25). *(D, upper left)* A filamentous angulate body lies adjacent to granular cell nucleus. *(Upper right)* Complex cytoplasmic vesicles contain lamellar figures and smaller vesicles and granules. *(Lower left)* Several complex vesicles nesting in a bed of intracytoplasmic filaments. *(Lower right)* Several granular cells contain pleomorphic dense granules; complex vesicles and a myelin figure surround a muscle fiber *(arrow)*. (Dolman PJ, Rootman J, Dolman CL: Infiltrating orbital granular cell tumour: A case report and literature review. Br J Ophthalmol 71:47, 1986)

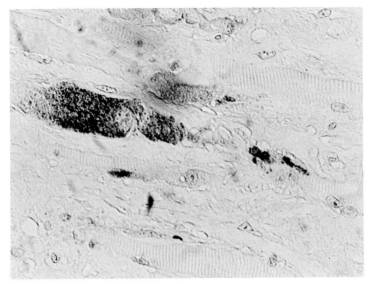

C

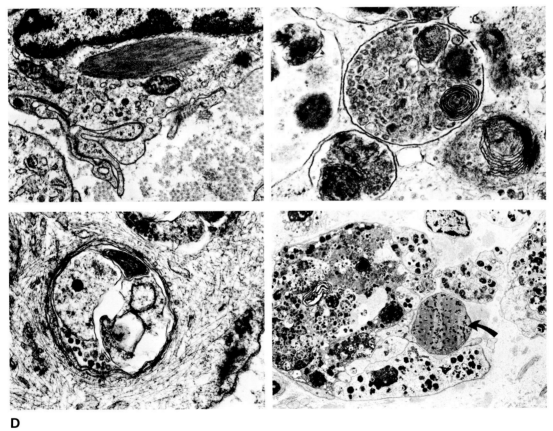

D

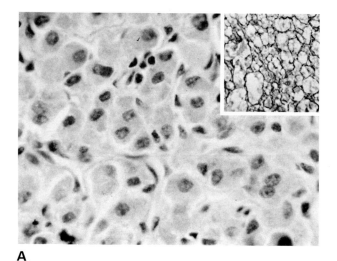

A

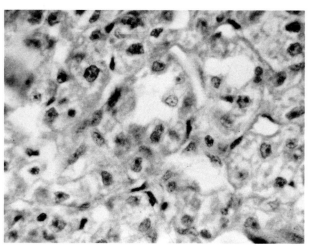

B

FIGURE 12-49. *(A)* Histopathology of an orbital paraganglioma shows nests of plump, regular eosinophilic cells surrounded by reticulin *(inset)* (H&E, original magnification × 40, *inset* × 10). *(B)* Orbital paraganglioma demonstrates a more organoid arrangement (H&E, original magnification × 40). *(C)* Orbital paraganglioma demonstrates nests of vacuolated cells, some of which resemble lipoblasts (H&E, original magnification × 40). *(A – C,* courtesy Dr. Zhang.)

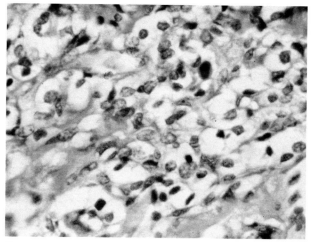

C

They are made up of sheets of small cells and may or may not have rosettes. They are frequently mistaken for other small cell tumors. Ultrastructurally, they have dense core (neurosecretory granules) and neuritic processes. Olfactory rosettes differing from the Homer-Wright type may be seen in those that demonstrate olfactory differentiation. These are lined by pseudostratified columnar cells with central mucin in the lumina. Neuroblastomas have been divided into two groups: those without olfactory differentiation and those with olfactory differentiation. The latter group may include ganglioneuroblastomatous differentiation (olfactory neurocytoma). Those with olfactory neuroblastomatous differentiation occur in patients of mean age 50 years, and the less differentiated neuroblastomatous type occurs in patients with a mean age of 20 years.

Rakes and co-workers have emphasized the common occurrence of ophthalmic manifestation in these tumors, noting that 53% of their cases had ocular manifestations at presentation and an additional 21% developed them later. Indeed, many of the different tumors of the sinus have ocular manifestations at the time of presentation and a small percentage of these patients may present to the ophthalmologist. The common ocular complaints are periorbital pain, lacrimation, and visual disturbance, which usually reflect a tumor in a more advanced stage than a tumor with primary nasal or nonocular symptoms. Additional ocular complaints include periorbital edema, ptosis, injection, and proptosis.

These tumors have been staged according to site of confinement: those in the nasal cavity are group A; those involving the paranasal sinuses are group B; and tumors extending beyond the sinuses into the cranium or orbit are group C. Elkon and co-workers have noted 5-year survival rates of 75% (group A), 68% (group B), and 28% (group C). Levine in a recent report of 26 cases has noted a dramatic increase in survival with the advent of aggressive craniofacial surgery and adjunctive radiotherapy and chemotherapy. They recommended combined preoperative radiotherapy and craniofacial resection for stage A and B disease and the addition of preoperative and postoperative antineoplastic drugs (vincristine and cyclophosphamide) for stage C disease.

Primary Neuroblastoma and Ganglioneuroma

Primary neuroblastoma and ganglioneuroma are thought to arise from the neuroblasts of the sympathetic nervous system. Neuroblastoma is the second most common orbital malignancy of childhood and is overwhelmingly metastatic in origin; thus, it will be discussed in the section on metastatic tumors. Systemically, ganglioneuromas are three times more common than neuroblastomas but occur at an older age (average 10 years) and in the posterior mediastinum and retroperitonium, in contrast to the younger age occurrence and adrenal site of neuroblastoma. They are by definition well-circumscribed, benign tumors that contain a histologically uniform population of cells. Scattered nests of mature ganglion cells are seen within a matrix of Schwann cells. Histologically confirmed primary occurrence of this lesion in the orbit has not been described, but a single case of secondary extension from the sinus has been noted.

PRIMARY ORBITAL MELANOMA

Primary melanoma of the orbit is a rare tumor and must be distinguished from the more common occurrence of metastases and secondary melanomas arising from the globe, lid, and conjunctiva. Late recurrence of uveal melanoma has been reported even 42 years after enucleation. Nevertheless, primary melanomas deep within the orbit do occur. They originate from melanocytes of the leptomeninges, ciliary nerves, and emissaria or from ectopic rests. They may arise *de novo* or in association with ocular and oculodermal melanocytosis. The oculodermal melanocytosis may be of a limited variety, and features of dermal pigmentation in the first and second divisions of the fifth nerve should be carefully sought. According to Hidano, up to the 65% of patients with the nevus of Ota will have evidence of pigmentation of the ocular tissues.

The clinical onset of primary orbital melanoma is usually described as a rapidly growing tumefaction, which may or may not be infiltrative. CT scans in cases described demonstrate a well-defined enhancing mass with variable low-density or cystic areas in some.

At surgery, they are usually pigmented and may even be black and necrotic, making gross distinction from a hematoma difficult. Histologically, primary melanomas usually consist of a mixture of spindle and epithelioid cells with a high mitotic index. Some melanomas may be mostly spindle cell or epithelioid in character and amelanotic. If associated with a nevus of Ota, scattered melanocytes in the remaining orbital tissues or rests of a cellular blue nevus may be identified.

These tumors have a uniformly grim prognosis because of their propensity to escape the local confines by means of the adjacent foramina or the bloodstream. Treatment is by exenteration, although a few cases of low-grade tumors have been locally resected.

RETINAL ANLAGE TUMOR (PIGMENTED RETINAL CHORISTOMA)

Retinal anlage tumor is a curiosity that characteristically occurs in the head and neck (usually in the upper or lower jaw) of an infant in the first year of life. Its interest to the ophthalmologist lies in its characteristic morphology, which reflects features of the retinal pigment epithelium and neuroblastic cells. In addition, this tumor occasionally involves the orbit by contiguity. Diverse names have been given, including pigmented neuroectodermal tumor of infancy, melanotic progonoma, congenital melanocarcinoma, melanotic adamantinoma, and pigmented epulis of infancy, reflecting differing theories of histogenesis. The consensus of opinion is still somewhat unsettled and lies between neural crest or neuroectodermal origin. Zimmerman has emphasized the characteristic morphologic features of the pigment within the tumor cells as being of retinal pigment epithelial type, and has proposed the name *pigmented retinal choristoma*.

The tumor usually presents as a mass involving the upper or lower jaw. Characteristically, the mass is radiolucent and may be locally destructive. Other sites include the skin, ovary, uterus, brain, and epididymis. In the head and neck, they may be locally recurrent in about 10% to 15% of cases. Multifocal lesions have been described and about 4% have been malignant with metastases.

The typical histopathologic feature is the presence of alveolar spaces lined by pigmented cuboidal cells. In addition, nests of nonpigmented, small, round cells may be seen within the alveoli or the surrounding fibrous stroma. Neurofibrillary material may be seen in association with these cells, which resemble benign neuroblasts.

Treatment is complete local excision of the involved bone and soft tissue.

ECTOMESENCHYMAL TUMORS

Because the mesenchyme of the head and neck is largely of neural crest origin (ectomesenchyme, mesectoderm), some tumors derived from these tissues may recapitulate a mixture of fibroblastic, muscle cell, and schwannian elements. Thus, schwannian tumors may have evidence of striated muscle components. More complex admixtures of pigmented, fibroblastic, and myoblastic tissues in these unusual tumors may be noted. Although these have been described in the head and neck region and in the globe, primary occurrence in the orbit is practically unknown.

■ MESENCHYMAL TUMORS

Jack Rootman and Jocelyn S. Lapointe

All of the lesions in this section can be grouped under a broad umbrella of mesenchymal and fibro-osseous tumors by suggesting that a primitive mesenchymal stem cell is capable of developing into a variety of cell types. These cell lines may undergo developmental arrest at varying stages of maturation and produce benign or ma-

lignant proliferations with differences in biologic behavior. The components of the orbit that are of mesenchymal origin include striated and smooth muscle, fibrous tissue, fat, cartilage, and bone. The embryologic derivation of orbital connective tissue is from the neural crest (ectomesenchyme or mesoectoderm). Because of their common progenitor, most of the mesenchymal tumor lines may share a continuum of histologic features. In addition, many of the mesenchymal tumor lines have a variable pattern and may be composed of cells and single cell lines expressing different functional states, for example, a collagenizing fibroblast, a myofibroblast, or a fibroblastic histiocyte. Myofibroblasts have features of both fibroblasts and smooth muscle cells. Similarly, osteoblasts and chondroblasts share features noted in both cartilaginous and bone-producing tumors.

We have seen 43 mesenchymal lesions of the orbit comprising 3% of all orbital cases and 16% of neoplasia. The undifferentiated embryonal mesenchymal tumors and tumors of muscle are classified together on the basis of either similar histology, clinical behavior, or features of myopathic differentiation. They include embryonal sarcoma, rhabdomyosarcoma, and rare smooth muscle tumors. Despite the wealth of cellular anlage, adipose and fibrous tissue tumors of the orbit are rare. In contrast, the fibrous histiocytomas appear to have an orbital predilection. The largest group of mesenchymal lesions derive from bone and include dysplasias, reactive lesions, and neoplasia.

Striated Muscle Tumors

RHABDOMYOSARCOMA

Jack Rootman and Ka Wah Chan

Rhabdomyosarcoma is the quintessential example of fulminant orbital malignancy in childhood. Clinically, its occurrence involves the differential diagnosis of acute and subacute proptosis of childhood, and pathologically, the differential diagnosis of small, round, and spindle cell tumors of the orbit in childhood. It has a distinctive age and site predilection as well as pathologic appearance. Changes in therapy over the last 20 years have markedly improved the prognosis, particularly in orbital cases.

Rhabdomyosarcoma is the most common soft tissue malignancy of childhood, representing 3.4% of all childhood malignancies and 19% of all sarcomas. In the orbit it is the most common primary malignant tumor in children. In our series it constituted 2% of orbital neoplasia. Seventy percent occur in the first decade and it has been reported from birth to the seventh decade. There is a bimodal peak depending on histology, with the embryonal and alveolar types occurring in childhood and adolescence, respectively, and the pleomorphic variety in older persons. Overall, there is a 3 : 2 male to female preponderance with a ratio of 5 : 3 when in the orbit.

The histogenesis of rhabdomyosarcoma is thought to reflect the embryogenesis of muscle. The tissue of origin for juvenile rhabdomyosarcomas is thought to be the pluripotential mesenchyme that normally differentiates into striated muscle. This theory is supported by a tendency for these to occur in the orbital soft tissue of juveniles and not in the extraocular muscles. The embryonal type corresponds to developing muscle at the 7-week to 10-week fetal stage and the alveolar type to the hollow tube stage. The pleomorphic type is thought to arise *de novo* as a result of dedifferentiation of adult muscle. The age at occurrence and location of these types tends to reflect this concept of histogenesis.

Most rhabdomyosarcomas arise spontaneously although familial occurrences, associations with congenital malformations, and trauma have been cited epidemiologically.

Clinical Presentation

The majority of orbital rhabdomyosarcomas present acutely, reflecting the fulminant growth pattern and virulence of this tumor. The most common presentation is rapidly developing exophthalmos, frequently associated with injection and swelling of the lids and a downward and outward displacement of the globe. Jones noted that 50% are retrobulbar, with 25% above and 12% below the globe. About one quarter of the patients have a palpable mass and one third have ptosis at diagnosis. Pain and decreased vision are uncommon presenting signs.

Because of the acute and subacute onset of exophthalmos, swelling, and injection, these tumors may be confused with inflammatory syndromes or related to spurious trauma, which may further delay diagnosis.

Cell Types

Although single rhabdomyosarcomas vary in histologic appearance, most can be classified in one of four general categories as suggested by Horne and Enterline. The stringency of histopathologic definition tends to vary somewhat depending on the view of the histopathologist. Enzinger has emphasized that some form of microscopic, immunohistochemical, or electron-microscopic demonstration of rhabdomyoblasts is central to the diagnosis. Cross striations are seen on the average in 50% to 60% of embryonal-type lesions and in only 30% of alveolar-type lesions. On the other hand, rhabdomyoblasts may be identified without necessarily demonstrating cross striation. Rhabdomyoblasts are characterized by an abundant eosinophilic cytoplasm containing fibrillary material or cells of spindle, irregular, tadpole, racquet, or angulated shape (see Figs. 12-50C, 12-53, 12-54A). They may have a markedly vacuolated cytoplasm suggesting the appearance of a spider web (see Fig. 12-54B).

Histochemistry using Masson trichrome, phosphotungstic acid – hematoxylin (PTAH), and periodic acid – Schiff (PAS) with and without diastase confirm empiric features of acidophilia and glycogen deposition in rhabdomyoblasts. Immunoperoxidase techniques help by identifying desmin, myoglobulin, and actin (see Fig. 12-50D). Myoglobulin is a more specific marker. Ultrastructurally, the degree of differentiation of the tumor varies greatly, with the least differentiated cells demonstrating thin (actin) myofilaments (60–80 nm) and the more differentiated thicker (myosin) filaments (120–150 nm) (see Figs. 12-51C, 12-52B). More obvious characteristics of muscle may be noted with A and I banding and Z lines (Fig. 12-51B). The cytoplasm may also contain a prominent Golgi apparatus, polyribosomes associated with myofilaments, glycogen, lipid, lysozomes, and incomplete basal lamina with pinocytotic vesicles.

Classification of Microscopic Features

There is some overlap with varying degrees of differentiation in rhabdomyosarcomas, but there are three major histopathologic subtypes: embryonal (including the botryoid type), alveolar, and pleomorphic. Embryonal and alveolar types have been grouped together by some authors as *juvenile rhabdomyosarcoma*. Table 12-5 summarizes the major features of the different types.

Embryonal Rhabdomyosarcoma

Embryonal rhabdomyosarcoma (Figs. 12-50 to 12-54), seen in two thirds of cases, has a histologic spectrum with major features consisting of patterns of loose (myxoid) and compact cellularity. There are varying numbers of densely eosinophilic, hyperchromatic rhabdomyoblasts. Pleomorphism is also variable with mitotic figures frequently noted. The least differentiated types consist of small spindle, round, or oval cells with hyperchromatic nuclei and small nucleoli. With increasing degrees of differentiation, larger round or oval rhabdomyoblasts with eosinophilic fibrillar cytoplasm, intracellular glycogen (some spider web cells), and fusiform or spindle cells are noted. Strap-shaped rhabdomyoblasts with peripheral myofilaments and cross striations may be noted in more differentiated tumors. The stroma is frequently mucoid with little collagen.

Botryoid embryonal rhabdomysarcoma is a variant that occurs when the tumor is immediately adjacent to mucosal surfaces where growth is unrestricted. This leads to a polypoid tumor with an abundant myxoid stroma and a densely cellular submucosal (cambium) layer. If light and electron microscopy and immunohistochemistry fail to demonstrate striated muscle differentiation,

TABLE 12-5.
TYPES AND MAJOR FEATURES OF RHABDOMYOSARCOMAS

Embryonal Sarcoma	Embryonal Rhabdomyosarcoma	Alveolar Rhabdomyosarcoma	Adult Pleomorphic Rhabdomyosarcoma
Major Loci			
Head and neck	Orbit	Head and neck	Peripheral skeletal muscle
Orbit	Head and neck		
Pelvic	Botryoid: Pelvic (urogenital)		
Epidemiology			
Children	Children (average) 7.8 years	Children and adolescents	Adults
Histogenesis			
Primitive mesenchyme	Primitive mesenchyme	Primitive mesenchyme	Dedifferentiation of adult striated muscle
	Muscle at the 7–10 week fetal stage	Muscle at the hollow tube stage	
Histology			
Resemble poorly differentiated embryonal rhabdomyosarcoma but no demonstration of striated muscle origin	Varying loose (myxoid) and compact cellularity	Poorly differentiated trabecular pattern	Larger; tadpole, strap, and racquet-shaped
	Least differentiated; spindle, round, or oval	Central cells degenerated	
	Better differentiated; larger, oval with fibrillar cytoplasm; fusiform and spindle; ± glycogen	Frequent mitosis	Cross striations may be present
	Strap-shaped with cross striations	Rhabdomyoblasts adjacent to or in septae	
	Botryoid–polypoid with cambium layer	Multinucleated giant cells	

but the overall pattern is one of embryonal rhabdomyosarcoma, the diagnosis of embryonal sarcoma is made. The prognosis for this lesion is the same as for embryonal rhabdomyosarcoma.

Alveolar Rhabdomyosarcoma

Alveolar rhabdomyosarcoma (Fig. 12-55) consists of poorly differentiated tumor cells arranged in a characteristic trabecular pattern resembling the alveoli of the lung. The cells immediately adjacent to the alveolar septae are generally well defined, whereas the central space contains degenerating free-floating cells. It is not unusual to note more densely cellular areas within these tumors. Most of the cells tend to be oval or round with minimal cytoplasm and there are frequent mitotic figures. Larger neoplastic rhabdomyoblasts are less common in alveolar rhabdomyosarcomas and are usually seen adjacent to or within the septae. Multinucleated giant cells are often present in alveolar rhabdomyosarcomas as opposed to embryonal types (see Fig. 12-55). This distinct histologic pattern is also noted in the metastases of alveolar tumors. Zimmerman has suggested that this type is more common in the inferior orbit. The overall prognosis is poorest with this histology.

Adult Pleomorphic Rhabdomyosarcoma

In all sites adult pleomorphic rhabdomyosarcoma is the least common, constituting 1% of rhabdomyosarcomas. In the orbit they occur in older patients and are intimate to muscle. Histologically, they are made up of deeply eosinophilic, loosely arranged, and variably sized pleomorphic cells. Larger tadpole, strap-type, and racquet-shaped rhabdomyoblasts with either granular or vacuolated cytoplasm may be noted. Cross striations are unusual and glycogen is frequently present. The occurrence of this type of tumor in the orbit as elsewhere is somewhat controversial, and its distinction from other pleomorphic sarcomas is difficult.

New Classification

Palmer and co-workers have proposed a new pathologic classification system for rhabdomyosarcoma. Three subtypes have been defined based on cytology. Anaplastic rhabdomyosarcoma (ANA) is characterized by the presence of enlarged, bizarre mitotic figures, diffuse nuclear hyperchromatism, and pleomorphism, all of which may be present focally. The second subtype, monomorphous round cell rhabdomyosarcoma (MRC), consists of uni-

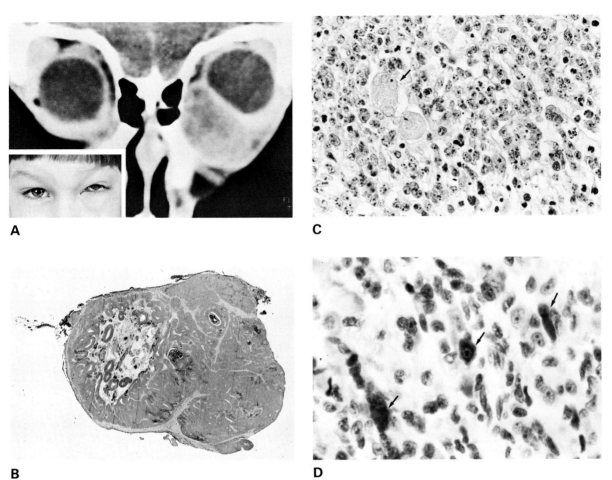

FIGURE 12-50. *(A)* A 7-year-old boy with an embryonal rhabdomyosarcoma presented with a mass involving the left lower lid and orbit. The mass had developed over a 5-week period. On palpation it was firm, slightly nodular, and had a tan-pink subconjunctival component. The coronal CT scan demonstrates a solid tumor with areas of low density. The tumor indents and displaces the globe upward. *(B)* At orbitotomy, a circumscribed, slightly nodular, pale tan mass was excised. Histologically, there were areas of loose (myxoid) and compact cellularity and distinct perivascular mantles of tumor. The myxoid areas correspond to the low-density foci noted on CT scan (H&E, original magnification × 2). *(C)* The cell population consisted of pleomorphic round and oval cells with hyperchromatic nuclei and dense nucleoli. In addition, there were large rhabdomyoblasts with eosinophilic fibrillar cytoplasm *(arrow)* (H&E, original magnification × 40). *(D)* Immunoperoxidase stains for myoglobulin demonstrate a highly positive reaction in the cytoplasm of the large cells in particular *(arrows)* (immunoperoxidase, original magnification × 100). The patient was treated with combined chemotherapy (modified VAC) and radiotherapy (4140 rad), and is alive and well 2 years later.

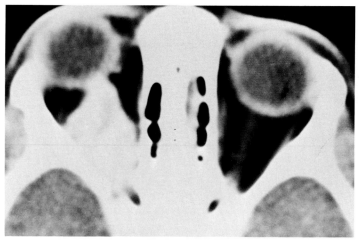

A

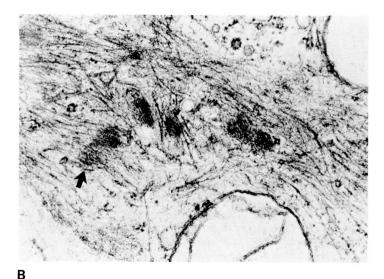

B

FIGURE 12-51. *(A)* Contrast-enhanced axial CT scan demonstrates a slightly nodular intraconal mass extending toward the orbital apex. This occurred in a 4-year-old boy who developed rapid prominence of the eye over a 1-week period. *(B)* Electron microscopic features from biopsy of the mass in *A.* Note myofilamentary structure with Z-band densities *(arrow).* These features suggest early sarcomeric organization substantiating a diagnosis of rhabdomyosarcoma. The patient was treated with VAC therapy and 4500 rad of radiotherapy. He is alive and well 2½ years after treatment (original magnification × 41,750). (Electron micrograph courtesy J. Dimmick, M.D.)

form sized, rounded cells with constant cytologic features. The final type, mixed rhabdomyosarcoma (MX), includes all the other rhabdomyosarcoma variants. Overall, the mixed rhabdomyosarcomas are seen in about 80% of tumors and constitute the most favorable histology. The anaplastic and monomorphous round cell variants are believed to be prognostically unfavorable.

Differential Diagnosis

Clinically, the differential diagnosis of rhabdomyosarcoma includes progressive, rapidly developing tumors and inflammatory conditions of childhood; these include neuroblastoma, chloroma, lymphangioma, infantile hemangioma, dermoid cysts, cellulitis, and nonspecific inflammatory diseases. The histopathologic differential diagnosis of childhood round cell tumors includes neuroblastoma, neuroepithelioma, Ewing's sarcoma, angiosarcoma, synovial sarcoma, malignant melanoma, granulocytic sarcoma, and malignant lymphoma. Granular cell tumor and alveolar soft part sarcoma may also be included in the histopathologic differential diagnosis. We have recently encountered a case of rhabdoid tumor of the orbit, a poorly differentiated sarcoma (usually seen in the kidney) that resembles rhabdomyosarcoma. It should be noted that focal myoblastic differentiation can occur as part of other types of tumors such as the neuroectodermal neoplasia. In addition, some inflammatory conditions may resemble it, including nodular fasciitis and destructive inflammations affecting muscle.

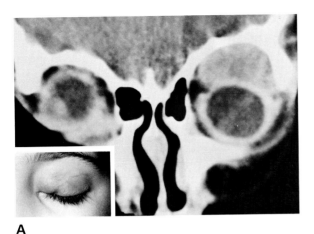

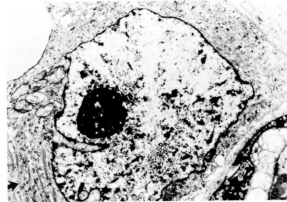

A

B

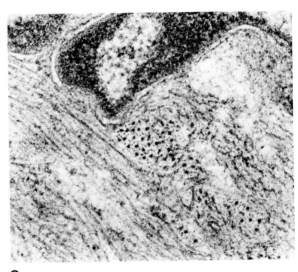

C

FIGURE 12-52. *(A)* An 8-year-old child presented with a mass that had developed in the left superior orbit over a 3- to 4-week period. Coronal CT scan demonstrates a large, well-delineated, slightly inhomogeneous superior orbital mass indenting and depressing the globe. *(B)* Electron microscopy of the biopsy specimen from the above mass demonstrates small thin and thick filaments *(arrow)* and a large vesicular nucleus, typical of a rhabdomyoblast. Final diagnosis was an embryonal rhabdomyosarcoma (original magnification × 9100). *(C)* Electron micrograph shows cross sections of filaments of thick and thin types (original magnification × 117,500). (*B* and *C* courtesy J. Dimmick, M.D.)

Management

Rhabdomyosarcoma is an example of the success of modern therapy in the management of poorly differentiated tumors of childhood. In all sites the prognosis for survival has improved from 20% to 65%, and in the orbit to 95% over 5 years. Prognosis is more specifically related to the location and staging of the disease than to histopathology alone. Orbital rhabdomyosarcomas have a distinctly favorable prognosis because of early presentation and lack of lymphatic drainage. There is some degree of controversy with regard to specific staging of rhabdomyosarcomas and differences exist depending on the particular study outline. The intergroup rhabdomyosarcoma study staging shown in Table 12-6 describes four groups and reflects the general trend in clinical classification of rhabdomyosarcoma. Most orbital rhabdomyosarcomas are groups I and II.

TABLE 12-6.
STAGING OF RHABDOMYOSARCOMA (INTERGROUP RHABDOMYOSARCOMA STUDY)

Group I: Localized disease, completely resected

Group II: Regional disease, with or without lymph nodes involved, grossly resected

Group III: Incomplete resection or biopsy with gross residual disease

Group IV: Distant metastases (lung, bone marrow, brain, distant nodules)

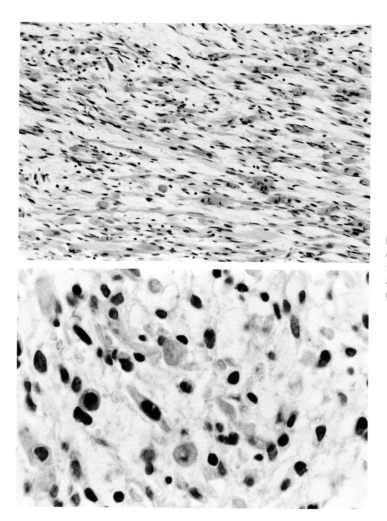

FIGURE 12-53. Photomicrographs of areas of embryonal rhabdomyosarcomas with varying features show elongated, straplike rhabdomyoblasts as well as some rounded, plump cells (H&E, original magnifications *top* × 10, *bottom* × 40).

Treatment is initiated after an urgent tissue diagnosis and metastatic workup to stage the disease. Metastases from orbital sites are to lung and bone with very rare lymphatic extension, in contrast to embryonal rhabdomyosarcoma elsewhere, which is one of the rare sarcomas with a predilection for node metastases. Local recurrence may extend into the intracranial and nasal cavities. Treatment protocols consist of a combination of limited surgical removal of the tumor, radiation therapy, and combined adjuvant chemotherapy with variations depending on location and stage of the disease. Currently, the most frequently used chemotherapy is a combination of vincristine, dactinomycin (Actinomycin-D), and cyclophosphamide (VAC). Patients with groups I and II disease are no longer given postoperative radiotherapy, as it has been shown that adjuvant Actinomycin-D and vincristine alone may be as efficacious as the full, standard VAC regimen. With only microscopic residual disease in the orbit, it is suggested that radiation therapy, limited to 4000 rad, with concomitant chemotherapy is sufficient to achieve local control; those with gross residual tumor require a dosage of 5000 rad. Surgery is limited to gross total removal of small tumors and exenteration, reserved for local failures.

The use of potent chemotherapy and radiotherapy is not without significant morbidity in the growing child, including structural and symptomatic abnormalities. The structural abnormalities include cataracts, corneal changes, retinal problems, ptosis, enophthalmos, and lacrimal duct stenosis. Cataracts, corneal changes, and retinal changes occur in 80%, and 75% of patients have impairment or loss of vision. A high incidence of facial asymmetry and bone hypoplasia has been noted as well. The symptomatic problems include keratoconjunctivitis, photophobia, conjunctivitis, and dry eye. Late complications of chemotherapy include leukemia and behavioral

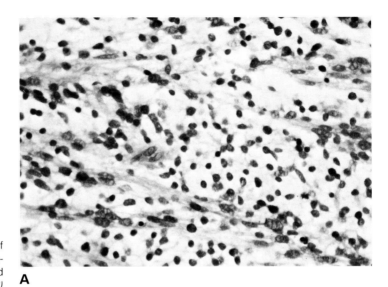

A

FIGURE 12-54. *(A)* Histopathologic features of an embryonal rhabdomyosarcoma with an admixture of loosely arranged cells and some elongated strap cells (H&E, original magnification × 25). *(B)* Rhabdomyoblasts with a central tumor cell demonstrating vacuolated cytoplasm secondary to lysis of glycogen ("spider web" cell) (H&E, original magnification × 100).

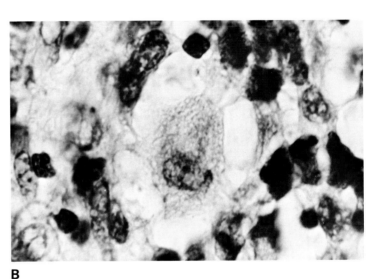

B

problems. Recent trends suggest a reduction in numbers of agents and amount of radiotherapy for earlier stage rhabdomyosarcomas. Some treatment centers are now advocating gross total excision or debulking and chemotherapy exclusively.

In summary, rhabdomyosarcoma is the most common primary orbital sarcoma of childhood. It is characterized by a fulminant onset frequently mimicking inflammatory conditions. Early diagnosis is imperative to facilitate appropriate treatment. Histopathologic characteristics are reasonably well defined with some overlap, and newer electron-microscopic and immunohistochemical methods are allowing more specific diagnosis.

Advances in multimodality therapy have dramatically altered the prognosis in this disease.

RHABDOMYOMA

Rhabdomyoma is an exceedingly rare tumor that has three morphologic varieties: adult, fetal, and genital. It remains a somewhat controversial tumor and may in fact be a hamartomatous lesion. In the orbit, the occurrence of a true rhabdomyoma has not been clearly identified and agreed upon by multiple authorities.

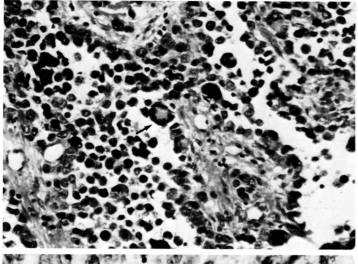

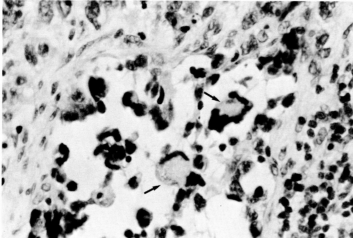

FIGURE 12-55. Histopathologic features of an alveolar rhabdomyosarcoma demonstrate rhabdomyoblasts immediately adjacent to the alveolar septae with central "free-floating" cells. Note giant cells *(arrows)* typical of this pattern (H&E, original magnifications *top* × 25, *bottom* × 40).

Smooth Muscle Tumors

Orbital smooth muscle tumors may arise from vessels, the smooth muscle overlying the inferior orbital fissure, and the capsulopalpebral muscles of Müller. Both the benign and malignant variants are exceedingly rare.

LEIOMYOMA

Although several cases of orbital leiomyoma have been reported, they are a curiosity and may be confused with angioleiomyomas. Leiomyomas are well-encapsulated, slowly progressive, isolated orbital tumors that occur in the third and fourth decades. Histologically, these solid tumors consist of bundles of palisading cells. The cytoplasm characteristically stains intensely with trichrome and contains filaments. There is a prominent vascular component. They can be excised in toto, and recurrence reflects incomplete excision. Because leiomyomas may demonstrate collagen deposition, confusion with nerve sheath tumors and fibrous histiocytomas is common.

LEIOMYOSARCOMA

Cases of leiomyosarcoma have been reported by several authors. It is a rare orbital tumor with varying degrees of malignancy. Several of the cases reported have had both local recurrence and metastases. Leiomyosarcoma either occurs *de novo* in older individuals (sixth decade) or as a radiation-induced sarcoma. Clinically, it is a relatively rapidly developing, usually infiltrative mass lesion. The histologic diagnosis rests on the demonstration of smooth muscle origin (i.e., cytoplasmic filaments on trichrome stain or electron-microscopy). It should be noted that this is a difficult and sometimes controversial histopathologic diagnosis. The lesions are characteristically vascular and densely cellular, and demonstrate foci of necrosis, mitoses, or nuclear pleomorphism. Because of their usual infiltrative nature, the treatment of choice is exenteration; however, several cases have been managed successfully by local excision, which was in one instance followed by radiotherapy.

A highly aggressive mesoectodermal leiomyosarcoma arising from the antrum and invading the orbit has been reported by Jakobiec and co-workers.

Adipose Tumors

Although the retrobulbar fat volumetrically constitutes the largest component of the orbit, unequivocal lipomas and liposarcomas are exceedingly rare in this site.

LIPOMA

The frequency of lipomas in orbital series varies from 0% to 9% of orbital tumors, and generally is closer to 0% where strict histopathologic criteria govern reporting.

A lipoma by definition should exist as an independent mass within the orbit, and growth would displace rather than insinuate into other soft tissues. A few cases of spindle cell lipoma have been documented in the orbit and proptosis has been reported with disseminated benign lipomas of lipomatosis. Clinically, lipomas develop slowly without infiltration, and at surgery appear circumscribed and appear slightly more yellow than normal orbital fat. Because of their circumscription, lipomas can be treated by simple excision.

LIPOSARCOMA

According to Enzinger, liposarcoma is the most common soft tissue sarcoma of adult life (16%–18%); however, it is distinctly rare in the orbit. In his series, only 1% of liposarcomas occurred in the face; the overwhelming majority were retroperitoneal or involved the thigh. It is believed to develop from undifferentiated mesenchyme and not primarily from fat. There are four histologic types: well-differentiated, myxoid, round cell, and pleomorphic liposarcoma. Overall, prognosis is largely related to size and site of the initial lesion and to pathologic type and grade. The pleomorphic and round cell variants are more locally aggressive and likely to metastasize.

The cases described in the orbit have usually presented as slowly developing mass lesions and were often difficult to diagnose from a clinical and pathological viewpoint. Central to the pathologic diagnosis is the demonstration of lipoblasts, which may vary in appearance from bloated, vacuolated cells to signet ring or round cells with lesser amounts of fat. A preoperative diagnosis is unlikely and is compounded by the possibility that these lesions may be quite circumscribed in appearance.

Management is governed by the location and possible circumscription of the tumor. Most are infiltrative and should be treated by radical excision, which usually implies exenteration. Some circumscribed and low-grade tumors have been successfully excised. Elsewhere, liposarcomas have been regarded as radiosensitive and in selected cases, adjunctive radiotherapy has been advocated. We have seen a case of metastatic liposarcoma to the orbit (Fig. 12-56). Since completing this series we have seen a primary liposarcoma. This myxoid liposarcoma was slow growing (8 years). CT scan showed low-density infiltrations of the extraocular muscles, representing the lesion's fat-containing component.

Fibrous Tissue Tumors

Although fibrous tissue tumors constitute an important aspect of the soft tissue lesion systemically, a limited number of them affect the orbit.

FIBROMA

The fibroma is the least common and most differentiated fibrous tissue tumor of the orbit. In fact, the diagnosis in a modern setting is of questionable validity and this lesion may be of historical significance only. It has been characterized as a clinically slow, noninfiltrative mass most commonly seen in men and in the medial orbit. Histologically, it is a paucicellular lesion with dense interwoven collagen bundles and few vessels with no evidence of inflammation. There may be areas that are more loosely arranged and some slightly more cellular foci. The major histologic differential diagnosis is keloid and severe fibrosis following a nonspecific orbital inflammatory disorder. They are relatively well circumscribed. Treatment is by excision, and they recur if it is incomplete.

NODULAR FASCIITIS

Nodular fasciitis is one of the most common fibrous tumors elsewhere in the body, usually involving the upper limb and trunk and presenting as a rapidly developing (weeks to months), tender, solitary mass in young adults. Head and neck lesions are rare and generally occur in children. In the orbital region, it usually affects the adnexa or conjunctiva. Few occur in the deeper orbit.

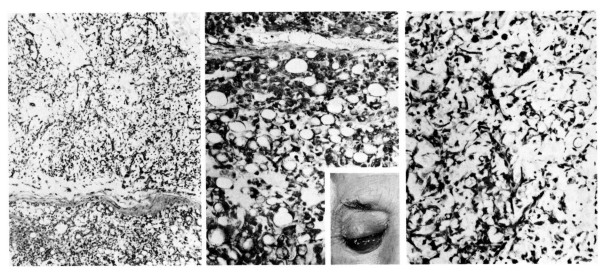

FIGURE 12-56. Photomicrographs of a myxoid liposarcoma from the retroperitoneum show a mixed pattern consisting mainly of myxoid areas with typical arborizing vessels and lipoblasts with a "signet-ring" appearance. The central photomicrograph demonstrates a more solid portion of the mass containing many bloated lipoblasts and some round cells. *(Inset)* A 65-year-old man in whom a myxoid liposarcoma had metastasized to the orbit (H&E, original magnifications *left* × 10, *center* × 25, *right* × 25). (Courtesy A. Worth, M.D.)

Grossly, they are nodular or well-circumscribed lesions. Histologically, there is a richly cellular, loosely arranged, reactive process. The basic cell population is a plump myofibroblast with a stellate appearance (resembling fibroblasts in tissue culture). Nodular fasciitis may be more cellular and less differentiated, and the diagnosis is based more on the architecture of the lesion, which often has central necrosis and peripheral "reactive" features. Myxoid areas and mitoses are noted, and account for the frequent confusion with fibrosarcoma. However, nodular fasciitis is less cellular, and has better differentiated cells and normal mitotic figures. More ancient lesions may have foci of collagen deposition. Treatment is by complete excision with an overall recurrence rate of 1% to 2%, according to Enzinger.

FIBROMATOSES

The fibromatoses are a complicated group of fibrous soft tissue lesions affecting primarily the musculoaponeurotic tissues; they are distinctly rare in the head. Their biologic behavior places them clinically and histopathologically between benign fibrous lesions and fibrosarcoma. Many subtypes have been defined based on sites of occurrence and histopathology. Overall, because they are locally infiltrative and often rapidly growing, distinction from fibrosarcoma may be difficult. Generally, however, they are less cellular, have focal maturation and collageniza-

tion, none or few mitotic figures, and benign-appearing fibroblasts (Fig. 12-57).

The most common type affecting the orbit are the extra-abdominal variants of deep (musculoaponeurotic) fibromatoses. They may develop rapidly and involve the orbit by contiguity or as a primary site. Histologically, they are poorly circumscribed and made up of slender, spindle-shaped, uniform cells with abundant collagen.

The fibromatoses occur twice as often in men. There are some differences based on age, with certain types characteristically occurring in childhood and infancy, including the infantile form of deep fibromatosis (desmoid type) and infantile myofibromatosis (congenital generalized fibromatosis). The infantile fibromatosis behaves in a fashion similar to the deep fibromatosis of the adult, but may be more rapid in development. Histopathologically, they are made up of well-differentiated fibroblasts with a varying spectrum of maturity from primitive to more mature-appearing fibroblasts. The infantile myofibromatosis is most often multiple, with a tendency to local aggressiveness and recurrence. These usually have a benign course and tend to regress unless they involve vital viscera. Half the cases are solitary, whereas the remainder have multiple or generalized lesions. The histologic spectrum ranges from dense collagenous to more cellular lesions. Microscopically, the lesions resemble smooth muscle tissue; electron-microscopically, they consist of an admixture of fibroblasts and myofibroblasts containing intracytoplasmic myofilaments.

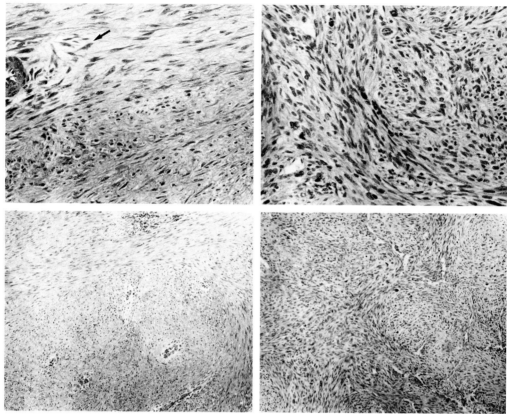

FIGURE 12-57. Photomicrographs comparing a fibromatosis *(left)* to a fibrosarcoma *(right)*. The fibromatosis has smaller cells, more collagen, and a looser matrix with some cells demonstrating a pattern typical of fibroblasts in tissue culture *(arrow)*. In contrast, the fibrosarcoma is more compactly arranged, has less collagen, and has larger cells with some mitotic figures and nuclear atypia (H&E, original magnifications *top* × 25, *bottom* × 10). (Courtesy A. Worth, M.D.)

Treatment of the fibromatoses is wide surgical excision because of a high recurrence rate (overall 25% to 65%). Adjunctive radiotherapy has been recommended, but carries a risk of sarcomatous degeneration. In addition, radiotherapy may be of limited use and its main value may be to cause cessation of growth. Steroids may be helpful in slowing the growth of these lesions. In instances where the pathology is more aggressive, these are best thought of as low-grade fibrosarcomas. Spontaneous regression and maturation of fibromatoses may occur.

FIBROSARCOMA

Fibrosarcoma has been overdiagnosed in the past, resulting in an exaggerated incidence. The introduction of new concepts and terminology such as *malignant fibrous histiocytoma, fibromatoses,* and numerous other spindle cell

tumors has made it an extremely uncommon lesion. Occurrence in the head and neck is distinctly rare other than in the nasal cavity.

The orbit may be involved primarily or by contiguity. When they occur in the orbit, fibrosarcomas tend to have a relatively short history measured in months. Although some may be circumscribed, they usually are infiltrative and insinuate themselves posteriorly, engulfing adjacent structures, and causing functional deficits. They may occur anywhere in the orbit and when primary in that site are more common in the elderly.

Microscopically, these neoplasms are made up of interwoven, fasciculated, densely packed, parallel, spindle cells. The degree of differentiation varies and correlates with both local aggressiveness and a tendency to metastases. Secondary histopathologic features may occur, such as osseous and cartilaginous metaplasia as well as mucoid deposition. These secondary features were more

(Text continues on p. 348.)

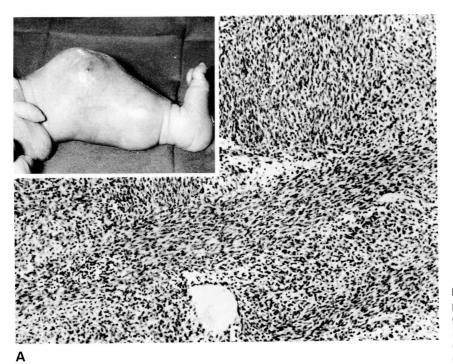

A

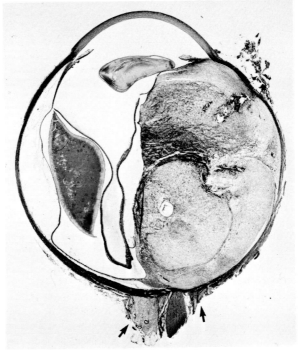

B

FIGURE 12-58. *(A)* Low-power photomicrograph of a primary congenital fibrosarcoma of the leg *(inset)* occurring at birth. Note the dense zones of interwoven bundles of spindle cells (H&E, original magnification × 10). *(B)* Gross specimen of globe enucleated 2 years after the primary tumor. There was a uveal metastasis with a temporal serous detachment and orbital extension of the tumor around the optic nerve *(arrows)* (H&E, original magnification × 4).

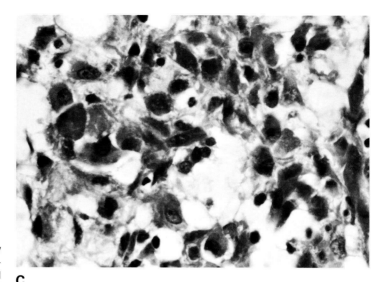

C

FIGURE 12-58 *(Continued).* *(C)* Histopathology of the ocular lesion showing an area of poorly differentiated cells with round, plump nuclei and abundant eosinophilic cytoplasm (H&E, original magnification × 100). *(D)* Low-power electron micrograph of the ocular metastasis, which had features identical to the original biopsy from the leg. The cells are spindle shaped and do not have basement membrane. Intracisternal and extracellular electron-dense deposits and extracellular fibrils *(arrow)* are present. The lack of basement membrane, presence of abundant rough endoplasmic reticulum, poorly developed desmosomes, and the electron-dense deposits suggest an immature fibroblastic origin. The patient is alive and well 7 years after exenteration (original magnification × 3000).

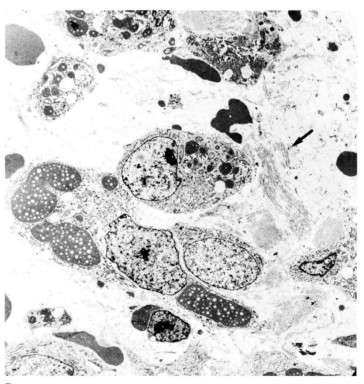

D

commonly reported in the older literature, and when present should invoke the possibility of a malignant fibrous histiocytoma rather then fibrosarcoma. Although the smaller tumors are grossly circumscribed, they often have satellite lesions accounting for recurrence after apparent total excision.

Fibrosarcomas are locally aggressive lesions. They are commonly incompletely removed and tend to be clinically more aggressive following recurrence. The greater the degree of differentiation, the slower the clinical development. In any site, 50% recurrence is not uncommon and can be greatly reduced by radical excision. Patients and surgeons both are less inclined to radical therapy when this lesion occurs in the orbit, making recurrence, extension, and metastases common. Exenteration or wide local excision with margins is the recommended therapy.

Postirradiation fibrosarcomas may arise in the soft tissues or bone of the orbit, particularly as second tumors in patients with the genomic mutation of retinoblastoma. In this circumstance, fibrosarcoma is second only to osteogenic sarcoma in incidence. These second tumors usually occur in patients who have been irradiated, but they may also appear *de novo* in this group. Postirradiation fibrosarcomas tend to be histologically more bizarre and aggressive.

CONGENITAL AND INFANTILE FIBROSARCOMA

Congenital and infantile fibrosarcoma is a rare, rapidly growing, usually congenital sarcoma with a low incidence of metastasis (0%–8%). Histologically, the tumor is composed of uniform spindle cells arranged in interwoven bundles and the more differentiated lesions show a characteristic herringbone pattern. Electron-microscopy has shown that the cells are embryonic fibroblasts that contain electron-dense material (Fig. 12-58). We have had a single case of a metastasis of a congenital fibrosarcoma to the globe with extension posteriorly into the orbit. Overall, these tumors have a considerably better prognosis than the adult counterpart, and treatment is by radical local excision.

MYXOMA

The diagnosis of myxoma in the orbit and elsewhere in the body is complicated by the large number of soft tissue tumors that can have a myxoid appearance. Malignant myxoid lesions must be ruled out, including malignant fibrous histiocytoma, liposarcoma, myxosarcoma, and rarely rhabdomyosarcoma or chondrosarcoma. Careful analysis of the entire specimen is necessary to substantiate this diagnosis. True orbital myxomas are exceed-

ingly rare, and the few that have been described have been characterized by a clinical picture of indolence and noninfiltrative features despite the lack of a true capsule. This probably reflects on the soft consistency of the tumor. Histologically, it is made up of a population of stellate or spindle cells dispersed in a rich mucinous matrix of hyaluronic acid derived from altered fibroblasts. At the time of surgery, these lesions are apparently indistinctly separated from adjacent tissues, which accounts for a significant risk of recurrence. All the reported cases have remained isolated to the orbit.

Histiocytic Tumors and Tumor-like Lesions

FIBROUS HISTIOCYTOMA

Fibrous histiocytomas are mesenchymal tumors that involve fascia, muscle, and soft tissues of the body. They were first well described in the 1960s, and the orbit was identified as site of predilection by Zimmerman in 1967. In fact, fibrous histiocytoma is the most common adult mesenchymal tumor of the orbit.

It is seen in middle adult life, with equal occurrence in males and females. The most common location is in the upper nasal quadrant of the orbit. The pathophysiology runs the gamut from rapidly growing, locally aggressive tumors to relatively benign mass effect. The major presenting clinical signs are proptosis, mass effect with decreased vision, and less frequently diplopia, pain, lid swelling, tearing, ptosis, and restriction of extraocular movements.

This neoplasm is usually characterized by infiltrative features with a tendency to local recurrence and very rare metastases. The specific biology parallels the underlying histopathology such that the slower growing, less bulky tumors reflect a benign variant and the fast growing, locally aggressive large tumors a malignant variant. Between the two is an intermediate group that is characterized primarily by locally aggressive behavior. Thus, duration of symptoms, size, frequency and rapidity of local recurrence, and tendency to metastatic or widespread local aggressive behavior parallels the underlying histopathologic characteristics.

These tumors are made up fundamentally of fibrous-appearing histiocytic cells that tend to form a characteristic cartwheel or storiform pattern. The benign type is the most common, and histologically is well circumscribed or has a fine capsule and is made up of benign-looking histiocytic cells with occasional well-differentiated multinucleated histiocytes (Fig. 12-59). Necrosis and mitoses are not major features. Within the benign group a more cellular subtype has been noted. The locally aggressive or intermediate fibrous histiocytoma is characterized by in-

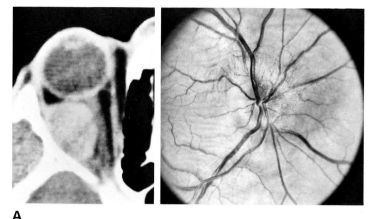

A

FIGURE 12-59. *(A)* CT scan and retinal photograph of a 38-year-old man who had a history of decreasing vision on the right side for 6 months. He had noted increasing prominence of the eye for 6 weeks. The vision was reduced to 20/70 and there was 5 mm of proptosis. The fundus demonstrates nasal choroidal folds and elevation of the superior margin of the disk. The axial CT scan shows a well-circumscribed homogeneous lateral orbital mass that displaces the optic nerve medially. *(B)* Low-power and high-power photomicrographs of the lesion shown in *A*. Note the characteristic cartwheel or storiform pattern of a fibrous histiocytoma. The patient is well with no recurrence 6 years after removal of the tumor. Diagnosis was confirmed with electron microscopy and on review by Ramon Font (H&E, original magnifications *top* × 10, *bottom* × 25).

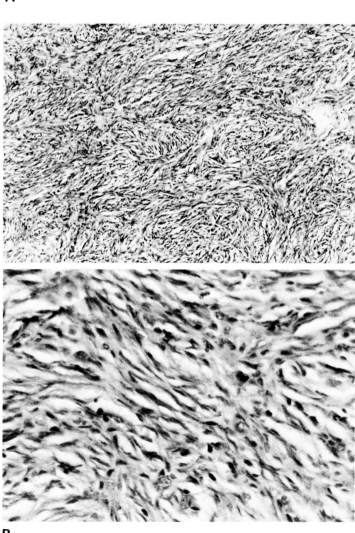

B

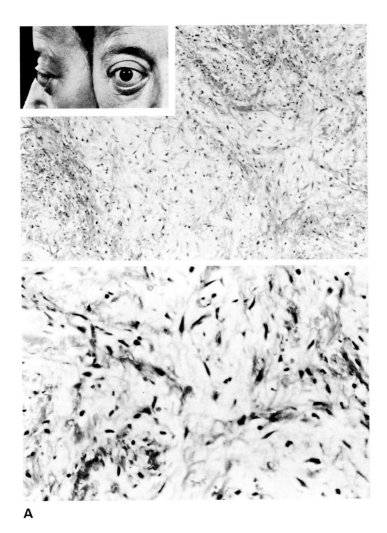

FIGURE 12-60. *(A)* An intermediate fibrous histiocytoma in a 38-year-old woman who presented with severe right proptosis. She underwent excisional biopsy of a rather loosely arranged intraconal vascular tumor. Histopathologically, it demonstrated a myxoid stroma with stellate fibrous histiocytic cells (H&E, original magnifications *top* × 10, *bottom* × 25).

A

creased cellularity without significant pleomorphism and an infiltrating margin. Mitotic figures are generally few and typical in appearance (Fig. 12-60). Both the benign and the intermediate group may have areas with myxoid patterns, and about one third of the tumors show marked vascularity. The least frequent variant is the malignant fibrous histiocytoma, which has the hallmarks of malignancy including necrosis, mitotic activity with abnormal mitoses, tumor giant cells, and pleomorphism (Figs. 12-61, 12-62). The cellular pattern may be either storiform, pleomorphic, or myxoid. Some of the cells may be vacuolated and contain fat, and the myxoid areas contain acid mucopolysaccharide sensitive to hyaluronidase.

The management of fibrous histiocytoma is essentially surgical and should be aimed at complete resection of local disease to prevent recurrence, because there is

some potential (particularly in the intermediate group) to undergo malignant transformation on repeat recurrence. Usually this can be accomplished by removal of the tumor alone. However, if there is widespread infiltration it may require more radical exenteration of tissues. The majority of tumors will fall into the benign and intermediate groups, and recurrences from the intermediate group tend to occur over relatively long periods of time. The management of recurrences should be governed by the biological behavior, that is, the more rapidly occurring should be treated more aggressively. Radiotherapy is of no benefit and chemotherapy has not been assessed.

The malignant fibrous histiocytoma in the orbit usually arises *de novo*. However, there is a group of malignant fibrous histiocytomas that tend to occur following orbital radiotherapy, particularly in children, with the

FIGURE 12-60 *(Continued)*. *(B)* Axial noncontrast *(top, right)* and contrast-enhanced *(top, left)* CT scans show an isodense, uniformly enhancing, sharply demarcated retrobulbar mass molding to the shape of the globe, sparing the apex, and herniating through the previous lateral orbitotomy defect. Ultrasonography *(inset)* reveals a somewhat irregular mass directly behind the globe with marked sound wave attenuation. Diagnosis of a locally aggressive myxoid fibrous histiocytoma was confirmed by electron microscopy *(bottom)* and on review by Ramon Font (H&E, original magnifications × 2.5 *left,* × 10 *right*).

B

genomic mutation of retinoblastoma. We have seen two cases of malignant fibrous histiocytoma, both following radiotherapy in the orbital region. One was in a child with retinoblastoma (see Fig. 12-61), and the other was in an adult who had been previously treated for lymphoma of the head and neck by radiotherapy and chemotherapy (see Fig. 12-62). In addition to the usual sites of orbital occurrence, fibrous histiocytoma has been described in the lacrimal sac, and we have seen a single case originating in the lacrimal gland (Fig. 12-63). This was an unusual, low-grade, spindle cell sarcoma that had developed over a long period of time. Histologically, it had some of the features of a fibrous histiocytoma but was not absolutely diagnostic for it. The differential diagnosis was fibrous histiocytoma, low-grade angiosarcoma, fibrosarcoma, and hemangiopericytoma.

JUVENILE XANTHOGRANULOMA

The histogenesis of juvenile xanthogranuloma is debatable, with some favoring true neoplasm and others an unusual reactive process. The basic cell resembles a histiocyte, and it has been suggested that this is a regressing fibrous histiocytoma of infancy. The most common manifestation is cutaneous nodules in the head and neck region of infants. The usual ocular presentation is iris lesions and spontaneous hyphema. Visceral involvement is rare. Few cases of orbital involvement have been described. The histopathology is characteristic with presence of multinucleated Touton giant cells in a background of histiocytes, lymphocytes, plasma cells, and eosinophils. This lesion characteristically responds to

(Text continues on p. 354.)

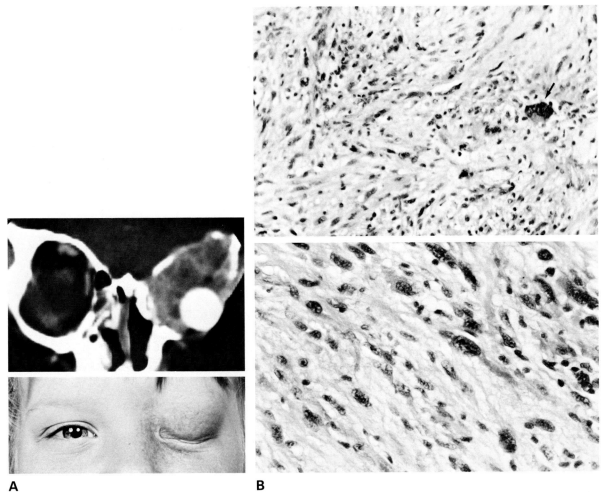

A   **B**

FIGURE 12-61. *(A)* A 6-year-old boy presented with progressive displacement of the implant in his anophthalmic left orbit. He had been treated 3 years earlier for a retinoblastoma with extrascleral extension by enucleation and postoperative radiotherapy. Coronal CT scan demonstrates a large infiltrating soft tissue mass in the posterior, superior, and medial portion of the orbit with displacement of the prosthesis. Permeative destruction of the orbital roof and medial and lateral orbital walls was present. *(B)* Histopathology of the biopsy taken from the patient shown in *A*. There is a highly anaplastic spindle cell tumor with some multinucleate cells and considerable pleomorphism. The cytoplasm of the histiocytic cells is slightly foamy. The final diagnosis was a malignant fibrous histiocytoma (H&E, original magnifications *top* × 10, *bottom* × 100).

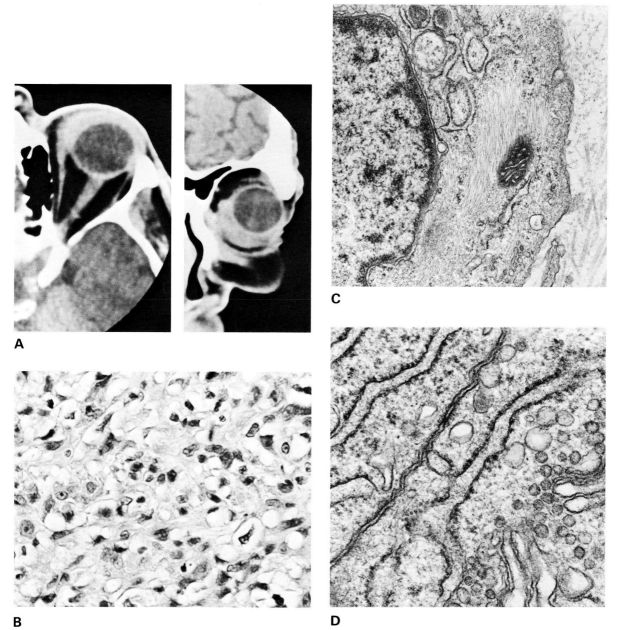

FIGURE 12-62. *(A)* Axial and coronal CT scans of a left orbit demonstrate a well-defined soft tissue mass on the anterior, inferior, and medial portion of the globe extending into the medial rectus and inferior rectus muscles. The patient was a 64-year-old farmer who had been aware of increasing left ocular irritation and a "growth" on the sclera. He had been treated 5 years earlier with chemotherapy and prophylactic central nervous system irradiation for a diffuse, poorly differentiated lymphocytic lymphoma involving the cervical nodes, pleura, and lung. *(B)* Biopsy revealed a malignant spindle-cell soft tissue tumor. Note the sworling arrangement of anaplastic cells in a collagen matrix. The cytoplasm of the fibrous histiocytes is slightly foamy (H&E, original magnification × 40). *(C)* Electron micrograph demonstrates intracytoplasmic filaments consistent with procollagen as well as some adjacent stromal collagen (H&E, original magnification × 43,200). *(D)* Electron micrograph demonstrates interdigitating spindle cells without basement membrane and few intracytoplasmic organelles. The histopathologic and electron microscopic features are consistent with the diagnosis of malignant fibrous histiocytoma (original magnification × 94,000).

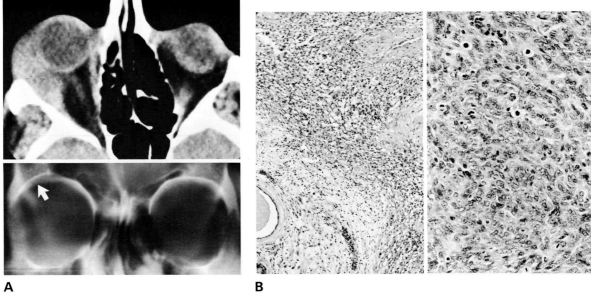

A   **B**

FIGURE 12-63. *(A)* Axial CT scan demonstrates a large right lacrimal gland mass with adjacent excavation of bone confirmed on tomography *(arrow)*. It occurred in a 47-year-old man who had a long-standing history of a lacrimal mass. *(B)* Excisional biopsy of the mass revealed a spindle-cell tumor infiltrating the lacrimal gland. The mass proved to have some of the immunohistochemical and electron microscopic features consistent with the diagnosis of fibrous histiocytoma. The overall differential diagnosis includes a low-grade angiosarcoma, fibrosarcoma, and hemangiopericytoma (H&E, original magnifications *left* × 10, *right* × 25).

systemic steroids, although occasionally adjunctive radiotherapy is necessary.

Orbital Tumors Originating in Bone

Jack Rootman, Ewan Kemp, and Jocelyn S. Lapointe

Tumors whose apparent site of origin is orbital bone are quite rare, constituting between 0.6% and 2% of lesions in this site. In our own series, 30% of orbital neoplasms involved bone and 12% of these originated from bone. Overall, 2% of all the orbital lesions we saw originated in bone. However, when viewed in the broadest context, neoplastic, structural, and inflammatory lesions involving bone constituted 9.8% of all orbital disease in our series. Table 12-7 summarizes the incidence and character of both primary and secondary orbital lesions seen in the University of British Columbia Orbital Clinic and provides a contextual framework for differential diagnosis.

Primary tumors of bone are difficult to categorize because considerable controversy exists concerning nosology and definition. Yet from a clinical viewpoint, they appear to have fundamental patterns of presentation and

CT findings that suggest origin in the bone. Probably the most characteristic clinical feature of lesions that originate in bone and affect the orbit is their propensity to cause nonaxial displacement and to affect adjacent facial structures.

In analyzing our experience, three clinical patterns emerge, all of which are dominated by mass effect. The first is a slowly progressive, noninfiltrative mass effect with proptosis, nonaxial displacement, and dystopia frequently associated with facial disfigurement. This pattern was due to benign and slow-growing noninfiltrative lesions originating in bone, such as fibrous dysplasia, osteoma, and low-grade chondrosarcoma. The second pattern is one of sudden, occasionally catastrophic orbital soft tissue displacement usually reflecting hemorrhage within a dysplastic or reparative lesion. Tumefactions in this category include reparative granuloma, aneurysmal bone cyst, reactive xanthomatous lesions, and brown tumor of hyperparathyroidism. Finally, there are lesions characterized by relentless progression (over months) of mass effect with infiltrative features (*i.e.,* sensory change, optic neuropathy, and restrictive myopathy) reflecting soft tissue entrapment. This is brought about by aggressive neoplasia like osteogenic sarcoma, Ewing's sarcoma, malignant fibrous histiocytoma, histiocytosis-X, lym-

TABLE 12-7.
NEOPLASTIC, STRUCTURAL, AND INFLAMMATORY LESIONS OF BONE, UNIVERSITY OF BRITISH COLUMBIA ORBITAL CLINIC, 1976–1986

Tumor Type	Number of Lesions	Total
Bone tumors		31
Fibrous dysplasia	9	
Osteoma — ossifying fibroma	5	
Reparative granuloma and aneurysmal bone cyst	3	
Reactive xanthomatous lesion	2	
Brown tumor of hyperparathyroidism	1	
Histiocytosis-X	3	
Lymphoma	2	
Plasmacytoma	2	
Ewing's sarcoma	2	
Osteogenic sarcoma	1	
Malignant fibrous histiocytoma	1	
Metastatic and secondary tumors of orbital bones		
Metastatic		9
Breast	2	
Prostate	2	
Unknown	2	
GI	1	
Thyroid	1	
Neuroblastoma	1	
From sinus		26
Epithelial	20	
Melanoma	1	
Malignant schwannoma	2	
Rhabdomyosarcoma	1	
Lymphoma	1	
Neurofibroma	1	
Intracranial		15
Sphenoid wing meningioma	15	
Structural lesions of bone		51
Dermoid cysts	27	
Mucoceles	24	
Inflammatory lesions with bone destruction		9
Chronic sinusitis	7	
Wegener's granulomatosis	2	
Total for all lesions of bone		141

phoma, and plasmacytoma. Although our series does not include all of the possible bony lesions of the orbit, these three clinical patterns incorporate the potential primary tumors.

From another perspective, the bony lesions can be defined along pathophysiologic lines as dysplastic, reactive, and neoplastic. This simplification allows characterization of each clinically and pathologically. The dysplasias and related fibro-osseous tumefactions include fibrous dysplasia, osteoma, ossifying fibroma, and osteoblastoma, all of which are associated with slowly developing noninfiltrative mass effect with or without facial disfigurement or orbital dystopia. The reactive lesions,

on the other hand, include a group of entities with similar behavior and some shared histologic features reflecting their tendency to sudden hemorrhagic episodes. Although several are difficult to define histopathologically, they bear sufficient similarity to blur distinctions between them. They affect adjacent bone and soft tissue structures primarily by displacement. Their major difference from dysplastic lesions is their tendency toward erosion of adjacent bone, loose vascularity, hemorrhage, and local recurrence in some instances. The reactive lesions in our series included reparative granuloma, aneurysmal bone cyst, brown tumor of hyperparathyroidism, and xanthomatous tumor. In spite of their tendency to involve adjacent bone, all of these displace rather than infiltrate soft tissues; this feature provides a major distinction from the more aggressive malignant lesions.

The neoplasms include many primary tumors, which fall into two broad clinical groups. Both categories produce unrelenting, progressive mass effect; the major difference is the presence or absence of infiltrative features reflecting biologically more aggressive tumor growth. Neoplasms such as chondrosarcoma and chordoma may be extremely slow growing and noninfiltrative. On the other hand, the more aggressive tumors such as Ewing's sarcoma, malignant fibrous histiocytoma, osteogenic sarcoma, lymphoma, plasmacytoma, and histiocytosis-X characteristically infiltrate surrounding soft tissue structures, producing restrictive and compressive effects.

The primary tumors must be distinguished from secondary lesions of bone. These include structural tumefactions like dermoid cysts and mucoceles, neoplasms such as meningiomas, tumors of the sinuses, and metastases deposited in and extending from bone (see Table 12-7). In addition, certain inflammatory lesions like Wegener's granulomatosis characteristically involve bony structures and encroach on the orbital soft tissues.

The primary infiltrative neoplasms are most difficult to differentiate from secondary and metastatic tumors involving bone. We have seen nine metastases to orbital bone from a total of 29 orbital metastases. All were characterized by a significant infiltrative effect. However, a particular subgroup that can be readily distinguished is the cicatrizing orbital metastases. In contrast to primary tumors of bone, the cicatrizing metastases lead to enophthalmos rather than proptosis. In addition, the noncalcifying soft tissue component helps to differentiate metastases from primary tumors of bone, which more often have foci of calcification.

Epithelial malignancies originating from the sinuses can also be distinguished on clinical grounds by their propensity to arise in the maxillary sinus and involve adjacent sensory structures leading to infraorbital paresthesia and pain. Radiologically, the major noncalcifying soft tissue component of these lesions lies within the sinuses and erodes through bone rather than having an epicenter within bone. Nevertheless, in some instances it may be impossible to distinguish these prior to biopsy.

Another important secondary neoplasm affecting the orbital bones is the sphenoid wing meningioma. This tumor often leads to hyperostosis and expansion of the paraorbital bones. Radiologically and clinically, it may be difficult to distinguish from fibrous dysplasia. However, it is the typical enhancing en plaque soft tissue component that allows differentiation. From a clinical point of view, orbital dystopia, nonaxial displacement, and major facial deformity are less frequently features of meningioma. Meningiomas are also more likely to compress the superior orbital fissure, leading to soft tissue swelling from venous obstruction. Also, fibrous dysplasia is more often a disease of childhood in contrast to the midlife occurrence of meningioma.

The structural lesions of bone, such as dermoid cysts and mucoceles, are readily distinguished from the primary bone tumors in most instances because of their cystic nature, fat density in the case of dermoid cysts, and sinus involvement in the case of mucoceles. In addition, mucoceles tend to have very well-defined margins and on ultrasonography are characteristically echolucent. Chronic sinusitis with bone destruction and Wegener's granulomatosis both have overriding features of inflammatory character and systemic associations that distinguish them from neoplasms. Nevertheless, there may be circumstances in which absolute differentiation is impossible without biopsy.

From a pathologic point of view, we were struck by the similarities between many of the primary bone tumors rather than clear-cut differences, particularly the groups we have classified as dysplasias and reactive tumefactions. Fibrous dysplasia, for example, is defined histologically as foci of osteoid and immature woven bone formation within a fibrous mesodermal matrix. Yet variations in the classical pattern are common, including some osteoblastic rimming, psammomatoid features, foci reflecting recurrent hemorrhage, fibroproliferation, and reparative phenomena. Similarly, reparative granuloma and solid aneurysmal bone cyst are dominated by reactive fibroplasia with an admixture of giant cells and features of recurrent hemorrhage. But these lesions are often associated with dysplastic bone formation and in some respects reflect features just described in fibrous dysplasia. Osteomas also appear to have a spectrum of pathologic findings that relate to fibrous dysplasia. Classically, they are described as solid tumors with compact or cancellous bone formation. However, within osteomas areas of osteoid, dysgenetic bone, mesodermal fibroplasia, giant cells, and even psammomatoid change may be noted. In many respects, the distinction between the dysplasias, osteomas, and reactive lesions may be difficult, and numerous authors have suggested they may be part of a spectrum of dysplastic bone formation. Certainly, the reactive and dysplastic lesions as defined in our series have a fundamental biologic difference from neoplasia; that is, their tendency to remain isolated to bone and not infiltrate soft tissue structures.

In summary, the major clinical features of lesions originating in bone and affecting the orbit are slow expansion with displacement of orbital structures and associated facial deformity with dystopia (dysplasias and noninfiltrative tumors), sudden orbital displacement (reactive lesions), or orbital displacement with infiltrative features (aggressive neoplasia).

DYSPLASIAS AND RELATED FIBRO-OSSEOUS LESIONS

Fibrous Dysplasia

Fibrous dysplasia is a benign disorder of indeterminate nature characterized by replacement of normal bone with immature bone and osteoid in a cellular fibrous matrix. This condition can be monostotic (single site) or polyostotic (multiple sites). The polyostotic form may be associated with endocrine abnormalities and cutaneous pigmentation as part of Albright's syndrome. The overwhelming majority of cases involving the orbit are monostotic, but may transgress local boundaries and involve several bones of the skull. Fibrous dysplasia is a disease of childhood and young adult life. It is frequently progressive but is thought to be self-limited with a variable end point in the second and third decades. It is important to differentiate it from more aggressive disorders such as meningioma and osteosarcoma. Of 33 bone tumors seen in our clinic, nine were fibrous dysplasia.

The major clinical signs and symptoms reflect displacement, distortion, and compression of orbital and facial structures. The frontal bone is most commonly involved in the orbital region, leading to dystopia and proptosis (Fig. 12-64). Dysplasia of the anterior ethmoid and maxillary region causes lateral or upward displacement, and posterior ethmoid or sphenoid involvement may lead to narrowing of the optic canal. Progressive stricture of the optic canal can cause compressive optic neuropathy but this is not always the case, even in the presence of anatomic narrowing. Involvement of the sella may affect the chiasm. Additional problems include cranial nerve palsies, trigeminal neuralgia, and raised intracranial pressure.

In our experience, the major clinical features of fibrous dysplasia were changes in facial contour (7), pain (7), proptosis (7), and horizontal or vertical displacement (6). The pain is either localized to the orbit or described as a diffuse headache on the ipsilateral side. Involvement of the maxilla and nasolacrimal system may lead to epiphora (Fig.12-65). Three of our cases had reduced visual acuity

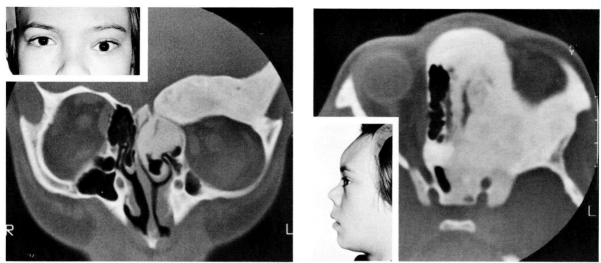

FIGURE 12-64.   This 13-year-old boy presented with downward displacement of the left globe. It had been noted for 1 year but had increased during the last month. His vision was 20/20 on the left side, and psychophysical and electrophysiologic functions were within normal limits. There is orbital dystopia and frontal bossing. Coronal and axial CT scans demonstrate fibrous dysplasia involving the frontal ethmoid complex of bones. Axial view shows the posterior end of the left optic canal, which appears of normal size. Follow-up examination after 18 months of observation revealed no progression of visual or physical deficit.

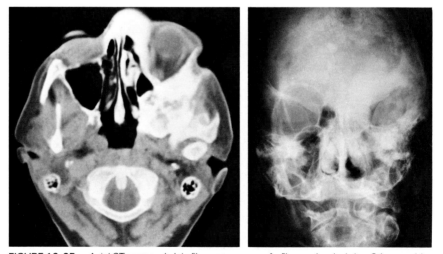

FIGURE 12-65.   Axial CT scan and plain film appearance of a fibrous dysplasia in a 34-year-old woman with known disease for 7 years. She had undergone previous maxillectomy and had suffered with epiphora and recurrent dacryocystitis. Ocular functions were entirely normal. CT scan demonstrates (residual) maxillary, mandibular, and ethmoid involvement. X-ray shows the typical ground-glass appearance of fibrous dysplasia with resulting distortion and decreased size of the orbit. Follow-up studies over a 7-year period have demonstrated no progression of the disease, but persistent pain has plagued the patient. She underwent left external ethmoidectomy and Jones tube insertion to cure the epiphora.

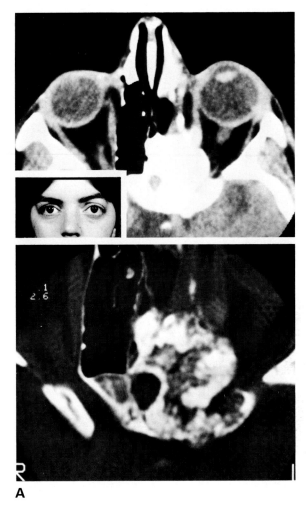

A

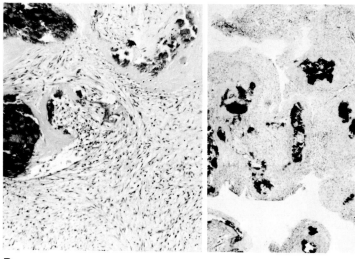

B

FIGURE 12-66. *(A)* Clinical photograph *(inset)* shows a 19-year-old woman who presented with outward displacement of the left globe in 1977. Onset was over a 2-week period, by history, and ocular function was normal. X-rays and CT scans done at that time (not shown) demonstrated involvement of the ethmoid sinus by an irregular, diffuse, inhomogeneous bony lesion. She underwent external ethmoidectomy and debulking, and was found to have fibrous dysplasia and a chronic sinusitis, which was drained. Over the next 6 years, her disease progressed, and she had debulking procedures on two separate occasions. Axial CT scans on standard and bone settings show the nodular inhomogeneous (pagetoid) appearance in 1983. At that time, she presented with a 2-month history of reduced visual acuity that occurred in the latter months of pregnancy, 9 years after the initial diagnosis. Her vision was 20/200, and she had slight temporal pallor on the left side. She underwent combined craniotomy–orbitotomy and radical removal of the dysplastic bone affecting the ethmoids, sphenoids, and optic canal, which led to improvement of vision to 20/60. She has remained stable for 3 years. *(B)* The histopathology of this lesion shows immature, woven, partially calcified bone within a fibrous matrix with absence of osteoblasts (H&E, original magnification × 10 *left,* × 2.5 *right*).

on presentation to 6/24, 6/36, and 6/60, respectively. Surgical decompression of the apex of the orbit or optic canal have improved two of these to 6/9 or better. The third has only improved from 6/60 to 6/18, as irreversible compressive optic neuropathy had already been established (Fig. 12-66). In the 2 months prior to presentation, this patient had noted reduction of visual acuity in the latter months of pregnancy 9 years after initial diagnosis. Previously, the patient had undergone several debulking procedures for ethmoidal involvement, but relentless progression of the dysplastic process led to encroachment on the optic canal and compressive optic neuropathy. She underwent combined craniotomy–orbitotomy to remove the dysplastic bone affecting the ethmoids, sphenoids, and optic canal. Another patient with acute reduction of vision developed a sudden hemorrhage within a cystic cavitation of fibrous dysplasia causing downward displacement and compression of the globe (Fig. 12-67). She underwent orbitotomy and evacuation of the cyst lining and contents with full recovery of acuity. The remaining patient with optic neuropathy had a lesion of the frontal, ethmoid, maxillary, and sphenoid bones (Fig. 12-68). The ethmoid and maxillary component had caused a compressive neuropathy which was successfully treated by anterior orbitotomy and resection of the offending lesion. On investigation he was found to have polyostotic disease with involvement of the ribs and femur.

The main radiographic features of fibrous dysplasia are expansion of bone with two basic patterns. About half of the cases have a sclerotic, homogeneous, dense, ground-glass appearance. The remainder may show alternate areas of lucency and increased density (pagetoid lesion). Although the dysplasias in this region are mainly unilateral, they may cross the midline and they do not respect suture lines. Some of the lytic areas within the dysplasia may contain fluid and debris, producing a linear interface (see Fig. 12-67A). The radiologic differential diagnosis includes hyperostotic meningiomas, Paget's disease, histiocytosis-X, and a number of bony tumors.

The extent and distribution of orbital wall involvement is variable. It is, however, worthy of note that eight of our nine cases had involvement of midline structures, seven affected the sphenoid bone, six affected the ethmoid, and five had a frontal component. Only three of our cases affected a single bone; one, the sphenoid (Fig. 12-69), one frontal, and one ethmoid. In all instances, even when a single bony region was involved, the lesion appeared to transgress suture lines and had irregular borders.

Pathologically, the tissue is composed of spicules of immature woven bone and osteoid within a matrix of cellular fibrous stroma (see Fig. 12-66B). The bone is lined by fibrous spindle cells rather than osteoblasts, reflecting an arrest in bone maturation. There may, however, be areas of osteoblastic bone formation, psammomatoid change, and reactive components with features of recurrent hemorrhage in addition to the typical fibrous dysplasia (see Fig. 12-67B).

Management is directed towards curing the facial deformity and preventing ocular and optic nerve complications. The recommended modality is surgery because radiotherapy may induce malignant degeneration, although this can very rarely occur without radiotherapy. Malignant degeneration (usually to osteogenic sarcomas) is said to occur in 0.5% to 1% of all cases of fibrous dysplasia, but fibrosarcomas, chondrosarcomas, or mixtures have been reported. Surgical management has consisted of debulking the lesion, because accurate definition of borders for resection has been difficult and reconstructive procedures unavailable. Some fibrous dysplasias may be highly vascular and extremely hemorrhagic at the time of surgery; thus, preoperative cross matching is advised. Recently, craniofacial surgical teams have developed more aggressive and earlier treatment approaches that include immediate orbital and cranial reconstruction. Moore and co-workers reported that 10 of 16 cases had a good cosmetic result on follow up more than 1 year after craniofacial surgery. In most circumstances, total excision is impossible and repeat surgical procedures may be necessary, but the goal remains to remove as much affected bone as possible and anticipate spontaneous arrest. When the bones surrounding the optic canal are involved and there is progressive visual loss, resection of the dysplasia can reverse or arrest the progression of visual deficit, but carries a risk of surgically induced visual loss.

Osteoid Osteoma, Ossifying Fibroma, and Osteoblastoma

Osteoid osteoma, ossifying fibroma, and osteoblastoma probably represent a spectrum of clinically and pathologically similar fibro-osseous lesions. Differences are based on degree of maturation of bone and size of lesions.

Osteoma

Osteomas represent 1% to 2% of orbital tumors, are benign, and arise within the sinuses. The order of incidence is frontal, ethmoid, maxillary, and sphenoid with the large majority occurring in the frontoethmoid complex. Male predominance has been noted in most series, and they are usually symptomatic in the second to fifth decades of life.

There are three theories of origin: developmental, traumatic, and infectious. The developmental theory suggests that they arise at sites of fusion of membranous and cartilaginous bone. The traumatic and infectious theories are based on a clinically high incidence of stated trauma and associated sinus infection. No single theory appears to explain all features of osteoma.

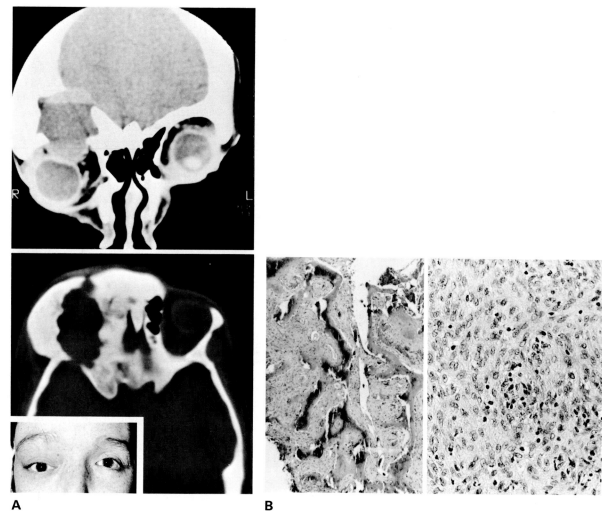

A

B

FIGURE 12-67. *(A)* This 24-year-old woman with cavitary fibrous dysplasia presented with a 1-month history of right proptosis, visual blurring, and pain following a whiplash injury. Crouzon's disease had been diagnosed 12 years prior to presentation, and she stated that the right side had been abnormal since birth. Vision was 20/60 on the right, with downward and outward displacement of the globe and limitation of upgaze. VEP was delayed because of the optic nerve compression. Coronal and axial CT scans show fibrous dysplasia involving an extensive portion of the frontal and ethmoid bones. In the center of the dysplasia was a large cyst that shows a fluid interface in the coronal scan and indentation of the globe by the portion extending into the orbit. The coronal scans were obtained with a "hanging head" position, so the denser dependent blood appears superior on the image. The axial image is photographed to maximize bone detail. The clinical diagnosis was fibrous dysplasia with "aneurysmal bone cyst." The patient underwent surgical drainage of xanthochromic fluid and debris in the cyst, with removal of the lining and immediately adjacent bone. Her vision returned to 20/20, and there was no recurrence at 6-month follow-up examination. *(B)* Histopathology of the lesion removed from the patient shown in *A*. The lining of the cyst consisted of a reactive fibrous component shown on the right. The margins of the lesions were dysplastic bone *(left)* (H&E, original magnifications × 2.5 *left,* × 25 *right*).

FIGURE 12-68. This 20-year-old man presented with a 4-month history of proptosis and 8 months of reduced vision on the left side. On physical examination, his vision was 20/60, he had left papilledema with a full range of ocular movements, elevation of the left globe, and proptosis. Psychophysical and electrophysiologic functions revealed a field reduction and a delayed VEP. Retrospective study of photographs showed that changes had been present for at least 5 years. The coronal CT scan photographed on bone settings demonstrates both basic patterns of fibrous dysplasia with areas of lucency and sclerosis (pagetoid lesion) involving the maxilla and lesser wing of sphenoid and the ground-glass sclerotic pattern affecting the greater wing of sphenoid. These changes have resulted in compression of the apex of the orbit. The patient underwent an orbitotomy and maxillectomy to decompress the orbital apex. His vision had returned to 20/20, and the papilledema had disappeared without recurrence when he was seen at 18-month follow-up examination. Systemic investigation revealed fibrous dysplasia involving the rib cage and femur, but normal endocrine function.

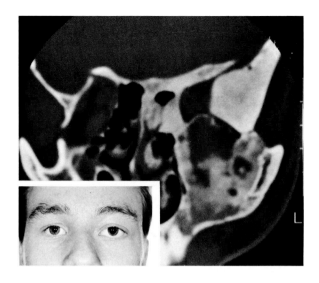

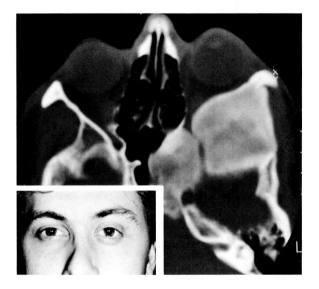

FIGURE 12-69. A 24-year-old man presented with an 8-month history of vague aches in the left temporal region. On physical examination, he had completely normal ocular functions with fullness of the left temporalis fossa and proptosis. Retrospective photographic documentation revealed proptosis of 4 years' duration. Axial CT scan on bone settings demonstrates the sclerotic type of fibrous dysplasia involving primarily the sphenoid bone and sinus. No progression was seen at 1-year follow-up examination.

These slow-growing masses produce symptoms on the basis of sinus obstruction and intracranial or intraorbital extension. The symptoms of sinus obstruction are pain and recurrent sinusitis. Rhinorrhea may occur with significant ethmoidal or maxillary involvement. In the past, intracranial extension was associated with a risk of infection and abscess formation, a rare occurrence in a modern setting.

The most common orbital symptoms are proptosis and displacement, particularly downward and outward. When anteriorly located, a palpable mass may be noted; when posteriorly located, a visual deficit, papilledema, pain on extraocular movement, and amaurosis have been described. In our series of five cases, all had proptosis, two had vertical or horizontal displacement, four had pain, and two had changes in facial contour. One of our patients had painless proptosis with subluxation of the globe on manipulation of the lids due to a large osteoma of the ethmoid sinus extending into the orbit (Fig. 12-70). Another case involving the ethmoid had painful proptosis with secondary opacification and obstruction of the frontal sinus due to interruption of the normal frontoethmoid drainage. This patient also had reduced acuity, which improved to normal levels after resection

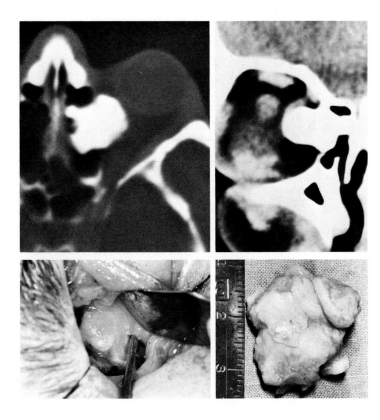

FIGURE 12-70. Axial and coronal CT scans *(top)* show a compact (ivory) osteoma involving the left ethmoid sinus (axial scan reversed) and extending into the orbit with displacement of the medial rectus muscle. This 23-year-old man had suffered two episodes of subluxation of the globe in a 12-month period. Ocular function was within normal limits aside from proptosis and lateral displacement. He underwent an anterior orbitotomy with excision of a well-defined bosselated osteoma (operative and surgical specimen photographs, *bottom*), and has had normal follow-up examinations over a 2-year period.

of the lesion (Fig. 12-71). The three remaining osteomas in our series were in the frontal sinus. One presented with ptosis and supraorbital paresthesia due to a secondary mucocele extending into the orbit from the lateral portion of the frontal sinus (Fig. 12-72). Another had acute orbital cellulitis and a history of recurrent sinusitis. The final frontal osteoma was in a patient who presented with proptosis and medial displacement of the globe (Fig. 12-73). Osteomas may be associated with multiple polyposis of the bowel (Gardner's syndrome: osteomata, cutaneous cysts, and fibromatosis). One of our patients had this syndrome with an additional small osteoma of the skull noted on CT scan.

Radiologically, osteomas are well-defined, round to oval, sometimes bossilated, densely sclerotic, solitary masses that can occlude the frontal or ethmoid sinus and may project into the orbit (3/5). On bone settings of CT scans, areas of lesser density may be noted centrally in the lesion. It is important to look for sinus opacification, mucocele formation, or intracranial extension to determine the extent, local effects, and most appropriate therapeutic approach.

Pathologically, these tumors are multilobulated, ivory-colored masses covered with a fine membranous lining originating from the sinuses. Three microscopic variants have been described: ivory, mature, and fibrous. Ivory osteomas consist of dense bone and a hypocellular fibrous stroma (see Fig. 12-73B), whereas the mature osteoma is made up of narrower lamellae and more cellular stroma (see Fig. 12-71C). The fibrous osteoma has osteoblasts surrounding the lamellar trabeculae of bone and a rich cellular fibrous stroma (Fig. 12-74). This form may bridge the histologic gap between the osteoblastoma, ossifying fibroma, and fibrous dysplasia.

Treatment is surgical and is indicated on the basis of symptoms, extension, or associated infection. The route is governed by the location of the tumor delineated preoperatively. Anterior localized masses can be removed by a direct percutaneous route or by a coronal flap. Evidence of intracranial extension necessitates a transfrontal or combined approach. In either instance, a multidisciplinary team is necessary. The tumor mass may be sessile or pedunculated. There is usually a plane of cleavage between normal bone and that of the osteoma allowing for separation by chiselling, drilling, and rocking. In difficult circumstances, the core of the lesion may be evacuated using high-speed drills and the wall may be collapsed and removed piecemeal. Associated sinus infection or mucocele formation requires resection of the affected mucosa and reestablishment of drainage.

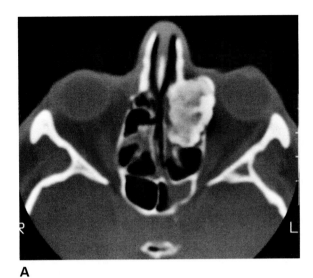

A

FIGURE 12-71. *(A)* The CT appearance of a mass in the anterior ethmoid complex in a 32-year-old man who presented with a history of 3 months of painful left proptosis. In retrospect, the proptosis had been noted for 10 years. Vision was 20/70 OS and the remaining ocular functions were normal. The mass shown on bone settings had a dense cortex with a more lucent central component. The patient underwent ethmoidectomy for removal of the tumor affecting the anterior ethmoids and frontoethmoid canal. The mass was removed piecemeal by coring the central portion out and collapsing the walls. *(B)* The histopathology of the dense portion of this osteoma shows thick bone with a haversian system and a more fibrous trabecular core (H&E, original magnification × 2.5). *(C)* A portion of the mass with a more trabecular appearance and a vascular stromal component is shown *(left)*. Note osteoblasts lining the bony trabeculae (H&E, original magnifications × 2.5 *left,* × 10 *right*).

B

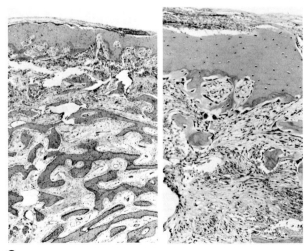

C

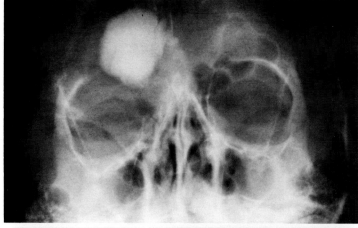

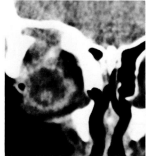
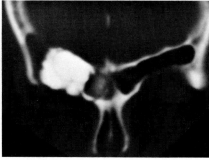

FIGURE 12-72. Plain film appearance *(top)* of a large ivory osteoma involving the medial portion of the right frontal sinus and ethmoids. This 68-year-old man presented with a 5-month history of right ptosis and paresthesia of the frontal region. In retrospect, he had always noted a drooping right upper lid. On physical examination he had slight restriction of upgaze and 5 mm downward displacement of the globe. Coronal CT scan *(bottom right)* shows a dense, bony lesion in the medial portion of the right frontal sinus with a soft tissue mass expanding the lateral portion of the sinus and extending into the orbit through a bony defect *(bottom left)*. The osteoma had a bosselated appearance. The mucocele and osteoma were excised by a right frontoethmoidectomy route. He has had an uneventful recovery with a 2-year follow-up.

Ossifying Fibroma (Fibro-osseous Dysplasia)

The clinical and histopathologic distinction of ossifying fibroma, a rare tumor, from other fibro-osseous lesions (in particular, from fibrous dysplasia) may be difficult. Some authors believe it is a variant of fibrous dysplasia or of osteoblastoma. Sufficient number of cases have been collected to suggest it is a distinct entity. It is believed to be a true benign neoplasm that most commonly occurs in the second and third decades of life, with a female preponderance. The pattern of growth is one of a slowly progressive, localized mass leading to displacement of orbital structures. Radiologically, it is a monostotic lesion with a homogeneous central matrix (which may be patchy), has a distinct sclerotic thin margin, and expands adjacent bone.

The major histologic features are a cellular, whorled, frequently vascular stroma that may contain lamellar bone with a rim of osteoid and osteoblasts. These bony spicules may resemble psammoma bodies (in the psammomatoid variant) leading to the differential diagnosis of a psammomatous meningioma.

The major differential diagnosis is fibrous dysplasia, but additional lesions include giant cell tumor of bone,

osteoblastoma, aneurysmal bone cyst, reparative granuloma, blistering meningioma, and intradiploic dermoid. In contrast to ossifying fibroma, fibrous dysplasia is most often discovered in the first decade of life, has no sex predilection, and frequently involves more than one bone of the skull with a slowly progressive irregular lesion. Radiologically, it has a ground-glass appearance with indistinct margins. Histologically, the major components reflect an arrest in bone maturation with fibro-osseous metaplasia. The immature woven bone of fibrous dysplasia is not surrounded by osteoblasts as it is in ossifying fibroma. The differences between fibrous dysplasia and ossifying fibroma have been summarized by Khalil and are listed in Table 12-8.

Because of its slow biologic growth and distinct margins, ossifying fibroma can be excised completely with a very low rate of local recurrence. In contrast, the lack of distinct margins and the slowly progressive biology of fibrous dysplasia make complete surgical excision frequently impossible.

Margo and co-workers have emphasized that the psammomatoid variant of ossifying fibroma is often misdiagnosed as fibrous dysplasia and is characterized by more aggressive local behavior. Psammomatoid ossifying

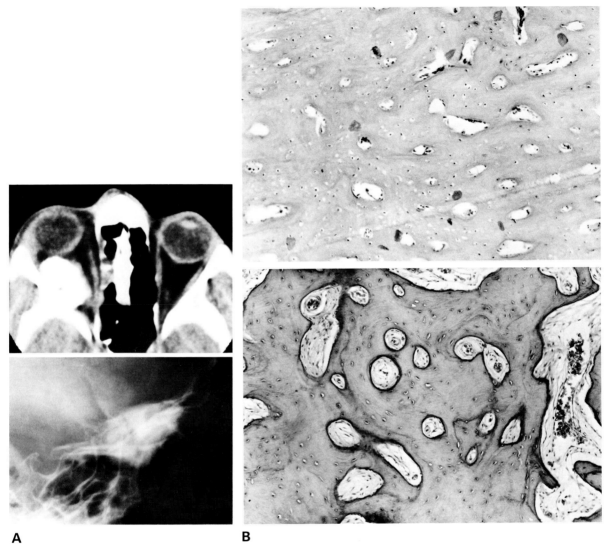

A   **B**

FIGURE 12-73. *(A)* Lateral plain film and axial CT scan of an osteoma originating in the posterolateral orbit and the posterior edge of the frontal sinus. This 17-year-old man presented with a 1-year history of right proptosis and swelling of the lid. Lateral gaze was slightly restricted. He underwent orbitotomy by coronal incision in anticipation of possible craniotomy because of the involvement of the orbital roof. A bosselated bony mass was completely excised intact. A 3-year follow-up has revealed no recurrence. *(B)* These photomicrographs demonstrate an ivory osteoma consisting of dense bone and a hypocellular fibrous stroma (H&E, original magnifications × 10 *top,* × 25 *bottom*).

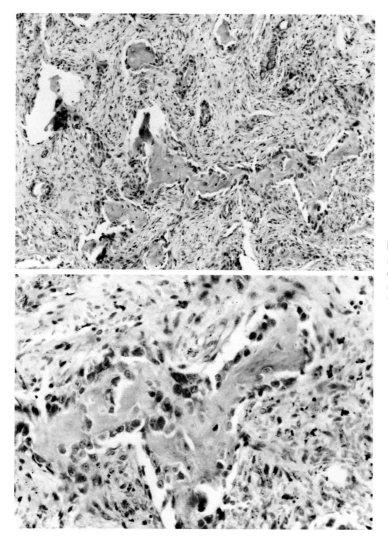

FIGURE 12-74. Photomicrographs demonstrate a more fibrous portion of an osteoma with a cellular stroma and narrow bony lamellae surrounded by osteoblasts (H&E, original magnifications × 10 *top,* × 25 *bottom*).

fibromas have been described in the orbital plate of the frontal bone and in the ethmoid sinus (Fig. 12-75). Histopathologically, 50% of the tumor is made up of small round ossicles (resembling psammoma bodies) embedded in a fibrous stroma. On CT scan the bulk of the lesion consists of a variably mottled radiolucent and radiodense tissue, which often has a shell. Because this tumor may behave in an aggressive fashion and recur, careful complete excision and follow up are indicated.

Osteoblastoma

Benign osteoblastoma is a rare bone tumor with a slight male preponderance, a peak incidence in the second to third decades, and a propensity to affect long bones or the spinal column. Only 15% to 20% of cases involve the skull and few (three reported) have been described in the orbital bones. Pathologically, it resembles osteoid osteoma sufficiently to be considered a giant osteoid osteoma; the major distinction between the two is size and vascularity, the osteoblastoma measuring more than 1 cm in diameter and containing a highly vascular central core. Immature lesions consist of osteoblasts forming irregular trabeculae of woven bone or osteoid, giant cells, and an active fibrous stroma with many thin-walled, endothelial-lined vascular channels. More mature lesions show increasing osteoid and bony trabeculae, especially peripherally. The histopathologic differential diagnosis includes osteosarcoma, giant cell tumor, aneurysmal bone cyst, and osteogenic sarcoma. The significant vascular component accounts for friability and a propensity to bleed on curettage and excision.

Radiologically, these are well-circumscribed tumors

TABLE 12-8.
DIFFERENTIATION BETWEEN FIBROUS DYSPLASIA AND OSSIFYING FIBROMA

	Fibrous Dysplasia	Ossifying Fibroma
Pathogenesis	Congenital defect Arrest in bone maturation Fibro-osseous metaplasia	True neoplasm — benign
Age of manifestation	More common in first decade	More common in second, third decades
Sex	No sex predilection	More common in females
Rate of growth	May be progressive	Slow growing
Site	Cranial bones, long bones	Cranial bones, rarely long bones Predilection for the mandible
Form	Monostotic, polyostotic Albright's syndrome	Monostotic, rarely multiple
X-ray	Ill defined	Well circumscribed
Type of bone	Woven (fiber) bone No evidence of maturation No osteoblastic rimming	Lamellar bone Rimming osteoblasts
Cement line	Feathery borders	Smooth regular borders
Polarized light	Random birefringence	Parallel lines birefringence
Type of stroma	No whorling	Parallel rows and whorls
Reticulin stain	Tangled masses of fibers Borders irregular and tangled	More vascular Regular, more parallel lines Border regular
PAS stain	Slightly positive	Of no value
At surgery	Cannot be shelled out Trimming or resection for cosmetic reasons or orbital decompression	Easily shelled out

(Kahlil MK, Leib ML: Cemento-ossifying fibroma of the orbit. Can J Ophthalmol 14:195, 1979)

that may have a radiolucent center with foci of calcification. The well-defined margin is clearly separable from the surrounding soft tissues. The radiologic differential diagnosis includes osteogenic sarcoma, chondrosarcoma, and osteoma.

Few cases have occurred in orbital bones, particularly in the midline, ethmoid, and sphenoid structures. Essentially, they cause noninfiltrative mass effects. Treatment is by excision when possible or by curettage. The large size and location govern the specific approach, and may require a combined otorhinolaryngology, ophthalmology, and neurosurgery team for en bloc excision and reconstruction. Overall throughout the body, the recurrence rate for osteoblastoma is 9.8% to 15.4%, a quarter of which have been sarcomatous. None of the sarcomas have been reported in the orbital region.

REACTIVE LESIONS

Although reactive lesions might be a slightly controversial grouping, it seems to us that they bear enough resemblance in clinical and biologic terms to treat them as related. In addition, reparative granuloma and aneurysmal bone cyst could be considered to be part of a histologically indistinct spectrum of reactive giant cell lesions. However, some authorities treat the two as separate entities.

Giant Cell Reparative Granuloma

Giant cell reparative granuloma is a benign lesion said to be related to trauma and intraosseous hemorrhage. It generally occurs in the mandible and affects patients in the first and second decades of life. Maxillary, ethmoid, and sphenoid involvement have been described. The biologic course of the disease is benign and associated with healing by new bone formation following surgical curettage. Rarely, it may be large and locally aggressive.

This lesion is characterized by lysis of bone, erosion of the cortex, and recurrent bleeding within the matrix of the mass. Sudden bleeding may lead to a catastrophic clinical onset, as in a 24-year-old man who had sudden proptosis and downward displacement of the left globe due to a reparative granuloma in the roof of the orbit (Fig. 12-76). On CT scan it was an inhomogeneous, enhancing soft tissue mass with indistinct margins and focal destruction of adjacent bone. No calcification or bony expansion was present.

(Text continues on p. 371.)

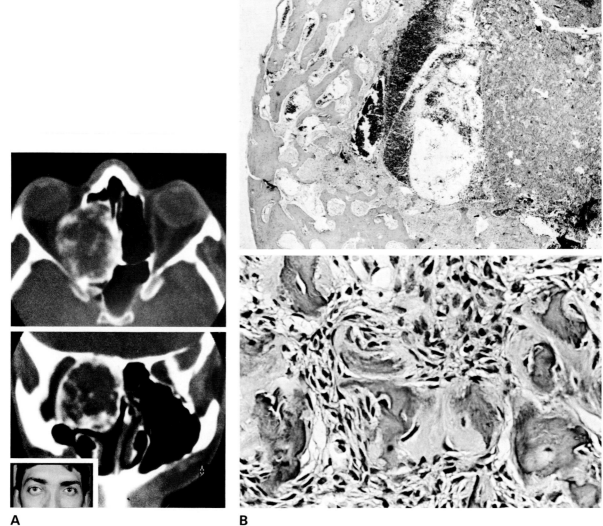

A   **B**

FIGURE 12-75. *(A)* This 25-year-old man presented with a 15-year-history of lateral displacement of the right globe. He had previously undergone ethmoidal and sphenoidal surgery for removal of an ossifying fibroma. He had a 1-year history of increasing headache on the right side. On physical examination there was lateral displacement and proptosis of the right globe with some restriction of abduction. Psychophysical findings were normal. The mass was debulked by an ethmoidectomy (lateral rhinotomy route), with improvement of physical appearance. He had remained stable for 1 year, with some residual tumor noted on CT scan. Axial and coronal scans on bone settings emphasize the expansion of the right ethmoid sinus, the corticated shell, and the mixed inner pattern of the tumor. *(B, top)* A portion of the mass shows a central, dense hypercellular vascular core and an outer cortex of lamellar bone. *(Bottom)* A high-power photograph shows a fibrous stroma with bony ossicles, suggesting a diagnosis of psammomatoid ossifying fibroma. The patient is currently being observed, and will undergo complete combined excision if the mass grows (H&E, original magnifications × 2.5 *top,* × 25 *bottom*).

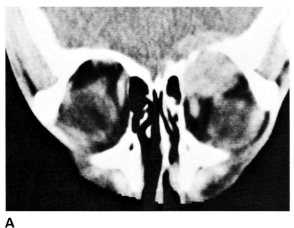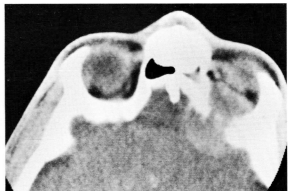

A

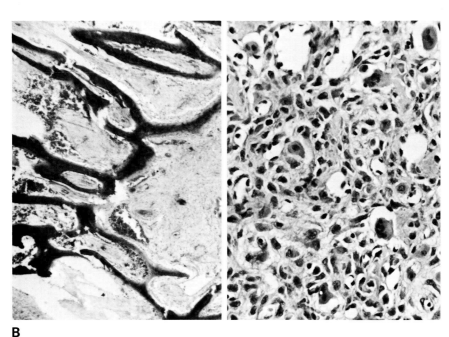

B

FIGURE 12-76. *(A)* Coronal and axial CT scans demonstrate a superior left orbital mass eroding the roof and extending into the anterior cranial fossa. This 24-year-old man presented with sudden onset of painless proptosis, downward displacement of the left globe, and diplopia over a 24-hour period. The lesion had irregular borders with adjacent destruction of bone, and was originally thought to be a malignancy with intralesional hemorrhage. Only blood was obtained on needle aspiration biopsy, and the patient underwent excision of the lesion by a combined craniotomy–orbitotomy. A hemorrhagic mass was removed from the roof of the orbit and some abnormal adjacent bone was noted at the time of surgery. *(B)* Biopsy specimen revealed two elements. The bulk of the lesion consisted of a spindle-cell stroma containing scattered osteoblastic giant cells, deposits of hemosiderin, and small vascular spaces *(right)*. At the margin of the lesion, spicules of osteoid and new bone formation were noted *(left)*. The diagnosis was reparative granuloma. The patient has been observed for 7 years without recurrence (H&E, original magnifications × 2.5 *right*, × 25 *left*).

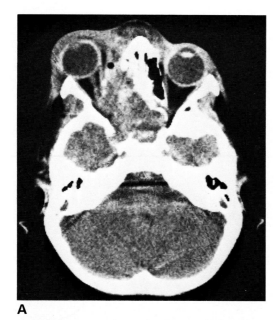

A

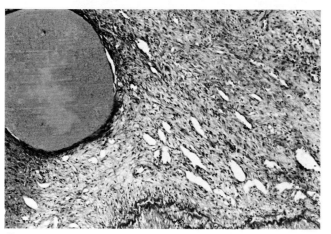

B

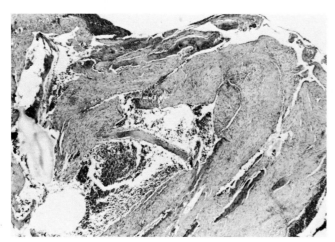

C

FIGURE 12-77. *(A)* Axial CT scan of an 8-year-old boy who presented with reduced right visual acuity associated with swelling, proptosis, and mild ptosis of 1 month's duration. He had 5 mm of downward and 3 mm of outward displacement of the globe with paresthesia involving the right cheek. A mixed-density mass lesion expanding and destroying bone was noted. It involved the ethmoid, maxillary, and sphenoid complex. He underwent a combined procedure with excision and curettage of the mass following frozen-section biopsy. *(B, C)* The bulk of the mass consisted of a stellate reactive fibroblastic tissue with large vascular spaces and spicules of bone and osteoid consistent with a diagnosis of solid aneurysmal bone cyst. The patient has been observed for 4 years without recurrence.

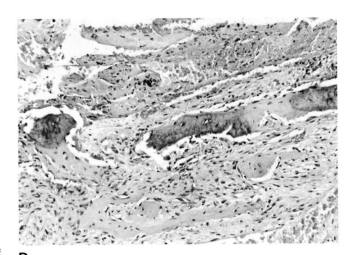

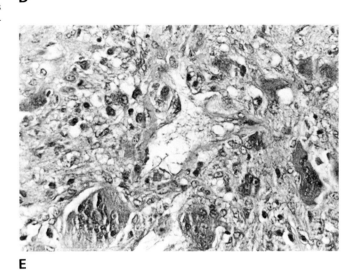

FIGURE 12-77 *(Continued).* *(D)* A higher-power view of bone spicules in a fibrous stroma. *(E)* Reactive fibrous stroma with osteoclastic giant cells (H&E, original magnifications × 10 *B*, × 2.5 *C*, × 10 *D*, × 25 *E*).

D

E

Pathologically, giant cell reparative granulomas are soft hemorrhagic masses with a spindle cell stroma containing scattered osteoblastic giant cells and deposits of hemosiderin. Spicules of osteoid and new bone formation may be noted at the margins (see Fig. 12-76*B*).

Orbital involvement has usually been secondary to extension from maxillary and ethmoid sinuses with displacement of adjacent soft tissues. Radiologically, an area of bone lysis is noted and contrast-enhanced CT scans may show patchy or rim enhancement with irregular bony margins. The majority of these lesions can be managed by surgical curettage. In some instances, however, they may behave in a more aggressive fashion and require extensive curettage followed by radiotherapy. Our patient was treated by complete curettage of the lesion and resection of the adjacent bony margin. He is cured without recurrence for 4 years.

Aneurysmal Bone Cyst

The pathologic difference from giant cell reparative granuloma is the presence of large, blood-filled channels in aneurysmal bone cyst (Fig. 12-77*B*, *C*, *D*, *E*). Some aneurysmal bone cysts are more solid and appear indistinguishable from reparative granuloma. In addition, aneurysmal bone cystlike areas may be seen in numerous other conditions, including fibrous dysplasia and giant cell tumor.

The overwhelming majority of aneurysmal bone cysts have been described in the second decade of life, but some have also been seen in young children. It is a benign reactive fibro-osseous lesion that usually affects the long bones, with more rare occurrence in the skull. Several theories of pathogenesis have been proffered, including abnormal hemodynamics, alteration of preexisting bony lesions, faulty bone formation, and organization of hemorrhage. The course can be either a slowly developing paraorbital tumefaction or sudden mass effect secondary to intralesional hemorrhage.

In the orbital region, most cases described presented with either slowly or rapidly developing ocular displacement. The majority have been in the superior orbit, but some have been seen in the medial, lateral, and posterior orbit with and without intracranial extension. The ocular signs and symptoms include diplopia, proptosis secondary to displacement of the eye, cranial nerve palsies, and papilledema due to raised intracranial pressure. In addition, a case of compression of the optic nerve with visual loss as a result of a midline lesion has been described.

We have had two cases that fit into the category of solid aneurysmal bone cyst, both of which have been midline lesions (Fig. 12-78; also see Fig. 12-77). In each instance, the clinical presentation was characterized by relatively rapid orbital displacement and visual deterioration due to optic nerve compression. Both were relatively extensive, central lesions that responded without recurrence to aggressive excision and curettage by a neurosurgical–orbital–otorhinolaryngologic team.

On routine radiography, the findings are not specific but usually involve destruction of bone or expansion of orbital walls. The CT findings include irregular expansion and destruction of bone with patchy or rim enhancement.

Surgically, these lesions consist of rather friable, pinkish masses with evidence of both serous and serosanguinous cavitation as well as some tissue with a granular texture. Histologically, they are composed of fibrous stroma containing reactive giant cells, histiocytes, and hemosiderin-laden macrophages with both osteoid and bone formation (see Fig. 12-77C, D, E). In addition, there are numerous large vascular spaces without evidence of endothelium, smooth muscle, or pericytes (see Fig. 12-77B).

Treatment is by local curettage and is usually effective. However, incomplete resection can cause recurrence within 6 months. Radiotherapy has been advocated for resistant lesions, but it carries the risk of radiation-induced sarcomas.

Reactive Xanthomatous Lesions

Two lesions seem to us somewhat difficult to distinguish histopathologically in their end stages; both of them are characterized by a reactive, xanthomatous, hemorrhagic stromal component. They are end-stage cholesteatoma and cholesterol granuloma. They may have originated from a primary epithelial lesion (cholesteatoma) or perhaps from a focal hemodynamic upset that led to a local reaction. Parke suggests that lesions containing epithelium are epidermoid cholesteatomas and nonepithelial

lesions are cholesterol granulomas. Because the provoking cause may be impossible to demonstrate histologically, we have grouped them as *xanthomatous reactive lesions of bone.*

We have encountered two clinically and histopathologically similar cases in this category (Figs. 12-79, 12-80). These male patients presented in the third decade of life with the sudden onset of downward inward displacement of the globe due to a mass lesion in the superotemporal region of the orbit. CT scan showed expansile, lytic lesions arising in the frontal bone and thinning both the outer and inner tables. The lesions were associated with a noncalcifying soft tissue mass projecting into the orbit. Both patients underwent surgical excision and curettage. Histopathologically, the tissues consisted of foci of reactive xanthogranulomatous infiltrate, cholesterol clefts, giant cells, and hemosiderin surrounded by a fibrous capsule. In one case, a small focus of metaplastic bone formation was noted within the peripheral matrix of the fibrous and vascular tissue (see Fig. 12-79C). Neither patient has had a recurrence after follow-up periods of 12 months and 3.5 years, respectively.

Brown Tumor of Hyperparathyroidism

Primary or secondary hyperparathyroidism may produce either diffuse demineralization of bone or focal reactive tumors simulating a neoplasm. These so-called *brown tumors* may be multiple or solitary. The biologic process consists of bone resorption by osteoclasts, replacement by reactive fibrous tissue, and concomitant bone formation (see Fig. 12-81B, C). These focal areas of resorption and bone formation are associated with intralesional hemorrhages and their sequelae. Osteoblastic activity with osteoid and woven bone formation at the margin of the lesion may produce focal calcification and a radiodense shell. Histopathologically, the admixture of multinucleated giant cells, features of hemorrhage (hemosiderin, cholesterol clefts, and blood), and a fibrous background may make this lesion indistinguishable from giant reparative granuloma and giant cell tumor of bone. The latter two tend to occur in a younger age group. The presence of these pathologic findings should prompt investigation for elevated serum calcium, depressed serum phosphorus, a parathyroid hormone assay, and a radiologic bone survey.

Paraorbital involvement has been rarely described. In a case that we saw, an isolated tumor mass suddenly appeared in the roof of the orbit of a 69-year-old woman (Fig. 12-81). No other lesions were noted and on operative resection a firm, rather fibrous, localized mass was identified. CT scan had disclosed a well-demarcated lytic lesion associated with a uniformly enhancing soft tissue mass and a calcific rim. The partially calcified rim was punctate and on some cuts had a radiating pattern. Histo-

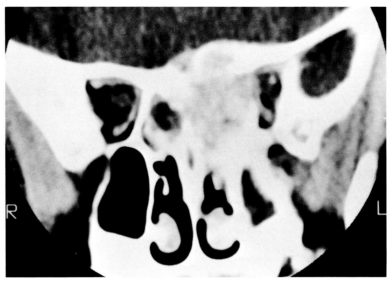

A

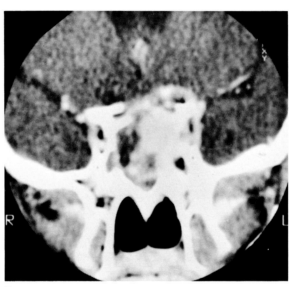

B

FIGURE 12-78. *(A, B)* Coronal CT scans of the posterior ethmoid and sphenoid region in an 11-year-old girl who presented with a 2-week history of pain in the left periocular region. She had been treated 2 years earlier for acute lymphoblastic leukemia and was currently on antimetabolite therapy. The vision on the left side was 20/30, and there was a superior temporal quadrantic visual field defect. A destructive lesion involving the sphenoid sinus, dorsum sella, and posterior ethmoid air cells was noted. Transnasal biopsy revealed a solid variant of aneurysmal bone cyst. Attempted treatment with steroids and radiotherapy failed to lead to regression of the lesion, and her vision dropped to counting fingers only. The patient underwent a combined craniotomy – orbitotomy with resection of the lesion. Her vision has returned to 20/80 with 4 months' follow-up; there has been no recurrence.

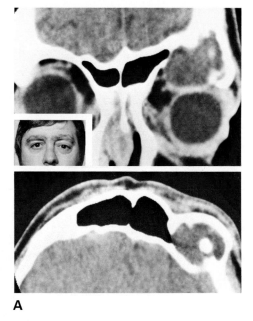

A

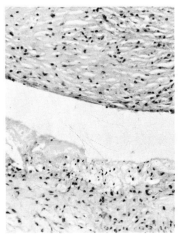

B

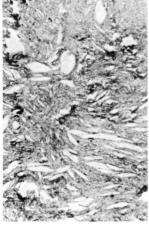

FIGURE 12-79. *(A)* This 35-year-old man presented with a 4-week history of diplopia on upgaze and an 8-week history of left ptosis. He had 5 mm downward displacement, 5 mm proptosis, a delayed VEP with a vision of 20/20, and acute choroidal striae. Coronal and axial CT scans revealed a soft tissue mass invading the superolateral orbit, eroding bone and expanding the diploic spaces of the left frontal bone. A posterior portion of the tumor extended through the roof into the anterior cranial fossa. The central portion appeared more radiolucent. This hemorrhagic mass was excised by a combined craniotomy–orbitotomy. (The hemorrhage was not acute, so the blood is of decreased density on CT scan.) *(B)* The bulk of the tumor consisted of a fibrous lining with many lipid-laden histiocytes in the wall *(left)*. In addition, there were large areas of cholesterol granuloma (H&E, original magnifications × 10 *left*, × 2.5 *right*). *(C)* At the margin of the lesion, there were some spicules of osteoid within a fibrovascular stroma, which suggested reactive bone or a possible origin of the lesion from dysplastic bone or aneurysmal bone cyst (H&E, original magnifications × 10 *left*, × 25 *right*).

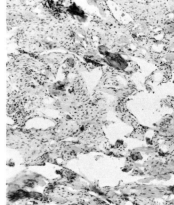

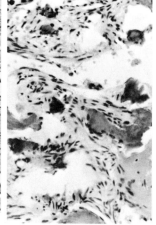

C

pathologically, it was a giant cell tumor with a fibrous stroma and bony shell. Subsequent systemic evaluation revealed raised serum calcium, lowered serum phosphorus, and an increased parathormone level due to a parathyroid tumor.

Removal of the parathyroid adenoma leads to spontaneous repair and resorption of the bony lesion.

NEOPLASMS

Chondroma

Chondromas are tumors of mature hyalin cartilage arising from cartilage or bones of cartilaginous origin. Because the orbital walls are made up of membranous bone, true benign chondromas are extremely rare and may include some cases with areas of cartilaginous metaplasia in fibrochondromas. A case has been described arising from the trochlea. Pathologically, these are lobulated tumors made up of a cartilaginous matrix containing mature chondrocytes. These tumors may be difficult to distinguish from chondrosarcoma and some cartilaginous types of chordoma. Calcification may occur along clefts, and cellularity is minimal. Treatment is by surgical excision.

Chondrosarcoma

Overall, chondrosarcomas are the second most frequent primary malignant tumors of bone, following osteogenic sarcoma. They usually occur in the metaphyseal end of long bones, but in the head and neck they arise from cartilage and cartilaginous rests in the paranasal sinuses. In the orbital region, chondrosarcomas are most frequently seen nasally and inferiorly. Biologically, they are nonmetastasizing, extremely slow-growing, locally aggressive tumors that cause proptosis and lateral displacement of the globe. Obstruction of the nasal lacrimal duct may lead to epiphora, and associated intranasal and sinus extension may cause nasal obstruction, rhinorrhea, or epistaxis.

Both chondrosarcomas that we have seen had a protracted onset. One patient presented with diffuse headache, counting fingers vision, hypertelorism, and bilateral compressive neuropathy with atrophy (Fig. 12-82). The other presented with left proptosis and lateral displacement, and a blocked left nasal passage (Fig. 12-83).

Routine radiography may show areas of bony destruction or a mottled, thickened area of bone. CT scan demonstrates an expansile, lytic lesion with a permeative pattern. The lesions contain amorphous, punctate, dense, irregular calcification with variable enhancement of the soft tissue component.

Pathologically, the tumor tends to have a firm granular texture and histologic features of hyalinized cartilage

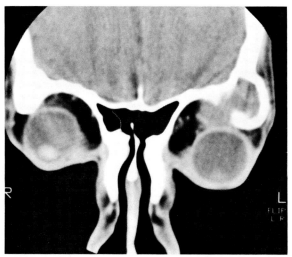

FIGURE 12-80. Coronal CT scan demonstrates a mass in the left superolateral orbit with erosion of bone and downward displacement of the eye. Note the radiolucent central portion. This 42-year-old man presented with a 5-week history of left proptosis and downward displacement. Attempted aspiration prior to referral revealed blood. The lesion involved the diploë of the frontal bone, leading to thinning of the external table with extension into the orbit. The mass was removed by anterolateral orbitotomy. Histologically, it consisted of a fibrous lining with large areas of cholesterol granuloma. No evidence of abnormal bone formation, aneurysmal bone cyst, or epithelial lining was noted. A diagnosis of cholesterol granuloma (xanthomatous lesion) was made. There has been no recurrence after an 8-month follow-up.

admixed with fibrous or even myxoid stroma (see Fig. 12-83B). The presence of myxoid stroma may suggest malignancy. The major features of malignancy are cytologic with variation in the shape and staining properties of the chondrocytes as well as the appearance of binucleate or multinucleate cells within lacunae. There may be areas of focal necrosis and calcium deposition. Malignancy may be graded on the basis of increasing cellularity, mitoses, and the development of sarcomatous myxoid stroma from grade I through grade III.

The problems in management of chondrosarcomas are governed by the frequently large size, poorly defined margins, and inaccessibility of these tumors. Nevertheless, the only means of adequate treatment is complete surgical excision, although excision with radiotherapy has been advocated. Many cases are characterized by a relentless, progressive, recurrent course over a long period leading to intracranial extension, nasal obstruction, and death. Both of our patients underwent radical debulking of the tumor by a multidisciplinary team, followed by radiotherapy; there has been no recurrence after 8 months' and 4 years' follow up, respectively.

(Text continues on p. 379.)

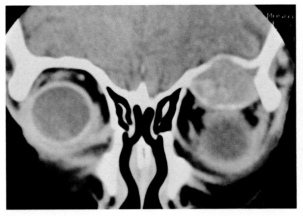
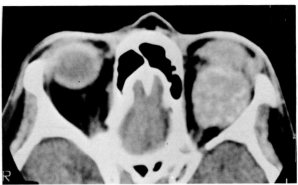

A

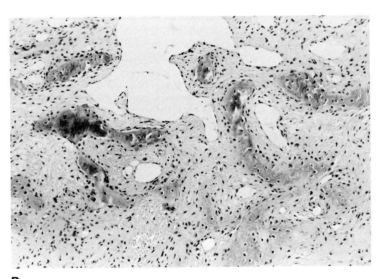

B

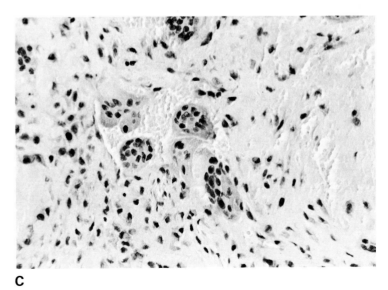

C

FIGURE 12-81. *(A)* Coronal and axial CT scans demonstrate a mass in the roof of the left orbit with erosion of the bone. The patient was a 69-year-old woman who had a 1-month history of painful swelling of the left upper lid. The tumor consisted of a uniformly enhancing soft tissue mass with a calcific rim and central punctate foci of calcification. *(B, C)* The mass was extirpated. Histologically, it consisted of a fibrous stroma with large vascular channels, many osteoclastic giant cells, and foci of bone formation. The findings led to a suspicion of brown tumor of hyperparathyroidism, which was confirmed on systemic evaluation. The parathyroid adenoma was removed. There has been no recurrence after a 1-year follow-up (H&E, original magnification × 10 *B*, × 25 *C*).

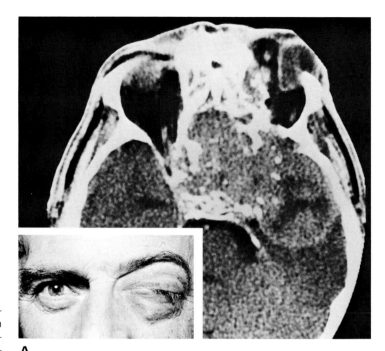

FIGURE 12-82. *(A, B)* This 56-year-old man presented with 13 years of progressive loss of vision on the left, increasing proptosis, and a firm infraorbital mass. On referral he had counting fingers vision on the left, with marked proptosis and optic atrophy. A massive lesion of the skull was noted on axial and coronal CT scans. It appeared lytic with amorphous, punctate, dense, irregular, calcific foci. Biopsy revealed a low-grade chondrosarcoma. The patient underwent combined multidisciplinary debulking of the tumor, followed by radiotherapy. There has been a 5-month follow-up to date, with no recurrence.

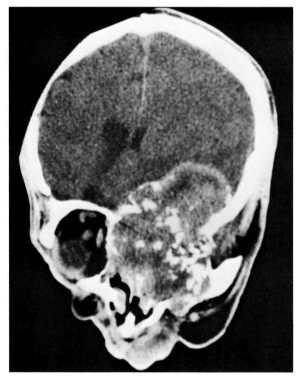

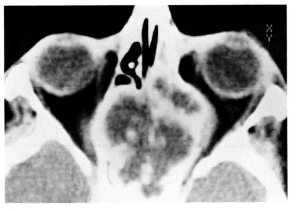

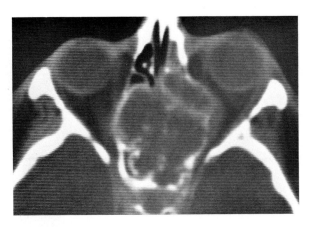

A

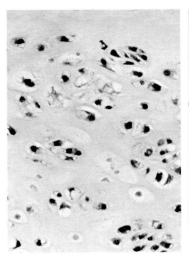

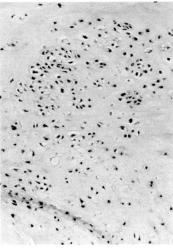

B

FIGURE 12-83. *(A)* Axial CT scan demonstrates an expansile, lytic lesion involving the ethmoid and sphenoid sinus with left proptosis and lateral displacement (standard and bone settings). This 44-year-old woman had a 5-month history of proptosis. Transnasal biopsy revealed a low-grade chondrosarcoma, and she underwent a multidisciplinary debulking of the tumor, followed by radiotherapy. There has been no recurrence after a 4-year follow-up. *(B, C)* The pathology of the low-grade chondrosarcoma. Note chondrocytes within lacunae (H&E, original magnifications × 25 *B, left;* × 10 *B, right;* × 40 *C*).

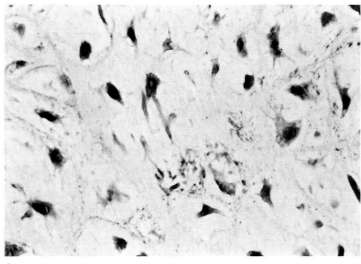

C

Extraskeletal Mesenchymal Chondrosarcoma

Extraskeletal mesenchymal chondrosarcomas are rare tumors occurring throughout the body three times more frequently in bones than in soft tissue. When originating in bone, they have a propensity to involve the jaws and ribs, whereas the principal soft tissue sites are in the head and neck, especially the soft tissues of the orbit. These tumors occur in the second and third decades and have a female preponderance. Extraskeletal mesenchymal chondrosarcomas are highly malignant with both locally infiltrative and metastasizing potential.

Pathologically, they are multilobular, fleshy, poorly circumscribed tumors with foci of bluish cartilage. They sometimes have areas of necrosis and hemorrhage. Histologically, the two major cellular elements are mesenchyme and cartilage with foci of calcification and ossification. The stromal elements consist of spindle or round cells with minimal cytoplasm and hyperchromatic nuclei, which may be arranged in sheets or around dilated vascular channels in a pattern similar to hemangiopericytoma. The cartilage is usually distinct, but may have more poorly defined areas fusing with the mesenchymal cells.

The clinical presentation in the orbit reflects the relentless local growth potential and infiltrative nature of the neoplasm. Patients present with both mass and infiltrative effects leading to displacement of the globe and functional (visual, sensory, and motor) effects. Treatment is by radical, local, and systemic therapy. Late metastases are not uncommon and occur most frequently in the lung. The usual clinical course is rapid with early metastases.

Chordoma

Chordoma is a rare, relentless, slow-growing, locally malignant midline neoplasm that arises in the dorsum sella and clivus from remnants of the embryonic notocord and grows intracranially or into the nasopharynx. When it originates from the caudal portion of the notocord, it results in a sacral or pelvic mass. Its clinical behavior is determined by the rate and direction of growth; the majority extend upward and cause raised intracranial pressure, chiasmal compression, or palsies of the third, fourth, and sixth cranial nerves. It may also extend anteriorly, obstructing the nasal cavity. Therefore, orbital and ocular involvement reflects progressive mass effect, which, when apical, leads to compression of the optic nerve or the structures in the superior orbital fissure. With massive midline anterior growth, proptosis and hyperteloric displacement of one or both orbits may occur. Growth down the clivus leads to marching cranial nerve palsies.

Radiologically, this tumor causes both expansile and destructive midline bony changes, and on CT scan appears as a nodular inhomogeneous mass. Fine osseous trabeculae and calcification may be seen. Pathologically, chordomas are smooth, multilobular, gray/blue or reddish masses with indistinct or infiltrative bony margins. The distinguishing features are the presence of physaliferous cells, which are round to oval and have central nuclei and mucin-filled cytoplasmic vacuoles. The large cells group as nests, cords, and alveoli within a mucin-rich stromal matrix. In the cervical area, a cartilaginous variant of this tumor may be difficult to distinguish from a chondrosarcoma.

Ideal treatment is complete surgical excision; this goal is rarely achieved because of the tumor's location and indistinct margins. The slow growth is compatible with long survival, particularly when the tumor is anterior, but the general prognosis is poor. Adjunctive radiotherapy has been advocated.

Osteogenic Sarcoma

Jack Rootman and Ka Wah Chan

Osteogenic sarcoma is the most common primary malignant neoplasm of bone. It occurs twice as frequently as chondrosarcoma and three times more frequently than Ewing's sarcoma. The majority arise *de novo,* but some occur secondarily to irradiation or predisposing conditions such as Paget's disease, fibrous dysplasia, giant cell tumor, and osteochondromas. They are a common second tumor in patients with the genomic mutation of retinoblastoma, wherein their behavior is particularly aggressive. They usually occur in the second decade, with the majority affecting long bones. Between 5% and 9% occur in the head and neck region, predominantly affecting the jaw and maxilla. Osteogenic sarcomas are extremely rare elsewhere in the skull. Orbital involvement is most commonly due to maxillary disease, which may or may not be associated with soft tissue infiltration depending on the grade of the primary tumor. Those occurring in the jaw are slightly different in histology, with more chondroid components and a slow, rather chronic course when compared to osteogenic sarcoma in the extremities. Routine radiography usually discloses massive destructive lesions with areas of calcification. On CT scan the bones demonstrate lytic and sclerotic changes with adjacent soft tissue infiltration and sometimes focal areas of calcification. Serum alkaline phosphatase is elevated in 50% of cases. Three to four percent of osteogenic sarcomas occur in extraosseous sites, and a single case has been described in the orbit.

We have seen one patient with osteogenic sarcoma. He presented with quite severe pain and marked reduction in visual acuity that developed over a 3-week period (Fig. 12-84). He had undergone multiple surgeries over

(Text continues on p. 382.)

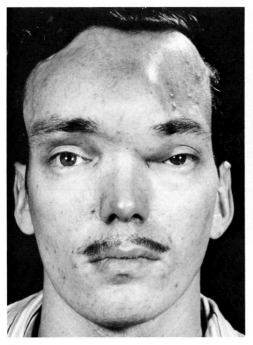
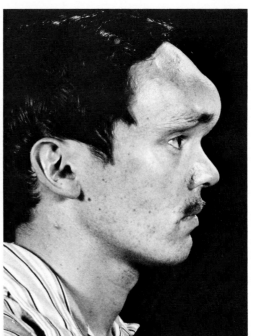

A

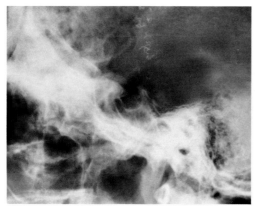
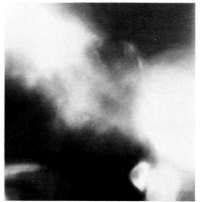

B

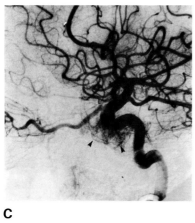
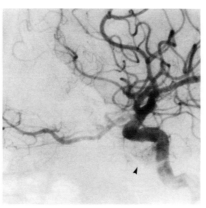
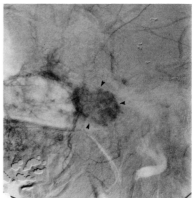

C

FIGURE 12-84. *(A)* This 41-year-old man presented with severe orbital pain and reduction in right visual acuity to no light perception. It occurred over a 3-week period and was associated with paresthesia. The AP and lateral photographs demonstrate his appearance 15 years earlier, prior to surgery for cosmetic deformity. He had had multiple surgeries over the previous 14 years for fibrous dysplasia. A massive lytic lesion involving the lateral wall, frontal bone, temporal fossa, sphenoid ridge, and orbital soft tissues with intracranial extension was noted. A diagnosis of osteogenic sarcoma was made, and the patient was treated palliatively. Within 1 month the left orbit became involved, and he died 6 months after onset. *(B)* Lateral view of skull and lateral tomogram show pagetoid fibrous dysplasia of the orbital roof, demineralization of the sella, and a destructive lesion of the sphenoid bone. The CT scan (not shown) also demonstrated a massive lytic lesion involving the lateral wall, frontal bone, temporal fossa, sphenoid ridge, and orbital soft tissues with intracranial extension. *(C)* Left *(left photo)* and right *(middle photo)* internal carotid angiography shows a leash of vessels around the carotid siphon representing hypertrophied branches of the inferolateral trunk and a tumor blush in the venous phase *(right photo),* indicating a very vascular mass. *(D)* Gross features at the time of autopsy revealed a whitish mass extending into the right orbit. *(E)* Histologic analysis shows a poorly differentiated osteogenic sarcoma with foci of osteoid. The electron micrograph demonstrates osteoid formation in the tumor (H&E, original magnification *top* × 10, *bottom* × 40, electron micrograph × 1520).

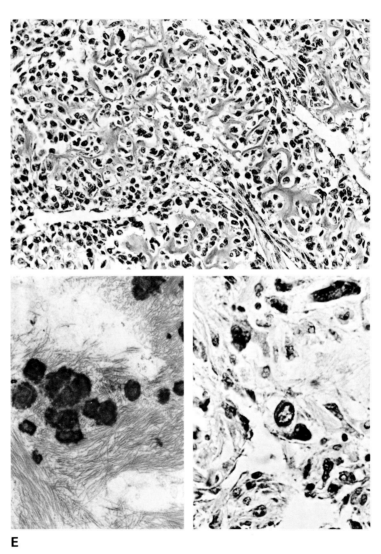

D

E

the previous 14 years for fibrous dysplasia of the skull, which had been static for approximately 6 years when the symptoms developed. There had been no previous radiotherapy. The tumor was extensive and involved all aspects of the lateral wall of the orbit, the frontal bone, the temporal fossa, the sphenoid ridge, and orbital soft tissues with intracranial extension in adjacent sites.

Histologically, the diagnosis is established by the demonstration of osteoid within a variably anaplastic sarcomatous stroma (see Fig. 12-84E). These stromal cells may also produce cartilage and fibrous tissue. Osteogenic sarcomas of the head and neck, particularly those of the jaw and maxilla, tend to be of lower grade than those seen in extrafacial sites.

The prognosis for patients with osteosarcoma arising in the skull is considered poor because late diagnosis and early intracranial extension limit the extent of surgical excision. Following surgery and postoperative irradiation, a 5-year survival rate of approximately 10% has been reported. During the past decade, significant progress has been made in treating primary osteosarcoma of the extremities based on combined chemotherapy and surgery. Rosen and co-workers reported that 82% of their patients survived for 5 years. These improved results serve as a model for more effective treatment of tumors arising in the cranial bones, especially because modern surgical techniques allow wide resections of tumors of the calvaria as well as of the base of the skull. The current therapy consists of high-dose methotrexate ($8–12$ g/m^2) followed by folinic acid rescue given weekly for 6 to 8 weeks, before definite surgery (sometimes multiple resections) is performed. Postoperative chemotherapy includes doxorubicin (Adriamycin), bleomycin, cyclophosphamide, dactinomycin and in the absence of major histologic response of the primary tumor (less than 90% necrosis), cisplatin substitutes for high-dose methotrexate. Radiation therapy should be administered to the site of residual disease after surgery. Chemotherapy can be discontinued 8 to 10 months after surgery. Using such a program, a 3-year survival rate of 50% has been reported.

Rare Tumors of Orbital Bones

Ewing's Sarcoma

Jack Rootman and Ka Wah Chan

Ewing's sarcoma is a highly malignant, small, round cell tumor. It represents up to 10% of all malignancies of bone. The majority arise in the lower extremity and pelvis, but they may occasionally originate from soft tissue (extraskeletal Ewing's sarcoma). There is a slight male predominance, and the overwhelming majority occur before age 30 years with a racial predilection for whites. The

incidence in the head and neck is 4%, with lesions usually affecting the maxilla or mandible. Maxillary tumors may be associated with exophthalmos or nasal obstruction.

Orbital Ewing's sarcoma is generally metastatic, and a diagnosis of a primary should not be made until the patient has undergone a complete skeletal survey. We encountered two cases of primary Ewing's sarcoma involving the orbital bones, with ages of onset at 6 and 10 years, respectively. Both patients presented with proptosis and nonaxial displacement; one was downward and outward due to a tumor of the nasopharynx, and the other was upward due to a maxillary tumor (Fig. 12-85). Both had a 4-week history of symptoms and had reduced visual acuity.

On CT scan, a permeative or moth-eaten pattern of bone destruction associated with soft tissue mass was noted. Neither enhanced with contrast injection.

Histopathologically, Ewing's sarcoma may be difficult to differentiate from the other round cell tumors of childhood. Characteristic features include PAS-positive, diastase-resistant, glycogen-rich cytoplasmic vacuoles. On electron microscopy, the cells contain few subcellular organelles, have cell membrane junctions and the cytoplasm is filled with pools of glycogen (see Fig. 12-85B, C).

Combination chemotherapy and radiation therapy are efficacious in improving the prognosis of Ewing's sarcoma. Cyclophosphamide, vincristine, doxorubicin (Adriamycin), and dactinomycin are currently used in combination to control micrometastases early after diagnosis. Induction chemotherapy is given for 6 to 12 weeks prior to the treatment of the primary tumor. Radiation therapy is used for local disease control, traditionally with 5500 to 6500 cGy encompassing the whole bone. This may be modified for tumor involving the skull according to the volume of brain that will be exposed to radiation. Good local disease control (exceeding 90% of cases) can be achieved. The effect of irradiation may be enhanced by adjuvant chemotherapy, but there are reports of an increased rate of late complications on the normal tissues. It has been suggested that the dose of irradiation may be reduced, although a dosage of less than 4000 cGy is not recommended at the present time. The current approach to local disease control involves surgical resection of the primary tumor after 9 to 12 weeks of induction chemotherapy. Resections with clear surgical margins do not require radiation therapy, and these patients have a superior disease-free survival compared to those treated only by radiation to the primary tumor site.

The use of multiagent chemotherapy with either local radical radiation or surgery has improved 5-year survival from 10% to 60% to 79%. About one fifth of these patients, however, have gone on to produce second primaries, in particular, osteogenic sarcoma. It is also impor-

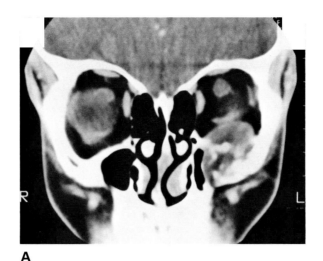

A

FIGURE 12-85. *(A)* Coronal CT scan demonstrates a destructive lesion of the left maxillary sinus and floor of the orbit, and a well-circumscribed soft tissue component invading the orbit. It was seen in a 12-year-old boy who had a 6-week history of a puffy left lower lid. His vision was reduced to 20/60, and there were 6 mm of elevation, 2 mm of proptosis, and a palpable mass in the left lower lid. He underwent incisional biopsy, with frozen section diagnosis of a poorly differentiated round-cell tumor. *(B)* Histopathology of his biopsy demonstrates a densely packed cellular tumor with PAS-positive, diastase-resistant cytoplasmic vacuoles (H&E, original magnification × 100). *(C)* Electron micrograph demonstrates the primitive cells with no junctions, large nuclei, scant organelles, and pools of glycogen typical of Ewing's sarcoma. The patient was treated with chemotherapy and radiotherapy, and is alive and well with no local or systemic recurrence on 2 years' follow-up (× 11,750). (*C*, courtesy J. Dimmick, MD.)

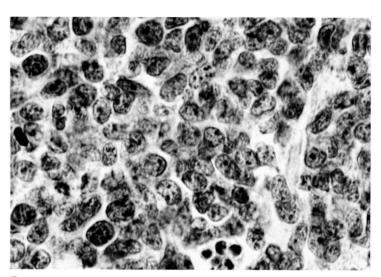

B

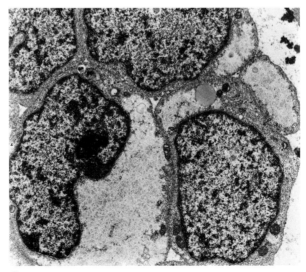

C

tant to emphasize that these patients are prone to late recurrence of disease and need scrupulous follow up for 5 years at a minimum. Both of our patients were treated with radiotherapy and chemotherapy and have achieved full remission after follow up periods of 8 months and 6 years, respectively.

Malignant Fibrous Histiocytoma

We encountered a single case of malignant fibrous histiocytoma involving bone 4 years after radiation of an orbit post enucleation for retinoblastoma (see Fig. 12-61). The patient had a large orbital mass that extended along the roof and medial wall and extended intracranially, elevating the carotid artery. On CT scan there was a lytic, permeative pattern of bone destruction of the orbital margin and expansion of the orbit with an associated ill-defined soft tissue mass surrounding the prosthesis. The patient died 6 months after presentation from local extension of his tumor. Fibrous histiocytoma is discussed in detail earlier in this chapter.

Lymphomas and Hematopoietic Malignancies

Lymphoma.   Lymphoma affecting paraorbital bones was seen in two of our patients, both previously diagnosed and treated for B-cell lymphocytic lymphomas in other sites with apparent remission. The relapse in both instances had an epicenter in orbital bone. Little pain was associated with these two tumors, although proptosis and alteration of globe position were quite evident. One affected the maxillary, ethmoid, and frontal bones with medial orbital involvement. The tumor was in the orbital apex, sphenoid bone, and cavernous sinus and led to a third nerve palsy and a compressive optic neuropathy (Fig. 12-86). CT scan showed an enhancing soft tissue mass associated with a small area of bone destruction in the sphenoid sinus in one instance and a large soft tissue mass with bony erosion of the maxillary and ethmoid sinus in the other. The involved area did not have the classic moth-eaten or permeative pattern seen in primary lymphoma of bone originating in long bones, but was consistent with the cortical breakthrough described with lesions of the mandible and maxilla. Local tumor regression was achieved by a combination of radiotherapy and chemotherapy in both instances with follow up of 2 months and 2.5 years, respectively.

Plasmacytoma.   We have encountered two cases of plasmacytoma affecting the paraorbital bones. Although multiple myeloma is the most common malignant tumor of the skeleton, occurrence in the paraorbital region is relatively rare. Both cases and their management have been described in Chapter 10. The CT scans showed lobulated, densely enhancing, well-defined soft tissue masses that had destroyed adjacent bone. A permeative or moth-eaten pattern of bone destruction was not present adjacent to the lesions, but in the instance of known myelomatosis, multiple "punched-out" lesions of the skull were noted.

Histiocytosis-X.   Histiocytosis-X is also discussed in detail in Chapter 10. Histiocytosis-X has a propensity to involve bones, and the orbit and paraorbital region are not uncommon sites. We have encountered three cases, all under the age of 6 years. Two had proptosis due to shallow orbits and all three had dramatic soft tissue swelling. CT scans demonstrated either a small lytic area associated with adjacent enhancing soft tissue masses, or extensive destruction of the bony walls of the orbit. Two of the cases had intracranial involvement on presentation. The remaining case presented with a soft tissue mass extending through the upper lid and originating in the underlying frontal bone. Treatment is governed by degree of involvement and consists of radiotherapy with or without chemotherapy. All three of our cases are currently in remission with an average follow up of 30 months.

Vascular Tumors of Bone

Frontal or maxillary intraosseous cavernous hemangiomas may affect the orbit. Radiologically, they are well-circumscribed areas of rarefaction that may be honeycombed with striated margins. Histologically, they are noninfiltrative cavernous hemangiomas. They can be treated by surgical excision. A single case of hemangioendothelioma has been reported. It was a locally aggressive infiltrative lesion that produced lysis of adjacent bone and recurred after incomplete excision.

Miscellaneous Tumors of Bone

Other bone tumors including myxomas, lipoma of the frontal bone, giant cell tumor, and angiosarcoma have been described, but they are distinctly rare in this region. A myriad of potential primary bone lesions that have not occurred in the orbit will, no doubt, be documented eventually in this region.

■ TUMORS OF THE LACRIMAL GLAND

Jack Rootman and Jocelyn S. Lapointe

Although the main focus of this section will be a discussion of primary epithelial malignancies of the lacrimal gland, it is important to consolidate knowledge of these tumors within the context of all space-occupying lesions of the lacrimal fossa. Throughout, this text has emphasized the correlation of clinical pattern, pathophysiology, investigative features, and pathology of diseases affecting the orbit. Nowhere is it more important to have a synthesized knowledge base than in the practical identification and management of lesions of the lacrimal fossa. The main categories of tumefaction here include inflamma-

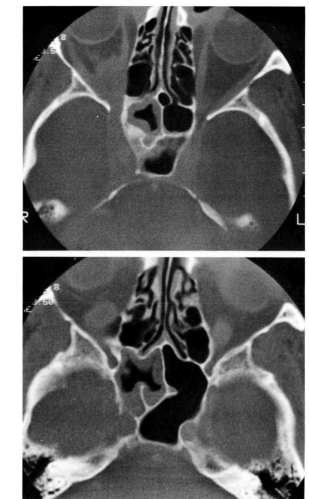

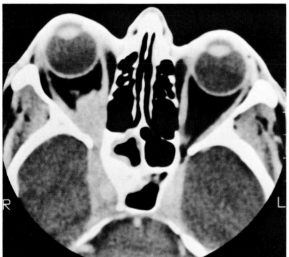

A   **B**

FIGURE 12-86.   Axial CT scans on standard *(A)* and bone *(B)* settings show a right apical soft tissue mass extending into and enlarging the right cavernous sinus. Mucosal thickening of the sphenoid sinus, subtle bone destruction of the lateral wall of the posterior right sphenoid air cells, and some mottled sclerosis are visible. This lesion occurred in a 65-year-old man who presented with a 6-month history of diplopia, ptosis, and increasing proptosis. In addition, he had recently become aware of reduced visual acuity on the right side with some desaturation of color vision. Six years previously, the patient had a paraspinal vertebral B-cell lymphoma. He had been treated with radiotherapy at that time and chemotherapy for a systemic recurrence 4½ years later. On physical examination he had a right afferent pupillary defect, a narrow interpalpebral fissure, chemosis, 2 mm of downward displacement, 4 mm of proptosis, and limitation of elevation, abduction, and adduction. In addition, he had raised intraocular pressure on the right side and papilledema. Aspiration needle biopsy demonstrated a lymphoma. He responded dramatically, with resolution of his ocular and orbital symptoms following local radiotherapy and chemotherapy.

TABLE 12-9.
SPACE-OCCUPYING LESIONS OF THE LACRIMAL FOSSA, UNIVERSITY OF BRITISH COLUMBIA ORBITAL CLINIC, 1976–1986

Type of Lesion	Intrinsic	Extrinsic
Neoplastic	20	5
Inflammatory	18	5
Structural	9	7
Total	47	17

TABLE 12-10.
SPACE-OCCUPYING LESIONS OF THE LACRIMAL FOSSA, UNIVERSITY OF BRITISH COLUMBIA ORBITAL CLINIC, 1976–1986

Tumor Type	Number of Lesions	Total
Intrinsic		
Neoplastic		
Epithelial		12
Adenoid cystic	4	
Adenoid cystic basaloid	1	
Pleomorphic Adenoma	4	
Malignant mixed	1	
Mucoepidermoid	2	
Lymphoma		7
Small cleaved	3	
Plasmacytoid small cell	1	
Small cell	2	
Benign lymphoproliferative	1	
Nonepithelial		
Spindle cell sarcoma	1	
Inflammatory		18
Infections		
Bacterial	1	
Viral (zoster)	1	
Noninfective		
Idiopathic	11	
Specific	5	
Sjögren's 1		
Sarcoidosis 3		
Wegener's 1		
Structural		9
Lacrimal cysts 9		
Extrinsic		
Neoplastic and Reactive		5
Myeloma	2	
Hodgkin's	1	
Eosinophilic granuloma	1	
Brown tumor (hyperparathyroidism)	1	
Inflammatory		5
Granulomatous	2	
Reactive xanthomatous lesion of bone	2	
Nonspecific sclerosing inflammation	1	
Structural		7
Dermoid	3	
Mucocele	3	
Implantation	1	

tory, neoplastic, and structural disorders. Appropriate management of lacrimal tumors demands clinical and investigative accuracy in order to define the correct method of surgical intervention. The core issue is to identify the characteristic clinical and investigative presentation of benign mixed tumors of the lacrimal gland so that complete extirpation is the initial management. Surgical intervention for diagnostic purposes in all other lesions of the lacrimal fossa except well-defined, noninfiltrative lesions (including dermoid cysts, other cysts, and solid benign tumors) should be incisional biopsy. To develop a contextual picture for masses in the lacrimal fossa, I have chosen to consolidate our experience in this area.

Incidence and Pathophysiology

Overall we have seen 64 lesions in the lacrimal fossa, 47 of which were intrinsic and 17 extrinsic to the lacrimal gland. The major tumefactions were neoplastic, inflammatory, and structural in character (Tables 12-9, 12-10). All exerted a mass effect clinically. The most easily defined clinicopathophysiologic differences were between those with and without inflammatory features. The most characteristic presentation involved acute and subacute inflammations with abrupt onset (days to weeks), accompanied by pain, localized tenderness, injection, S-shaped deformity of the lid, pouting of the lacrimal ducts, localized chemosis, and mild to moderate tumefaction. Chronic inflammatory processes were dominated by mass effect with more subtle features of inflammation and could not readily be distinguished on clinical grounds from intrinsic and extrinsic neoplasms of the lacrimal fossa; thus, they required histopathologic identification.

INFLAMMATIONS

Intrinsic Inflammations

The intrinsic inflammatory lesions of the lacrimal gland can be divided by etiology into infective and noninfective causes.

Infective Lesions

The infective lesions include bacterial and viral dacryoadenitis. These patients present with all of the features of acute and subacute inflammation of the lacrimal gland and may also show suppuration, preauricular and cervical adenopathy, and systemic features of malaise, upper respiratory infection, fever, and leukocytosis. CT scan reveals a diffuse lacrimal tumefaction with irregular margins, frequently demonstrating contrast enhancement

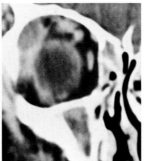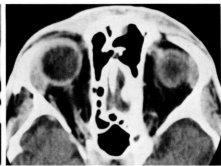

FIGURE 12-87. Coronal and axial CT scans of a patient who presented with acute suppurative dacryoadenitis due to a staphylococcal infection. Clinically, the lateral portion of the lid was tender and swollen and the lacrimal gland was tense. The patient was a debilitated alcoholic and had a concurrent maxillary sinusitis visible on the coronal CT scan. The right lacrimal gland is increased in size and partially obscures the lateral margin of the globe. He was treated with systemic antibiotics and recovered uneventfully.

(which may be patchy) and no bony defect (Fig. 12-87). Ultrasonography may show features suggestive of inflammation, including irregular margins and echolucent zones. Bacterial dacryoadenitis may require aspiration from the local site or regional lymph node to identify the organism for appropriate antibiotic therapy.

Dacryoadenitis may occur secondarily to infectious mononucleosis, herpes zoster, and mumps with their characteristic associated systemic abnormalities. Acute dacryoadenitis may progress to chronic disease. In addition, a number of specific infections (such as trachoma, syphilis, and tuberculosis) may affect the lacrimal gland and produce chronic inflammations.

Noninfective Lesions

Nonspecific Inflammations. The noninfective inflammatory lesions of the lacrimal gland constituted the largest number of inflammations seen at the University of British Columbia Orbital Clinic. They could be divided into nonspecific idiopathic and specific inflammatory categories. The nonspecific idiopathic inflammations of the lacrimal gland have been discussed in Chapter 9. These patients presented with a typical syndrome of pain, tenderness, injection, and an S-shaped deformity of the lateral lid. In this group, two were bilateral and four had a recurrent episodic presentation. The majority had no other associated abnormalities, but two had organ-specific inflammatory disease. Orbital imaging by CT revealed a compressed and molded enlargement of the lacrimal gland with obscuration of the lateral aspect of the globe and enhancement including on occasion the adjacent sclera (Fig. 12-88). Ultrasonography showed in some cases an echolucent area posterior to the scleral shell with thickening of the adjacent muscle. Motility is involved only minimally and generally reflects the mass effect alone.

Specific Inflammations. There are a number of specific inflammations of the lacrimal gland that bear identification and management. Five of our cases were in this category. The first was a case of Sjögren's syndrome presenting with bilateral subacute dacryoadenitis, de-

creased tearing, and punctate keratitis associated with xerostomia. Biopsy suggested Sjögren's syndrome, and the patient was managed with appropriate systemic steroidal and nonsteroidal anti-inflammatory agents following systemic evaluation (Fig. 12-89). Because of the potential association of autoimmune inflammatory disorders and lymphoma, patients with this syndrome should be followed prospectively for life. Three patients had sarcoid involving the lacrimal gland, two of which were bilateral. A relatively acute onset was noted in one patient and chronic tumefaction in the remaining two. All had characteristic hilar lymphadenopathy. Biopsy confirmed the diagnosis and led to specific treatment. The final case of specific inflammation involved both lacrimal glands along with CT evidence of midline destruction of nasopharyngeal and sinus structures. Biopsy showed features of a necrotizing vasculitis characteristic of Wegener's granulomatosis. This patient was successfully treated with systemic prednisone and cyclophosphamide.

In summary, the acute nonspecific inflammatory lesions of the lacrimal gland have a distinctive clinical and investigative picture. They can be appropriately categorized and treated. Failure of resolution, a subacute or chronic picture, bilateral involvement, or systemic associations implies the need for incisional biopsy. An important feature that may help distinguish intrinsic inflammation from either extrinsic or neoplastic lesions is the overall tendency for lacrimation to be affected with these lesions, but not with the structural or neoplastic tumefactions.

Extrinsic Inflammations

We have seen five cases of extrinsic inflammation in the lacrimal fossa. All of them presented with tumefaction as their major clinical feature. Two reactive xanthomatous lesions of bone with associated bony defects had sudden onset due to hemorrhage within the tumor and required excisional biopsy. Two extrinsic lesions were granuloma-

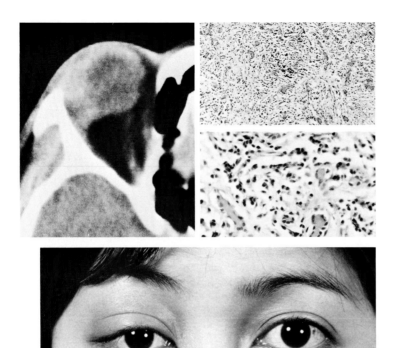

FIGURE 12-88. This 25-year-old woman had a 1-month history of swelling, injection, and tenderness of the right upper lid with downward and inward displacement of the globe. The axial CT scan demonstrates a mass in the lacrimal fossa. The biopsy shows a diffuse polymorphous chronic inflammatory infiltrate with sclerosis and destruction of the lacrimal gland and preservation of some ductal structures. This nonspecific inflammatory lesion responded clinically to treatment with systemic corticosteroids (H&E, original magnifications *top* × 2.5, *bottom* × 10).

tous inflammations of a nonspecific variety affecting the anterior orbit and soft tissues adjacent to the gland. The remaining extrinsic inflammatory lesion in the lacrimal fossa was a nonspecific sclerosing inflammation.

STRUCTURAL ABNORMALITIES

Intrinsic Lesions

The only structural abnormality with tumefaction in the lacrimal gland area was lacrimal cysts. All of the lesions were ductal in origin. They characteristically are blue-domed, cystic swellings visible through the conjunctiva, and they transilluminate. By definition, they involve the excretory ducts and are usually localized, but they can be multiple or even bilateral. Their appearance is distinctive, and management requires a limited careful microscopic excision with caution to avoid other lacrimal ducts. Occasional cases of cysts arising in the orbital lobe of the lacrimal gland have been described and are usually of congenital origin. (See Chapter 13.)

Extrinsic Lesions

The extrinsic structural lesions we encountered were dermoid cysts, mucoceles, and implantation cysts. The majority of dermoid cysts occurring temporally are exter-

nally visible and involve the lateral extrinsic portion of the orbit. These superficial dermoids do not constitute a serious differential diagnostic problem in this area. However, we saw three cases of deep dermoids with tumefaction in the lacrimal fossa. They characteristically occur in a young age group (usually the first two decades), and are well-defined, smooth, painless masses that may have a palpable anterior portion. The bulk of the tumor, however, is deep in the lacrimal fossa. A major differentiating feature on investigation is the sharp demarcation of the lower margin corresponding to the frontozygomatic suture line. The bony margins are frequently thinned and rarely sclerotic. When they contain a significant amount of fat, they have a central lucency on CT scan and on ultrasonography may be defined as cystic. Extension through the suture line may be associated with a tumor on both sides of the bone (the so-called "dumbbell" dermoid). Ruptured dermoid cysts may lead to fistulization or granulomatous destruction of the bone (Fig. 12-90). The associated well-defined lower demarcation at the frontozygomatic suture in this instance was strong presumptive evidence of dermoid cyst.

A second type of extrinsic structural lesion we encountered in this locale was three mucoceles. All developed in the lateral part of the frontal sinus as a result of an antecedent fracture. CT scan showed thinning and corti-

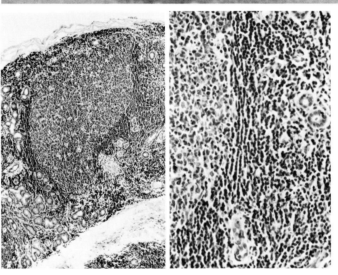

FIGURE 12-89. Axial CT scan demonstrates bilateral enlargement of the lacrimal glands in a 50-year-old woman who had a 3-month history of bilateral nontender masses and dry-eye syndrome. The biopsy demonstrates a dense lymphocytic infiltration and follicular centers with destruction of the lacrimal gland. On systemic investigation, the patient had right submandibular salivary gland enlargement and bilateral effusions of her knee joints. A diagnosis of Sjögren's syndrome was made, and the patient was treated with systemic prednisone, which led to improvement in tear secretion and reduction of lacrimal masses (H&E, original magnifications *left* × 2.5, *right* × 25).

cation of the bone with a large cystic mass extending into the lateral superior portion of the orbit, and evidence of an old fracture (Fig. 12-91). The third type of extrinsic structural lesion was an implantation cyst that presented as a mass in the lateral portion of the lid associated with a cystic lesion of the conjunctiva in the fornix. On CT investigation a well-demarcated mass containing calcification and enlarging the lacrimal fossa was indentified (Fig. 12-92).

NEOPLASMS

Intrinsic Lesions

The two major groups of intrinsic neoplasms of the lacrimal gland are epithelial and lymphoproliferative lesions. Broadly speaking, they can be divided on the basis of the known biology. Lymphomas for the most part appear in a slightly older age group, are clinically pain free, and often have a characteristic pink, fish-flesh subconjunctival component. The majority appear as primary lesions of the lacrimal gland (without known systemic lymphoma). There was one instance of bilateral lacrimal involvement in a previously diagnosed systemic lymphoma. The six primary lesions were all low grade (three small cleaved cell, one plasmacytoid small cell, and two small cell). Five of the six had a bilateral lacrimal lymphoma. On CT scan they characteristically molded to the adjacent structures without invading soft tissue, excavating bone, or flattening the globe (Fig. 12-93). On ultrasonography they had features suggestive of the "lymphoma pseudotumor" category.

The remaining intrinsic tumors of the lacrimal gland were primary epithelial neoplasms. The epithelial tumors

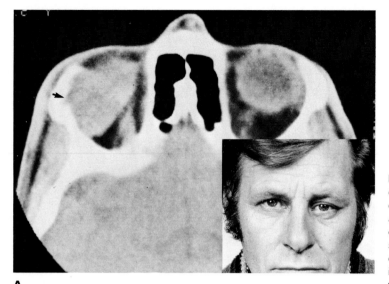

A

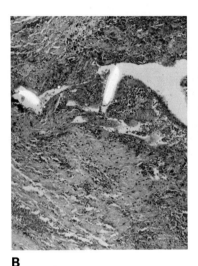

B

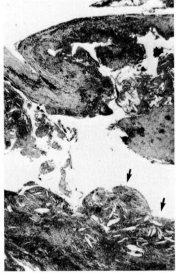

C

FIGURE 12-90. This case demonstrates the clinical features, CT findings, and histopathology of an extrinsic lesion of the lacrimal gland in the adjacent fossa, which proved to be a dermoid cyst. *(A)* This 41-year-old man presented with a sudden onset of downward inward displacement of the left globe following an apparently minor injury. However, retrospective photographs revealed orbital asymmetry that had been present for many years. The axial CT scan demonstrates a smooth posterior margin to this slightly inhomogeneous mass with irregular erosion of the bone adjacent to it *(arrow)*. At surgery, the bone in the lacrimal fossa was thin and had a yellowish discoloration. *(B, C)* Histologically, the lesion consisted of a cyst filled with lipid and inflammatory debris. The wall of the cyst also contains numerous hairs (clearly noted using polarized light; *B*) and cholesterol clefts *(arrows)* (H&E, original magnifications *B* × 10, *C* × 2.5).

are the subject of the remainder of this chapter, but in terms of the differential diagnosis a number of features may help to distinguish these tumors. They are characterized by relentless, progressively increasing mass effect. The benign variants have noninvasive features that correlate with a history of gradual onset (greater than 1 year), painless progression, and evidence of excavation without infiltration of bone. All of the intrinsic tumors lead to deformation of adjacent soft tissue structures, but the benign mixed tumors do not have clinical or investigative evidence of infiltration of either soft tissues or bone. In contrast, the malignant tumors have a slightly shorter course of onset (under 1 year) and are characterized by pain in about 40% of instances (variable depending on the series studied). In addition, they may have features of bony infiltration radiologically as well as irregular or serrated margins on CT scan. Calcification may suggest malignancy; however, in our experience it also occurs with several other lesions, including dermoid and implantation cysts, plasmacytoma, lymphoma, and choristoma.

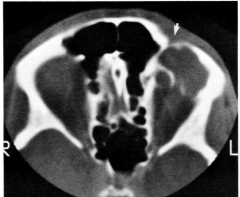
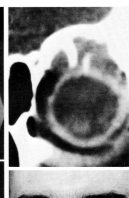
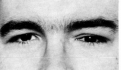

FIGURE 12-91. A mucocele arising in the lateral portion of the left frontal sinus presented as a mass in the superolateral orbit affecting the lacrimal fossa. Clinically, this 34-year-old man presented with downward displacement of the left eye and diplopia in upgaze. The axial and coronal CT scans demonstrate a mucocele arising lateral to a fracture site *(arrow)* in the frontal sinus and extending inferiorly into the orbit.

The only other intrinsic tumor of the lacrimal gland that we encountered was a unique case of low-grade spindle cell sarcoma with the differential diagnosis of a fibrous histiocytoma, fibrosarcoma, low-grade angiosarcoma, and hemangiopericytoma. This tumor had all of the clinical features of a benign mixed tumor of the lacrimal gland. There are numerous other slowly progressive soft tissue tumors that may occur in the lacrimal gland, including cavernous hemangiomas, melanomas, and peripheral nerve tumors. The biology of cavernous hemangiomas, melanomas, and peripheral nerve tumors in this location parallels that described for other locales within the orbit and is discussed elsewhere.

Extrinsic Lesions

The extrinsic tumefactions of the lacrimal fossa included four different entities: myeloma, sclerosing Hodgkin's lymphoma, eosinophilic granuloma, and parathyroid tumor. The myelomas were characterized by profound osteolytic defects of bone involving the lateral orbit and adjacent skull. One had known multiple myeloma and many osteolytic lesions of bone, whereas the other was a primary presentation of an extramedullary plasmacytoma of bone.

The single case of sclerosing Hodgkin's disease had the features of a chronically expanding localized lesion of the lacrimal fossa, which made it indistinguishable on clinical and radiologic grounds from a slow-growing tumor of the lacrimal fossa. Extirpative biopsy was planned on a presumptive basis for an intrinsic tumor of the lacrimal gland, but a lesion adjacent to and separate from the lacrimal gland was encountered. Because of known systemic Hodgkin's disease frozen sections at

biopsy aided in making the correct diagnosis. The lesion was removed and the patient treated with local radiotherapy.

We had one case of eosinophilic granuloma in this region that progressed rapidly by eroding through adjacent bone and lid.

The final case was a brown tumor of hyperparathyroidism with a very sudden onset due to bleeding within the mass, causing downward and inward displacement of the globe and a palpable tumor. On CT scan it appeared to involve more of the roof of the orbit than the lacrimal fossa and was irregularly calcified.

The foregoing summarizes our experience with tumors in this area and serves as a basis for understanding the intrinsic epithelial tumors of the lacrimal gland, and the problems in differential diagnosis.

Epithelial Tumors of the Lacrimal Gland

Epithelial neoplasms of the lacrimal gland were collectively classified as *mixed tumors* until 1954, when Forrest applied the classification of salivary gland tumors developed by Foote and Frezel to the lacrimal gland, and so distinguished benign from malignant types. This classification, with minor modification, has allowed a more clear-cut definition of the biology and expected clinical behavior of these tumors. The relative frequency of epithelial tumors (averaged from many series) is approximately 50% benign mixed tumor (pleomorphic adenoma) and 50% carcinomas. Half of the carcinomas are adenoid cystic with the remaining divided between malignant *(Text continues on p. 394.)*

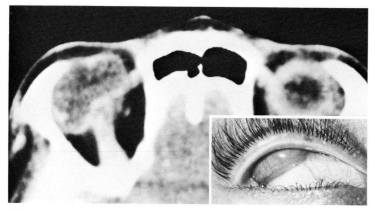

A

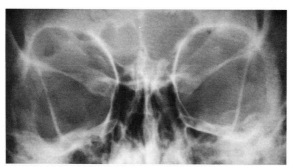

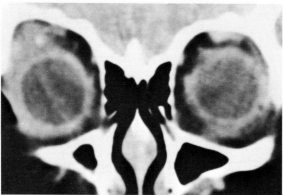

B

FIGURE 12-92. *(A)* A large implantation cyst in the right superolateral fornix and orbit. The axial CT scan demonstrates an inhomogeneous cystic mass with focal areas of calcification in the wall *(arrow)*. *(B)* Plain radiograph and coronal CT scan of the same lesion showed the excavation of the lacrimal fossa due to pressure erosion. A punctate area of calcification in the lesion can be seen on CT scan.

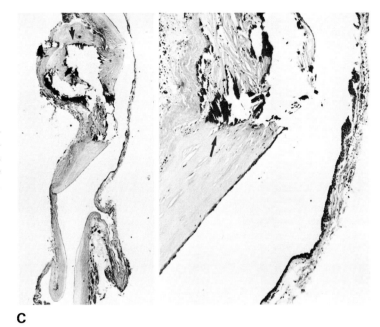

FIGURE 12-92 *(Continued).* *(C)* The histopathologic features of this lesion demonstrate a collapsed cyst with thin epithelial lining and focal areas of calcification in the surrounding fibrous capsule *(arrow)* (H&E, original magnification *left* ×2.5, *right* ×10).

C

FIGURE 12-93. A 78-year-old man presented with bilateral lacrimal gland enlargements. The axial CT scan demonstrates the relatively smooth contours, which mold to the orbital structures. Histologically, it was a small cell lymphoma and was associated with widespread lymphadenopathy and hepatosplenomegaly (H&E, original magnification ×25).

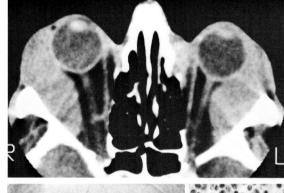

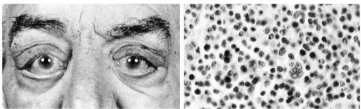

TABLE 12-11.
INCIDENCE OF PRIMARY EPITHELIAL TUMORS OF THE LACRIMAL GLAND

Authors	Number of Cases	Benign Mixed	Malignant Mixed	Adenoid–Cystic	Other Carcinomas
Font and Gamel	265	136 (51%)	34 (13%)	70 (27%)	25 (9%)
Henderson	41	13 (32%)	10 (24%)	12 (29%)	6 (15%)
Ashton	54	30 (55%)	2 (4%)	13 (24%)	9 (17%)
Wright, 1968–1981	54	30 (55.5%)	3 (5.5%)	11 (20%)	10 (19%)
Total	414	209 (50%)	49 (12%)	106 (25%)	54 (13%)

mixed tumors and other carcinomas (Table 12-11). Our series represents the experience of a single clinician with a relatively stable referral base in which epithelial tumors of the lacrimal gland constituted 5% of orbital neoplasia. Various authors report incidences ranging from 3% to 8%.

The majority of the epithelial tumors arise from the orbital lobe of the lacrimal gland, thus tending to reach a relatively large size before presentation. The clinical picture is dominated by mass effect leading to a downward and inward displacement of the eye with varying degrees of proptosis. Characteristically, the gland continues to function and the remaining ocular and orbital structures reflect mass effect leading to indentation of the globe, choroidal folds (Fig. 12-94), and mechanical limitation of movement in the direction of the mass. Temporal development roughly parallels the underlying character of the neoplasm. Benign mixed tumors are noninfiltrative, slow-growing masses, whereas the malignant tumors are

either silent masses or are characterized by features of infiltration including pain (due to perineural and bone invasion), a relatively rapid onset (generally less than 1 year), and soft tissue entrapment. The distinction between malignant and benign neoplasms is based on the clinical features described as well as orbital imaging studies. Benign tumors tend to show excavation of adjacent bone without frank infiltration, a feature more common in malignancies (Figs. 12-95 to 12-97; compare with Fig. 12-103). Other findings suggesting malignant rather than benign epithelial lesions include the presence of calcification in the tumor, and serrated or irregular margins between the tumor and surrounding tissue (see Fig. 12-103). Ultrasonography may delineate a condensation or pseudocapsule in the benign masses and may also help to distinguish between solid epithelial tumors and the lymphoproliferative group. The clinical and investigative features do not necessarily provide distinct and universal differentiation, and individual cases can cross boundaries. For instance, in the young patient, because of plasticity of bone, excavation rather than erosion may occur more readily in malignant tumors, mimicking benign mixed tumor. Nevertheless, the large majority of these lesions can be diagnosed with available technology prior to management.

Studies on the histogenesis of epithelial lacrimal gland tumors suggest that they are of ectodermal origin. In particular, both Dardick and Iwamoto suggest that benign mixed tumors are derived from cells of the epithelium with potential for multidirectional differentiation.

PLEOMORPHIC ADENOMA (BENIGN MIXED TUMOR)

Pleomorphic adenoma is the term used in the World Health Organization classification of epithelial tumors of the lacrimal gland. It accurately describes the nature of the neoplasm with its widely varying histologic picture, although the traditional term *benign mixed tumor* remains popular. They usually occur in the second to fifth decades, with the peak incidence in the fourth. However,

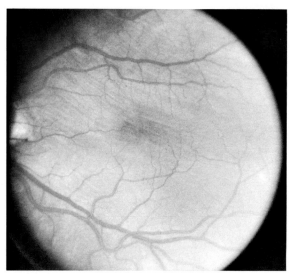

FIGURE 12-94. Superotemporal choroidal folds seen in a patient with a benign mixed tumor of the lacrimal gland.

they have been described in a range from childhood through the eighth decade. There is a slight male to female preponderance of 1.5–2:1. They commonly present as slow-growing tumors with a progressive, painless downward and inward displacement of the globe and axial proptosis (see Fig. 12-95). The degree of proptosis varies with the size of the mass posterior to the equator. Symptoms are usually present for over 12 months and are unassociated with any features of inflammation. On investigation, there is evidence of enlargement or expansion of the lacrimal fossa due to pressure erosion (see Figs. 12-95 to 12-97). The lesion itself appears well-circumscribed and may have a slightly nodular configuration. On standardized A-mode echography there may be a definable pseudocapsule. Large tumors may be associated with blurring of vision, diplopia, retinal and choroidal striae (see Fig. 12-94), and very occasionally, swelling of the optic nerve head.

On gross pathologic examination they appear as grayish-white, bosselated, solitary masses that are well circumscribed by a pseudocapsule (see Figs. 12-95, 12-96). The pseudocapsule is a deceptive component of the lesion, and histology shows excrescences invading this condensation (see Fig. 12-95B). It is this feature that has led to a high incidence of recurrence when a margin of normal tissue is not removed with the tumor at the time of excision. Pleomorphic adenomas also have a propensity to recur when the capsule is incised for direct biopsy (32% compared to 3% recurrence without incisional biopsy).

Histologically, these tumors have a diverse pattern. Although the histogenesis is believed to be epithelial, there are two morphologic components. One is composed of cells resembling ductal epithelium, whereas the other consists of stellate, spindle cells streaming in a loosely arranged stroma (see Figs. 12-95 to 12-97). The ductal cells tend to be arranged as irregular islands, tubules, anastomosing ducts, and as the lining of mucus-containing cysts (see Figs. 12-95, 12-97). The stromal component may be myxoid, hyalinized, pseudocartilaginous, or calcified and occasionally demonstrates bone formation. Occasionally, the spindle cell population may dominate the picture. The epithelial component may undergo metaplasia, forming squamous cysts and eddies (see Fig. 12-97C). Some of the areas may be densely cellular. An important feature is the presence of microscopic nodular extensions into the pseudocapsule, which account for the tendency to recurrence when appropriate margins are not taken (see Fig. 12-95B).

Management and Prognosis

The prognosis of pleomorphic adenomas is excellent, and if one studies combined series it approaches 99% survival. Nevertheless, when not properly handled, the morbidity of this tumor can be significant. A number of studies have emphasized the high recurrence rate following incomplete excision or incisional biopsy. In addition, authors have noted the importance of careful surgical excision without capsular rupture. It is important to establish the specific diagnosis prior to surgical intervention. It has also been emphasized that recurrence following incomplete excision may take a long time (up to 30 years) and may be associated with malignant transformation.

Effective management implies extirpative biopsy by a modified lateral orbitotomy. Important aspects are a wide surgical exposure, microscopic dissection of the lid and lateral portion of the levator aponeurosis to identify and excise the palpebral lobe, an extraperiosteal approach on the lateral portion of the tumor, and an excision of a margin of orbital fat medially. The extension of the palpebral lobe can be excised with an ellipse of conjunctiva where the lacrimal ducts open into the fornix. When care is taken to remove this tumor, the incidence of recurrence drops to virtually zero.

CARCINOMA AND PLEOMORPHIC ADENOMA (MALIGNANT MIXED TUMOR)

Jack Rootman and Peter Dolman

The reported frequency of malignant mixed tumors ranges from 4% to 24% and averages 12%. Early series reported no sex predilection for malignant mixed tumors; however, Font and Gamel found different sex ratios for subtypes of malignant mixed tumors. Adenocarinoma arising in a benign mixed tumor was three times more common in males, whereas adenoid cystic carcinoma in benign mixed tumor was twice as common in females and overall malignant mixed tumor was almost twice as common in males. The age range is from 15 to 80 years with an average of 50 years.

Clinical and Pathologic Features

Malignant mixed tumors have the histologic features of a benign mixed tumor with areas of malignant change (Fig. 12-98). The latter are usually poorly differentiated adenocarcinoma, but may have areas of adenoid cystic change or even squamous or sarcomatoid degeneration. When noninvasive, the anaplastic foci may in fact be carcinoma in situ. On the other hand, these tumors may appear as infiltrative and invasive lesions extending into the surrounding soft tissues and bone, particularly when they arise in recurrent incompletely excised tumors. The malignant areas are generally believed to arise from transformation either in a primary lacrimal gland pleomorphic

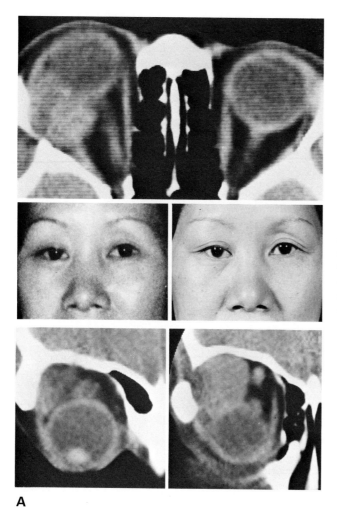

FIGURE 12-95. *(A)* This 50-year-old woman presented with a long-standing history of progressive right proptosis, which was evident on retrospective photographs taken 5 years earlier *(left)*. On axial *(top)* and coronal *(bottom)* CT scans, she shows a multilobular well-defined mass with smooth excavation of the adjacent orbital roof and a focal absence of the lateral orbital wall.

A

adenoma or in its recurrence. There are three clinical circumstances in which malignant mixed tumors arise. The first is a sudden expansion of an indolent long-standing lacrimal mass reflecting a malignant transformation. The second presentation parallels those seen in other varieties of lacrimal epithelial malignancies, and includes pain, bony infiltration, and rapid growth. The third clinical situation is a sudden recurrence of a previously excised mixed tumor of the lacrimal gland.

Management and Prognosis

As with the other rare malignant epithelial neoplasms, the management remains controversial. When preoperative evaluation indicates a malignant tumor, recommended therapy is surgical and involves a protocol of percutaneous perseptal biopsy followed by radical en bloc orbitectomy as defined for adenoid cystic carcinoma.

On the other hand, when these tumors arise as a component of a benign mixed tumor they are usually approached by lateral orbitotomy and en bloc excision. If malignant transformation is discovered locally within the mass, a wider excision of adjacent tissues should be carried out, and some would argue for more radical orbitectomy. The role of radiotherapy has not been clearly established in the treatment of this tumor. The average recurrence rate of malignant mixed tumor following surgery from a combined series is 72%. Roughly 70% of these recurrences were restricted to the orbit, whereas the remaining 30% were divided among orbital bones, paranasal sinuses, and intracranial cavity. About half of the patients had died at the time of publication, and Font

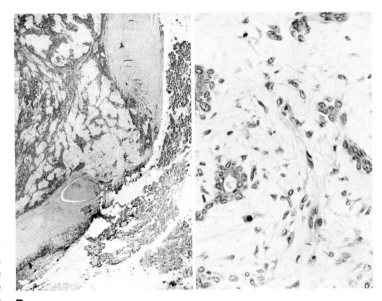

B

FIGURE 12-95 *(Continued).* *(B)* Histopathology of this benign mixed tumor was obtained from a complete excision of the mass and adjacent lacrimal gland. Note the two typical morphologic components of a loosely arranged stroma containing stellate cells and islands or tubules surrounded by ductal epithelium. The low-power photomicrograph *(left)* demonstrates an excrescence extending through the pseudocapsule (H&E, original magnifications *left* × 2.5, *right* × 25). *(C)* Electron micrograph obtained from the same tumor shows ductular structures with a distinct lumen (L), junctional complexes, and secretory granules. There are also outer spindle-shaped cells and loose stroma. *(Inset)* Cytoplasmic tonofilaments suggest squamous differentiation (original magnifications × 4170, *inset* × 32,500).

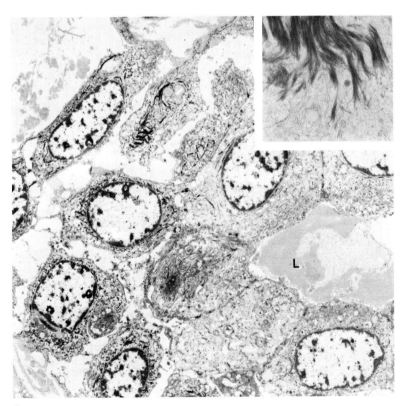

C

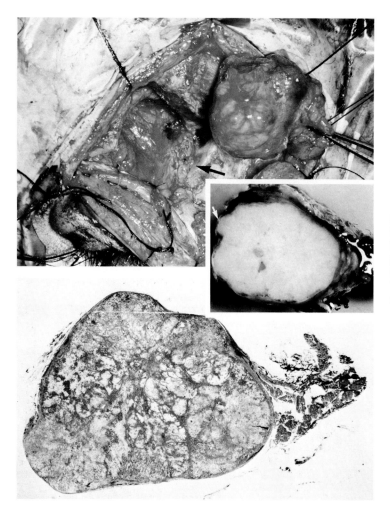

FIGURE 12-96. This composite demonstrates the surgical, gross, and low-power microscopic features of a benign mixed tumor of the lacrimal gland. Note the bosselated surface with corresponding excavation of bone *(arrows)* and the "mixed" nature of the tumor (H&E, original magnification × 2).

and Gamel report that 30% of their patients had died of tumor at 5 years, 45% at 10 years, and 50% by 12 years. These rates are better than *de novo* adenoid cystic carcinoma and adenocarcinoma, but are considerably worse than the benign mixed tumor. At the time of death, roughly 50% of patients had intracranial extension of the tumor and a further 30% had distant metastases to lung, chest wall, or bone. Because recurrence can occur over a very long period of time and most cases in the literature had been followed for less than 10 years, many could succumb to recurrence and metastases later, worsening the mortality statistics. Overall, it would appear that patients with carcinoma in situ have a better prognosis than those with extension beyond the capsule or those with occurrences in areas of recurrent benign mixed tumor.

ADENOID CYSTIC CARCINOMA

Adenoid cystic carcinoma is the most common epithelial carcinoma of the lacrimal gland. It occurs in either sex with a peak in the fourth decade. Wright has suggested a bimodal distribution for this tumor with a peak in the second and fourth decades. Again, these tumors are dominated by mass effect with a more rapid temporal sequence (under 1 year) when compared to the benign mixed tumor (over 1 year). In addition, because of the propensity of this tumor to invade perineurally and into adjacent bone, pain and more rarely paresthesia may be associated with this tumor. The incidence of pain is reported between 40% and 9% in different series. Radiographs may show areas of pressure erosion, bony destruc-

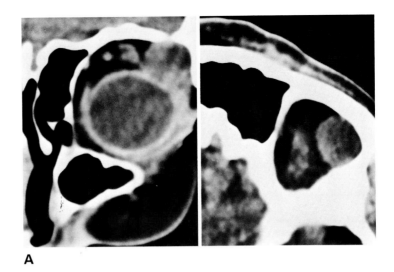

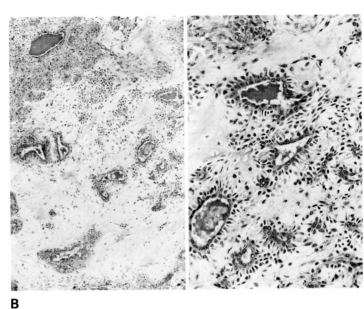

FIGURE 12-97. CT and histologic features of a benign mixed tumor of the lacrimal gland. *(A)* CT scan shows well-defined margins associated with excavation of the adjacent bone. *(B)* Histologically, this lesion had both the cuboidal and stellate component with a myxoid stroma. *(C)* Focal area of squamous metaplasia in a benign mixed tumor of the lacrimal gland (H&E, original magnifications *B, left* × 2.5; *B, right* × 10; *C* × 25).

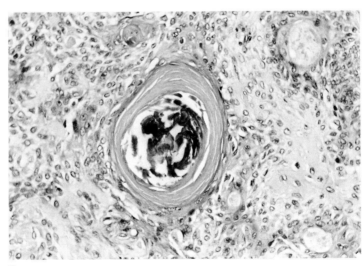

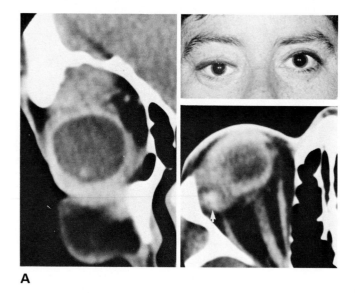

A

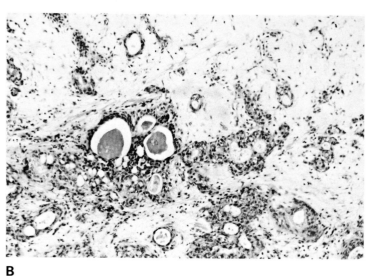

B

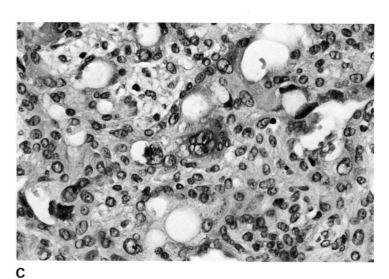

C

FIGURE 12-98. *(A)* This 35-year-old woman presented with a 5-year history of downward displacement of the right eye, increased tearing, and double vision in extreme right gaze. On physical examination, she had a firm, nodular mass protruding just behind the junction of the outer one third and inner two thirds of the superior orbital rim. The globe was 1 mm inward, 6 mm downward, and 3 mm proptosed. CT scan showed a soft tissue mass with focal calcification *(arrow)* and excavation of adjacent bone. The patient underwent an excisional biopsy of the tumor, lacrimal gland, and adjacent soft tissues with gross total removal within the capsule. *(B)* Histopathologically, the lesion had the typical features of a benign mixed tumor of the lacrimal gland, but in focal areas *(C)* there was evidence of malignant transformation with large anaplastic cells. Thus, the final diagnosis was benign mixed tumor of the lacrimal gland with *in situ* malignant transformation (H&E, original magnifications *B* × 10, *C* × 40).

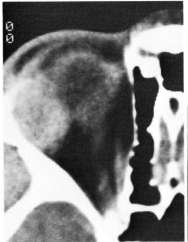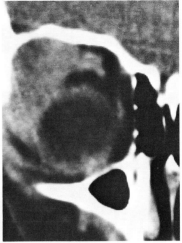

FIGURE 12-99. Axial and coronal CT scans demonstrate a large, well-defined anterolateral orbital mass with excavation of adjacent bone in a 14-year-old boy. Histologically, it proved to be an adenoid cystic carcinoma, and was treated by radical en bloc orbitectomy. Excavation in youth can be a misleading sign because the bone at that age is more easily and more rapidly sculpted by a tumor.

tion, or calcification in the lacrimal fossa. The tumor mass may be less well circumscribed on CT scan and can extend toward the orbital apex. The most distressing aspect of the fundamental pathology of this carcinoma is its tendency to perineural invasion, which may extend centimeters beyond the apparent margins of the solid mass. This feature has been well documented in similar tumors of the parotid gland and is a dominant factor in the prognosis. In fact, cases have been described of relatively well-defined, apparently localized tumors showing clinical features of extension well beyond the apparent margins (i.e., cavernous sinus involvement). We should point out that because this tumor has a tendency to occur in young persons, the investigative features suggesting invasion of adjacent structures may not be obvious because the youthful orbital bones may have a tendency to undergo localized expansion more readily than the less pliable adult orbit (Fig. 12-99). We have noticed this feature in two children, one aged 11 years and the second aged 14 years, who presented with adenoid cystic carcinomas of the lacrimal gland.

Pathology

Grossly, adenoid cystic carcinoma is grayish-white with a firm, nodular surface, and there may be a suggestion of an incomplete capsule. Microscopically, the cell population consists of densely packed hyperchromatic small cells with scant cytoplasm. These cells appear to proliferate around cystic spaces that contain a mucicarmine-positive material (Fig. 12-100). The cystic spaces vary considerably in size and number and may be so numerous as to give it a typical "Swiss cheese" pattern. On the other hand, the tumor may be dominantly cellular, forming solid cords. The border of the epithelial components is usually sharply demarcated from dense surrounding con-

nective tissue. The tumor tends to spread along the adventitia of orbital nerves and vessels and invade adjacent structures. Five histologic patterns have been described: Swiss cheese (cribriform), sclerosing, basaloid (solid), comedocarincomatous, and tubular (ductal). Each of these may constitute only a part of the tumor itself, and in the case of lacrimal gland adenoid cystic carcinoma only one pattern has a suggested prognostic implication. The presence of a solid basaloid component to the tumor is believed by Font and co-workers to worsen the prognosis (Fig. 12-101). On the other hand, Waller and colleagues have noted no specific correlation with histologic patterns.

Management and Prognosis

The prognosis for adenoid cystic carcinoma remains dismal, and the clinical course is one of painful local and regional recurrence followed by systematization. The course is not infrequently prolonged and extremely distressing. Often the die is cast at the time of presentation, the tumor having clearly escaped the bounds of surgical extirpation. Biologically, it is a tumor demanding complete excision, because radiotherapy has not been clearly shown to be efficacious. However, because of the involvement and immediacy of the cranial nerves, the bounds of excision may have been breached. Nevertheless, when the tumor appears to be confined to the orbital tissues the recommended therapy is en bloc excision of the orbit and its contents by a multidisciplinary team (orbital surgeon, neurosurgeon, and craniofacial surgeon). Excision should include the orbital roof, the lateral wall, the lids, and the anterior portion of the temporalis muscle where the zygomaticofrontal and zygomaticotemporal nerves extend. Radical radiotherapy is often recommended as an adjunctive measure, but

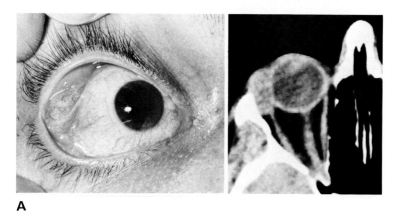

A

FIGURE 12-100. *(A)* Clinical photograph and axial CT scan of a patient who presented with a focal palpable tumor mass in the lacrimal fossa with slight flattening of the globe. There were no features of orbital infiltration or sensory loss. The lesion was removed totally by lateral orbitotomy. *(B)* Histopathologically, the mass proved to be an adenoid cystic carcinoma with a typical "Swiss cheese" pattern. Note cords of epithelial cells surrounded by dense connective tissue. In view of the diagnosis, a wide local excision of the adjacent bone and soft tissues (excluding the extraocular muscles and eye) was done. There has been no recurrence to date (4-year follow-up) (H&E, original magnifications *left* × 2.5, *right* × 10).

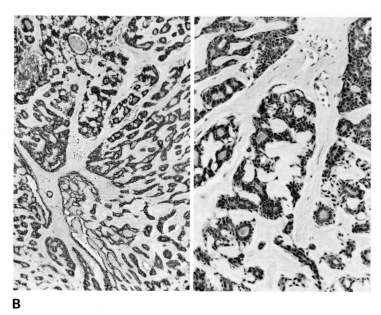

B

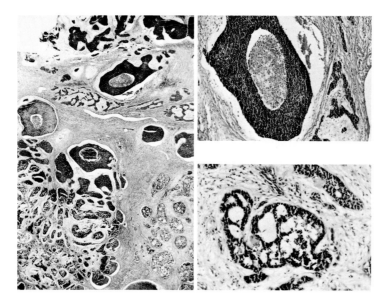

FIGURE 12-101. Histopathologic features of an aggressive, widely infiltrating, rapidly growing basaloid adenoid cystic carcinoma of the lacrimal gland. Note cords of solid tumor cells with central foci of necrosis and focal area of a more typical adenoid cystic pattern *(bottom right)* (H&E, original magnifications *left* × 2.5, *right* × 10).

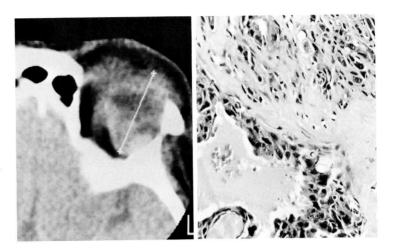

FIGURE 12-102. A well-defined, slow-growing lacrimal mass that on axial CT scan demonstrates excavation of the adjacent orbital wall and inhomogeneous pattern. This mucoepidermoid carcinoma was completely excised along with the adjacent lacrimal gland. It had a dense capsule containing cords of both mucin-producing and epidermoid cells. Note pools of mucin (H&E, original magnifications × 10).

is not of clearly proven efficacy. Although slightly encouraging results have been reported recently, the overall prognosis remains poor.

ADENOCARCINOMA

Adenocarcinomas may arise *de novo* or within a benign mixed tumor. In Font and Gamel's series, those arising *de novo* constituted 7% of cases. Clinically, they are aggressive, rapidly growing masses that often exceed the limits of adequate surgical excision at the time of presentation. Henderson has noted a tendency for them to extend below the horizontal raphe and deeply within the orbit. The clinical features parallel those of adenoid cystic carcinoma, which is, after all, a subgroup of adenocarcinomas in general.

Histologically, they consist of proliferating bundles of cells with varying degrees of anaplasia; the nuclei vary in size, staining properties, and nuclear-to-cytoplasmic ratio. In addition, frequent mitoses and a sparse connective tissue stroma are noted. With increasing degrees of malignancy the tendency to glandular differentiation is less evident.

Prognosis and Management

Adenocarcinomas share the poor prognosis of adenoid cystic carcinoma. They tend to occur in an older age group (fifth and sixth decades) and most commonly in males (74% versus 26%). Management is directed towards wide en bloc surgical excision when possible. Radiotherapy as an adjunct has been advocated, but is not of proven efficacy. The overall survival is around 25% to 30%.

MUCOEPIDERMOID CARCINOMA

Mucoepidermoid carcinoma is believed to arise from the ductal epithelium of the lacrimal gland. It occurs more commonly in minor salivary glands and is rare in the lacrimal gland. Histologically, it is classified as either low or high grade depending on the degree of differentiation and the amount of mucin production. The low-grade tumors have larger numbers of mucin-producing cells and variable epidermoid cells (Fig. 12-102). High-grade tumors are dominated by epidermoid cells with less frequent mucus-secreting cells, which may be identified using special stains (Fig. 12-103). Thus, specimens must include multiple sections with the use of histochemical and immunohistochemical stains to identify mucoid and squamous differentiation.

Prognosis and Management

It is suggested that the prognosis of mucoepidermoid carcinoma parallels the histologic grading, but there are so few described in the literature it is difficult to draw conclusions. We have seen two such tumors that appear to span the spectrum. One was a rapidly developing, massively infiltrating tumor in an older patient. The tumor was treated by debulking, local bone resection, and radiotherapy in 1981 (see Fig. 12-103). The patient is currently disease free 4 years following therapy. The second tumor of this variety had all of the cardinal clinical features of a benign mixed tumor and appeared histologically to be well encapsulated and well differentiated (see Fig. 12-102). It was treated surgically as a benign mixed tumor with wide, local extirpation and the patient has been disease free since 1982. Generally speaking, treatment ought to parallel the biologic behavior as inferred from the histology of this rare tumor.

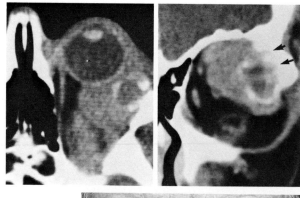

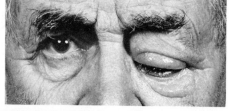

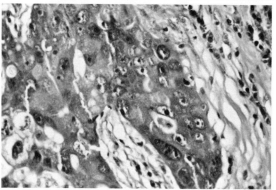

FIGURE 12-103.   Axial and coronal CT scans and histopathologic features of a rapidly developing infiltrative tumor of the lacrimal gland. It proved to be a poorly differentiated mucoepidermoid carcinoma. This 77-year-old man presented with 13 mm of proptosis, marked limitation of ocular movements, counting fingers vision, marked swelling, and firm tumefaction of the superolateral orbital soft tissue. Irregular erosion of adjacent bone *(arrows)* due to invasion by the tumor and calcification within favor a malignancy (H&E, original magnification × 25).

SQUAMOUS CARCINOMA

A squamous carcinoma involving all of the lacrimal gland is a rare entity and is more often a feature of focal metaplasia. Nevertheless, it has been described as a tumor of the lacrimal gland. The cellular features are those of squamous differentiation with infiltrative margins, variable keratinization, and varying degrees of differentiation. It shares the poor prognosis of the other types of carcinomas of the lacrimal gland and is treated in a similar manner.

Regardless of the technique of treatment, the prognosis with lacrimal gland malignancies is dismal. The major factors governing the poor prognosis are intimacy to surrounding structures, relatively late presentation, and the ease of penetrating the tissue planes of the orbit.

Overall Management Protocol

The major steps in management of tumors of the lacrimal area consist of accurate clinical and investigative categorization into inflammatory, structural, and neoplastic processes. The acute inflammatory diseases are generally well defined on the basis of dramatic onset and localized features of inflammation. Once specific etiology is ruled out, idiopathic acute inflammation can be treated with a short course of corticosteroids. Failure to resolve over a short period of time (days to weeks) should lead to incisional biopsy. Lesions with a subacute or chronic onset and investigative features that suggest a nondestructive localized infiltration assuming the contours of the adjacent structures should lead to incisional biopsy and appropriate management based on the histology.

In the area of neoplasia, the fundamental problem consists of differentiating epithelial from nonepithelial malignancies. The large majority of the nonepithelial lesions are lymphoproliferative and characterized by insidious, painless onset in an older age group and associated conjunctival involvement. In addition, they are frequently bilateral and on investigation have a tendency to contour to, rather than indent, adjacent structures. The core of the management problem in epithelial malignancies consists of differentiating between benign mixed tumor of the lacrimal gland and carcinomas. Generally speaking, benign mixed tumor is dominated by mass effect without invasive features and a long-standing painless history. In contrast, the carcinomas have a more aggressive temporal sequence, are associated with pain in about one third of cases, and orbital imaging suggests infiltration of adjacent structures, destruction of bone, and calcification.

A synthesis of the constellation of features described both clinically and on investigation provides a rationale for managing these complex and diverse lesions, and frequently yields accurate diagnoses. Nevertheless, I can think of no other focus within the orbit in which the diagnostic gray areas have such profound and important consequences to the patient. Marginal or elusive cases plague and humble the physician; it is these cases in which early accurate identification remains an urgent goal.

■ METASTATIC AND SECONDARY TUMORS OF THE ORBIT

Jack Rootman

Orbital Metastasis

Jack Rootman, Joseph Ragaz, Roy Cline, and Jocelyn S. Lapointe

Metastasis of solid tumors to the orbit appears to be increasing in frequency, reflecting the change in natural history and prolonged longevity of cancer patients treated with modern modalities. This longevity may contribute to an increasing number of occurrences in rare metastatic sites such as the orbit. In addition, the eye and central nervous system, because they are pharmacologic sanctuaries, are more frequent sites of metastatic disease.

The major pathophysiology of orbital metastases reflects the nature of the site and the character of the underlying neoplasm. This varies from rapidly developing masses, often with adjacent tissue infiltration or bone destruction or both, to slow cicatrization of soft tissues. The characteristic clinical features of most metastases is their unrestricted growth, which leads to local infiltra-

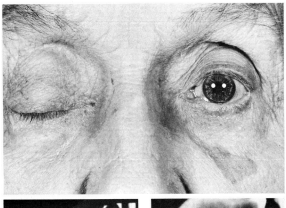
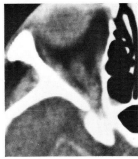
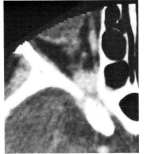

FIGURE 12-104. This 81-year-old woman suddenly developed ptosis on the right side, and complete ophthalmoplegia over several weeks. It was associated with a decrease of vision to hand movements, a fixed pupil, 3 mm of proptosis, and reduced sensation of the first and second division of the fifth nerve. The CT scan shows a well-demarcated, enhancing apical orbital mass that extends into the optic canal and minimally through the superior orbital fissure. A complete systemic survey with a potential diagnosis of metastatic disease disclosed no primary tumor. She died within 2 months of widespread carcinomatosis; a primary was not identified.

tion and entrapment of structures. Thus, the major clinical signs and symptoms in the orbit are proptosis and displacement due to the mass effect, and functional deficits reflecting infiltration and pressure effects (Fig. 12-104). Metastatic masses cause firm axial proptosis when retrobulbar (50% in our series) or solid palpable lumps (Fig. 12-105; also see Fig. 12-114) when anteriorly located. Enophthalmos may be the result of cicatrization (25% of our patients) (Fig. 12-106). The functional deficits include motor abnormalities with diplopia, limitation of movement, and ptosis (Fig. 12-107), whereas the sensory abnormalities include the common occurrence of a dull, aching pressure-like pain, paresthesia, and visual loss (especially if located apically). More rarely, neoplasia may be prone to sudden changes, like necrosis and hemorrhage (neuroblastoma is a classic example; Fig. 12-108), and catastrophic onset with either ecchymosis or inflam-

(Text continues on p. 409.)

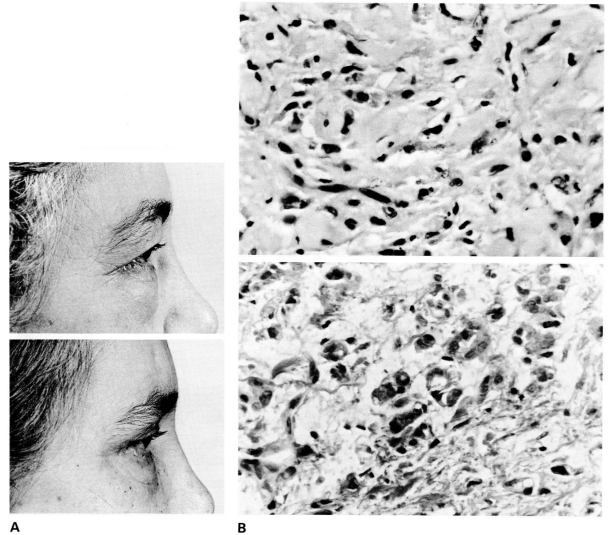

A   **B**

FIGURE 12-105. *(A)* This 62-year-old woman presented with a 4-month history of progressive tender swelling of the right lower lid anteceded by pain. She had had a mastectomy 1 year earlier for carcinoma of the breast, and she had known metastases to bone. The mass was firm, tender, and associated with local hypoesthesia and upward displacement of the globe. CT scan showed an inferior diffuse infiltrative orbital mass (not shown). *(B)* An attempted aspiration biopsy was negative, but a small open biopsy revealed diffuse cords of relatively poorly differentiated adenocarcinoma insinuated between tissue planes and associated with desmoplasia *(top)*. The tumor cells had mucin-positive vacuoles and a pseudoglandular arrangement *(bottom)*. Because this was the patient's only good eye, she was treated with 2000 rad in five fractions and had a good local response *(A, bottom)*. She lived for 18 months after treatment without local recurrence.

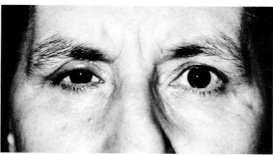

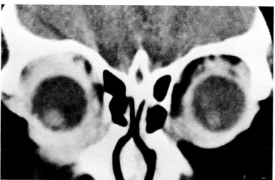

FIGURE 12-106. This 53-year-old woman was referred with a history of right ptosis associated with blurring of vision occurring over a 6-month period. She had reduced extraocular movements, a firm orbit, a narrow interpalpebral fissure, slightly injected firm skin, and an enophthalmos of 3 mm on the right side. Coronal and axial CT scans demonstrated an infiltrative mass involving the anterior orbit, encasing the globe, and extending into the upper lid. The patient had a carcinoma of the breast diagnosed 3 years earlier. Biopsy revealed a scirrhous carcinoma with ductal features that was estrogen-receptor positive. The lower photograph was taken 1 year after diagnosis and following radiotherapy, chemotherapy, and hormonal therapy. There is marked improvement in local symptoms and signs.

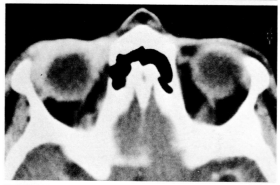

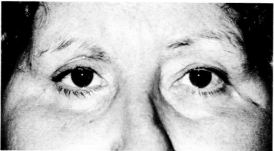

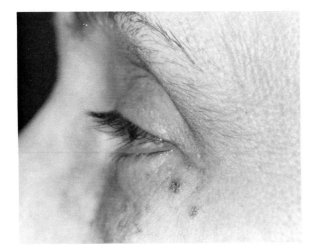

FIGURE 12-107. This 53-year-old woman presented with left enophthalmos 4 months after a diagnosis of metastatic breast carcinoma to bone. She had a firm cicatrized orbit with reduced extraocular movements due to breast metastasis.

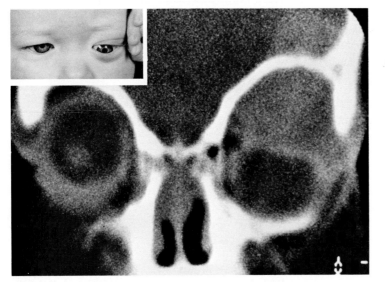

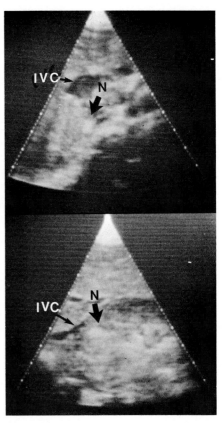

A   **B**

FIGURE 12-108. *(A)* This 1-year-old child was admitted in 1980 with a 2-week history of redness and crusting of the left eye associated with gradual protrusion and downward displacement. A contrast-enhanced coronal CT scan demonstrated a large, irregularly enhancing orbital mass flattening the globe and extending through the orbital roof (area of bone destruction not shown) into the anterior cranial fossa. In the section shown, the orbital roof is slightly bowed superiorly and the anterior cranial fossa mass is seen. *(B)* Ultrasonography demonstrated a 3-cm to 4-cm mass (N) in the region of the right adrenal gland *(top,* transverse scan; *bottom,* coronal scan). A tumor was also noted in the region of the vena cava (IVC). The bone marrow biopsy revealed heavy infiltration with neuroblastoma, and bone scan demonstrated a metastatic lesion in the left femur. The patient was treated with systemic chemotherapy and orbital radiotherapy, but died of stage IV neuroblastoma within 1 year.

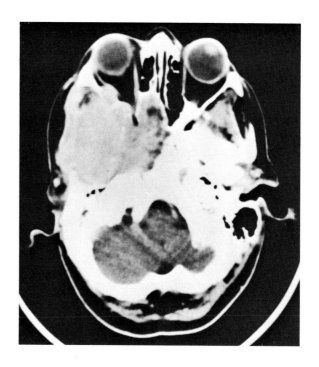

FIGURE 12-109. CT scan shows a large right inferotemporal, parapharyngeal, and nasopharyngeal enhancing mass lesion. It demonstrated patchy, irregular, inner areas of decreased density, and had destroyed the medial aspect of the right skull base, the base of the sphenoid bone, the posterolateral wall of the orbit, and the posterior margin of the nasal aperture. It was seen in a 67-year-old woman with a 1-month history of reduced vision. On physical examination she had no light perception, an afferent pupillary defect, 6 mm of proptosis, and 4 mm of downward displacement of the right eye. In addition, ocular movement was limited. The patient had a history of a follicular carcinoma of the thyroid gland diagnosed 6 years earlier, with known metastases to the occipital region of the skull treated 1 year prior to this presentation.

matory signs. Another rare phenomenon is pulsation due to increased vascularity of some tumors (thyroid and renal cell carcinoma) or bone destruction with transmission of cranial pulsation (Fig. 12-109). Simultaneous or consecutive bilaterality is not unheard of, and in our experience occurred in 14% of cases (Fig. 12-110). At initial presentation, 7% to 9% of patients with orbital metastases may have bilateral disease; Henderson has emphasized that this incidence will double with follow up and disclosure of subsequent contralateral involvement. In addition, simultaneous ocular metastasis may rarely occur (Fig. 12-111). All of these factors may produce misleading signs and symptoms that should raise the clinician's index of suspicion. In our series, these signs and symptoms include reduced extraocular movements (60%); proptosis (55%); ptosis (35%); nonaxial displacement of the globe (35%); lid mass (30%); pain (25%); enophthalmos (25%); and reduced visual acuity (14%). Nontender inflammation of the orbit (Figs. 12-112, 12-113; also see Fig. 12-106) may also be a feature of orbital metastases (14%) along with unusual signs such as ecchymosis and pulsation. Overall, the major distinguishing clinical features of orbital metastases are the constellation of relentless, relatively rapid progression (generally months) and associated motor and sensory symptoms.

An unusual feature of orbital metastases that bears specific mention is the occurrence of enophthalmos (Fig. 12-114; also see Fig. 12-107). This is brought about by cicatrization, which causes retraction as the collagen matures and the myofibroblasts contract. The overwhelming majority of enophthalmic orbital metastases are caused by breast carcinoma, but cicatrization has also been noted with GI, lung, and prostate carcinomas. In fact, GI carcinomas frequently present with metastases and occult primaries. Enophthalmos is an insidious and gradual process that leads to ptosis, restricted extraocular movements, and reduced corneal sensation. Characteristically, the orbit is "rock hard," vision is frequently reduced, and there may be surprisingly little pain. Because of the insidious and gradual onset, both patients and physicians are frequently unaware of the development of the signs and symptoms.

Other important factors to consider are epidemiology and specific variations depending on tumor types. In our series, metastases constituted 10.5% of orbital tumors. In the literature, incidence varied from 2% to 10% depending on the particular bias of the study. Metastases in most circumstances occur in patients with known malignancies, as was the case in 80% of those seen in our clinic. But they can be either a very late manifestation (i.e., even after many years) or a presenting symptom in some patients (30% according to Henderson, 20% according to Rootman). Thus, careful historical questioning is necessary in the first circumstance and accurate tissue diagnosis in the latter. Sex and age are also relevant because the malignancies commonly metastasizing to the

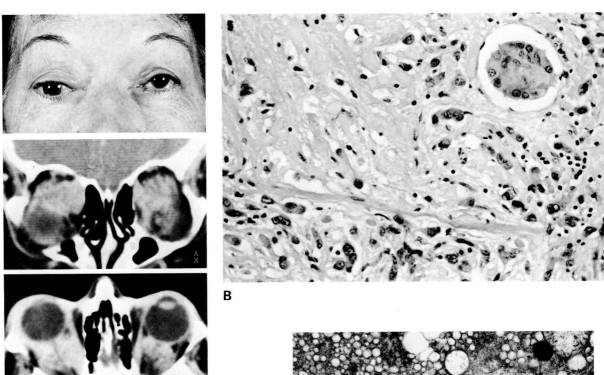

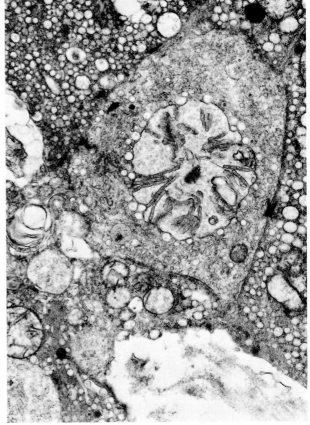

A

B

C

FIGURE 12-110. *(A)* This 63-year-old woman presented with an 8-month history of progressive right ocular and retrobulbar pain accentuated by ocular movement. She had also become aware of diplopia present for about 4 months. In addition, the left lower lid began to swell 3 months prior to presentation. On physical examination, she had bilaterally narrowed interpalpebral fissures with solid nodular fixed masses involving the lid, and the superior and inferior orbital rims. There was 3 mm of downward displacement of the right eye, limited levator function, and slight right proptosis. She also had a 15-D right hypotropia and marked limitation of movement bilaterally. Coronal and axial CT scans showed enhancing soft tissue densities in the retro-orbital space bilaterally, surrounding the optic nerves and extending around both globes to varying degrees. The infiltrations were confluent with the extraocular muscles and the right globe was proptotic. Biopsy revealed a firm, fibrous mass. *(B)* Histologic examination revealed a poorly differentiated cicatrizing adenocarcinoma with some focal glandular differentiation (H&E, original magnification × 25). *(C)* Electron microscopy revealed a columnar cell with brush border and cytoplasmic secretory vacuoles consistent with an adenocarcinoma (original magnification × 12,200). Systemic investigation failed to reveal a primary, but the patient subsequently developed liver metastases suggesting a primary source in the abdomen.

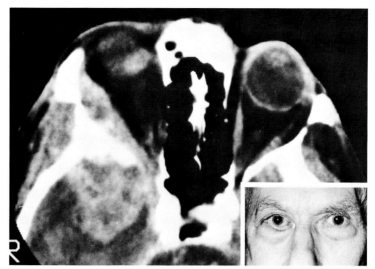

FIGURE 12-111.   This 80-year-old man was referred 6 months after having an "adenocarcinoma" of the right parotid excised. He had developed a prominent right eye with periorbital pain and infraorbital numbness. On physical examination, he had a right tarsorrhaphy, reduced vision on the right side to 20/200, 3 mm of inward displacement, and 3 mm of downward displacement, with 9 mm of right proptosis. In addition, he had a right afferent pupillary defect and on fundus examination had five choroidal metastases on the right and two on the left. A contrast-enhanced axial CT scan demonstrates a right-sided mass involving the lateral orbital wall, associated with hyperostosis and soft tissue components in the temporalis fossa and in the middle cranial fossa. Note choroidal metastasis on the right side. The bone appears irregular and partially destroyed, and the soft tissue density in the orbit obscured the lateral rectus muscle. On retrospective investigation, the patient was noted to have had a carcinoma of the prostate diagnosed on cystoscopy 4 months prior to his referral. Review of the original tissue specimen led to a diagnosis of metastatic prostatic carcinoma to parotid with extension into the infratemporal fossa, right orbit, and right middle cranial fossa as well as bilateral uveal metastases.

orbit have distinct relationships to these factors (compare Tables 12-12 to 12-15). Overall, childhood metastases are from undifferentiated sarcomas and adult metastases are from postembryonal carcinomas.

Breast carcinoma is the most common orbital metastasis in most series. Thus, female predominance is noted. Lung cancer is more frequent in men, as are gastrointestinal cancers and kidney tumors. The increasing frequency of lung cancers in women may alter this in the future. Prostate is, of course, exclusively male and is later in occurrence (generally in the late seventh decade). As to the relationship of age to metastases, most solid cancers occur in the fifth, sixth, and seventh decades with the exception of neuroblastoma (childhood) and some forms of breast cancer (see Tables 12-14 and 12-15). In fact, the prognosis of some cancers, such as neuroblastoma and Wilms' tumor, may relate to specific age subgroups (younger is generally better) and to the staging of the disease.

In our experience, the diagnosis is frequently unsuspected on referral (50% of cases) and the prevailing attitude may be somewhat hopeless with regard to management. It is worthwhile to note that half of our patients developed orbital metastases within 1 year of their primary. In spite of this, many patients fail to mention the past occurrence of cancer; thus, a thorough medical history is important in achieving a diagnosis.

The final factor of major importance is the primary histology. Carcinomas far outweigh sarcomas in orbital metastases, and the fundamental tumor biology affects the course and management of these lesions. For instance, as stated, carcinoma of the breast, gastrointestinal tract, and occasionally lung and prostate may be of a cicatrizing type producing enophthalmos (often not clinically recognized) and entrapment as primary signs. The cicatrizing type of breast carcinoma is often associated with clinical inflammatory features reflecting the underlying scarring and inflammation. Certain neoplasms re-

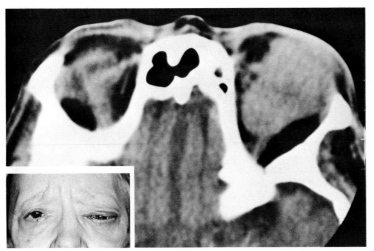

FIGURE 12-112. This 75-year-old woman was referred from a long-term care facility because they had noted recent swelling of her left eye. The swelling had been present for an unknown period of time. Physical examination revealed a left ptosis of 4 mm with reduced levator function, downward displacement of the globe, and 2 mm of proptosis. The upper lid appeared somewhat injected and swollen, and she had chemosis with restriction of upgaze. On palpation there was an indurated mass in the left upper lid and the orbit felt firm. The axial CT scan demonstrates a homogeneous mass in the superior orbit with well-defined, relatively smooth borders. A biopsy was done through a superior fornix incision. Histologically, the tumor consisted of a poorly differentiated small cell malignancy that had a trabecular pattern and was associated with considerable tumor cell necrosis. Cytologically, both on section and imprint, the tumor was most consistent with a poorly differentiated small cell carcinoma. Electron microscopy confirmed the epithelial nature of the tumor, and many cells contained uniform dense core granules. The findings were consistent with a small cell carcinoma, in particular metastatic oat cell carcinoma. Chest x-ray showed a mass in the right hilum with a probable parenchymal nodule in the right lobe.

spond to specific therapies based on their biology; for example, breast and prostate may respond significantly to hormonal manipulation (Fig. 12-115). Some cancers may have a tendency to metastasize to certain structures, such as skin melanoma and breast carcinoma to extraocular muscle (Figs. 12-116, 12-117) and prostatic carcinoma to bone. Other neoplasms have specific systemic associations, such as carcinoids with secretion of 5-hydroxytriptamines, producing the carcinoid syndrome. Some have bizarre and unusual features such as hypernephroma wherein the resection of a primary may lead to regression of the metastases. Seminoma may cause a nonmetastatic reversible proptosis.

Specification of particular tumor types is important and may require a biopsy with special immunohistochemical or tumor marking studies. The studies include the use of monoclonal antibodies for specific tumor types, cytology, histochemistry, and electron microscopy (Table 12-16; see Fig. 12-110).

Imaging studies also reflect the fundamental biology of these tumors. CT examination reveals infiltrative or circumscribed masses that may be related to specific structures, such as the lacrimal gland, or more often to the extraocular muscles (see Figs. 12-116, 12-117). Frequently there is widespread encasement of the globe or retrobulbar soft tissues (see Fig. 12-110), and there may be extension into the sinuses or the intracranial cavity associated with direct bone destruction (Fig. 12-118). In addition, extension may occur through the superior and inferior orbital fissures into the cavernous sinus. While bone destruction is not infrequent, calcification of metastases is rare. Areas of necrosis within a tumor may present as low-density foci. With intravenous contrast the metastases may enhance, a useful adjunct to detect intracranial spread of the tumor. Contrast is also helpful in detecting small lesions that are strategically located, for example, in the orbital apex (see Fig. 12-104), superior orbital fissure, or in the cavernous sinus. Ultrasonography may confirm the solid nature and infiltrative margins of these tumor masses.

In addition to imaging studies, a careful systemic evaluation is mandatory and would include radiologic investigation of the chest and abdomen, bone scans, and in some circumstances bone marrow biopsy. Because the orbit has no lymphatics, all metastases are hematologic and, therefore, must transit through the lung. Thus, the lung is a particularly important site to investigate. In addition, tumor-associated antigens such as carcinoembryonic antigen (CEA) may help detect unsuspected primaries and assess tumor load. As stated earlier, special histochemical and immunohistochemical techniques will help to delineate more specifically the tumor type and aid in planning therapy (see Tables 12-15, 12-16).

It should be noted that in the patient subpopulation presenting with metastases of an undifferentiated type, the primary source may be found in one third or less of patients, despite complete and often time-consuming assessment. Overall, this group of patients has a 2-year survival rate of about 10%; therefore, one ought to weigh the advantage and likelihood of specific diagnosis against the time, and the emotional and physical expenditure necessary to achieve a diagnosis when the quality of life may be at its best and is likely to rapidly deteriorate.

With longer duration of survival and improved methods of treatment, it is important to recognize these tumors and to institute treatment promptly to enhance the quality of life of these patients. Many patients, espe-

(Text continues on p. 422.)

TABLE 12-12.
SITE OF ORIGIN AND CLINICAL FEATURES OF ORBITAL METASTASIS, UNIVERSITY OF BRITISH COLUMBIA ORBITAL CLINIC, 1976–1986

Tumor Type	Number of Lesions
Breast	12
Gastrointestinal	4
Stomach 2	
Bowel 2	
Prostate	3
Lung	2
Unknown primary	3
Thyroid	1
Melanoma (skin)	1
Ovary	1
Liposarcoma	1
Neuroblastoma	1
Total	29
Bilateral	4
Breast 3	
GI 1	
Bone involved	9
Breast 2	
Prostate 2	
Unknown 2	
GI 1	
Thyroid 1	
Neuroblastoma 1	
Sex	
Female	20
Male	9
Enophthalmos	7
Breast 5	
Stomach 2	

TABLE 12-13.
COMBINED SERIES OF ORBITAL METASTASES

Tumor Type	Number	Percentage
Breast	81	39.9
Unknown primary	28	13.8
Lung	25	12.3
Neuroblastoma	18	8.9
Prostate	11	5.4
GI	10	5.0
Stomach 5		
Bowel 5		
Kidney	9	4.4
Melanoma (skin)	6	2.9
Thyroid	3	1.5
Miscellaneous	12	5.9
Testes 2 (1.0%)		
Adrenal 2		
Carcinoid 2		
Ovary 1 (0.5%)		
Hepatoma 1		
Liposarcoma 1		
Pancreas 1		
Parotid 1		
Hemangiopericytoma (costal) 1		
Total	203	

Font RL, Ferry AP: Carcinoma metastatic to the eye and orbit: III. A clinocopathologic study of 28 cases metastatic to the orbit. Cancer 38:1326, 1976

Henderson JW, Farrow GM: Orbital Tumors, 2nd ed, p 67. New York, Brian C Decker, 1980

Hou PK, Garg MP: Tumors of the orbit: A report of 193 consecutive cases. In Blodi FC (ed): Current Concepts in Ophthalmology, Vol 2, p 176. St Louis, CV Mosby, 1982

Jakobiec FA: Presentation, pathology and management of orbital metastatic disease. Presented at 5th International Symposium on Orbital Disorders. Amsterdam, September 1985

Jensen OA: Metastatic tumours of the eye and orbit. A histopathological analysis of a Danish series. Acta Pathol Microbiol Scand [Suppl] 212:201, 1970

Kennedy RE: An evaluation of 820 orbital cases. Trans Am Ophthalmol Soc 82:134, 1984

Rootman J: Orbital Metastatic disease. Presented at 5th International Symposium on Orbital Disorders. Amsterdam, September 1985

Shields JA, Bakewell B, Augsburger JJ et al: Classification and incidence of space-occupying lesions of the orbit. Arch Ophthalmol 102:1606, 1984

TABLE 12-14.
SUMMARY OF ORBITAL METASTASIS

General Clinical Features

Temporal features	Generally occur within 6 months of primary
	Relentless development over 3–4 months
	Rarely acute
General physiologic features	Infiltrative effects
	Motor—ptosis, decreased extraocular movements
	Sensory—pain
	Structural—mass effect or enophthalmos
Age occurrences	Children and infants
	Undifferentiated sarcomas
	Neuroblastoma
	Ewing's sarcoma
	Wilms' tumor
	Medulloblastoma
	Adults
	Postembryonal carcinoma
Sex	Male predominance
	Neuroblastoma (in children)
	Lung
	GI
	Hypernephroma
	Testicle
	Prostate
	Female predominance
	Breast
	Adrenal
	Thyroid

Special Features of Histologic Types in Orbit

Orbital propensity	Neuroblastoma
	Breast
	Ewing's sarcoma
Cicatrizing subgroup (± enophthalmos)	Breast
	GI
	Prostate
	Lung
Bone metastases	Breast—osteolytic > osteoblastic
	Prostate—osteoblastic > osteolytic
	Thyroid—osteolytic
Vascular with pulsation	Thyroid
	Hypernephroma
Bilateral	Breast
	Stomach
	Neuroblastoma (40%)
Particularly painful	Mucin-secreting adenocarcinoma
Muscle metastases	Skin melanoma—smooth contour on CT
	Breast—irregular and focal enlargement
	Oat cell
Hemorrhage and necrosis (ecchymosis)	Neuroblastoma
Orbital metastases as a presenting sign	Neuroblastoma (8%)
	Prostate
	Stomach
	Lung
	Kidney
	Gall bladder
	Pancreatic
	Testicular
	Undifferentiated
Nonmetastatic proptosis	Seminoma

TABLE 12-15.
ORBITAL METASTASIS BY COMMON TYPE IN ORDER OF FREQUENCY (COMBINED SERIES)

Tumor Type	Clinical Features				Management
	Age	Sex	Clinical Presentation	CT Findings	
Breast	5th decade	F	Infiltration Enophthalmos Pain 4.5–6.5 yr after primary	Infiltrative Muscle — irregular border	Radiotherapy Hormone therapy, ER-positive ± Combination chemotherapy
Lung	45–60 yr	M > F	Short presentation (4 mo) Eye and orbit at same time May be occult	Infiltrative or circumscribed	(Oat) Small cell carcinoma — radiotherapy; combination chemotherapy Nonsmall cell lung carcinoma — radiotherapy; chemoresistant
Neuroblastoma	Mean 2 yr	M > F	40% bilateral 15% orbit metastases, primary presentation 20% ocular — orbit > Horner's syndrome > opsoclonus Ecchymosis	Frequently involves lateral bone	Radiotherapy — highly responsive Combination chemotherapy — cyclophosphamide, dacarbazine (DTIC), and vincristine
Prostate	Late 7th decade	M	May be occult	Bone metastases frequent — osteoblastic	Radiotherapy Hormone therapy — ablation ± peripheral blockade Chemotherapy if hormone failure
GI	6th decade	M > F	May be occult Painful if mucinous May be bilateral	Infiltrative, may have bone metastases	Colorectal carcinoma — radiotherapy; fluorouracil (5-FU) infusion Stomach — radiotherapy, combination chemotherapy — chemoresistant
Kidney Renal carcinoma (hypernephroma)	5th decade	M > F	May be occult May pulsate	May be circum- scribed	Radiotherapy ± Immune modulators
Melanoma			To extraocular muscle	Frequently involves muscle with smooth contour	Radiotherapy Chemotherapy — chemoresistant Immunomodulators
Thyroid	6th decade	F > M	May pulsate	May be bone metastases May be circum- scribed	Radiotherapy Radioactive iodine — well differentiated Chemotherapy if nonrespon- sive
Carcinoid	5th–6th decades	F = M	May have carcinoid syndrome if liver metastasis 2–4 yr survival	Can be circumscribed	Radiotherapy — less effective Carcinoid syndrome — androgenic blocking agents, inhibition of serotonin synthesis Combination chemotherapy
Seminoma	5th decade	M	May have proptosis without orbital secondary		Radiotherapy — highly responsive Chemotherapy — cisplatin, vinblastine, and bleomycin
Ewing's sarcoma	10–25 yr		Long bone or trunk Primary in orbit, usually soft tissue		Radiotherapy — highly responsive Combination chemotherapy improves local control VAC (vincristine, actinomy- cin-D, cyclophosphamide) + doxorubicin (Adriamycin)

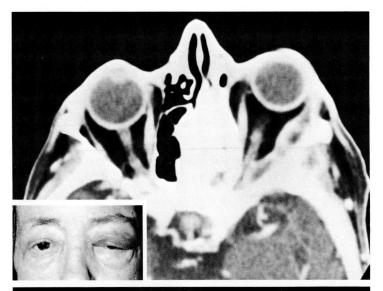

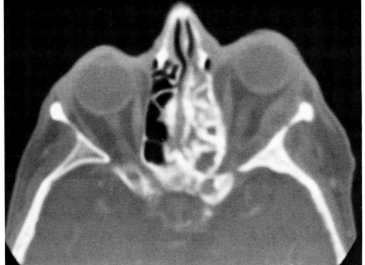

A

FIGURE 12-113. *(A)* This 85-year-old woman presented with swelling of the left eye for approximately 4 months. It was associated with mild intermittent supraorbital ache and some diplopia. On physical examination, she had a left afferent pupillary defect with a vision of 20/40. The lid was edematous and injected, and she had superior chemosis with a narrow interpalpebral fissure. There was 5 mm of proptosis and marked limitation of movement, especially in abduction and elevation. The left temporalis fossa appeared slightly fuller than the right. The axial CT scans (soft tissue and bone windows) demonstrate left proptosis with sclerotic changes in the greater sphenoid wing and ethmoid sinus. This is associated with a soft tissue mass in the lateral, posterior, and apical portion of the orbit. The mass is predominantly low-density, but had some rim enhancement medially. In addition to bony sclerosis, there is soft tissue opacification of the ethmoid and sphenoid sinuses. The patient had no systemic complaints on admission to hospital, but soon developed some abdominal distress with distention.

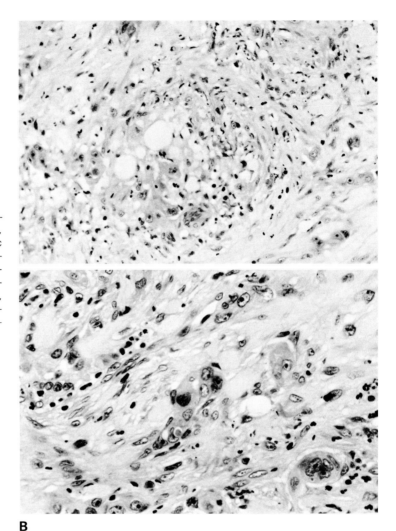

FIGURE 12-113 *(Continued).* *(B)* She underwent a small percutaneous biopsy of the orbit, which revealed dense, focally inflamed fibrotic tissue extensively infiltrated by a poorly differentiated mucin-secreting adenocarcinoma consistent with a metastatic colonic carcinoma. Systemic investigation revealed a rectal tumor, which on biopsy proved to be an adenocarcinoma (H&E, original magnification *top* × 25, *bottom* × 40).

B

FIGURE 12-114. This 77-year-old man had noted a firm swelling of the left upper and lower lids for several months, associated with slight pigmentation. On physical examination he had a narrow interpalpebral fissure, limitation of upgaze, and woody, firm lids. Biopsy revealed a mucin-secreting, poorly differentiated adenocarcinoma. Systemic investigation revealed diffuse sclerotic bone metastases and a mass in the antrum of the stomach consistent with a carcinoma (H&E, original magnification × 40).

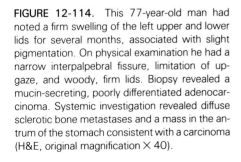
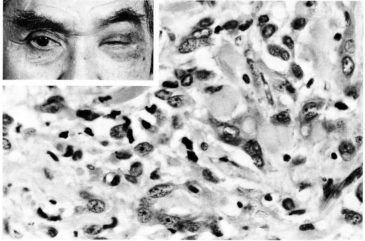

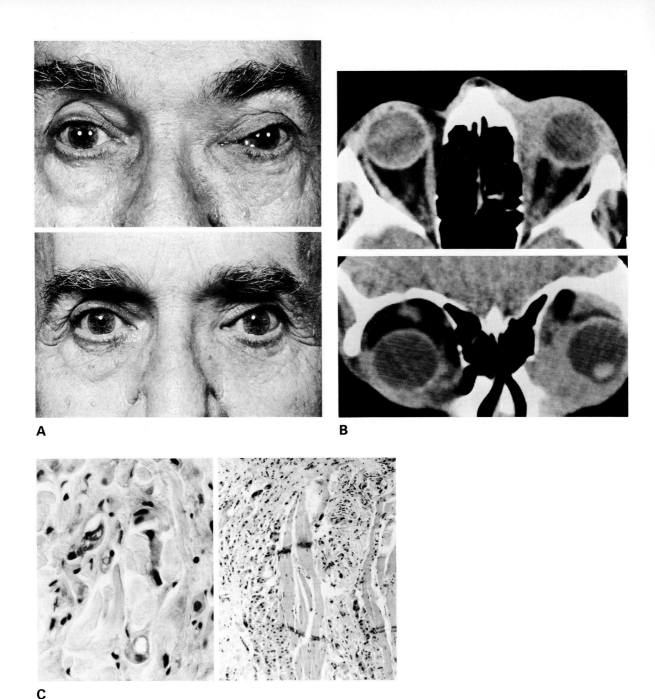

C

FIGURE 12-115. *(A, top)* This 65-year-old man presented with a history of chronic progressive epiphora on the left side. He had become aware of a ptosis and thickening of the lid for about 1 year. On physical examination, he demonstrated 4 mm of lateral displacement of the globe with 3 mm of proptosis, and a solid infiltration of the medial orbit and upper and lower lids. It was associated with a limitation of upgaze. *(B)* Axial CT scan demonstrates a diffuse medially located infiltrating mass involving the anterior and medial portion of the left orbit and lid, whereas the coronal scan shows that the involvement surrounds the left globe. *(C)* Biopsy revealed an infiltrating adenocarcinoma characterized by small cords and irregular pseudoglandular arrangement associated with a marked desmoplastic response. The tumor cells demonstrated mucin secretion within the glandlike structures as well as some intracytoplasmic mucin. Systemic investigation revealed an enlarged prostate, and biopsy confirmed a poorly differentiated diffusely infiltrating adenocarcinoma. The patient was treated with diethylstilbestrol (Stilbestrol), and had a dramatic response. *(A, bottom)* The appearance of the patient 1 year after initiation of therapy demonstrates almost total resolution of local infiltrative disease. He is alive and well 4 years following diagnosis.

FIGURE 12-116. Axial and coronal CT scans show an infiltrative mass involving the medial rectus, adjacent orbital fat, and optic nerve. The patient was a 64-year-old woman with carcinoma of the breast diagnosed 14 years earlier. She had suffered for 4 years from bone pain and, 1 year prior to presentation, had bony metastases diagnosed. She presented with a 3-month history of a firm lump in the inner canthus of the left eye. Physical examination revealed a superomedial mass with 3 mm of enophthalmos, reduction in upgaze, and in abduction due to an orbital metastasis.

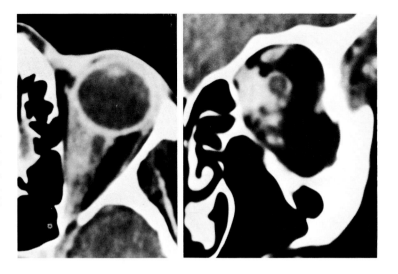

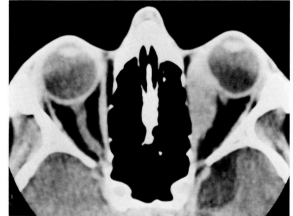

FIGURE 12-117. This 30-year-old man with a known diagnosis of metastatic melanoma of skin presented with left retrobulbar pain accentuated by eye movement and associated with increasing injection of the medial portion of the globe. Axial and coronal CT scans reveal a homogeneous, enhancing mass due to the metastatic melanoma. The mass involved the medial rectus muscle without infiltration of the adjacent fatty tissues.

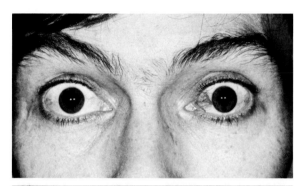

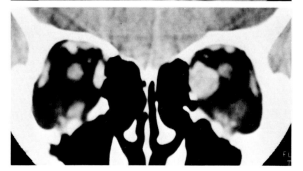

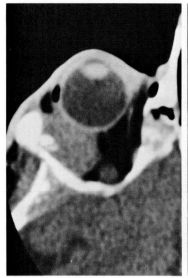
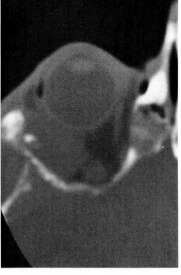

A

FIGURE 12-118. *(A)* Axial CT scans (soft tissue and bone windows) demonstrate a soft tissue mass in the lateral wall of the right orbit and middle cranial fossa. The mass has displaced the globe forward and is associated with local destruction of bone. It was seen in an 82-year-old man who presented with a 2-month history of right proptosis and a 4-month history of diplopia. On physical examination he had marked limitation of abduction, elevation, and adduction with 7 mm of proptosis and 4 mm of downward displacement. A systemic examination was negative. *(B)* The patient underwent biopsy of a rather granular, firm, fibrotic lesion. The specimen consisted of bundles of coarse collagen with numerous clumped fibroblasts. Within this connective tissue, small islands of malignant cells with large nuclei that varied in shape, size, and staining property were found. The cells have abundant eosinophilic foamy cytoplasm. In several areas the cells appeared to be forming primitive glandular structures. The entire lesion tended to infiltrate spicules of bone, which were surrounded by an exuberant fibrous reaction. The malignant cells were slightly positive for PAS, but were negative for mucicarmine. Immunoperoxidase stains for prostatic-specific antigen and prostatic acid phosphatase were both negative. Systemic survey failed to reveal a primary lesion for this poorly differentiated adenocarcinoma (H&E, original magnifications *top* × 2.5, *bottom* × 40).

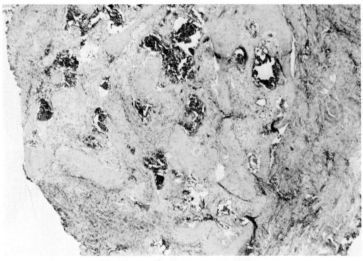

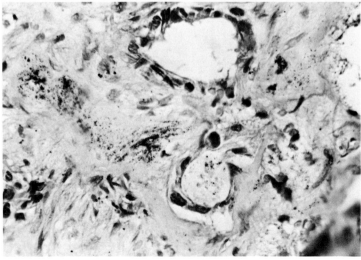

B

TABLE 12-16.
HISTOLOGIC, HISTOCHEMICAL, AND ELECTRON-MICROSCOPIC FEATURES OF COMMON ORBITAL METASTASES

Tumor Type	Histology — Usual	Histology — Variants	Distinguishing Features — Histochemical	Distinguishing Features — Immunohisto-chemical	Distinguishing Features — Electron Microscopy
Breast	Adenocarcinoma	Papillary, anaplastic, mucinous Histiocytoid—intracytoplasmic lumen + cicatricial —lobular carcinoma	Mucin, variably systemic CEA positive PAS-positive central "target" Alcian blue haloes	Estrogen receptor Immunohistochemistry for breast tumor-associated antigens and products	Mucus—secretory granules—intracytoplasmic lumens No features are specific
Lung	Oat cell May show necrosis with DNA in vessel walls + calcospherites	Undifferentiated oat cell (± carcinoid) Squamous carcinoma, adeno-carcinoma, mixed	Mucin—adenocarcinoma Carcinoid—Gremelius positive (argyrophilic)	Carcinoid oat cell group—neuron-specific enolase Serotonin	Electron-dense secretory granules—carcinoid oat cell group Mucin—adenocarcinoma—cytoplasmic inclusions Tonofilaments—squamous carcinoma
Neuroblastoma	Round cell neoplasm	Occasionally Wright's rosettes			Neurosecretory granules, neurotubules ± axons
Prostate	Tubuloalveolar adenocarcinoma	Undifferentiated	With or without mucin (usually without)	Prostate-specific antigen Prostatic acid phosphatase	
GI	Varies—adenocarcinoma—columnar	Acinar, papillary, mucinous ± mucin positive signet ring	Mucin, systemic CEA positive		Columnar, brush border with luminal aspect, terminal cytoplasmic filamentary webs
Kidney Renal carcinoma (hypernephroma)	Clear cell adeno-carcinoma (± granular)	Mixed, granular, and clear	Lipid—usually present		Abundant glycogen with lipid inclusions
Melanoma	Amelanotic epithelioid cells		With or without fontana	S-100 protein positive	Premelanosomes
Thyroid	Adenocarcinoma (follicular)	Varied types—follicular ± papillary Medullary (spindle component)		Calcitonin	Neurosecretory granules—in medullary
Carcinoid	Abundant granular cytoplasm and nuclear stippling	Commonly solid May be tubular, acinar, or rosette-like	Lipid, argyrophilic—lung > GI Argentaffin—GI > lung	Neuron-specific enolase Serotonin	Neurosecretory granules
Seminoma	Large pale syncytial cells + lymphocytes				
Ewing's sarcoma	Round cell neoplasm		PAS-positive, diastase-sensitive glycogen		Glycogen

cially those with biologically slow-growing tumors, can have very prolonged disease control from palliative measures alone.

The management of neoplasia, and especially metastatic tumors, is the domain of a multispecialty team. The team should include a medical oncologist, radiotherapist, pathologist, and ophthalmologist (see Figs. 12-105, 12-106, and 12-115). The goal of therapy in virtually all but rare circumstances is palliation. Long survival with control of disease is not infrequent and is an important aspect of management. In addition, there are some rare types of neoplasia that are known to be associated with solitary metastases, in which case total eradication of the disease may be considered. This, of course, would be guided by specific tumor type and a multidisciplinary decision.

In summary, orbital metastatic disease is an entity of increasing frequency associated with mass and infiltrative effects (pain, proptosis, reduced extraocular movements, ptosis) and has particular age, sex, and histologic associations. Metastases are clinically frequently unrecognized, may have special diagnostic considerations, and in a modern setting have increasing potential for adequate palliative treatment.

To illustrate the broad range and character of orbital metastases, the common features and variations of the nine most frequent metastatic solid tumors to the orbit will be discussed in greater depth. Tables 12-15 and 12-16 summarize these features and describe an additional group of rarer orbital metastases.

Metastatic disease affecting the orbit is incurable in all but a small minority of cases. Hence, the general aim of treatment is palliation. Therefore, asymptomatic, regional radiotherapy may be all that is required. If, on the other hand, as is the usual case, orbital disease represents dissemination and is not the only metastatic site, additional systemic chemotherapy or hormones are indicated, as discussed below.

BREAST CARCINOMA

Carcinoma of the breast is the most frequent cause of cancer death in women and the most common ocular and orbital metastasis. In Bullock's series, two thirds of metastases were ocular and one third were orbital. Forty percent of orbital metastases from a combined series shown in Table 12-13 were breast carcinoma. The orbital metastases usually occur in the fifth decade of life, and in up to 30% of patients may be the presenting symptom. The overwhelming majority, however, have evidence of a primary in the breast discovered either concomitantly with or antecedent to the orbital metastasis. In addition, the large majority of patients have widespread dissemination by the time orbital disease is discovered and may

have involvement of adjacent bony and intracranial structures. The average interval from primary to orbital metastasis varies from 4.5 to 6.5 years. Latency may be very long, as was demonstrated in one of our cases, which occurred 20 years after diagnosis of the primary tumor.

The characteristic presentation consists of firm infiltration of the orbit (with proptosis if posterior, see Fig. 12-116; and a palpable mass if anterior, see Fig. 12-105) with restricted extraocular movements, ptosis (see Fig. 12-106), and in about one quarter of instances enophthalmos (see Fig. 12-107). When metastatic breast carcinoma causes enophthalmos, it occurs in the right orbit in the majority of cases (76%) in contrast to the overall equal distribution of other types of orbital metastases. Another contrasting feature of metastatic cicatrizing breast carcinoma is that only 4% are bilateral compared to the 7% to 9% overall incidence of bilateral metastatic carcinoma. On CT scan, these are usually infiltrative tumors and have some propensity to metastasize to the extraocular muscles, in which instance an irregular reticulated pattern of adjacent orbital involvement is evident (see Fig. 12-116).

Pathologically, metastatic breast carcinoma is usually an intraduct adenocarcinoma (see Fig. 12-105B), and it may have varying patterns including papillary, mucinous, and anaplastic. The histiocytoid variant is characterized by the presence of intracytoplasmic lumina, and is often cicatricial with significant associated inflammation that correlates with a clinical syndrome of low-grade inflammatory infiltration of the orbit (Fig. 12-119). Histochemically, there may be evidence of mucin (mucicarmine) and PAS-positive central target cells as well as alcian blue haloes. When there is a significant tumor load, Bullock has emphasized that carcinoembryonic antigen (CEA) is usually elevated. Immunohistochemical tests may help in the diagnosis of breast tumor by identifying associated antigens and products. It is also important to remember that an undiagnosed orbital primary suspected of breast metastasis should be biopsied with estrogen receptor assay (ERA) studies in mind, because they may aid not only in diagnosis but also in selecting appropriate treatment. A positive response implies a greater chance of tumor regression following hormonal manipulation. Electron microscopy is not specific, but may show evidence of secretory granules and intracytoplasmic lumina.

Management

Hormones

For patients with estrogen receptor-positive or progesterone receptor-positive disease and for those with long disease-free survival, hormonal manipulation is the initial treatment of choice. In premenopausal patients, oophorectomy by either radiation or surgery is the first-choice

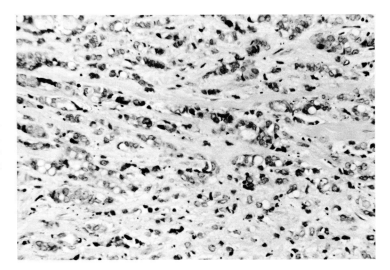

FIGURE 12-119.   An infiltrating signet cell carcinoma of the breast metastatic to the orbit. Note the typical "Indian file" arrangement of vacuolated cells with intervening fibrous stroma. It was seen in a patient with known breast carcinoma and metastatic disease who presented with a firm mass in the superior orbit.

hormonal treatment. Recent evidence suggests equivalence of tamoxifen and oophorectomy in premenopausal patients. In postmenopausal patients, tamoxifen is the first line of hormone therapy at a dose of 20 mg/day. The second line of hormonal therapy currently would include one of the progestational agents (megestrol acetate [Megace] 160 mg/day or medroxyprogesterone acetate [Provera] 300 mg/day). Treatment with medical adrenalectomy (aminoglutethimide and hydrocortisone) has shown its efficacy and comparability with surgical adrenalectomy or tamoxifen. Hence, some investigators use medical adrenalectomy with aminoglutethimide as a first hormone modality, particularly for bone metastases where a superior response has been noted. Androgens (fluoxymesterone [Halotestin]) are usually used for palliation when overall nutritional and bone marrow support are required. Hypophysectomy, very popular in the 1950s and 1960s, has been replaced by additive hormones. Nevertheless, very prompt relief of bone pain has been repeatedly documented after hypophysectomy, which, despite its interventional nature and a need for lifelong hormonal replacement, is still considered as one of the most effective hormonal manipulations.

If a response is observed to the first hormone, a reasonably good response can be expected with the second or third hormones at subsequent failures. However, if relapse occurs after the first hormone, indicating rapid progression, chemotherapy should be considered.

Chemotherapy

Breast cancer is a chemosensitive tumor and results of adjuvant chemotherapy indicate a clear reduction in mortality. The main indication for chemotherapy as a primary therapy for metastatic breast carcinoma is a more rapidly progressing systemic dissemination, usually (but not necessarily) with an estrogen receptor-negative tumor. In these instances, the slower onset of hormonal action will not bring early relief. Multiple painful bone metastases with or without hypercalcemia are common first metastatic sites. If orbital disease is present, it is often seen as a part of the overall complex involvement rather than a solitary lesion.

Combination regimens are superior to single agents, particularly for induction of a rapid response. However, most studies agree that chemotherapy for metastatic disease, albeit palliative, does not prolong overall survival. Chemotherapeutic agents with known efficacy in breast cancer include doxorubicin (Adriamycin [A], cyclophosphamide (C), methotrexate (M), fluorouracil (5-FU [F]), and vincristine (V). Currently, the most frequently used regimens are CMF (with or without vincristine) and prednisone with cyclophosphamide used by mouth every day, or alternatively as a bolus intravenously every 3 weeks. Recent evidence indicates superiority of doxorubicin-containing regimens. New generation anthracyclines (epirubicin, mitoxantrone) show promising results with similar response to doxorubicin, but significant reduction of cardiotoxicity and some reduction of bone marrow and GI side-effects. Most recent work emphasizes the overall importance of dose intensity in chemotherapy of breast cancer with autologous bone marrow transplantation as an ultimate example of the dose-intensity concept. Because of the complexity and toxicity of autologous bone marrow transplantations and high-intensity regimens in general, results of prospective controlled studies with the conventional regimens will be needed before the final verdict on the survival impact of the dose intensity in breast cancer can be made.

In summary, no therapy for metastatic disease of the breast has been shown to increase survival. Hence, treatment is always palliative and should be focused on optimum management of symptoms. This includes radiation to the orbit in the first instance, hormonal manipulation in estrogen receptor-positive or otherwise asymptomatic disease, and combination chemotherapy with or without hormones if disease onset is rapid (see Figs. 12-105, 12-106).

CARCINOMA OF THE LUNG

Carcinoma of the lung is a male-dominated disease occurring in the fourth through sixth decades. In contrast to breast carcinoma, metastatic carcinoma of the lung tends to have a relatively short course of presentation and development, reflecting a more rapidly growing and metastasizing neoplasm (see Fig. 12-112). Thus, the interval from primary to orbital metastases is shorter and occult primaries are more frequent. The clinical features reflect the rapid development of a mass with more evidence of displacement and less of infiltration, although infiltrative patterns may also occur. CT scan may demonstrate a relatively circumscribed mass with areas of necrosis and occasional calcification may be noted.

The most common pathologic type metastasizing to orbit and brain is the undifferentiated oat cell carcinoma. This group of carcinomas may have carcinoid variants. The two other common carcinomas of lung are squamous and adenocarcinoma, both of which have a low incidence of orbital metastasis compared to the oat cell variant.

Histochemically, mucin may be evident in adenocarcinomas and the carcinoids are argyrophilic. The carcinoid oat cell group may have evidence of neuron-specific enolase or serotonin on immunohistochemistry; on electron microscopy, it demonstrates dense secretory granules. The mucin-secreting adenocarcinomas will show cytoplasmic inclusions both histologically and on electron microscopy. Squamous carcinoma has tonofilaments, the presence of which should raise suspicion of a squamous cell carcinoma invading from an adjacent site rather than a hematogenous metastasis.

Treatment

The most important point in therapy for lung cancer is a correct histologic diagnosis, because different treatment regimens are used for oat cell, squamous, and adenocarcinomas. Virtually no long-term survival is expected in lung cancer once dissemination occurs. Hence, treatment is palliative; for patients not responding in the initial weeks of therapy, only supportive care is now indicated.

Small Cell Lung Carcinoma

Small cell lung carcinoma is an example of a malignancy with a short doubling time and high sensitivity to radio-

therapy and chemotherapy. Along with a short doubling time, however, an increased mutation rate towards resistance is noted and resistance to therapy may occur relatively early. Radiotherapy is effective, and is the primary treatment for orbital metastases. Chemotherapy will likely produce additional effective palliation; however, it is usually short-lived.

Trials in the early 1970s established the superiority of combination regimens over single agents. Currently, most chemotherapy for oat cell carcinoma includes a combination of cyclophosphamide, doxorubicin (Adriamycin), and vincristine (CAV regimen); alternating with methotrexate, mitomycin C, and lomustine (CCNU). More recently, etoposide (VP-16) and cisplatin are also being used routinely in most institutions. Clinical research in the management of oat cell carcinoma suggests that modification of dose intensity, duration of therapy, and alternation of active combinations may achieve more satisfactory control. Higher intensity drug schedules result in more complete responses, and even more extremes of high drug dose with autologous bone marrow rescue are being tested. Theoretical and experimental data suggest that early alternation of "non-cross resistant" combinations may prevent resurgence of resistant clones. Several studies show that although clear survival advantage has not yet been confirmed, improved responses and duration of responses nevertheless bring some validity to the concept. The additional advantage of alternating regimens may be a reduction of the total dose of individual agents, which could then be used at a later stage.

Nonsmall Cell Lung Carcinoma: Adenocarcinoma and Squamous Cell Carcinoma

Although chemotherapy is highly effective for small cell cancer, adjuvant trials for nonsmall cell lung carcinoma (NSCLC) show that patients will not benefit significantly from chemotherapy. Regimens of greatest efficacy in nonsmall cell lung carcinoma include cyclophosphamide, doxorubicin (Adriamycin), and cisplatin (CAP regimen). Responses are noted in 30% to 40% of patients.

NEUROBLASTOMA

Jack Rootman and Ka Wah Chan

Neuroblastoma is second only to rhabdomyosarcoma as the most frequent malignant tumor of the orbit in early childhood. In general orbital series, the incidence varies from 1% to 2%; in the combined series shown in Table 12-13, neuroblastoma accounted for 9%. Ophthalmic manifestations include proptosis and ecchymosis, Horner's syndrome, and opsoclonus–myoclonus. In a large study of neuroblastoma, Musarella has noted that 20% of patients have ophthalmic manifestations, three quarters of which are related to direct orbital metastases or ecchymosis, or both.

Neuroblastomas arise from primitive neuroblasts of the sympathetic system, most commonly in the abdomen (about 60%). In addition, they may occur in thoracic, cervical, or pelvic sites. Eight percent of neuroblastomas have ocular features as a presenting symptom. The median age of occurrence is 2 years, with 90% seen before the age of 5 years. There is a slight male predominance, and females have a better prognosis. Prognosis correlates with the stage of the disease and the age of the patient (the younger the patient, the better the prognosis).

The orbital presentation of metastatic neuroblastoma is characterized by sudden onset and dramatic progression (often over weeks) of proptosis, periorbital and lid swelling, ptosis, and ecchymosis (see Fig. 12-108). About 40% of the patients have bilateral orbital involvement. The overwhelming majority of orbital metastases (approximately 90%) originate from the abdomen. The fulminant nature and clinical features of orbital metastases make the differential diagnosis one of sudden inflammatory swellings of the orbit and other rapidly progressive neoplasia (including, in decreasing order of occurrence, rhabdomyosarcoma, Ewing's sarcoma, medulloblastoma, and Wilms' tumor). Seventy-five percent of neuroblastomas have the above ocular features as a manifestation of direct metastatic disease, which usually affects both the bone and soft tissues. The most common orbital site is the superolateral orbit and the zygoma with secondary extension, but any locus may be noted. On radiologic investigation, there may be evidence of bone destruction and other foci of cranial metastasis. Abdominal ultrasonography may disclose a retroperitoneal mass in the region of the adrenal gland (see Fig. 12-108B); abdominal x-rays may show calcification in this site. On CT scan, the orbital lesion may contain lucent areas reflecting necrosis.

The other ocular features of neuroblastoma include Horner's syndrome due to mediastinal involvement and opsoclonus–myoclonus, possibly due to an autoimmune factor. Musarella has emphasized the correlation between the type of ocular involvement and prognosis, noting a 3-year survival of 11.2%, 78.6%, and 100% for orbital metastases, Horner's syndrome, and opsoclonus–myoclonus, respectively.

Histologically, neuroblastoma consists of sheets or clumps of round cells with relatively well-defined hyperchromatic nuclei. Occasional Homer-Wright's rosettes with central neurofibrils may be noted. Both mitotic figures and necrosis are common. On electron microscopy neurosecretory granules, neurotubules, and axons are seen. Occasionally, more differentiated ganglion cells may be present, suggesting some degree of maturation.

The primary treatment for disseminated neuroblas-

toma is chemotherapy. Currently, the most effective agents are cyclophosphamide, vincristine, doxorubicin (Adriamycin), cisplatin, dacarbazine (DTIC), and teniposide (VM-26). When these agents are given in various combinations, 60% to 70% of patients respond with complete or partial resolution of metastatic lesions in 4 to 6 months. Local tumor control by surgery may then be attempted, with or without radiation therapy. Unfortunately, disease frequently recurs within 1 year and less than one tenth of patients will be disease-free survivors after 2 years. Palliative radiotherapy may be given for severe bone pain and periorbital lesions.

The dismal outlook of advanced neuroblastoma has not changed in the past 20 years, but innovative therapeutic approaches have been tried recently. High-dose combination chemotherapy along with supralethal doses of total body irradiation are given, followed by bone marrow rescue. Both histocompatible allogeneic marrow or autologous marrow, purged with specific monoclonal antibodies or chemotherapy, are effective in repopulating the marrow space and allowing hematopoietic recovery. Preliminary results are encouraging, provided the procedure is performed prior to disease progression. As many as 40% to 50% of the patient population may be cured. This approach also has been applied to patients who have relapsed after initial chemotherapy, but results have been less encouraging.

CARCINOMA OF THE PROSTATE

Carcinoma of the prostate is a frequent occult malignancy of late adult male life. Overall, its peak occurrence is in the seventh decade, which is later than most other carcinomas metastatic to the orbit. It has a propensity to metastasize to bone and is associated with an increase in serum acid phosphatase. It is an indolent neoplasm, and life expectancy is generally quite prolonged. Orbital spread can be to soft tissue or bone, or both. Bony metastasis may be associated with osteoplasia (sclerosis) with an adjacent soft tissue component (see Fig. 12-111). Soft tissue involvement may be seen as an expanding or cicatrizing lesion (see Fig. 12-115).

Histologically, it is an adenocarcinoma that can be very poorly differentiated. The cells may contain mucin in intracytoplasmic vacuoles (see Fig. 12-115). Dense and prolific fibroplasia may be noted in association with this tumor. Immunohistochemistry for prostate-specific antigen and prostatic acid phosphatase help in differentiating this tumor from other metastatic adenocarcinomas.

Prostatic carcinoma is a radiosensitive malignancy, and treatment for orbital metastasis is usually local radiotherapy. It is also sensitive to hormonal manipulation, which may lead to dramatic reversal of signs and symptoms (see Fig. 12-115).

Hormone therapy consists of ablation of androgen production, either by removing the source or by antiandrogen therapy. Androgen production is most frequently ablated by orchiectomy, or alternatively by excessive gonadotrophin stimulation with luteinizing hormone releasing factor (LHRH) agonists, which leads to depletion of testosterone. Peripheral antiandrogen therapy includes conventional estrogens, progestins, and more recently a new generation of antiandrogens, including cyproterone acetate and flutamide. Because of the high incidence of cardiovascular side-effects, estrogens are becoming increasingly less popular. A correlation between androgen receptors in prostatic carcinoma with subsequent response has been noted. Because of extragonadal sources of androgens (adrenal glands, liver, fat tissues) total androgen blockade is being suggested. In this, peripheral antiandrogen therapy is combined with ablation of hormone production. It has been shown that up to 40% of patients have complete or partial responses, with pain relief and improvement of performance status seen in an additional 35% to 40% of patients.

All hormonal therapies delay the development of metastases, but overall survival is not significantly prolonged. Chemotherapeutic agents for prostatic carcinoma are reserved for those patients who fail to respond to hormone therapy. A wide variety of agents is recommended, and investigationally synchronized hormone treatment and chemotherapy is being tested.

GASTROINTESTINAL CARCINOMA

Gastrointestinal carcinomas were the fifth most common metastatic carcinoma of the orbit (see Table 12-13). Usually they occur in the sixth decade with a slight male predominance. They are often occult, and up to 70% have evidence of regional or metastatic spread on initial diagnosis. When metastatic to the orbit, they may be particularly painful if they are mucin secreting. Orbital involvement may be directly to soft tissues or to the bone, which can lead to hyperostosis (see Fig. 12-113). The two primary GI sites are scirrhous carcinoma of the stomach and lower bowel adenocarcinoma. An unusual feature of GI carcinomas is a relatively high incidence of bilateral orbital metastasis from an occult primary, an occurrence which should invoke this as a possible diagnosis (see Fig. 12-110).

Histologically, these adenocarcinomas may have signet ring cells with mucin production or acinar and papillary structures (see Figs. 12-110B, 12-113B, 12-114B). Widespread systemic metastases are associated with elevation of CEA levels. Electron microscopy may show columnar cells with abundant brush borders and terminal cytoplasmic filamentary webs as well as intracytoplasmic vacuoles (see Fig. 12-110C).

Radiotherapy to the orbit remains the treatment of choice. The role of systemic therapy is strictly palliative. Colorectal carcinoma responds in up to 40% of patients to various schedules of fluorouracil (5-FU) and no clear advantage has been shown by adding other agents. Recent studies have shown increased efficacy of fluorouracil (5-FU) infusion compared to bolus therapy. Stomach cancer has been traditionally considered chemoresistant, but recent combination regimens have shown some promise (40% response rate). Agents of known effectiveness include fluorouracil (5-FU), doxorubicin (Adriamycin), mitomycin, and semustine (Methyl CCNU), and more recently, cisplatin and hydroxyurea. Chemotherapy may be considered only as a palliative measure in orbial metastases.

RENAL CELL CARCINOMA

Renal cell carcinoma is another tumor that has a male predominance, occurs in the fifth decade, and is often occult. An unusual feature of renal cell carcinoma is its tendency to develop rich vascularity, which in the case of the orbit may lead to pulsation. This tumor may exhibit somewhat bizarre behavior insofar as a single metastatic nodule can occur and excision is possible. In addition, removal of a primary renal cell carcinoma may lead to regression of the secondary. Histologically, it may be a clear cell adenocarcinoma with abundant lipid-rich vacuolated cells evident both histochemically and on electron microscopy.

Renal cell carcinoma is radiosensitive; thus, radiotherapy is the mainstay of orbital therapy. This tumor is not responsive to traditional chemotherapy, but recent studies of immune modulating agents, particularly with interferon and interleukin 2, show great promise.

MELANOMA

In looking at a combined series of orbital metastases (see Table 12-13), the incidence of skin melanoma metastatic to orbit is striking. The intriguing feature of this tumor is it has a propensity to metastasize to extraocular muscles, rather than infiltrate the orbital tissues, producing a generalized enlargement of the muscle (see Fig. 12-117). On CT scan, rather than demonstrating the infiltrative margins of a carcinoma, the metastatic melanoma causes a smooth enlargement of the muscle. Histologically, the cells may be amelanotic and epithelioid in character; thus, histochemical stains for melanin and its precursors, as well as electron-microscopic evidence of premelanosomes, may be useful in distinguishing this tumor.

Satisfactory palliation for metastatic melanoma can be achieved with radiotherapy. This is traditionally considered a chemoresistant tumor, and responses to the usual agents are poor and generally of short duration. Immunotherapy has been of some value and recent studies with interferon and immunomodulators show some encouraging results, underlining the importance of immunity in the natural history of melanoma.

THYROID CARCINOMA

Metastatic thyroid carcinoma has a peak occurrence in the sixth decade and is more common in women than in men. Epidemiologic data indicate a definite increase in the incidence of thyroid cancer in the last three decades. Behavior of this carcinoma tends to reflect the underlying histology. The low-grade well-differentiated papillary or follicular carcinomas metastasize regionally and develop slowly, with distant metastases being much less frequent (see Fig. 12-109). The poorly differentiated anaplastic thyroid carcinomas are highly aggressive, tend to metastasize to bone, and show increased vascularization. In the orbital region, this may lead to pulsation. An unusual variant of thyroid carcinoma, with a longer median survival, is medullary carcinoma, known to produce thyrocalcitonin measurable by radioimmunoassay.

External beam irradiation is used for symptomatic metastases. In addition, when tumors concentrate iodine (well-differentiated papillary and follicular carcinomas), radioactive iodine is used. Chemotherapy is used for carcinomas not responsive to radioactive iodine. Chemotherapeutic agents include doxorubicin (Adriamycin) and more recently cisplatin, vindesine, and bleomycin. The most important fact affecting survival in this carcinoma is the primary histology.

CARCINOID

Carcinoids are unusual neoplasms arising from argentaffin cells in the gastrointestinal (GI) tract. When significant hepatic metastatic load exists, the clinical symptoms of carcinoid syndrome (vasomotor disturbances, intestinal hypermotility, bronchoconstrictive attacks, right-sided cardiac involvement, hepatomegaly) may occur due to hormone production by the tumor. Orbital metastases are rare and have been described as being circumscribed. Histologically, they have a typical abundant granular cytoplasm with nuclear stippling and may be distinguished with the use of special stains (argentaphilic, argyrophilic). Immunohistochemistry may identify neuron-specific enolase or serotonin, and on electron microscopy there may be evidence of neurosecretory granules.

Treatment for orbital metastases is radiotherapy, although these tumors are not greatly sensitive. The carcinoid syndrome is treated with specific therapy against suspected or documented vasoactive substances. This in-

cludes androgenic blocking agents and inhibition of serotonin synthesis. For extensive metastatic disease, combination chemotherapy using streptozocin, fluorouracil (5-FU), doxorubicin or (Adriamycin) is added.

Secondary Tumors of the Orbit

Jack Rootman

Secondary tumors of the orbit include all lesions that extend from adjacent primary sites including the sinuses, nasopharynx, intracranial cavity, bone, lids, conjunctiva, globe, and lacrimal sac. The incidence and type of lesions arising from these sites are outlined in Table 12-17.

TABLE 12-17.
INCIDENCE AND TYPE OF SECONDARY TUMORS OF THE ORBIT, UNIVERSITY OF BRITISH COLUMBIA ORBITAL CLINIC, 1976–1986

Tumor Type	Number of Lesions	Total
Nasopharynx and sinus (epithelial and soft tissue)		26
Epithelial	20	
Melanoma	1	
Malignant schwannoma	2	
Rhabdomyosarcoma	1	
Lymphoma	1	
Neurofibroma	1	
Bone		24
Fibrous dysplasia	8	
Osteoma	4	
Myeloma	3	
Ewing's sarcoma	2	
Chondrosarcoma	2	
Histiocytosis X	3	
Fibrohistiocytic sarcoma	1	
Osteogenic sarcoma	1	
Intracranial		17
Sphenoid wing meningioma	15	
Dural melanoma	1	
Medulloblastoma	1	
Lid		9
Basal cell	4	
Squamous cell	3	
Melanoma	1	
Meibomian (sebaceous)	1	
Conjunctiva		10
Melanoma	7	
Squamous carcinoma	3	
Lacrimal sac		4
Transitional carcinoma	2	
Squamous carcinoma	1	
Meningioma	1	
Ocular		4
Melanoma	3	
Retinoblastoma	1	
Total		94

TABLE 12-18.
SECONDARY TUMORS OF THE ORBIT INVOLVING THE SINUS AND NASOPHARYNX, UNIVERSITY OF BRITISH COLUMBIA ORBITAL CLINIC, 1976–1986

Tumor Type	Number of Lesions	Total
Carcinomas		18
Squamous cell	9	
Well differentiated 3		
Moderately differentiated 2		
Poorly differentiated 4		
Transitional	3	
Well differentiated 1		
Poorly differentiated 2		
Adenoid cystic	3	
Adenocarcinoma	1	
Basal cell	1	
Neuroendocrine	1	
Mesenchymal		17
Fibrous dysplasia	7	
Osteoma	4	
Chondrosarcoma	2	
Ewing's sarcoma	2	
Rhabdomyosarcoma	1	
Osteogenic sarcoma	1	
Others		7
Schwannoma	2	
Myeloma	2	
Lymphoma	1	
Neurofibroma	1	
Melanoma	1	
Total		42

Tumors of mesenchymal and neurogenic origin have been discussed as separate entities earlier in the chapter. The main emphasis of this section will be orbital extension of lesions of epithelial origin (lid, sinus, conjunctiva, and lacrimal sac) and selected tumors arising from the eye and intracranial cavity. We had 95 secondary tumors in our series, or about one third of orbital neoplasia; thus, they are an important aspect of orbital disease.

NEOPLASIA OF THE SINUS AND NASOPHARYNX

Malignant neoplasms of the sinus account for 0.2% to 0.8% of all systemic malignancies, about 3% of malignancies involving the upper aerodigestive tract, and 6% of head and neck cancers (Table 12-18). In Godtfredsen and Lederman's combined Scandinavian–British series of 673 patients with primary nasopharyngeal tumors, 36% (240) had ophthalmoneurological manifestations. Smith and Wheliss found eye and orbital abnormalities in 55% (29) of 53 patients with histologically proven nasopharyngeal tumors.

Epithelial Malignancies of the Sinus and Nasopharynx

Epithelial malignancies of the paranasal sinuses frequently spread to the orbit. Conley has noted that 75% have extension beyond the sinus with 45% orbital inva-

TABLE 12-19.
SITE AND HISTOLOGY OF EPITHELIAL MALIGNANCIES OF ORBIT AND SINUS/NASOPHARYNX

	Maxillary	Ethmoid	Nasopharynx and Nose	Diffuse	Total Histologic Types
Squamous	4 (25)*	2	2	1	34
Transitional		2 (3)	1 (1)		7
Adenoid cystic	3 (3)				6
Adenocarcinoma	1 (3)	(1)			5
Mucoepidermoid carcinoma	(1)				1
Basal cell carcinoma			1		1
Neuroendocrine carcinoma		1			1
Melanoma		1			1
Total sites	40	10	5	1	56

* Data from Johnson study in parentheses.
Combined data from University of British Columbia Orbital Clinic and Johnson LN, Krohel GB, Yeon EB et al: Sinus tumors invading the orbit. Ophthalmology 91:209, 1984.

TABLE 12-20.
STAGING AND CLASSIFICATION OF ANTRAL CARCINOMA

Staging of Antral Carcinoma*

T1 Tumor confined to the antral mucosa of the infrastructure with no bone destruction

T2 Tumor confined to the suprastructure mucosa without bone destruction or to the infrastructure with destruction of the medial or inferior walls only

T3 More extensive tumor invading the cheek, orbit, anterior ethmoid air cells, or pterygoid muscles

T4 Massive tumor with invasion of cribriform plate, posterior ethmoid air cells, sphenoid sinus, nasopharynx, pterygoid plates, or base of skull

Classification of Sinus Carcinoma by Tumor Spread[†]

T1 Tumor limited to antral mucosa with no bone erosion

T2 Bony erosion without evidence of involvement of skin, orbit, pterygopalatine fossa, or ethmoid labyrinth

T3 Bony erosion with involvement of above structures

T4 Tumor extension into the nasopharynx, sphenoid sinus, cribriform plate, or pterygopalatine fossa

---

* From the American Joint Committee on Cancer: Staging of Cancer of Head and Neck Sites and of Melanomas, pp 30–31. Chicago, 1980
† Modified from Harrison DF: Ann Otol Rhinol Laryngol 87:3, 1978

---

sion. In a recent study by Johnson and Krohel, 47 of their 79 patients with known sinus and nasal tumors had orbital involvement. Of these, 37 were epithelial in origin. The specific site of origin and histologic types seen by us and by Johnson and Krohel are summarized in Table 12-19. Seventy percent originate from the maxillary sinus and 60% are squamous cell in type. Epithelial malignancies of the sinus and nasopharynx are classified according to the extent of local invasion and regional nodal spread (Table 12-20). Thus, by definition, orbital involvement reflects an advanced stage (T3 and T4).

The clinical hallmark of secondary epithelial tumors arising from the nasopharynx and sinuses is nonaxial displacement of the globe associated with infiltration of orbital and paraorbital structures, leading to pain, paresthesia, decreased vision, and reduced extraocular movements (Fig. 12-120). It is these features of chronic relentless pain, paresthesia, and nonaxial displacement that help to clinically distinguish secondary epithelial malignancies from practically every other tumefaction of the orbit. In our experience, metastatic disease was painful only in about 25% of cases and proptosis was usually axial. In contrast, the secondary malignancies were associated with pain and paresthesia in 74% of cases and nonaxial displacement in 53% (Table 12-21). Only 2 of the 19 patients in our series had proptosis without nonaxial displacement (11%). The major nasal symptoms experienced were obstruction or epistaxis. The frequency and severity of ocular and orbital symptoms attest to the

TABLE 12-21.
SIGNS AND SYMPTOMS OF SINUS AND NASOPHARYNGEAL CARCINOMAS, UNIVERSITY OF BRITISH COLUMBIA ORBITAL CLINIC, 1976–1986

Symptoms	Number of Patients*
Ocular and Orbital	
Facial pain and paresthesia	14
Globe displacement	12
Proptosis 2	
Nonaxial displacement + proptosis 10	
Decreased vision	9
Extraocular muscle restriction	9
Diplopia 5	
Lid and conjunctival edema	9
Tearing	8
Lid mass (firm)	3
Ocular invasion and glaucoma	1
Total patients with some ocular symptoms	15
Nasal	
Obstruction	6
Nodes in neck	4
Epistaxis	3
Gum ulcer	1
Chronic sinusitis	1
Total patients with some nasal symptoms	13
Other	
Headache	1

---

* Total number of patients participating in study: 19.

---

relatively silent origin and late stage of presentation reflected by orbital invasion.

Generally, in studies of nasopharyngeal tumors, men outnumber women two to one and the peak age range is between 40 and 60 years. The site of origin is reflected in the dominant orbital signs. Because the majority arise within the maxillary sinus, upward displacement of the globe, fullness of the lower lid, infraorbital pain or paresthesia, and distortion of the maxilla are the major clinical signs. In contrast, lesions arising from the ethmoid complex are characterized by outward and downward displacement of the globe (Fig. 12-121). Although in all of these instances inflammatory signs may be suggested by injection, chemosis, and some edema, tenderness, and significant rubor are unusual.

Radiologic findings consist of either focal or widespread destruction of the sinuses with invasion of the adjacent structures by a solid tumor mass. The mass is usually large (Fig. 12-122); however, sometimes it may be relatively small, yet have extended to adjacent structures, particularly in the case of adenoid cystic carcinoma. The sinus and orbit may be the only structures involved, but

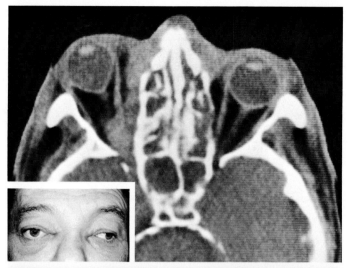

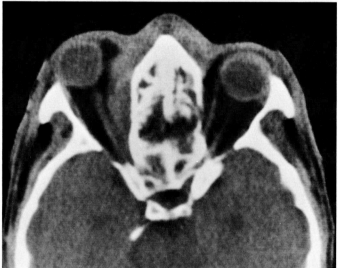

A

FIGURE 12-120. *(A)* This 47-year-old man presented with a progressive right ophthalmoplegia, restriction of medial rectus function, and swelling of the medial canthi and upper lids. In addition, he was aware of some retrobulbar pain and progressive loss of vision on the right. On examination he had vision of 20/200 OD with an afferent pupillary defect, limitation of abduction, and slight proptosis with notable thickening of the base of his nose and medial canthal region. CT scan demonstrates opacification of the ethmoids with multiple subtle focal areas of destruction of bone and infiltration of the right orbit and medial canthi bilaterally by a soft tissue mass. *(B)* Percutaneous biopsy revealed a diffuse, gritty, subcutaneous lesion consisting of cords of neoplastic cells surrounded by a desmoplastic and inflammatory reaction. It was a poorly differentiated neoplasm that had the tinctorial and electron microscopic features of a mucoepidermoid carcinoma. He underwent radiotherapy and systemic chemotherapy with regression of local disease, but died 1 year later of cerebral extension (H&E, original magnifications *left* × 10, *right* × 25).

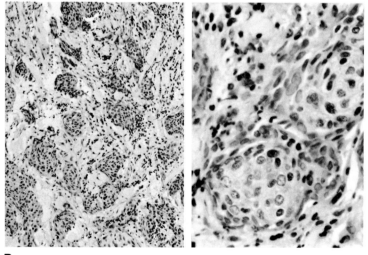

B

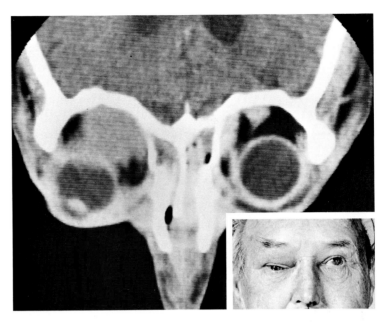

FIGURE 12-121. This 66-year-old man presented with the sudden development of a superior orbital mass on the right side and a known history of melanoma of the nasopharynx. He had previously been treated on the left side with radiotherapy and had lost vision. Coronal CT scan demonstrates midline involvement and extension of the lesion into the right superomedial orbit and residual tumor in left superolateral orbit. He was treated urgently with radiotherapy and had local regression of disease, but died 6 months later of disseminated melanoma.

there is frequently extension to the base of the skull (Fig. 12-123).

Batsakis has divided the epithelial malignancies into those that arise from metaplastic epithelium, including squamous cell carcinoma and "transitional" tumors, and those arising from the mucoserous epithelium, including adenocarcinoma and salivary gland neoplasia such as adenoid cystic carcinoma, mucoepidermoid carcinoma, and rare malignant salivary neoplasia.

Overall, the prognosis has been dismal with a 5-year survival of about 35%. Patients with T3 and T4 staging have had a survival rate of 31% and 10%, respectively.

Mortality is largely related to the inability to eradicate local disease. Flores and colleagues, reporting on the recent experience at the Cancer Control Agency of British Columbia, emphasize that during the last decade encouraging results have been obtained using a combination of radiotherapy and surgery in the treatment of epithelial malignancies of the sinuses. Their overall crude 5-year survival for all cases was 46%, and a combined treatment using irradiation and surgery in selected cases generated a 5-year survival rate of 74.4% as compared to 42.1% in cases receiving irradiation alone. They emphasize that the important factors in management consist of accurate sur-

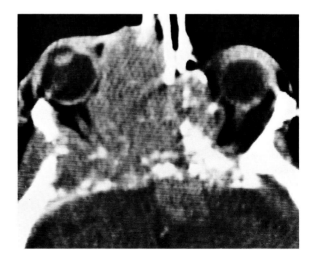

FIGURE 12-122. Contrast-enhanced axial CT scan shows a diffusely infiltrating destructive lesion arising in the nasopharynx and extending bilaterally into the orbits and intracranial cavity. It was seen in an 89-year-old woman who had a known nasopharyngeal carcinoma.

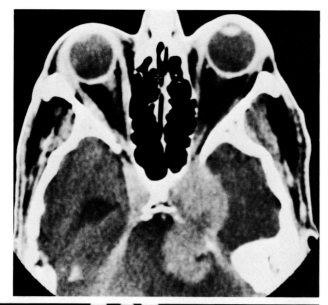

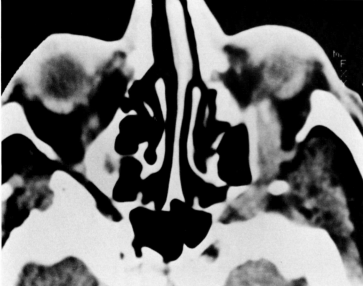

FIGURE 12-123. Contrast-enhanced axial CT scans demonstrate a large mass involving the left cavernous sinus and extending into the inferior orbit, the posterior fossa, and the pterygopalatine fossa. Subtle bone erosions are present. This was seen in a 38-year-old man with a known adenocarcinoma of the tongue. It subsequently involved the nasopharynx and surrounding structures. He presented with cranial nerve palsy and infraorbital numbness.

gical pathological staging, a combination of a full course of curative irradiation (6000 cGy in 25 treatments over 5 weeks or 5000 to 5500 cGy in 15 treatments in 3 weeks), with radical surgical resection as the treatment of choice for most paranasal sinus malignancies. In addition, patients with regional nodal disease but without distant metastases are potentially curable and should be treated aggressively. This individualized treatment based on a realistic knowledge of the exact extent of the disease has produced encouraging results in the management of these malignancies.

Squamous cell carcinomas of the paranasal sinuses do not declare themselves clinically until they have breached their sinus of origin in more than 90% of instances. Up to 80% arise within the maxillary sinus and the remainder originate from ethmoid, frontal, or sphenoid sinuses. The signs and symptoms of maxillary tumors are oral (pain in the teeth, trismus, a full alveolus, and palatal erosion); nasal (obstruction, epistaxis, chronic sinusitis); ocular (tearing, diplopia, displacement, pain, and exophthalmos); and facial (paresthesia, swollen cheek, pain, and facial asymmetry). Tumors arising from the posterior portion of the maxillary sinus have a worse prognosis because of the proximity to the orbit, cribriform plate, and pterygoid region. In fact, about 20% of squamous carcinomas have regional lymph node metastases on initial presentation. Progression and ultimate death are usually related to complications of local invasion, but about 18% develop distant metastases. The majority are histopathologically moderately well-differentiated keratinizing squamous carcinoma, but they may be anaplastic.

Transitional carcinomas originate from the schneiderian epithelium of the nasal cavity and paranasal sinuses. The majority of lesions of this histopathologic type are benign papillomas characterized by multiple and multifocal occurrence and local recurrence. Histologically, they may be either papillary (exophytic) or inverted. They may occasionally have ciliated or cylindrical cells. The large majority of schneiderian papillomas, although recurrent, remain benign but a small percentage undergo malignant transformation, particularly those of the lateral nasal wall or of the inverted type. Thus, transitional carcinomas invading the orbit characteristically arise from the ethmoid sinuses or nasopharynx. Treatment is both radical surgery and radiotherapy.

Adenoid cystic carcinomas of the nasopharynx and sinus parallel the behavior of those seen elsewhere. These are biologically locally aggressive tumors with extensive perineural invasion, sometimes far beyond the apparent limits of resection (evident in 75% of cases at presentation). Thus, although presenting as localized masses, they are characterized by a course of indolence and recurrence (sometimes extending over very long periods of time) and ultimately death, usually from spread to contiguous structures. Fourteen percent of these tumors spread to regional lymph nodes, whereas 40% develop hematogenous metastases. Overall, they are seen in a slightly younger age group than other sinus and nasopharyngeal tumors and are associated with less local reaction in the orbit and more indolent mass effect. In Henderson's series, 90% of the patients with adenoid cystic carcinomas of the sinuses were dead between 7 and 21 years after diagnosis, and the remaining patient had experienced nine recurrences over 32 years. The general trend in management is towards local, less aggressive surgery and radiotherapy to control local manifestations.

Adenocarcinomas usually occur higher in the sinuses and nasopharynx, typically in the ethmoids. They are seen in unusually high numbers in woodworkers. Their local behavior is similar to adenoid cystic carcinoma but they are less frequently well differentiated; thus, they develop more rapidly. Treatment is surgically aggressive because they are not significantly radiosensitive.

Melanomas rarely occur in the nasopharynx (3.5% of all sinonasal neoplasia; see Fig. 12-121). They tend to occur in the anterior part of the nasal cavity, presenting as bulbous masses with nasal obstruction and epistaxis. Five-year survival is from 17% to 38%.

The other rare epithelial malignancies include neuroendocrine carcinoma and esthesioneuroblastoma, which have been discussed separately. Odontogenic tumors (ameloblastoma, ameloblastic fibrosarcoma, and calcifying epithelial odontogenic tumor) and cysts may rarely involve the orbit. Ameloblastomas are locally invasive, benign (2% are malignant), epithelial tumors that arise from the mandible in 80% of cases. Among the remaining 20% that originate from the maxilla, local growth and extension may lead to orbital involvement. Treatment is by local resection, after which about one third may recur. Radiotherapy is palliative and not curative.

In summary, epithelial malignancies arising from the nose, nasopharynx, and sinuses are characterized by an infiltrative, nonaxial mass effect with significant neurosensory and motor deficit. They are occult neoplasms, and orbital involvement represents a late presentation with a grim prognosis.

EXTENSION OF INTRACRANIAL TUMORS

Meningioma is the most common intracranial tumor to extend into the orbit, and invasion by any other primary is exceedingly rare. Esthesioneuroblastomas arise from the olfactory structures and commonly invade the adjacent sinuses and orbit. (Neurogenic tumors have been discussed earlier in the chapter). The other rare occurrences of orbital invasion include high-grade astrocytomas, pituitary adenomas, chordomas (discussed earlier in the chapter), and ectopic meningiomas of the ethmoid sinus.

We have encountered a number of patients with intracranial tumors, either primary or metastatic (meningeal carcinomatosis, leukemia, and lymphoma), that have extended by means of the subarachnoid space into the optic nerve sheath or orbit, or both. One was a medulloblastoma that spread bilaterally into the optic nerve (Fig. 12-124). Another was seen in a woman who had a dural melanoma of the spinal cord that subsequently presented as a large mass extending into the orbit around the peripheral and optic nerve structures (Fig. 12-125).

ORBITAL EXTENSION OF LID TUMORS

Any of the primary tumors of the skin and adnexa may invade the orbit either because of late presentation or multiple recurrence following incomplete excision (as is the case with basal cell carcinoma), or because of more rapid and aggressive growth (as in some squamous cell carcinomas), or finally, because of an insidious onset that

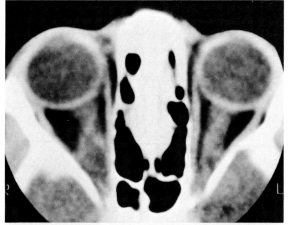

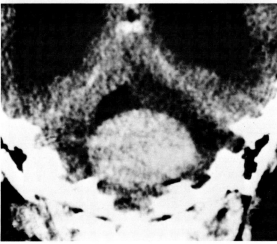

FIGURE 12-124. *(Top)* Axial CT scan demonstrates bilateral enlargement of the optic nerves. This occurred in a 5-year-old girl who had been treated (radiotherapy and resection) 6 months earlier for a medulloblastoma shown in the coronal CT scan *(bottom)*. She presented with hand movements vision and an afferent pupillary defect on the right and 20/30 vision on the left. In addition, there was right optic atrophy with some slight pallor of the left disk. Aspiration needle biopsy of the right optic nerve revealed the presence of medulloblastoma.

masquerades as some other condition (as in the case of meibomean carcinoma).

Although there is a large variety of unusual and rare adnexal tumors that may affect the skin of the lid and rarely invade the orbit, the above three carcinomas represent the most important and common epithelial malignancies of the lid that extend in this fashion.

Basal Cell Carcinoma of the Lid

Overall, basal cell carcinoma is the most common epithelial malignancy of the lid, yet in terms of frequency of orbital invasion it equals squamous cell carcinoma in most series. This is a reflection of the more aggressive nature of squamous carcinoma. The rather indolent painless course of basal cell carcinoma (median duration about 3 years at presentation for all basal cell carcinomas) may contribute to late presentation with orbital invasion (Fig. 12-126). Orbital invasion is usually a part of either advanced presentation, recurrence, or morpheic variant.

Basal cell carcinomas occur in the fifth to eighth decades with a male predominance. Overall, about 50% are seen in the lower lid, 25% the inner canthus, 10% to 15% in the upper lid, and 5% in the outer canthus.

Orbital extension is more common in medial canthal lesions for two reasons: the first is the anatomic intimacy of bone and lacrimal system, and the second is the propensity for surgeons to undertreat lesions in this locale to avoid damaging the lacrimal apparatus. With modern controlled techniques of management, orbital extension from this site is no more frequent than any other site.

The majority of basal cell carcinomas have a typical clinical picture starting as pearly raised nodules that develop central ulceration and characteristically extend radially. These ultimately can ulcerate and erode through adjacent tissues, producing grotesque local disfigurement (see Fig. 12-126), yet they do not metastasize.

There are a large number of histologic variants of basal cell carcinoma including solid (the majority), adenoid, keratotic, mixed, and sclerosing. It is the sclerosing

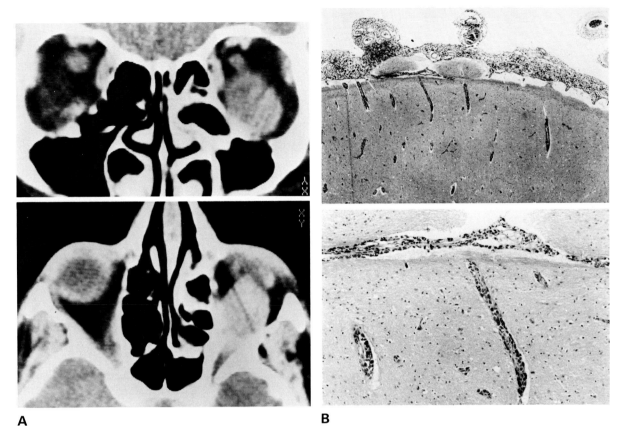

A   **B**

FIGURE 12-125.   *(A)* Coronal and axial CT scans demonstrate a large, well-defined left inferior orbital mass. The patient was a 45-year-old woman who presented with proptosis that had developed over a 2-month period. Several months earlier, she had undergone surgery for a dural melanoma of the spinal cord. Aspiration needle biopsy of the orbital tumor revealed cells consistent with the melanoma removed from the dura. The patient died within 1 week of diagnosis. *(B)* Autopsy showed diffuse involvement of the meninges with extension into the subarachnoid sheath of the optic nerve and around peripheral nerves of the orbit (H&E, original magnifications *top* × 10, *bottom* × 25).

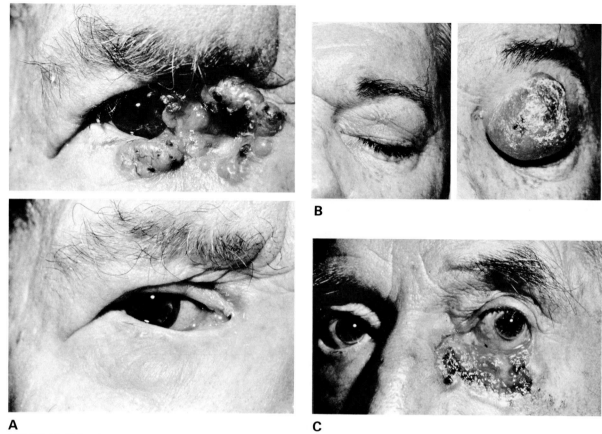

FIGURE 12-126.   Advanced basal cell carcinoma of the lid in three different patients. *(A)* This 71-year-old man presented in 1971 with an extensive ulcerated medial canthal lesion *(top)*. Note the large, nodular, pearly, raised edges. For the previous 3 years, he had noted a "boil" that constantly broke down and gradually increased in size. It was treated with 5,000 rad over 22 days *(bottom)*. The disease recurred in 1973, and he had local surgery. When last seen in 1977, he had no evidence of recurrent disease. *(B)* This 62-year-old man presented to the Cancer Control Agency of British Columbia in 1965 with a large adenoid cystic basal cell carcinoma *(right)*. He underwent radiotherapy with 4,000 rad over 10 days. He had no evidence of recurrence over the next 9 years, when he died of an unrelated esophageal stricture. Photograph on the *left* was taken 1 year after radiotherapy. *(C)* This 76-year-old chronic alcoholic presented with an ulcerated lesion of the left lower lid. It had been present for 20 years and ulcerated for 2 years. He received 4,500 rad over 23 days. He had no recurrence of local disease over the next 11 years, when he died of chronic obstructive pulmonary disease.

(morphea) variety that has a notorious reputation for extension, largely because they have clinically and pathologically indistinct margins. Clinically, the only clue to extension may be a tendency for the adjacent or overlying skin to appear very thin and slightly telangiectatic, and to have lost its adnexa (cilia). Histopathologically, they consist of minute chords of cells in a dense fibrous stroma.

Invasion of the orbit usually occurs after incomplete (often multiple) excision and is heralded by infiltrative features affecting the anterior structures, in particular, restriction of extraocular movements, cicatrization and induration of the lid structures, and fixation to adjacent bone. Orbital invasion is frequently antedated by long duration, yet is usually associated with very little pain until perineural involvement occurs. Henderson has noted that the soft tissues of the lid are frequently involved in a circumferential manner before deep orbital invasion occurs.

The management of basal cell carcinoma with orbital invasion demands a firm resolve to use radical therapy that incorporates the entire lesion. The most assured treatment is a surgical, and is best obtained by a multidisciplinary team of surgeon and pathologist. Wide excision should be controlled by pathologic confirmation of free borders and may require exenteration, bony removal, and even extirpation of dura. Reconstruction may involve a craniofacial surgical team.

Many centers have emphasized the efficacy and cost effectiveness of radiotherapy in the treatment of basal cell carcinoma, particularly primary lesions. Fitzpatrick has emphasized that individualized careful treatment planning gives a 5-year tumor control rate of 95%. More extensive lesions can be effectively treated providing the management team has the same resolve as outlined for surgery. Thus, detailed planning is necessary. Extensive surgical procedures may be anathema to many and particularly cruel for the elderly and frail; thus, radical radiotherapy may be the method of choice in these circumstances. When planned appropriately and delivered carefully, the complication rate is relatively low; however, complications do tend to occur more frequently in the extensive lesions. Luxemberg and Guthrie have reported encouraging results with cisplatin chemotherapy for advanced basal cell carcinoma.

Squamous Cell Carcinoma of the Lid

Squamous cell carcinoma is far less common than basal cell carcinoma of the lid by a factor of at least 12. Reifler and Hornblass, in a review of squamous cell carcinoma of the eyelid, noted that it accounts for about 9% of all eyelid malignancies. The major predisposing factor for the development of this malignancy is sun exposure in fair-skinned persons. Exposure to carcinogenic agents (hydrocarbons, arsenic, and irradiation) as well as genetic predisposition (xeroderma pigmentosum) are other important factors.

The clinical development of squamous cell carcinoma is faster than basal cell carcinoma (mean duration, 1 year) and consists of focal hyperkeratotic lesions that slowly extend and ulcerate. They are more common in the lower lid (Reifler reports 1.4:1.0) and at the lid margin. Rarely, papillary forms may be seen. Orbital extension of squamous cell carcinoma is usually preceded by a history of chronic and repeated recurrence of lesions following treatment or by long-term neglect by the patient (Fig. 12-127). Once the orbit is invaded, the tumor tends to spread along fascia and fatty planes relatively rapidly compared to basal cell carcinoma. In addition, in contrast to basal cell carcinoma, squamous cell carcinoma is capable of metastases, usually to the regional preauricular or submandibular nodes. Perineural invasion may occur and is associated with pain or ophthalmoplegia. The overall mortality rate from squamous cell carcinoma of the lid is about 15% in a modern setting; however, late-stage presentation is much more common in third world countries, where orbital invasion is the usual presentation. The incidence of regional spread varies greatly from 1.3% to as high as 21.4%, but is generally closer to the lower figure.

Management of squamous cell carcinoma of the lid is usually surgical, with care to obtain adequate controlled margins using frozen section or Mohs' technique. Fitzpatrick and colleagues report a control rate of 93.3% with

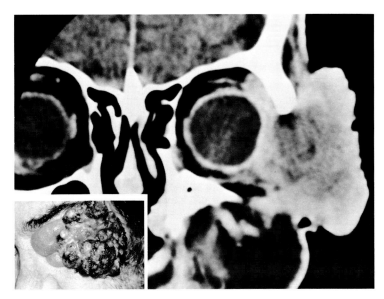

FIGURE 12-127. The patient was a 61-year-old chronic alcoholic with Korsakoff's syndrome. He presented with a fungating putrifying left temporal mass *(inset)* that extended into the adjacent orbit and flattened the globe, as shown on the coronal CT scan. It proved to be a squamous cell carcinoma of skin associated with cervical and mediastinal adenopathy. He underwent radical local radiotherapy, which led to regression of the local lesion.

radiotherapy. Squamous cell carcinoma is thought to be less sensitive to radiotherapy than basal cell carcinoma; thus, higher doses are usually recommended. Deep orbital invasion implies a need for radical therapy, usually by surgical excision by exenteration or radical radiotherapy in the circumstances outlined for basal cell carcinoma.

Malignant Melanoma of Skin

Malignant melanoma arising from skin of the lid is exceedingly rare, constituting 1% of all malignant eyelid lesions and less than 1% of orbital lesions. Conjunctival melanoma, on the other hand, is a more common precursor to orbital invasion perhaps because of later recognition and contiguity. In spite of the rarity, melanomas of the skin are important to recognize and understand because of their potentially lethal nature. We have seen only one melanoma arising from the skin of the lid that led to orbital invasion and required exenteration.

Most melanomas arise *de novo,* but a percentage are thought to develop in relationship to preexistent moles. There are three recognizable precursor lesions. The most important in terms of the lid is lentigo maligna (Hutchinson's melanotic freckle), with the dysplastic nevus syndrome (B-K mole syndrome) and giant nevocytic nevi being the other two. Giant nevocytic nevi are childhood lesions that rarely occur in the scalp and are readily recognized. The dysplastic nevus is a precursor to melanoma, occurs as a familial autosomal dominant trait, is seen first in childhood, and progresses throughout life. These patients are at high risk for developing cutaneous melanomas. The major differentiating features from other nevi are their multiple early occurrence, large size (generally over 5–10 mm), and flat irregular surface with haphazard pigmentation.

Melanomas in general are thought to undergo two phases of growth. The first is a radial intraepidermal pattern, which is followed by vertical growth into the deeper layers of skin. The radial growth phase is clinically and pathologically discernible in the biphasic melanomas (superficial spreading, lentigo maligna, acral lentiginous). In contrast, the nodular melanoma appears clinically to be monophasic and does not have a clinically discernible radial growth phase.

The cutaneous melanomas have been divided into four different types based on patterns of clinical development and histopathology. These include superficial spreading melanoma, lentigo maligna, acral lentiginous melanoma, and nodular melanoma (*de novo*). Superficial spreading melanoma can occur anywhere but is more common in the areas of the body exposed to intermittent and sudden bursts of sun, such as the lower legs of women and the chest and back of men. These appear as 2- to 3-cm raised nodules with bizarre coloration varying from black or brown to rose, white, gray, and blue. Characteristically, they have an irregular border. Lentigo maligna usually arises in middle-aged and elderly persons with sun-damaged facial skin. Clinically, they are usually large, irregular, pale brown patches with a fine peppered distribution of increased pigmentation. These lesions usually have a long history of radial extension, which may wax and wane. It is believed that about 25% to 30% undergo malignant transformation heralded by the development of nodular elevated dark brown or black areas. Acral lentiginous melanoma occurs primarily in the distal extremities or mucosal surfaces, particularly vaginal mucosa. Nodular melanoma, on the other hand, is a relatively rapidly developing focal tumor without clinically perceptible antecedent radial growth. It may be brown to black or amelanotic and can involve exposed areas of skin or mucous membrane. It invades more deeply than the other types of skin melanoma. The overall frequency of the different types of skin melanomas is 5% lentigo maligna, 70% superficial spreading melanoma, 16% nodular melanoma, and 9% other. The various kinds of malignant melanomas can be distinguished by their clinical history, appearance, and histology. The prognosis of melanoma correlates with depth of invasion as well as histologic type. Deeper invasion correlates with a worse prognosis, and according to Clark's classification, levels IV and V (reticular dermis and subcutaneous tissue) have 5-year survivals of 65% and 15%, respectively. Breslow has correlated tumor thickness with survival and reports that patients with tumors 0.76 mm thick have a 5-year survival of 100%, whereas patients with tumors 1.5 mm or thicker have a 5-year survival of less than 50%. The order of prognosis from worst to best according to type is nodular, superficial spreading, and lentigo maligna melanoma. Other factors in prognostication include degree of pigmentation (amelanotic is worse), mitotic activity (more mitoses are worse), and inflammation (less inflammation is worse).

With increasing awareness of epidemiologic factors such as the role of ultraviolet radiation, light skin and hair color, and the nature of melanoma types and premelanotic lesions, the emphasis in management is shifting to prevention and early identification. Because melanomas have a propensity to regional nodal metastases and widespread systemic metastases, treatment is by wide local excision, with or without nodal resection or systemic chemotherapy. The role of node dissection is controversial and chemotherapy remains palliative.

Sebaceous Carcinoma of the Lid

In contrast to sebaceous carcinoma elsewhere, the lid is a frequent site where carcinoma usually arises from the meibomian glands. In terms of incidence it runs a distant second or third to basal cell carcinoma depending on which series is studied (80% to 90% basal cell carcinoma versus 3% to 4% sebaceous carcinoma for all eyelid malignancies). In terms of orbital tumors in general, it constitutes less than 1% (0.4% in Henderson's series and 1% in Shields'). We have seen only one case of orbital extension of sebaceous carcinoma of meibomian origin, representing 0.4% of all of our tumors and 1% of secondary invasions (see Table 12-17). It is, however, interesting to note that of epithelial malignancies invading the orbit from the eyelid, about one third are sebaceous carcinomas. There are some racial predilections, and Chinese may be more prone to developing this lesion. Rao and colleagues suggest that this carcinoma was second only to basal cell in frequency in a study done at the Armed Forces Institute of Pathology (AFIP). The upper lid is the usual site with two thirds noted here, about 20% in the lower lid or diffusely, and a small percentage in the caruncle. These incidences vary slightly depending on the series studied. It is characteristically a lesion of the elderly, with a maximum occurrence in the seventh decade and a slight female predominance.

Sebaceous carcinoma has achieved a notorious reputation because of failure to recognize it early. The tumor may masquerade as chronic chalazion, blepharoconjunctivitis, basal cell carcinoma, keratoconjunctivitis, or very rarely as a primary orbital tumor. Delay in diagnosis significantly affects mortality, with a duration of greater than 6 months associated with 43% mortality, compared to 13% when duration is less than 6 months. Another cause for confusion has been pathologic misdiagnosis, most commonly as basal cell or squamous cell carcinoma. Increasing awareness of the characteristic presentation, with earlier and more accurate clinical and pathologic diagnosis, has improved the mortality of this tumor. The blepharoconjunctivitis associated with this lesion is the result of an intraepithelial (pagetoid) spread of sebaceous carcinoma. The usual clinical appearance is a thickening of the conjunctiva associated with frank injection in areas of invasion. A careful biomicroscopic examination will reveal yellowish, plaque-like foci within the affected epithelium.

The incidence of orbital extension varies from 6% in Ginsberg's series to 35% in the review of Doxanas. Orbital invasion is associated with 70% mortality rate. This tumor has a propensity to spread to the lymphatic system and subsequently to lung, liver, brain, or skull. Those that extend into the orbit have about a 70% association with preauricular cervical or submaxillary adenopathy compared to an overall incidence of around 19% for all sebaceous gland carcinomas of the lid and adnexa.

The pathologic diagnosis is based on evidence of sebaceous origin. These carcinomas are usually lobular or consist of cords of cells with a varying degree of sebaceous differentiation and infiltration. The degree of differentiation tends to progress from the periphery toward the center of lobules, recapitulating the normal pattern of sebaceous glands. Cells that are differentiated have a foamy or vacuolated, slightly basophilic cytoplasm (Fig. 12-128). In contrast, the less differentiated tumors have cells that are more deeply basophilic, anaplastic, and display more mitotic figures. The peripheral location of the basophilic, less vacuolated cells produces a pattern that is similar to basal cell carcinoma, but the cells are more anaplastic. Sebaceous carcinomas have a propensity to invade the basal layer of skin and mucous membranes in a radial fashion due to pagetoid spread, which correlates with the chronic blepharoconjunctivitis syndrome. These tumors characteristically contain fat; therefore, frozen sections and fat stains are useful in the diagnosis and at the time of controlled resection. The large AFIP series has correlated various clinical and pathologic features with mortality; these are summarized in Table 12-22.

Sebaceous carcinoma of the lid is best managed by surgery. Doxanas and Green have emphasized the improvement in mortality based on earlier recognition and wide excision with frozen section control. Although microscopically controlled excision may be attempted in instances of orbital invasion, this circumstance usually necessitates exenteration. The frequent association with lymphatic spread implies a need to assess spread, obtain histologic proof of involvement, and carry out a radical resection of the parotid, submaxillary, and cervical nodes. Several reports on radiotherapy indicate that when given in adequate doses, generally over 4500 rad, this tumor can be treated in patients who refuse excision or have contraindications for surgery. In addition, radiotherapy is a useful palliative modality.

Other Adnexal Carcinomas

The adnexa may give rise to rare apocrine and eccrine carcinomas of sweat gland origin that invade the orbit. This includes the mucinous sweat gland adenocarcinoma, which tends to occur in the elderly and may rarely invade the orbit and adjacent bony structures. They are usually locally aggressive and best managed by en bloc wide excision. An unusual and exceedingly rare eccrine adenocarcinoma with a tendency for orbital invasion is the infiltrating signet-ring carcinoma. Because of its histiocytoid appearance, metastases from other sites, in particular the breast, should be ruled out. Finally, apocrine gland carcinomas arise from the gland of Moll. Ni and co-workers have described a single case of orbital invasion by this locally invasive tumor.

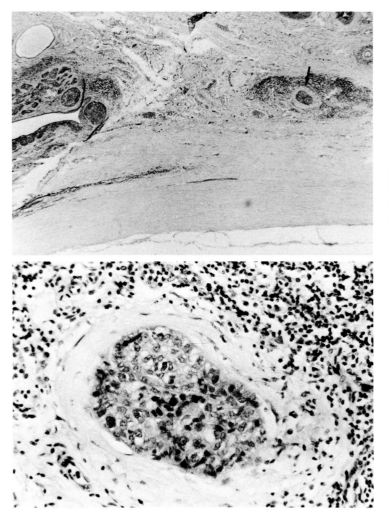

FIGURE 12-128. These photomicrographs are from an exenteration specimen in a patient who had a meibomian gland carcinoma involving the entire right upper lid and the lateral portion of the lower lid. *(Top)* The superior fornix with infiltration of the conjunctiva and adjacent forniceal structures. There is a distant focus of infiltration surrounded by inflammation in the anterior orbit *(arrow)*. *(Bottom)* A higher-power view of the orbital infiltration by this poorly differentiated meibomian gland carcinoma. Note the vacuolated anaplastic cells (H&E, original magnification *top* × 2.5, *bottom* × 25).

SECONDARY TUMORS ARISING FROM THE CONJUNCTIVA

Squamous Carcinoma of the Conjunctiva

Squamous cell carcinoma of the conjunctiva usually occurs at the limbus, arising in a preexisting carcinoma in situ, in solar keratosis, or in epithelial dysplasia. It is an indolent lesion seen primarily in men in the sixth and seventh decades and is believed to arise secondary to long-standing actinic exposure or chronic irritation; thus, in the tropics, it is more often seen in young adults. Additional factors that contribute to its more common occurrence in these areas are nutritional disorders, recurrent infection, and racial predilection. The initial clinical appearance is either one of a whitish, rough, dry, irregular, leukoplakic lesion or a telangiectatic gelatinous epibul-

bar mass. These tumors may rarely be papillary, exophytic, or fixed to the underlying sclera. When confined to the conjunctiva, it may masquerade as conjunctivitis. The usual course is one of superficial invasion and slow growth, because the majority are well-differentiated tumors. It can be a locally aggressive tumor and invade intraocularly in less than 10% of cases. In about an equal percentage, orbital invasion or nodal metastases may occur. Orbital invasion may be heralded by the development of a mass lesion with fixation of the globe. In addition, because these lesions are insidious in development, patients may present with apparent orbital cellulitis (Fig. 12-129), draining fistulas (Fig. 12-130), or plaque-like infiltrations of the conjunctiva, sclera, and adjacent orbital tissues associated with fixation (Fig. 12-131). Orbital invasion may follow multiple attempts at excision. In un-

TABLE 12-22.
CLINICAL AND PATHOLOGIC FEATURES INDICATIVE OF BAD PROGNOSIS IN SEBACEOUS CARCINOMAS OF OCULAR ADNEXA

Clinicopathologic Features	Total Number of Cases	Number of Fatal Outcomes	Percentage Mortality
Vascular invasion	3	3	100
Lymphatic invasion	6	5	83
Upper and lower lid involvement	6	5	83
Orbital invasion	17	13	76
Poor differentiation	10	6	60
Pagetoid invasion	17	10	59
Tumors larger than 10 mm	17	9	53
Highly infiltrative pattern	11	5	45
Multicentric origin	12	5	42
Duration of symptoms more than 6 months	34	13	38

(Rao NA, Hidayat AA, McLean IW et al: Sebaceous carcinomas of the ocular adnexa: A clinicopathologic study of 104 cases, with five-year follow-up data. Hum Pathol 13:113, 1982)

derdeveloped countries, higher rates of orbital invasion and metastases have been noted because of late presentation. Even with orbital invasion, death from metastases is exceedingly rare.

Histologically, the majority are well-differentiated squamous carcinomas (see Fig. 12-129B). There are two more aggressive variants: spindle cell carcinoma (Fig. 12-132) and mucoepidermoid carcinoma, both of which have a greater tendency to invade.

Local lesions of the conjunctiva can be treated adequately with histologically controlled conjunctival resection with or without superficial sclerectomy. In addition, local cryotherapy is useful in the management of these lesions. Massive conjunctivectomy may be necessary for more rapidly developing and diffuse lesions. Orbital extension is managed by exenteration. Evidence of regional nodal involvement should be managed by radical node dissection. Radical radiotherapy may be considered for the elderly or for extensive lesions.

Malignant Melanoma of the Conjunctiva

It is somewhat difficult to establish the incidence of melanoma of the conjunctiva invading the orbit, because our understanding of the natural history and management of this disease is undergoing significant change. We had seven patients with orbital invasion secondary to conjunctival melanoma; they constituted 0.5% of our overall series and 7.4% of secondary orbital invasions. Orbital extension of uveal melanomas appears to be a more significant component in most series. The incidence of orbital extension of conjunctival melanoma in several general series varied from 0.5% to 2% of all orbital lesions. With improved understanding of the natural history, progression, and management of these lesions, the likelihood of orbital extension ought to decrease.

Although theoretically, conjunctival melanomas may arise in the three different circumstances of primary acquired melanosis, preexistent nevi, and as *de novo* malignancies in both clinical and pathologic settings, it may be difficult to ascertain the specific precursor lesion in many instances. However, Folberg, McLean, and Zimmerman in their series have suggested that an acquired melanosis was present in 75% of their cases. Reese estimated that one quarter of conjunctival melanomas arose in nevi, one quarter as *de novo* lesions, and 50% in acquired melanosis; and the large series reported by Lederman and co-workers supports a similar incidence. In spite of the difficulty of exact determination of origin in many instances, categorization is useful from a clinical point of view.

Malignant Melanoma Arising in Acquired Melanosis

Primary acquired melanosis (PAM) is typically a lesion of middle-aged whites; it is rare in younger age groups. The natural history is one of development of a superficial, variegated, epithelial pigmentation with a characteristic

(Text continues on p. 445.)

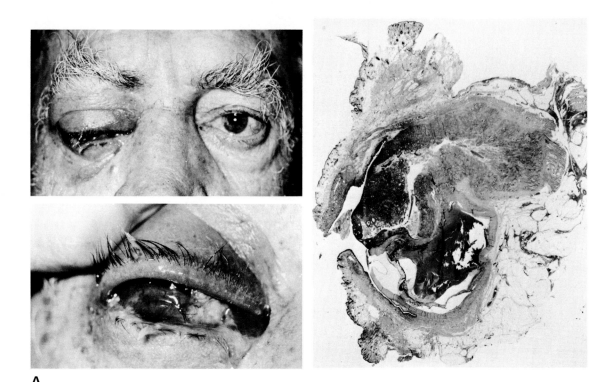

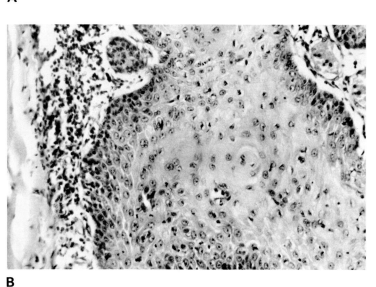

A

B

FIGURE 12-129. *(A)* This 64-year-old chronic alcoholic presented with a 4- to 5-day history of a painful right eye and proptosis. He claimed to have had no vision in his right eye for years and had recurrent infections in the same eye, which usually responded to minimal conservative treatment. On this occasion, in spite of local antibiotic treatment, there had been no response. On examination, there was 6 mm lateral, 8 mm inferior, and 9 mm axial displacement of the right eye with a fullness of the upper lid and erythema of the overlying skin. There was restricted extraocular movements, a purulent discharge, and a boggy, indurated, red, superior conjunctiva. Biopsy of the conjunctiva revealed a well-differentiated squamous cell carcinoma. The patient underwent exenteration after CT scan demonstrated orbital involvement, and he had no evidence of local lymph node or systemic disease. The photomicrograph demonstrates a well-differentiated squamous cell carcinoma infiltrating deeply into the orbit, and invading and perforating the globe (H&E, original magnification ✕ 2). *(B)* Higher-power photomicrograph demonstrates this well-differentiated squamous cell carcinoma. The patient has been observed without recurrence for 6 years (H&E, original magnification ✕ 25).

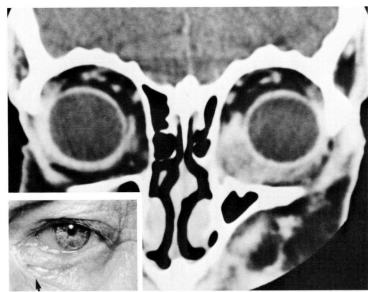

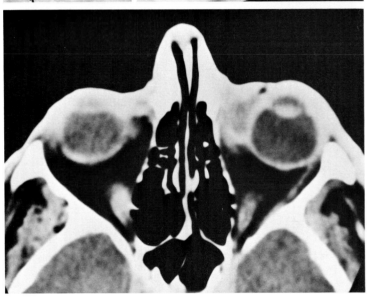

FIGURE 12-130. This 61-year-old man presented with a chronic fistula *(arrow)* of the left lower lid and medial canthal region. It was associated with limitation of abduction and a palpable mass in the inferomedial orbit. The coronal and axial CT scans demonstrate an inferomedial infiltrating orbital mass. On biopsy, it proved to be a poorly differentiated squamous cell carcinoma arising from mucous epithelium of either the conjunctiva or lacrimal sac. The patient refused exenteration, and underwent radical radiotherapy with regression of the lesion to date 1 year later.

FIGURE 12-131. Clinical photograph and axial CT scan of a patient presenting 3 years after excision of a squamous cell carcinoma of the left lower fornix demonstrate a recurrence that infiltrated the lower lid, conjunctiva, globe, and anterior orbit. She had originally presented 13 years earlier with a "white spot" on the surface of the left eye, which had been resected on a number of occasions. Carcinoma *in situ* was diagnosed 8 years before this presentation.

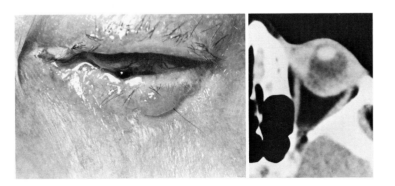

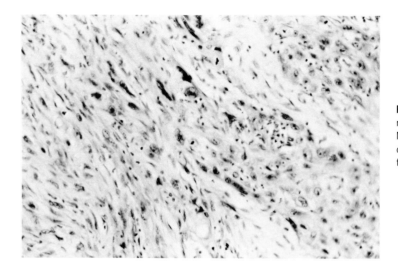

FIGURE 12-132. Photomicrograph of a squamous cell carcinoma that had infiltrated the orbit. Note the cords of moderately differentiated spindle-shaped squamous cells (H&E, original magnification × 25).

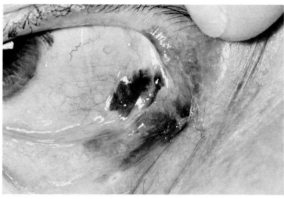

A

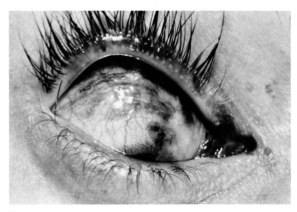

B

FIGURE 12-133. (A) An acquired melanosis (noted for 1 year) in the medial canthal region of a 63-year-old man. Biopsy demonstrated stage IB primary acquired melanosis with atypical melanocytic hyperplasia. It responded well to local cryotherapy. (B) This extensive pigmented lesion involving the superior conjunctiva, fornix, and lid was seen in a 33-year-old man who presented with a history of known conjunctival pigmentation present for at least 2 years. The caruncle and superior fornix were infiltrated by a thickened, nodular, blackish lesion. Biopsy revealed multiple foci of stage IIB malignant melanoma arising from primary acquired melanosis. The patient underwent exenteration, and is alive and well 4 years later.

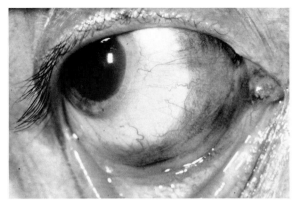

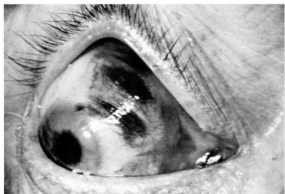

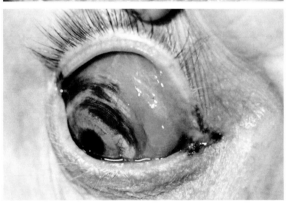

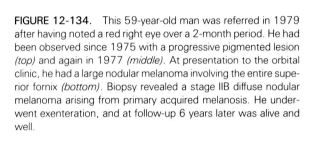

FIGURE 12-134. This 59-year-old man was referred in 1979 after having noted a red right eye over a 2-month period. He had been observed since 1975 with a progressive pigmented lesion *(top)* and again in 1977 *(middle)*. At presentation to the orbital clinic, he had a large nodular melanoma involving the entire superior fornix *(bottom)*. Biopsy revealed a stage IIB diffuse nodular melanoma arising from primary acquired melanosis. He underwent exenteration, and at follow-up 6 years later was alive and well.

pepper-like distribution of variegated pigment. These lesions can evolve over many years, extending in a radial fashion over larger and larger areas of conjunctiva and skin (Figs. 12-133, 12-134). In addition, they may wax and wane over time. Ultimately, nodular melanomas (Fig. 12-135) may arise within the primary acquired melanosis, invade deeper tissues, or extend into lymphatics and lymph nodes. Biopsy of primary acquired melanosis may help to predict those prone to progression. In particular, primary acquired melanosis with atypia (about 68% of Folberg's series) will progress to melanoma in approximately 50% of circumstances. The mortality rate due to

melanoma within PAM is about 25% and correlates with tumor thickness as well as evidence of pagetoid invasion of the epithelium (Table 12-23). Involvement of the caruncle, fornix, sclera, or orbit implies a greater likelihood of metastasis.

Zimmerman, Jakobiec, and others have championed information that has led to earlier recognition and management of conjunctival melanoma arising from primary acquired melanosis. Early recognition, biopsy, and treatment of potentially aggressive lesions ought to control this disease in many circumstances. In fact, even extensive conjunctival disease is amenable to removal of the

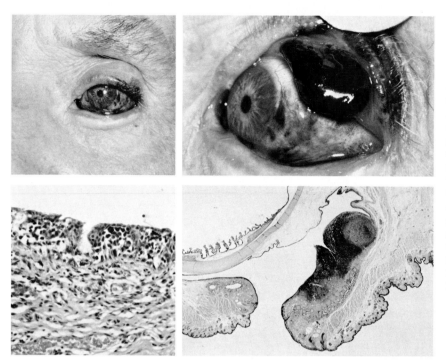

FIGURE 12-135. *(Top)* This 80-year-old man presented with massive conjunctival and adjacent lid involvement with a malignant melanoma arising from primary acquired melanosis. He underwent exenteration. *(Bottom, left)* The pathology photograph shows an intraepithelial component consisting of nests of loosely arranged malignant melanoma cells. *(Bottom, right)* Diffuse superior forniceal involvement with a large nodular melanoma is shown (H&E, original magnifications *left* × 10, *right* × 2).

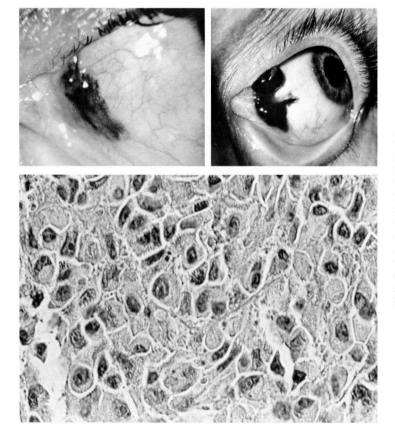

FIGURE 12-136. This 61-year-old man was referred with the lesion shown *(top, right)*. He had been aware for many years of a pigmented lesion in the medial canthal region. *(Top, left)* The lesion is shown 6 years earlier. At the time of referral, the lesion had been bleeding intermittently. It was a nodular malignant melanoma. He underwent resection, cryotherapy, and reconstruction of the medial canthal region. However, he developed a local recurrence 1 year later that required exenteration. He is alive and well with 4 years' follow-up. *(Bottom)* Histologically, the anaplastic lesion appeared to have arisen from a nevus, which is not shown (H&E, original magnification × 40).

nodular component and repeated local treatment with cryotherapy. Lederman and co-workers, in reviewing a series of 184 melanomas of conjunctiva treated by radiotherapy, have emphasized that with controlled, adequate, and individualized methods, radiotherapy may be possible in treating some of these lesions with minimal complications. They have suggested that site, macroscopic appearance (melanoma from limbal nevi do better; *de novo* melanomas not radiocurable and widespread malignant acquired melanosis less satisfactory than smaller lesions), and type of lesion bear significantly on method of treatment and likelihood of response. Frank or significant orbital invasion implies the necessity for exenteration. Subtotal exenteration can be carried out if there is no evidence of radial epithelial extension of the lesion to the skin of the anterior lid. Nodal involvement implies widespread metastatic disease in almost all circumstances, but occasionally cases have been restricted to the regional nodes and cured by node resection.

Malignant Melanoma Arising Within a Nevus

Melanomas arising from nevi usually appear as a change in known pigmented lesions of conjunctiva (Fig. 12-136). Nevertheless, it may be impossible to establish a clear-cut clinical history of a preexisting history of a nevus. However, at the time of excision of a melanoma, nevoid rests are seen histologically in one third of cases, and are noted in about one quarter of melanomas in primary acquired melanosis. Development of a melanoma may be heralded by increasing nodularity, variegated pigmentation, bleeding, or inflammation. Treatment of a localized lesion is wide excision with cryotherapy of the adjacent conjunctiva. Limbal melanomas arising from nevi appear to have a better prognosis than those in other conjunctival sites or when arising *de novo*. Orbital invasion implies the necessity for exenteration as described for melanomas arising in primary acquired melanosis.

Malignant Melanoma Arising de Novo

Melanomas arising *de novo* in conjunctiva parallel the so-called nodular melanoma of skin insofar as a clinically and histologically recognizable radial growth phase is not noted (Fig. 12-137). Epibulbar melanomas arising *de novo*, however, can be ulcerative, amelanotic, papillary, or fungating (Fig. 12-137).

In contrast to melanomas arising in acquired melanosis, those arising from nevi or *de novo* do not have clear-cut histologic risk factors. It is important to be aware of the possibility of local lymphatic spread in the conjunctiva and the appearance of satellite lesions, which should be sought carefully on a prospective basis (see Fig. 12-137).

Management is by wide local excision followed by local cryotherapy. Nodal involvement usually implies widespread disease, but occasional cases of patients

TABLE 12-23.

HISTOLOGIC CLASSIFICATION OF IDIOPATHIC PRIMARY ACQUIRED MELANOSIS OF CONJUNCTIVA

Stage I	Benign acquired melanosis
A	With minimal melanocytic hyperplasia
B	With atypical melanocytic hyperplasia
	(1) Mild to moderately severe
	(2) Severe (in situ malignant melanoma)
Stage II	Malignant acquired melanosis
A	With superficially invasive melanoma (tumor thickness less than 1.5 mm)*
B	With more deeply invasive melanoma (tumor thickness greater than 1.5 mm)*

* Selection of tumor thickness of 1.5 mm as a convenient measurable dividing line between Stages IIA and IIB is based on data provided by Silvers, Jakobiec, Freeman et al (1978). These investigators reported that regardless of method of treatment, patients who had lesions no thicker than 1.5 mm did well, whereas all lethal tumors measured more than 1.8 mm in thickness.

(Spencer WH, Zimmerman LE: Conjunctiva. In Spencer WH: Ophthalmic Pathology: An Atlas and Textbook, 3rd ed, Vol 1, p 201. Philadelphia, WB Saunders, 1985)

being salvaged by nodal resection have been reported. Orbital extension may require exenteration.

Of melanomas we saw that arose from conjunctiva and involved the orbit, two were *de novo* lesions, one appeared to develop from a nevus, and the remaining four were cases of extensive and invasive melanoma arising from primary acquired melanosis.

ORBITAL EXTENSION OF OCULAR MALIGNANCIES

Extrascleral and Orbital Extension of Uveal Melanoma

Uveal melanoma has a number of distinctive biologic characteristics that have made it the center of some controversy in recent years. Although much is known about the clinical and pathologic nature and evolution of this tumor, there are many unusual and unique characteristics that provide a focus for this controversy. The core of the controversy centers on the role of extirpation (whether by local resection, enucleation, or in the case of extrascleral extension, exenteration) in the management of this tumor. Zimmerman has summarized the major controversies regarding pathogenesis of spread, including (1) trauma of enucleation, and/or (2) decreased host resistance incurred by removal, and (3) increased virulence concomitant with appearance of clinical symptoms. This controversy has led to more "conservative" management in selected circumstances (including observation, local radiotherapy, and local resection), greater attention to atraumatic enucleation techniques, and prospective multicenter studies aimed at ultimately resolving these important issues.

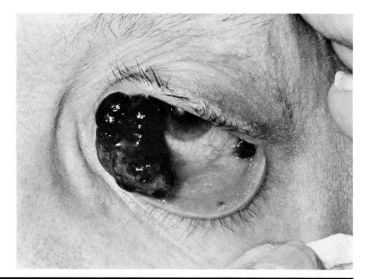

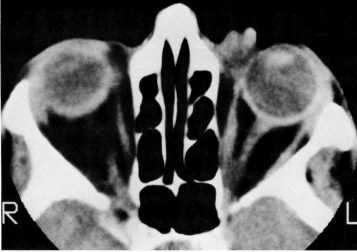

FIGURE 12-137. *(Top)* This 81-year-old woman had been aware of a pigmented lesion in the left caruncular region for 18 months. It was gradually increasing in size and had bled on several occasions. In addition, she was aware of a lump present for 6 weeks on the left side of her neck. On physical examination, she had vision of 20/200 on the left (compared to 20/40 on the right) and lateral displacement of the left globe with some limitation of abduction. This massive pigmented lesion was associated with thickening and induration of the tarsal conjunctiva and nodular satellite lesion in the temporal aspect of the inferior fornix due to local lymphatic spread. *(Bottom)* The axial CT scan demonstrates the irregularly shaped homogeneous density in the anterior orbit. The patient refused exenteration and was managed by local resection and cryotherapy with removal of involved nodes. Two of the 31 neck nodes were positive for metastatic disease. Subsequently, she presented with a nodular recurrence in the left jaw, and died 1 year after treatment without evidence of local recurrence.

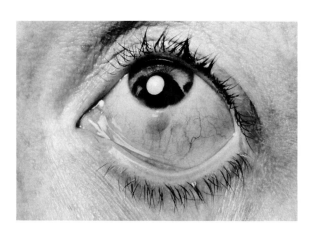

FIGURE 12-138. Anterior epibulbar extension of melanoma. This patient presented with an iris melanoma resected 8 years earlier. It had recurred at the base of the resection and extended through the sclera. She underwent local eye-wall resection and graft, and has no evidence of recurrence to date.

TABLE 12-24.
ORBITAL RECURRENCE RATES IN RELATION TO EXTRASCLERAL EXTENSION

Size and Appearance of Extrascleral Extension	Recurrence Rates (%)
No extraocular extension observed	0.7
All sizes and types	18
Very large	65
Small and medium	12
Nonencapsulated or surgically transected	50
Small and encapsulated	8

(After Starr JH, Zimmerman LE: Extrascleral extension and orbital recurrence of malignant melanomas of the choroid and ciliary body. Int Ophthalmol Clin 2:369, 1962)

(Zimmerman LE: Malignant melanoma of the uveal tract. In Spencer WH: Ophthalmic Pathology, Vol 3, p 2111. Philadelphia, WB Saunders, 1985)

Death from uveal melanoma increases with time; overall, it is 30% at 5 years, 50% at 10 years, and 2% per year thereafter for up to 25 years. The major negative factors affecting survival are larger intraocular tumor size, the presence of mixed or epithelioid cell type, and evidence of extrascleral extension. Melanomas gain access to the orbit by paraemissarial extension and less often by intraemissarial growth. The incidence of orbital recurrence is about 3% of patients enucleated for melanoma and increases to 18% when there is histologic evidence of extrascleral extension at the time of enucleation. Factors that increase orbital recurrence rates include larger tumor size, epithelioid, mixed or necrotic cell types, and nonencapsulated or surgically transected epibulbar tumors (Table 12-24). Transection of the tumor is associated with 50% orbital recurrence.

Extrascleral extension may present clinically as visible anterior nodules (Figs. 12-138 and 12-139), proptosis in patients with known intraocular tumor or with phthisis and unsuspected tumor, or as a mass in orbital recurrence (which has been described as late as 42 years after primary enucleation). Increasingly, the use of ultrasonography and CT scan may lead to preoperative detection of extrascleral nodules (Fig. 12-140). Finally, orbital extension may only become evident at the time of surgery (Figs. 12-141, 12-142).

The controversy over the management of orbital recurrence parallels that of intraocular melanoma. However, it does seem that by the time extrascleral and orbital extension is evident, other biological factors are already in play that dominate the grave mortality, which is about 80% in these circumstances. The role of exenteration has not yet been defined in a prospective controlled study. There is very strong retrospective evidence (most recently reviewed by Kersten and co-workers) suggesting that exenteration does not afford protection from metastases, except perhaps in the instance of frank transection or nonencapsulation at enucleation. Shields and co-workers

FIGURE 12-139. A small epibulbar extension of a large ciliary body melanoma.

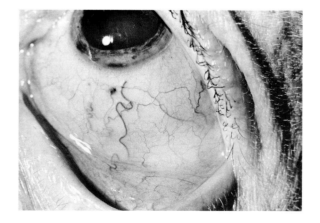

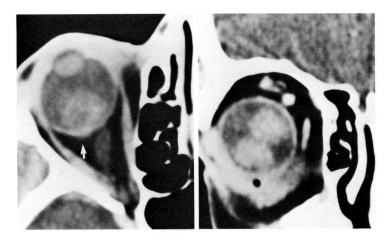

FIGURE 12-140. Axial *(left)* and coronal *(right)* CT scans demonstrate a large right intraocular melanoma with posterior extension *(arrow)*. It was seen in a 73-year-old woman who underwent primary subtotal exenteration and died 2 years later of metastatic disease.

have summarized their current management (Table 12-25). Essentially, the trend is towards resection only of adjacent tissues when the lesion is nodular, and exenteration (which can usually be subtotal) is reserved for instances where there is evidence of tumor transection at the time of enucleation. In these circumstances, exenteration may only be a palliative measure. The role of preoperative and postoperative radiotherapy has not been clearly determined. Orbital recurrence for similar reasons requires exenteration, although low-grade spindle cell tumors may be curable in such circumstances. The biological factors previously outlined appear to dominate the poor prognosis in orbital melanoma.

Orbital Extension of Retinoblastoma

Retinoblastoma is the most common intraocular tumor of childhood, accounting for 1% of childhood cancer deaths in the United States and 5% of blindness in children. The incidence has doubled in the last 50 years from 1 in 34,000 live births to 1 in 16,000 to 1 in 20,000 live births. This change in incidence is related to an increasing gene pool as a result of prolonged survival and increasing mutation rate related to environmental mutagens.

The common clinical presentation is leukokoria or strabismus; less frequently, ocular inflammation, hyphema, or glaucoma may be noted. The overall mortality for retinoblastoma has decreased from 95% 100 years ago to 10% to 20% in a modern setting. In underdeveloped countries, patients characteristically present with extensive local and widespread disease; thus, mortality rates range between 90% and 100%.

A major biologic characteristic of retinoblastoma, like all other malignancies, is the ability to invade and spread. Most retinoblastomas remain for a long time within the confines of the globe, except perhaps for blood-borne metastases, but the barriers to egress are ultimately penetrated. Depending on the site of the primary lesion, retinoblastoma may spread by means of the choroid to the adjacent orbital structures, by the optic nerve (particularly when the origin is peripapillary) to the central nervous system, and by the vascular system to distant metastatic sites.

Bruch's membrane initially resists invasion, but is eventually eroded, leading to choroidal growth. Once the tumor cells reach this choroidal network of fine vascular channels, growth appears to accelerate as evidenced by three clinical features: (1) rapid growth over a period of days or weeks; (2) high elevation on a narrow peduncu-

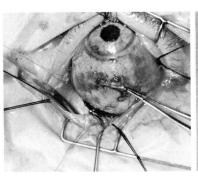
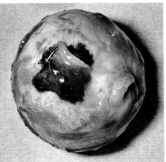

FIGURE 12-141. An epibulbar extension of melanoma noted at enucleation. The globe and adjacent Tenon's capsule were resected. *(Right)* The tumor after enucleation and removal of Tenon's capsule. The patient developed metastases 8 months following surgery.

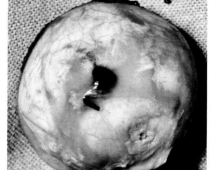
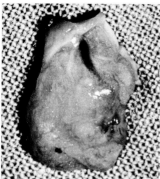
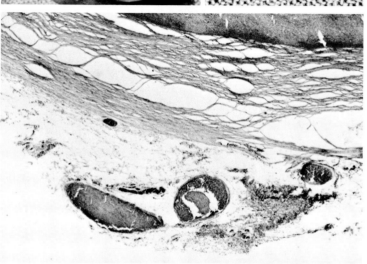

FIGURE 12-142. Enucleation specimen demonstrates an epibulbar extension of a malignant melanoma with growth into a vortex vein. *(Top, right)* The adjacent Tenon's capsule contains the remainder of the vortex vein with melanoma in it. *(Bottom)* The photomicrograph demonstrates the intravascular melanoma, which was histologically of mixed cell type. The patient developed liver metastasis 3 years after enucleation and local resection of involved tissues (H&E, original magnification × 10).

TABLE 12-25.
MANAGEMENT OF UVEAL MELANOMAS WITH EXTRASCLERAL EXTENSION

Type of Extrascleral Extension	Detected Clinically	Detected at Surgery	Detected Pathologically After Enucleation
Flat	1. Modified enucleation with tenonectomy 2. Plaque radiotherapy	1. Modified enucleation with tenonectomy 2. Plaque radiotherapy	1. External irradiation 2. Immunotherapy
Nodular (small)	1. Preoperative orbital radiation followed by modified enucleation with tenonectomy 2. Plaque radiotherapy	1. Modified enucleation with tenonectomy and postoperative orbital radiotherapy 2. Plaque radiotherapy	Tenonectomy with removal; ball implant followed by orbital radiotherapy
Nodular (large)	Preoperative orbital radiation followed by exenteration	Exenteration followed by orbital radiotherapy	Exenteration
Vortex vein		1. Vortex vein resection followed by modified enucleation or plaque radiotherapy 2. Postoperative chemotherapy or immunotherapy	Systemic chemotherapy or immunotherapy
Recurrence after enucleation	Preoperative orbital radiation followed by exenteration		

(Shields JA, Augsburger JJ, Corwin S et al: The management of uveal melanomas with extrascleral extension. Orbit 5:31, 1986)

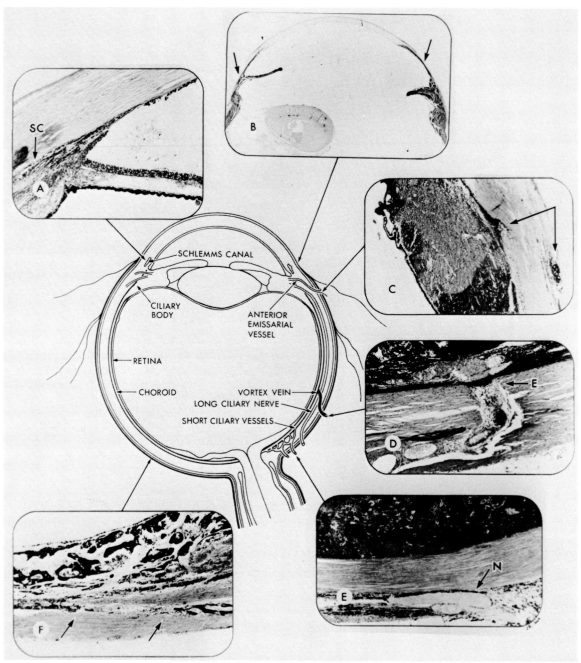

FIGURE 12-143. Spread of retinoblastoma from the globe to surrounding tissues. *(A)* By means of Schlemm's canal (SC) and the intrascleral venous plexus (H&E, original magnification × 10). *(B)* Buph-thalmic eye with direct erosion of the tunic *(arrows)* (H&E, original magnification × 4). *(C)* Ciliary body replaced by retinoblastoma with egress along anterior emissary *(arrow)*. Note episcleral retinoblastoma (H&E, original magnification × 6.3). *(D)* Early extension along emissary in region of the vortex vein (H&E, original magnification × 10). *(E)* Epibulbar nodules of retinoblastoma surrounding posterior ciliary vessel and nerve (N) (H&E, original magnification × 6.3). *(F)* Egress along posterior emissary from choroid *(arrows)* (H&E, original magnification × 6.3). (Rootman J, Ellsworth R, Hofbauer J et al: Orbital extension of retinoblastoma: A clinicopathologic study. Can J Ophthalmol 13:72, 1978)

lated stalk; and (3) a yellow color at the summit suggesting that the lamina vitrea has been pushed forward ahead of the tumor. Once in the choroid, the tumor spreads diffusely and rapidly in a lateral fashion.

When the mass of cells within the sponge-like network of choroidal vessels reaches a critical size, the chances of metastatic spread increase. Choroidal involvement is frequent in retinoblastoma, and metastases relate more closely to the critical mass of the tumor than to the mere presence of cells within the choroid.

As soon as Bruch's membrane is broken, egress from the confines of the globe follows (Fig. 12-143). An enucleated globe has three features that may suggest the possibility of orbital recurrence: spread in continuity to episcleral nodules; periemissarial retinoblastoma not extending to the surface; and significant invasion of the choroid. The loose periemissarial connective tissue provides a natural plane for tumor growth. Thus, massive posterior choroidal involvement has a greater opportunity for access to the many posterior emissaria (see Fig. 12-143).

Lateral growth from the adventitial coats of the intrascleral emissaria may also lead to lamellar separation of the sclera and ultimately destroy the ocular coats (Fig. 12-144). Once outside the globe, the orbit provides a rich, loose tissue plane and growth further accelerates, leading to a large orbital mass (Figs. 12-145, 12-146).

Retinoblastoma may gain direct egress by means of the optic nerve to the central nervous system. Access to the subarachnoid space occurs by growth along the optic nerve to the site of penetration of the central retinal artery and vein. However, other modes are evident from our study of optic nerve invasion. Although many cases had a central nervous system death, the tumors had not invaded much beyond the lamina cribrosa, but were noted to occupy the nerve immediately adjacent to the pial lining (Fig. 12-147G). Some of these cases also had evidence of pial erosion; thus, direct egress from the nerve into the subarachnoid space (see Fig. 12-147E,F). The degree of optic nerve extension has been correlated with prognosis (Table 12-26).

More unusual modes of egress into the central nervous system include the posterior ciliary circulation (see Fig. 12-147C,D,H). A tumor that involves the peripapillary choroid can also reach the subarachnoid space along the radicals of the posterior ciliary vessels that supply the optic nerve head and the pia-arachnoid of the distal optic nerve. Another unusual route of spread into the optic nerve is by means of the orbit into the subarachnoid space. Once in the CSF, the tumor spreads by the circulating CSF and sets up malignant rests even in the opposite optic nerve sheath.

Awareness of the significance of optic nerve invasion led to the development of adequate techniques of enucleation and improvement in survival in the last century. Although invasion up to but not beyond the lamina cribrosa has relatively little prognostic significance, invasion to the line of transection carries a poor prognosis and suggests the need for cytopathologic examination of the CSF and possibly additional therapy. Tumor beyond the lamina cribrosa but not to the line of transection may also carry a poor prognosis if it extends to the pia arachnoid, and implies a need for cytologic study of the CSF (see Table 12-26).

Retinoblastoma has widespread metastatic potential in addition to the capacity for local invasion (Table 12-27). The combination of potential for orbital, intra-

(Text continues on p. 456.)

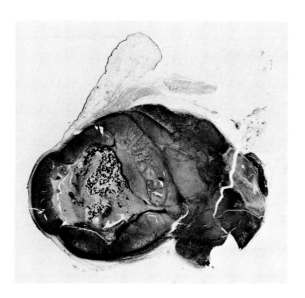

FIGURE 12-144. A retinoblastoma that had occupied the entire globe and eroded through it into the adjacent orbit (H&E, original magnification × 2).

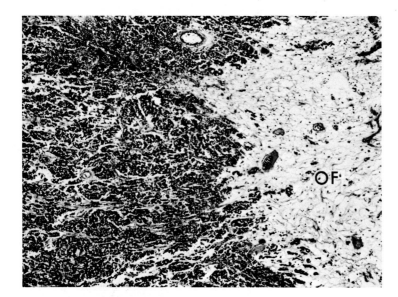

FIGURE 12-145. Orbital fat (OF) infiltrated by retinoblastoma (H&E, original magnification × 10).

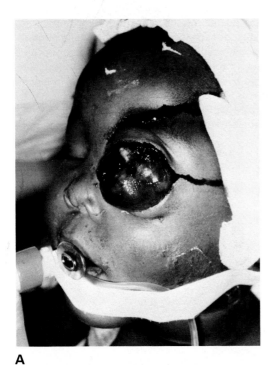

A

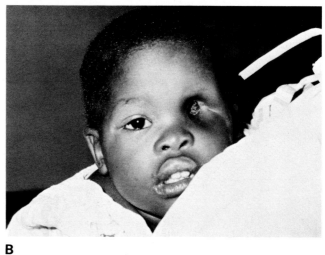

B

FIGURE 12-146. *(A)* Clinical photograph of a child with orbital extension of retinoblastoma. *(B)* Same child 14 months after exenteration, radiotherapy, and chemotherapy. She is alive and well 3.5 years after presentation. (Courtesy of Dr. H.L. Goldberg, Johannesburg, South Africa)

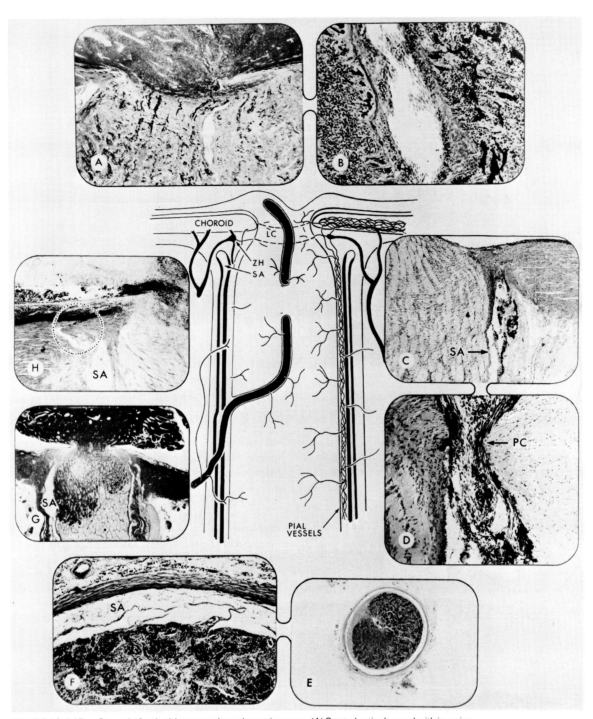

FIGURE 12-147. Spread of retinoblastoma along the optic nerve. *(A)* Central retinal vessel with invasion of the adventitia by retinoblastoma (H&E, original magnification × 6.3). *(B)* High-power view of subendothelial retinoblastoma (H&E, original magnification × 25). *(C)* Retinoblastoma adjacent to subarachnoid space (SA) (H&E, original magnification × 6.3). *(D)* Higher-power view of deeper section from *C* showing egress by means of posterior ciliary vessel (PC) (H&E, original magnification × 40). *(E)* Retinoblastoma eroding the pial and arachnoidal sheaths (H&E, original magnification × 2.5). *(F)* Higher-power view of specimen in *E* showing erosion of the pial sheaths adjacent to subarachnoid space (SA) (H&E, original magnification × 10). *(G)* Invasion of the optic nerve beyond the lamina cribrosa (LC). Tumor cells are immediately subjacent to the pia and arachnoid (H&E, original magnification × 6.3). *(H)* Peripapillary choroidal retinoblastoma; emissarial vessels *(circle)* in continuity with the small vessels of nerve head (H) (H&E, original magnification × 6.3). (Rootman J, Hofbauer J, Ellsworth R: Invasion of the optic nerve by retinoblastoma. Can J Ophthalmol 11:106, 1976)

TABLE 12-26.
SURVIVAL VERSUS OPTIC NERVE EXTENSION

	Overall (%)	Unilateral (%)	Zimmerman* (%)
Group I[†]	77	100	85
Group II	67	65	56
Group III	40	42	36

* Zimmerman LE: The registry of ophthalmic pathology: Past, present and future. Trans Ophthalmol Otolaryngol 65:88, 1961
† Group I = Invasion of the optic nerve up to the lamina cribrosa
Group II = Invasion beyond the lamina but not to the line of transection
Group III = Invasion to the line of transection
(Rootman J, Hofbauer J, Ellsworth R: Invasion of the optic nerve by retinoblastoma. Can J Ophthalmol 11:106, 1976)

cranial, and systemic spread determines the form of therapy following primary enucleation.

Spread from the orbit may reach regional lymph nodes. The incidence of local and nodal extension varies in different parts of the world. In modern medical centers the incidence is between 7.5% and 10%, but it can be up to 62.5% and even higher in undeveloped countries where presentation is usually with orbital extension.

The causes of death in Merriam's autopsy series were intracranial in 52.9%, generalized spread in 41.2%, and local disease in 5.9%. The sites of hematogenous spread are bone, especially the long bones and skull, and viscera (most often the liver; also the pancreas, kidney, spleen, testes, ovaries, and uterus). Lymph node involvement both regionally and widespread is noted at autopsy in 33% to 47% of cases.

Management following enucleation for retinoblastoma is based on the presence or likelihood of extraocular spread as determined by pathologic examination of the globe. Therapy consists of adjuvant combined chemotherapy with local orbital and central nervous system irradiation if central nervous system spread is confirmed. The pathologic criteria suggesting orbital or systemic spread and indicating treatment of the orbit as well as systemic chemotherapy are (1) extrabulbar retinoblastoma, (2) orbital recurrence, (3) massive, particularly posterior, choroidal extension with periemissarial invasion.

The pathologic criteria suggesting a need to investigate and treat the central nervous system are (1) tumor cells in the CSF; (2) extension in the optic nerve to the line of transection; and (3) extension beyond the lamina cribrosa with retinoblastoma adjacent to the pia arachnoid.

Orbital extension of the tumor has been associated with a mortality of 67% to 91%, although modern chemotherapeutic and radiotherapeutic techniques are now producing better results. Orbital recurrences of retinoblastoma are managed by an aggressive chemotherapeutic and radiotherapeutic regimen directed towards systemic and central nervous system spread.

Orbital Extension of Neuroepithelial Tumors of the Ciliary Body

The neuroepithelial tumors of the ciliary body can be divided into congenital and acquired tumors, either of which may be benign or malignant (Table 12-28).

Medulloepitheliomas

Medulloepitheliomas are embryonic tumors that arise from the neuroepithelium in the ciliary body region in children (mean age 5 years at diagnosis). More rarely, they occur adjacent to the optic nerve and extend into the nerve substance. Histologically, they are composed of cords of nonpigmented and pigmented cells resembling medullary epithelium, which may form structures resembling the optic vesicle or optic cup. In addition, they often have areas of undifferentiated cells that resemble retinoblastoma with Homer-Wright and Flexner-Wintersteiner rosettes. The tumor cells can elaborate vitreous-like material. Heteroplastic elements such as cartilage, brain tissue, and striated muscle may be noted in the so-called teratoid medulloepitheliomas. They may be divided pathologically into benign and malignant variants. In a series of 56 cases, Broughton and Zimmerman noted 66% had histologic evidence of malignancy. However, they emphasized the characteristic slow growth and locally invasive nature of the tumor. The single most im-

TABLE 12-27.
CAUSES OF TUMOR-RELATED DEATH IN RETINOBLASTOMA (% VALUES)

	Merriam*	Overall Literature	Carbjal[†]	Taktikos[‡]	Stannard et al[§]
CNS solely	47	45.8	75	29	48
Distant	53	54.2	25	71	52

* Merriam GR: Retinoblastoma: Analysis of seventeen autopsies. Arch Ophthalmol 44:71; 1950
† Carbajal UM: Metastasis in retinoblastoma. Am J Ophthalmol 48:47, 1959
‡ Taktikos A: Investigation of retinoblastoma with special reference to histology and prognosis. Br J Ophthalmol 50:225, 1966
§ Stannard C, Lipper S, Sealy R et al: Retinoblastoma correlation of invasion of the optic nerve and choroid with prognosis and metastasis. Br J Ophthalmol 63:560, 1979

TABLE 12-28.
CLASSIFICATION OF NEUROEPITHELIAL TUMORS OF THE CILIARY BODY

I. Congenital
  A. Glioneuroma
  B. Medulloepithelioma
    1. Benign
    2. Malignant
  C. Teratoid medulloepithelioma
    1. Benign
    2. Malignant
II. Acquired
  A. Nonpigmented
    1. Benign
      a. Pseudoadenomatous hyperplasia
      b. Adenoma
        (1) Solid
        (2) Papillary
        (3) Pleomorphic
    2. Malignant
      a. Glandular and papillary
      b. Pleomorphic, low-grade
      c. Pleomorphic with hyaline stroma
      d. Anaplastic
  B. Pigmented
    1. Benign
      a. Adenoma
      b. Vacuolated adenoma
    2. Malignant
      a. Adenocarcinoma
  C. Mixed pigmented and nonpigmented
    1. Benign
    2. Malignant

(Green WR: Retina. In Spencer WH: Ophthalmic Pathology: An Atlas and Textbook, 3rd ed, Vol 2, p 1246. Philadelphia, WB Saunders, 1985)

portant life-threatening prognostic factor was evidence of extraocular spread.

The typical presentations are poor vision, pain, leukocorea, and ciliary body mass in childhood. Eight of the 56 cases presented with proptosis or an orbital mass. Of the four tumor deaths, all had orbital extension; one developed nodal metastases and the remaining three died by local extension into the intracranial structures. Of the remaining cases of extraocular extension, the major factor in survival appeared to be complete local excision. Tumors occurring in the optic nerve region are more treacherous because of later identification and easier access to the orbital and intracranial structures.

Treatment is by wide local excision. Recent advances in combined craniofacial surgery and reoperative imaging may allow for clearer identification of extension and planned wider excision.

Acquired Neuroepithelial Tumors of the Ciliary Body

The majority of acquired neuroepithelial tumors are benign hyperplasias or adenomas, and malignant variants are rare. Malignant tumors vary from well-differentiated to pleomorphic tumors. The majority arise in previously traumatized, chronically inflamed eyes. Most tumor deaths are due to contiguous invasion, but widespread metastatic disease may occur. Treatment is by wide local excision.

ORBITAL EXTENSION OF LACRIMAL SAC TUMORS

Tumors of the lacrimal sac constitute a small but wide variety of lesions that may invade the orbit. They are best viewed within the context of mass lesions of the medial and inferomedial orbit, the large majority of which are secondary to sinus disease and have been discussed earlier. Neoplasia of the lacrimal sac must be differentiated from all other tumefactions in this region, including acute and chronic inflammations. About 25% of lacrimal sac tumors are, in fact, inflammatory lesions including granulomas and nonspecific inflammatory disease. The remaining tumors are true neoplasms, of which 75% are malignant. The large majority of neoplasms are of epithelial origin, but a number of nonepithelial tumors have been described, including fibrous histiocytoma, schwannoma, lymphomas, angiosarcomas, and melanomas.

From a clinical point of view, the most important neoplastic lesions of the lacrimal sac that ought to be identified are those that can be or are potentially malignant. The benign lesions have a tendency to slower growth, obstructive symptoms, and recurrent dacryocystitis that may mimic inflammation of the lacrimal sac. In contrast, the infiltrative character of malignancies dominates the higher risk category tumors, which tend to present with mass effect, local infiltration of the orbit and adjacent bony structures, occasional pain, a mass above the medial canthal ligament, telangiectasis of the skin, serosanguinous discharge or bloody reflux following irrigation, and an overall relentless progressive course. In addition, recurrence is a clinical feature of malignancy.

Epithelial Tumors

Ryan and Font have divided the epithelial malignancies into papillomas and de novo tumors. The papillomas display three growth patterns including exophytic, inverted, and mixed types. Additionally, they can be subdivided histologically into squamous, transitional cell, and mixed cell papillomas. The exophytic papillomas occur in any age group and have a tendency to multiple occurrence affecting the whole of the epithelium of the nasolacrimal system, particularly when they are of the transitional cell type (Fig. 12-148). The inverted papilloma is (Text continues on p. 460.)

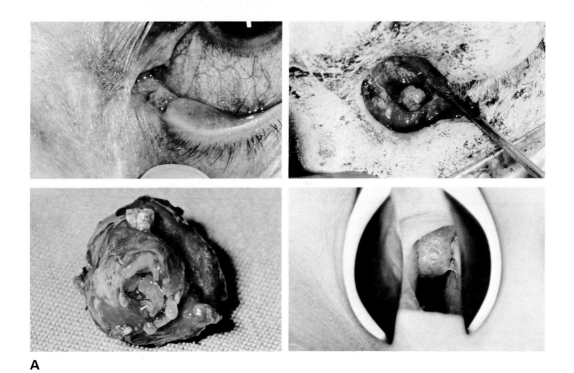

A

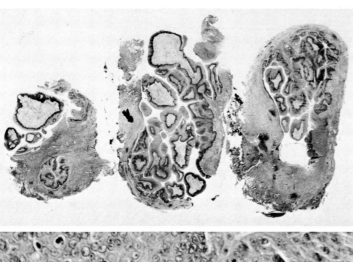

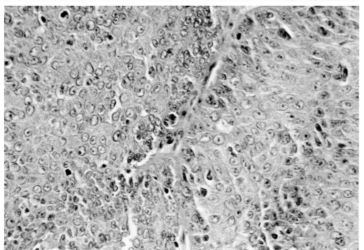

B

FIGURE 12-148. *(A)* The patient, a 69-year-old woman, presented in 1976 with a long-standing history of recurrent papillary lesions in the medial canthal region for which she had undergone multiple local resections. She had a palpable anterior inferior medial orbital mass. The medial canthal region and adjacent lacrimal sac were resected *en bloc (bottom, left)* and the nasolacrimal duct was also noted to be involved *(top, right).* A lateral rhinotomy with removal of the nasolacrimal canal was undertaken. On routine follow-up 5 years later, a papillary lesion of the nose was noted and an inferior turbinectomy was done. She is alive and well without recurrence 5 years after nasal surgery. *(B)* Histologically, the orbital lesion proved to be low-grade papillary transitional cell carcinoma with some inverted areas. *(Top)* The lacrimal sac and nasolacrimal canal; *(bottom)* the low-grade carcinoma (H&E, original magnifications *top* × 2, *bottom* × 25).

FIGURE 12-149. *(A)* CT scans demonstrate a left medial orbital mass in a 45-year-old man who presented in October 1986 with a history of epiphora. He had undergone dacryocystorhinostomy on two occasions prior to referral. On physical examination, he had a medial orbital mass with fixation of the medial rectus and outward upward displacement of the globe. The axial and coronal CT scans demonstrate the infiltrative mass, which involved the inferomedial orbit and adjacent dacryocystorhinostomy site. *(B)* The biopsy shows a moderately differentiated infiltrating squamous cell carcinoma, which had presumably arisen from the lacrimal sac. The patient refused exenteration and was treated with radical radiotherapy. Follow-up examination 1 year later showed no recurrence.

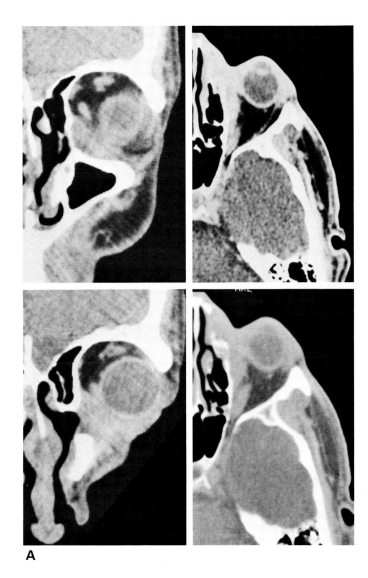

A

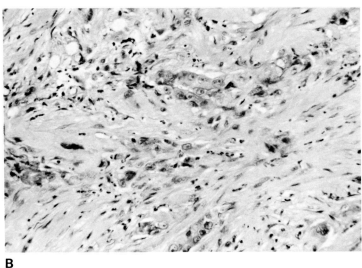

B

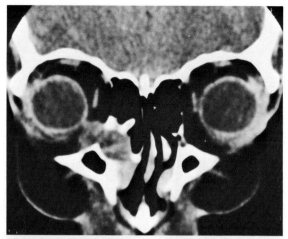

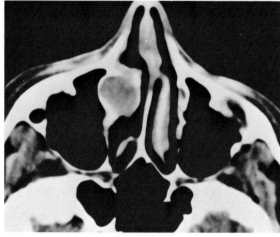

FIGURE 12-150. Coronal and axial CT scans demonstrate a mass lesion of the right lacrimal sac, nasolacrimal system, and nose in a 38-year-old woman who presented with a 2-year history of epiphora. She was noted to have a mass at the time of dacryocystorhinostomy. Biopsy of the mass revealed a spindle cell tumor consistent with fibrous histiocytoma. We undertook a medial orbitotomy and lateral rhinotomy to remove the entire lacrimal sac and involved medial nasal and sinus walls. The patient had a local recurrence 8 months later and underwent further resection.

much more prone to develop focally invasive carcinoma, which is usually of a low-grade variety.

De novo carcinomas have been divided into papillary and nonpapillary types on the basis of their gross pattern of involvement and into squamous, transitional cell, and adenocarcinomas. The majority are squamous carcinomas, and all of them arise in patients over 40 years of age (Fig. 12-149). In Ryan and Font's series, 7 of the 27 tumors were carcinomas arising in endophytic papillomas and were generally low grade. The remaining nine carcinomas were *de novo*; six were squamous cell, two were

transitional cell, and one was adenocarcinoma. In Ni and co-workers' report of lacrimal sac tumors from China, a much higher incidence of aggressive carcinomas was reported.

Management should be based on histopathologic type and degree of extension. The papillomas, especially of the inverted type and particularly when focal invasion is demonstrated, should be treated by total excision of the nasolacrimal system and carefully observed for any evidence of recurrence in the nose. More aggressive carcinomas should be treated by wide local excision including the bone of the nasolacrimal system. Adjacent orbit, and wall of the sinus. Postoperative radiotherapy is advocated for the more aggressive lesions and significant orbital involvement implies the need for exenteration.

Other Epithelial Tumors

A number of other epithelial tumors of the lacrimal sac may cause tumefaction in this region or invade the orbit. They include oncocytomas (the majority of which are benign, noninvasive lesions) and mucoepidermoid carcinoma, a rare locally aggressive tumor.

Nonepithelial Tumors

A wide variety of nonepithelial tumors of the lacrimal sac occur, and their management relates to the primary histology. In short, the locally infiltrative lesions such as fibrous histiocytoma (Fig. 12-150) should be widely excised; lymphomas should be treated by radiotherapy or chemotherapy based on systemic status; and the more malignant lesions should be treated by wide local excision with or without radiotherapy.

Lloyd and Leone have reported on malignant melanoma of the lacrimal sac. They emphasize the grim prognosis that it shares with other melanomas of respiratory mucosa.

Bibliography

OPTIC NERVE GLIOMA

Anderson DR, Spencer WH: Ultrastructural and histochemical observations of optic nerve gliomas. Arch Ophthalmol 83:324, 1970

Borit A, Richardson EP Jr: The biological and clinical behaviour of pilocytic astrocytomas of the optic pathways. Brain 105:161, 1982

Brand WN, Hoover SV: Optic glioma in children. Review of 16 cases given megavoltage radiation therapy. Childs Brain 5:459, 1979

Bynke H, Kagstrom E, Tjernstrom K: Aspects of the treatment of gliomas of the anterior visual pathway. Acta Ophthalmol 55:269, 1977

Chutorian AM, Schwartz JF, Evans RA, Carter S: Optic gliomas in children. Neurology 14:83, 1964

Danoff BF, Kramer S, Thompson N: The radiotherapeutic management of optic nerve gliomas in children. Int J Radiat Oncol Biol Phys 6:45, 1980

Dosoretz DE, Blitzer PH, Wang CC et al: Management of glioma of the optic nerve and/or chiasm: An analysis of 20 cases. Cancer 45:1467, 1980

Fazekas JT: Treatment of grades I and II brain astrocytomas. The role of radiotherapy. Int J Radiat Oncol Biol Phys 2:661, 1977

Fienman NL, Yakovac WC: Neurofibromatosis in childhood. J Pediatr 76:339, 1970

Glaser JS, Hoyt WF, Corbett J: Visual morbidity with chiasmal glioma. Arch Ophthalmol 85:3, 1971

Gombi R, Hullay J: Diagnosis and treatment of the optic glioma. Acta Neurochir [Suppl] (Wien) 28:405, 1979

Grimson BS, Perry DD: Enlargement of the optic disc in childhood optic nerve tumors. Am J Ophthalmol 97:627, 1984

Harper CG, Stewart-Wynne EG: Malignant optic gliomas in adults. Arch Neurol 35:731, 1978

Harter DJ, Caderao JB, Leavens ME et al: Radiotherapy in the management of primary gliomas involving the intracranial optic nerves and chiasm. Int J Radiat Oncol Biol Phys 4:681, 1978

Heiskanen O, Raitta C, Torsti R: The management and prognosis of gliomas of the optic pathways in children. Acta Neurochir (Wien) 43:193, 1978

Holman RE, Grimson BS, Drayer BP et al: Magnetic resonance imaging of optic gliomas. Am J Ophthalmol 100:596, 1985

Horwich A, Bloom HJG: Optic gliomas: Radiation therapy and prognosis. Int J Radiat Oncol Biol Phys 11:1067, 1985

Hoyt WF, Baghdassarian SA: Natural history and rationale for conservative management. Br J Ophthal 53:793, 1969

Hoyt WF, Meshel LG, Lessell S et al: Malignant optic glioma of adulthood. Brain 96:121, 1973

Imes RK, Hoyt WF: Childhood chiasmal gliomas: Update on the fate of patients in the 1969 San Francisco study. Br J Ophthal 70:179, 1986

Iraci G, Gerosa M, Scanarini M et al: Anterior optic gliomas with precocious or pseudoprecocious puberty. Childs Brain 7:314, 1980

Iraci G, Gerosa M, Tomazzoli L et al: Gliomas of the optic nerve and chiasm: A clinical review. Childs Brain 8:326, 1981

Jakobiec FA, Depot MJ, Kennerdell JS et al: Combined clinical and computed tomographic diagnosis of orbital glioma and meningioma. Ophthalmology 91:137, 1984

Karaguiosov L: Surgical treatment of gliomas of the optic nerve and chiasm. Acta Neurochir [Suppl] (Wien) 28:411, 1979

Klug GL: Gliomas of the optic nerve and chiasm in children. Aust NZ J Surg 47:596, 1977

Lewis RA, Riccardi VM: Von Recklinghausen neurofibromatosis: Incidence of iris hamartomata. Ophthalmology 88:348, 1981

Love JG, Dodge HW, Bair HL: Complete removal of gliomas affecting the optic nerve. Arch Ophthalmol 54:386, 1955

Lowes M, Bojsen-Moller M, Vorre P et al: An evaluation of gliomas of the anterior visual pathways: A 10-year survey. Acta Neurochir (Wien) 43:201, 1978

MacCarty CS, Boyd AS, Childs DS: Tumors of the optic nerve and optic chiasm. J Neurosurg 33:439, 1970

McDonnell P, Miller NR: Chiasmatic and hypothalamic extension of optic nerve glioma. Arch Ophthalmol 101:1412, 1983

Marejeva TG, Rostotskaya VI, Sokolova ON et al: Tumors of the optic nerve and chiasma in children: Diagnosis and surgical treatment. Acta Neurochir [Suppl] (Wien) 28:409, 1979

Marquardt MD, Zimmerman LE: Histopathology of meningiomas and gliomas of the optic nerve. Hum Pathol 13:226, 1982

Parker JC Jr, Smith JL, Reyes P et al: Chiasmal optic glioma after radiation therapy. J Clin Neuro Ophthalmol 1:31, 1981

Peyster RF, Hoover ED, Hershey BL et al: High resolution CT of lesions of the optic nerve. AJNR 4:169, 1983

Redfern RM, Scholtz CL: Long-term survival with optic nerve glioma. Surg Neurol 14:371, 1980

Reese AB: Bowman lecture: Expanding lesions of the orbit. Trans Ophthalmol Soc UK 91:85, 1971

Reese AB: Tumors of the Eye, 3rd ed, pp 141, 164. Philadelphia, Harper & Row, 1976

Richards RD, Lynn JR: The surgical management of gliomas of the optic nerve. Am J Ophthalmol 62:60, 1966

Richardson AE: Optic pathway tumors. Trans Ophthalmol Soc UK 96:424, 1976

Robertson AG, Brewin TB: Optic nerve glioma. Clin Radiol 31:471, 1980

Rothfus WE, Curtin HD, Slamovits TL et al: Optic nerve sheath enlargement. Radiology 150:409, 1984

Rush JA, Younge BR, Campbell RJ et al: Long-term follow-up of 85 histopathologically verified cases. Ophthalmology 89:1213, 1982

Spencer WH: Diagnostic modalities and natural behavior of optic nerve gliomas. Ophth AAO 86:881, 1979

Spoor TC, Kennerdell JS, Martinez AJ, Zorub D: Malignant gliomas of the optic nerve pathways. Amer J Ophthalmol 89:284, 1980

Stein BM: Surgical lesions of the intracranial optic nerves and optic chiasm. Ophthalmol AAO 86:308, 1979

Swenson SA, Forbes GS, Younge BR et al: Radiologic evaluation of tumors of the optic nerve. AJNR 3:319, 1982

Taveras JM, Mount LA, Wood EH: The value of radiation therapy in the management of glioma of the optic nerves and chiasm. Radiology 66:518, 1956

Tenny RT, Laws ER Jr, Younge BR et al: The neurosurgical management of optic glioma: Results in 104 patients. J Neurosurg 57:452, 1982

Tertsch D, Schon R, Ulrich FE et al: Pubertas praecox in neurofibromatosis of the optic chiasma. Acta Neurochir [Suppl] (Wien) 28:413, 1979

Woog JJ, Albert DM, Solt LC et al: Neurofibromatosis of the eyelid and orbit. Int Ophthalmol Clin 22:157, 1982

Wright JE, McDonald WI, Call NB: Management of optic nerve gliomas. Br J Ophthalmol 64:545, 1980

Zimmerman LE: Correspondence: Arachnoid hyperplasia in optic nerve glioma. Br J Ophthalmol 64:638, 1980

Zimmerman LE, Arkfeld DL, Schenken JB et al: A rare choristoma of the optic nerve and chiasm. Arch Ophthalmol 101:766, 1983

MENINGIOMAS

Crosby EC, Humphrey T, Lauer EW: Correlative Anatomy of the Nervous System. New York, Macmillan, 1962

Cushing H, Eisenhardt L: Meningioma. Their Classification, Regional Behavior, Life History and Surgical End Results, 1938. Springfield, IL, Charles C Thomas, 1962

Hendersen JW: Orbital Tumors, 2nd ed, p 472. New York, Brian C Decker, 1980

Reese AB: Tumors of the Eye, 3rd ed. Philadelphia, Harper & Row, 1976

Rubenstein LJ: Tumors of the Central Nervous System. Washington, DC, Armed Forces Institute of Pathology, 1972

Russell D, Rubenstein LJ: Pathology of Tumors of the Nervous System, 4th ed. London, Arnold, 1977

Intracranial, Intracanalicular, and Orbital Meningiomas

Als E: Intraorbital meningiomas encasing the optic nerve. Acta Ophthalmol 17:900, 1969

Bailey P, Bucy PC: The origin and nature of meningeal tumors. Am J Cancer 15:15, 1931

Boniuk M, Messmer EP, Font RF: Hemangiopericytoma of the meninges of the optic nerve. Ophthalmology 92:1780, 1986

Cophignon J, Lucena J, Clay C et al: Limits to radical treatment of spheno-orbital meningiomas. Acta Neurochir [Suppl] (Wien) 28:375, 1979

Craig WM, Gogela LJ: Intraorbital meningiomas. Am J Ophthalmol 32:1663, 1949

Crouse SK, Berg BO: Intracranial meningiomas in childhood and adolescense. Neurology 22:135, 1972

Dandy WE: Prechiasmal intracranial tumors of the optic nerves. Am J Ophthalmol 5:169, 1922

Deen HG Jr, Scheithauer BW, Ebersold MJ: Clinical and pathological study of meningiomas of the first two decades of life. J Neurosurg 56:317, 1982

Ehlers N, Malmros R: The suprasellar meningioma. Acta Ophthalmol [Suppl] 121:1, 1973

Grant FC, Hedges TR: Ocular findings in meningiomas of the tuberculum sellae. Arch Ophthalmol 56:163, 1956

Gregorius FK, Hepler RS, Stern WE: Loss and recovery of vision with suprasellar meningiomas. J Neurosurg 42:69, 1975

Hart M Jr, Burde RM, Klingele TG et al: Bilateral optic nerve sheath meningiomas. Arch Ophthalmol 98:149, 1980

Holden J, Dolman C, Churg A: Immunohistochemistry of meningiomas including the angioblastic type. J Neuropathol Exp Neurol 46(1):50, 1987

Horten BC, Urich H, Rubenstein LJ et al: The angioblastic meningioma: A reapprasal of a nosological problem. J Neurol Sci 31:387, 1977

Karp LA, Zimmerman LE, Borit A et al: Primary intraorbital meningiomas. Arch Ophthalmol 91:24, 1974

Kearns TP, Wagener HP: Ophthalmologic diagnosis of meningiomas of the sphenoidal ridge. Am J Med Sci 226:221, 1953

Kennerdell JS, Maroon JC: Intracanalicular meningioma with chronic optic disc edema. Ann Ophthalmol 7:507, 1975

Lapresle J, Netsky MG, Zimmerman HM: The pathology of meningiomas. Am J Pathol 28:757, 1952

Little HL, Chambers JW, Walsh FB: Unilateral intracranial optic nerve involvement. Arch Ophthalmol 73:331, 1965

MacMichael IM, Cullen JF: Primary intraorbital meningiomas. Br J Ophthalmol 53:169, 1969

Mehra KS, Khanna S, Dube B: Primary meningioma of the intraorbital optic nerve. Ann Ophthalmol 11(5):758, 1979

Mirra S, Miles ML: Unusual pericytic proliferation in a meningotheliomatous meningioma: An ultrastructural study. Am J Surg Pathol 6:573, 1982

Moore CE: Sphenoidal ridge meningioma with optic nerve metastases. Br J Ophthalmol 52:636, 1968

Muller J, Mealy J: The use of tissue culture in differentiation between angioblastic meningioma and hemangiopericytoma. J Neurosurg 34:341, 1971

Newell FW, Beamon TC: Ocular signs of meningiomas. Am J Ophthalmol 45:30, 1958

Popoff NA, Malinin TI, Rosomoff HC: Fine structure of intracranial hemangiopericytoma and angiomatous meningioma. Cancer 34:1187, 1974

Susac JO, Smith JL, Walsh FB: The impossible meningioma. Arch Neurol 34:36, 1977

Trobe JD, Glaser JS, Post JD et al: Bilateral optic canal meningiomas: A case report. Neurosurg 3:68, 1978

Walsh FB: Meningioma, primary within the orbit and optic canal. In Smith JL (ed): Neuro-ophthalmology Symposium of the University of Miami and the Bascom Palmer Eye Institute, Vol 5, 240–266. St. Louis, CV Mosby, 1970

Wilson WB: Meningiomas of the anterior visual system. Surv Ophthalmol 26, No. 3:109, 1981

Wilson WB, Gordon M, Lehman RAW: Meningiomas confined to the optic canal and foramina. Surg Neurol 12:21, 1979

Wolter JR, Benz SC: Ectopic meningioma of the superior orbital rim. Arch Ophthalmol 94:1920, 1976

Optic Nerve Meningioma

Alper MG: Management of primary optic nerve sheath meningiomas. Current status—therapy in controversy. J Clin Neuro Ophthalmol 1:101, 1981

Boniuk M, Messmer EP, Font RL: Hemangiopericytoma of the meninges of the optic nerve: A clinicopathologic report including electron microscopic observations. Ophthalmology 92:1870, 1985

Boschetti NV, Smith JL, Osher RH et al: Fluorescein angiography of optociliary shunt vessels. J Clin Neuro Ophthalmol 1:9, 1981

Cibis GW, Whittaker CK, Wood WE: Intraocular extension of optic nerve meningioma in a case of neurofibromatosis. Arch Ophthalmol 103:404, 1985

Craig WMcK, Gogela LJ: Intraorbital meningiomas: A clinicopathologic study. Am J Ophthalmol 32:1663, 1949

Daniels DL, Williams AL, Syvertsen A et al: CT recognition of optic nerve sheath meningioma: Abnormal sheath visualization. AJNR 3:181, 1982

Dunn SN, Walsh FB: Meningioma (dural endothelioma) of the optic nerve. Arch Ophthalmol 56:702, 1956

Eggers H, Jakobiec FA, Jones IS: Tumors of the optic nerve. Doc Ophthalmol 41:43, 1976

Ellenberger C: Perioptic meningiomas: Syndrome of long-standing visual loss, pale disk edema, optociliary veins. Arch Neurol 33:671, 1976

Frisen H, Hoyt WF, Tengroth BM: Optociliary veins, disc pallor and visual loss: A triad of signs indicating spheno-orbital meningioma. Acta Ophthalmol 51:241, 1973

Hart WM Jr, Burder RM, Klingele TG et al: Bilateral optic nerve sheath meningiomas. Arch Ophthalmol 98:149, 1980

Hollenhorst RW Jr, Hollenhorst RW Sr, MacCarty CS: Visual prognosis of optic nerve sheath meningiomas producing shunt vessels on the optic disc. Trans Am Ophthalmol Soc 75:141, 1977

Jakobiec FA, Depot MJ, Kennerdell JS et al: Combined clinical and computed tomographic diagnosis of orbital glioma and meningioma. Ophthalmology 91:137, 1984

Lloyd GAS: Primary orbital meningioma: A review of 41 patients investigated radiologically. Clin Radiol 33:181, 1982

Mark LE, Kennerdell JS, Maroon JC et al: Microsurgical removal of a primary intraorbital meningioma. Am J Ophthalmol 86:704, 1978

Marquardt MD, Zimmerman LE: Histopathology of meningiomas and gliomas of the optic nerve. Hum Pathol 13:226, 1982

Miller NR: Progressive visual loss: What type of mass lesion? Surv Ophthalmol 28:45, 1983

Rothfus WE, Curtain HD, Slamovits TL et al: Optic nerve/sheath enlargement: A different approach based on high-resolution CT morphology. Radiology 150:409, 1984

Rucker CW, Kearns TP: Mistaken diagnoses in some cases of meningioma: Clinics in perimetry no. 5 Am J Ophthalmol 51:15, 1961

Sibony PA, Krauss HR, Kennerdell JS et al: Optic nerve sheath meningiomas. Ophthalmology 91:11 1984

Smith JL, Vuksanovic MM, Yates BM et al: Radiation therapy for primary optic nerve meningiomas. J Clin Neuro Ophthalmol 1:85, 1981

Spencer WH: Primary neoplasms of the optic nerve and its sheaths: Clinical features and current concepts of pathogenetic mechanisms. Trans Am Ophthalmol Soc 70:490, 1972

Wright JE: Primary optic nerve meningiomas: Clinical presentation and management. Trans Am Acad Ophthalmol Otolaryngol 83:617, 1977

Wright JE: Call NB, Liaricos S: Primary optic nerve meningioma. Br J Ophthalmol 64:553, 1980

Zakka KA, Summerer RW, Yee RD et al: Opticociliary veins in a primary optic nerve sheath meningioma. Am J Ophthalmol 87:91, 1979

PERIPHERAL NERVE SHEATH TUMORS

Neurofibromatosis

Burrows EH: Bone changes in orbital neurofibromatosis. Br J Radiol 36:549, 1963

Canale DJ, Bebin J: Von Recklinghausen disease of the nervous system. In Vinken PJ, Bruyn GW (eds): Handbook of Clinical Neurology, Vol 14, p 132. New York, American Elsevier, 1968 (1972)

Crowe FW, Schull WJ, Neel JV: A Clinical, Pathological, and Genetic Study of Multiple Neurofibromatosis. Springfield, IL, Charles C Thomas, 1956

Enzinger FM, Weiss SW: Soft Tissue Tumors, p 580. St Louis, CV Mosby, 1983

Fialkow PJ, Sagebiel RW, Gartler SM et al: Multiple cell origin of hereditary neurofibromas. N Engl J Med 284:298, 1971

Guccion JG, Enzinger FM: Malignant schwannoma associated with von Recklinghausen's neurofibromatosis. Virchows Arch [A] 383:43, 1979

Gurland JE, Tenner M, Hornblass A et al: Orbital neurofibromatosis. Arch Ophthalmol 94:1723, 1976

Holt GR: ENT manifestations of Von Recklinghausen's disease. Laryngoscope 88:1617, 1978

Holt JF: Neurofibromatosis in children. AJR 130:615, 1978

Jackson IT, Laws ER, Martin RD: The surgical management of orbital neurofibromatosis. Plast Reconstr Surg 71:751, 1983

Jacoby CT, Go RT, Beren RA: Cranial CT of neurofibromatosis. AJR 135:553, 1980

Jakobiec FA, Font RL, Zimmerman LE: Malignant peripheral nerve sheath tumors of the orbit: A clinicopathologic study of 8 cases. Trans Am Ophthalmol Soc 83:17, 1985

Jones IS, Desjardins L: Management of orbital neurofibromatosis and lymphangiomas. In Jakobiec FA (ed): Ocular and Adnexal Tumors, p 735. Birmingham, Aesculapius, 1978

Kennedy RE: Pulsating exophthalmos: Orbital tumors in siblings. Trans Am Ophthalmol Soc 80:205, 1982

Kobrin JL, Blodi FC, Weingeist TA: Ocular and orbital manifestations of neurofibromatosis. Surv Ophthalmol 24:45, 1979

Lassmann H, Jurecka W, Lassmann W et al: Different types of benign nerve sheath tumors: Light microscopy, electron microscopy, and autoradiography. Virchows Arch [Pathol Anat] 375:197, 1977

Levi-Montalcini R: Growth control of nerve cells by a protein factor and its antiserum. Science 143:105, 1964

Lewis RA, Riccardi VM: Von Recklinghausen neurofibromatosis: Incidence of iris hamartomata. Ophthalmology 88:348, 1981

Lictenstein BW: Neurofibromatosis (von Recklinghausen's disease of nervous system): Analysis of a total pathologic picture. Arch Neurol Psychiatr 62:822, 1949

Lisch K: Ueber Beteiligung der Augen, insbesondere das Vorkommen von Irisknotchen bei der Neurofibromatose (Recklinghausen). Z Augenheilkd 93:137, 1937

Reed D, Robertson WD, Rootman J et al: Plexiform neurofibromatosis of the orbit: CT evaluation. AJNR 7:259, 1986

Rodriquez HA, Berthrong M: Multiple primary intracranial tumors in von Recklinghausen's neurofibromatosis. Arch Neurol 14:467, 1966

Schenkein I, Bueker ED, Helson L et al: Increased nerve-growth stimulating activity in disseminated neurofibromatosis. N Engl J Med 290:613, 1974

Woog JJ, Albert DM, Solt LC et al: Neurofibromatosis of the eyelid and orbit. Int Ophthalmol Clin 22:157, 1982

Zimmerman RA, Bilaniuk LT, Metzger RA et al: Computed tomography of orbital facial neurofibromatosis. Radiology 146:113, 1983

Zorab P, Edwards H: Spinal deformity in neurofibromatosis. Lancet 2:823, 1972

Solitary Neurofibromas

Coleman DJ, Jack RL, Franzen LA: Neurogenic tumors of the orbit. Arch Ophthalmol 88:380, 1972

Erlandson RA, Woodruff JM: Peripheral nerve sheath tumors: An electron microscopic study of 43 cases. Cancer 49:273, 1982

Francois J: Ocular aspects of the phakomatoses. In Vinken PJ, Bruyn GW (eds): Handbook of Clinical Neurology, p 624. New York, American Elsevier, 1972

Gogi R, Nath K, Kahn AA: Peripheral nerve tumors of the orbit (a clinicopathologic study). Indian J Ophthalmol 24:1, 1976

Krohel GB, Rosenberg MD, Wright JE Jr et al: Localized orbital neurofibromas. Am J Ophthalmol 100:458, 1985

Kuo PK, Ni C, Seddon JM et al: Orbital tumors among Chinese in the Shanghai area. Int Ophthalmol Clin 22:87, 1982

McDonald P, Jakobiec FA, Hornblass A et al: Benign peripheral nerve sheath tumors (neurofibromas of the lacrimal gland). Ophthalmology 90:1403, 1983

Amputation Neuromas

Blodi FC: Amputation neuroma in the orbit. Am J Ophthalmol 32:929, 1949

Messmer EP, Camara J, Boniuk M et al: Amputation neuroma of the orbit: Report of two cases and review of the literature. Ophthalmology 91:1420, 1984

Schwannoma

Ackerman LV, Taylor FH: Neurogenous tumors within the thorax. Cancer 4:669, 1951

Allman M, Frayer WC, Hedges TR: Orbital neurilemmoma. Ann Ophthalmol 9:1409, 1977

Chisholm IA, Polyzoidis K: Recurrence of benign orbital neurilemmoma (schwannoma) after 22 years. Can J Ophthalmol 17:271, 1982

Dahl I: Ancient neurilemmoma (schwannoma). Acta Pathol Microbiol Scand [A], 85A No. 6:812, 1977

Fisher ER, Vuzevski VD: Cytogenesis of schwannoma (neurilemmoma), neurofibroma, dermatofibroma, and dermatofibrosarcoma as revealed by electron miscroscopy. Am J Clin Pathol 49:141, 1968

Izumi AK et al: Von Recklinghausen's disease associated with multiple neurilemmomas. Arch Dermatol 104:172, 1971

Jakobiec FA, Font RL, Iwamoto T: Diagnostic ultrastructural pathology of ophthalmic tumors. In Jakobiec FA (ed): Ocular and Adnexal Tumors, p 359. Birmingham, Aesculapius, 1978

Messmer EP, Font RL: Applications of immunohistochemistry to ophthalmic pathology. Ophthalmology 91:701, 1984

Razzuk MA, Urschel HC, Martin JA et al: Electron microscopical observations on mediastinal neurilemmoma, neurofibroma, and ganglioneuroma. Ann Thorac Surg 15:73, 1973

Rootman J, Goldberg C, Robertson W: Primary orbital schwannomas. Br J Ophthalmol 66:194, 1982

Rottino A, Kelly AJ: Specific nerve sheath tumor of orbit. Arch Ophthalmol 26:478, 1941

Schatz H: Benign orbital neurilimmoma: Sarcomatous transformation in von Recklinghausen's disease. Arch Ophthalmol 86:268, 1971

Schmitt E, Spoerri O: Schwannomas of the orbit. Acta Neurochir (Wien) 53:79, 1980

Stefansson K, Wollmann R, Jerkovic M: S-100 protein in soft-tissue tumors derived from Schwann cells and melanocytes. Am J Pathol 106:261, 1982

Stout AP: The peripheral manifestations of specific nerve sheath tumor (neurilemmoma). Am J Cancer 24:751, 1935

Sun CN, White HJ: An electron microscopic study of a schwannoma with special reference to banded structures and peculiar membranous multiple-chambered spheroids. J Pathol 114:13, 1974

Weiss WS, Langloss JM, Enzinger FM: Value of S-100 protein in the diagnosis of soft tissue tumors, with particular reference to benign and malignant Schwann cell tumors. Lab Invest 49:299, 1983

MALIGNANT PERIPHERAL NERVE SHEATH TUMORS

D'Agostino AN, Soule EH, Miller RH: Primary malignant neoplasm of nerves (malignant neurilemmomas) in patients without manifestations of multiple neurofibromatosis (von Recklinghausen's disease). Cancer 16:1003, 1963

D'Agostino AN, Soule EH, Miller RH: Sarcomas of the peripheral nerves and somatic soft tissues associated with multiple neurofibromatosis (von Recklinghausen's disease). Cancer 16:1015, 1963

Duke-Elder S: System of Ophthalmology. London, Kimpton, 1974

Enzinger FM, Weiss SW: Soft Tissue Tumors, p 625. St Louis, CV Mosby, 1983

Ghosh BC, Ghosh L, Huvos AG et al: Malignant schwannoma: A clinicopathologic study. Cancer 31:184, 1973

Grinberg MA, Levy NS: Malignant neurilemmoma of the supraorbital nerve. Am J Ophthalmol 78:489, 1974

Guccion JG, Enzinger FM: Malignant schwannoma associated with von Recklinghausen's neurofibromatosis. Virchows Arch [Pathol Anat] 383:43, 1979

Harkin JC, Reed RJ: Tumors of the peripheral nervous system. In Atlas of Tumor Pathology, 2nd series, Fascicle 3. Washington, DC, Armed Forces Institue of Pathology, 1969

Henderson JW: Orbital Tumors, 2nd ed. New York, Brian C Decker (Thieme-Stratton), 1980

Jakobiec FA, Font RL, Zimmerman LE: Malignant peripheral nerve sheath tumors of the orbit: A clinicopathologic study of 8 cases. Trans Am Ophthalmol Soc 83:17, 1985

Jakobiec FA, Jones IS: Neurogenic tumors. In Jones IS, Jakobiec FA (eds): Diseases of the Orbit, p 371. Philadelphia, Harper & Row, 1979

Messmer EP, Font RL: Applications of immunohistochemistry to ophthalmic pathology. Ophthalmology 91:701, 1984

Mortada A: Solitary orbital malignant neurilemmomas. Br J Ophthalmol 52:188, 1968

Schatz H: Benign orbital neurilemmoma: Sarcomatous transformation in von Recklinghausen's disease. Arch Ophthalmol 86:268, 1971

Spencer WH: Ophthalmic Pathology: An Atlas and Textbook Vol 3, 3rd ed. Philadelphia, WB Saunders, 1986

Weiss WS, Langloss JM, Enzinger FM: Value of S-100 protein in the diagnosis of soft tissue tumors, with particular reference to benign and malignant Schwann cell tumors. Lab Invest 49:299, 1983

White HR: Survival in malignant schwannoma: An 18-year study. Cancer 27:720, 1971

Woodruff JM: Peripheral nerve tumors showing glandular differentiation (glandular schwannoma). Cancer 37:2399, 1976

Woodruff JM, Chernik NL, Smith MC et al: Peripheral nerve tumors with rhabdomyosarcomatous differentiation (malignant "Triton" tumors). Cancer 32:426, 1973

ALVEOLAR SOFT PART SARCOMA

Abrahams IW, Fenton RH, Vidone R: Alveolar soft-part sarcoma of the orbit. Arch Ophthalmol 79:185, 1968

Altamirano-Dimas M, Albores-Saavedra J: Alveolar soft part sarcoma of the orbit. Arch Ophthalmol 75:496, 1966

Bunt AH, Bensinger RE: Alveolar soft part sarcoma of the orbit. Ophthalmology 88:1339, 1981

Christopherson WM, Foote FW Jr, Stewart FW: Alveolar soft part sarcomas: Structurally characteristic tumors of uncertain histogenesis. Cancer 5:100, 1952

DeSchryver-Kecskemeti K, Kraus FT, Engleman BA: Alveolar soft part sarcoma—a malignant angioreninoma: Histochemical, immunocytochemical, and electron-microscopic study of four cases. Am J Surg Pathol 6:5, 1982

Font RL, Jurco S III, Zimmerman LE: Alveolar soft part sarcoma of the orbit. Hum Pathol 13:569, 1982

Grant GD, Shields JA, Flanagan JC et al: The ultrasonographic and radiologic features of a histopathologically proven case of alveolar soft part sarcoma of the orbit. Am J Ophthalmol 87:773, 1979

Lieberman PH, Foote FW, Stewart FW et al: Alveolar soft part sarcoma. JAMA 198:1047, 1966

Nirankari MS, Greer CH, Chaddah MR: Malignant nonchromaffin paraganglioma in the orbit. Br J Ophthalmol 47:357, 1963

Shipkey FH, Lieberman PH, Foote FW Jr et al: Ultrastructure of alveolar soft part sarcoma. Cancer 17:821, 1964

Unni KK, Soule ED: Alveolar soft part sarcoma: An electron microscopic study. Mayo Clin Proc 50:591, 1975

Varghese S, Nair B, Joseph TA: Orbital malignant nonchromaffin paraganglioma. Br J Ophthalmol 52:713, 1968

Welsh RA, Bray DM III, Shipkey FH et al: Histogenesis of alveolar soft part sarcoma. Cancer 29:191, 1972

GRANULAR CELL TUMOR

Armin A, Connelly E, Rawden G: An immunoperoxidase investigation of S-100 protein in granular cell myoblastomas: Evidence for Schwann cell derivation. Am J Clin Pathol 79:37, 1983

Chaves E, Oliveira AM, Arnaud AC: Retrobulbar granular cell myoblastoma. Br J Ophthalmol 56:854, 1972

Dolman PJ, Rootman J, Dolman CL: Infiltrating orbital granular cell tumour: A case report and literature review. Br J Ophthalmol 71:47, 1986

Drummond JW, Hall DL, Steen WH et al: Granular cell tumor (myoblastoma) of the orbit. Arch Ophthalmol 97:1492, 1979

Dunnington JH: Granular cell myoblastoma of the orbit. Arch Ophthalmol 40:14, 1948

Fisher ER, Wechsler H: Granular cell myoblastoma—a misnomer: Electron microscopic and histochemical evidence concerning its Schwann cell derivation and nature (granular cell Schwannoma). Cancer 15:936, 1962

Goldstein BG, Font RL, Alper MG: Granular cell tumor of the orbit: A case report including electron microscopic observations. Ann Ophthalmol 14:231, 1982

Gonzales-Almarez G, de Buen S, Tsutsumi V: Granular cell tumor (myoblastoma) of the orbit. Am J Ophthalmol 79:606, 1975

Ingram DL, Mossler J, Snowhite J et al: Granular cell tumors of the breast: Steroid receptor analysis and localization of carcinoembryonic antigen, myoglobin and S100 protein. Arch Pathol Lab Med 108:897, 1984

Karcioglu ZA: Granular cell tumor of the orbit: Case report and review of the literature. Ophthalmic Surg 14:125, 1983

Lack EE, Worsham GF, Callihan MD: Granular cell tumor: A clinicopathologic study of 110 patients. J Surg Oncol 13:301, 1980

Miettinen M, Lehtonen E, Lehtola H et al: Histogenesis of granular cell tumor: An immunohistochemical and ultrastructural study. J Pathol 142:221, 1984

Morgan G: Granular cell myoblastoma of the orbit. Arch Ophthalmol 94:2135, 1976

Morgan LR, Fryer MP: Granular cell myoblastoma of the eye: Case report. Plast Reconstr Surg 43:315, 1969

Moriarty P, Garner A, Wright JE: Case report of granular cell myoblastoma arising within the medial rectus muscle. Br J Ophthalmol 67:17, 1983

Obayashi K, Yamada Y, Kozaki M: Granular cell myoblastoma in the orbit. Folia Ophthalmol Jpn 20:566, 1969

Rode J, Dhillon AP, Papadaki L: Immunohistochemical staining of granular cell tumor for neurone-specific enolase: Evidence in support of a neural origin. Diagn Histopathol 5:205, 1982

Sakamaki Y: A case of intraorbital myoblastoma. Jpn J Clin Ophthalmol 17:883, 1963

Shimoyama I: Granular cell myoblastoma in the orbit. Neurol Med Chir (Tokyo) 24:355, 1984

Singleton EM, Nettleship M: Granular cell tumor of the orbit: A case report. Ann Ophthalmol 15:881, 1983

Stefansson K, Wollmann RL: S-100 protein in granular cell tumors (granular cell myoblastomas). Cancer 49:1834, 1982

Timm G, Timmel H: Zum Myoblastenmyom am Auge. Klin Monatsbl Augenheilkd 148, 665, 1966

CHEMODECTOMA (PARAGANGLIOMA)

Deutsch AR, Duckworth JK: Nonchromaffin paraganglioma of the orbit. Am J Ophthalmol 68:659, 1969

Fisher ER, Hazard JB: Nonchromaffin paraganglioma of the orbit. Cancer 5:521, 1952

Glenner GG, Grimley PM: Tumors of the extra-adrenal para-ganglion system (including chemoreceptors). An Atlas of Tumor Pathology, 2nd series, Fascicle 9. Washington, DC, Armed Forces Institute of Pathology, 1974

Kadoya M, Amemiya T: A case of orbital paraganglioma. Acta Soc Ophthalmol Jpn 83:359, 1979

Zhang RY et al: Orbital paraganglioma: A report of ten cases. Chin J Ophthalmol 20:197, 1984

PRIMARY ORBITAL CARCINOID

Godwin JD 2nd: Carcinoid tumors: An analysis of 2837 cases. Cancer 36:560, 1975

Riddle PJ, Font RL, Zimmerman LE: Carcinoid tumors of the eye and orbit: A clinicopathologic study of 15 cases with histochemical and electron microscopic observations. Hum Pathol 13:459, 1982

Robbins SL, Cotran RS, Kumar V: Pathologic Basis of Disease, 3rd ed. Philadelphia, WB Saunders, 1984

Zimmerman LE, Stangl R, Riddle PJ: Primary carcinoid tumor of the orbit. Arch Ophthalmol 101:1395, 1983

NEUROEPITHELIAL TUMORS

Neuroepithelioma

Bolen JW, Thorning D: Peripheral neuroepithelioma: A light and electron microscopic study. Cancer 46:2456, 1980

Howard GM: Neuroepithelioma of the orbit. Am J Ophthalmol 59:934, 1965

Seemayer TA, Thelmo WL, Boland R et al: Peripheral neuroectodermal tumors. Perspect Pediatr Pathol 2:151, 1975

Olfactory Neuroblastoma

Chaudhry AP, Haar JG, Koul A et al: Olfactory neuroblastoma (esthesioneuroblastoma): A light and ultrastructural study of two cases. Cancer 44:564, 1979

Elkon D, Hightower SI, Lim ML et al: Esthesioneuroblastoma. Cancer 44:1087, 1979

Homzie MJ, Elkon D: Olfactory esthesioneuroblastoma: Variables predictive of tumor control and recurrence. Cancer 46:2509, 1980

Kadish S, Goodman M, Wang CC: Olfactory neuroblastoma: A clinical analysis of 17 cases. Cancer 37:1571, 1976

Levine PA, McLean WC, Cantrell RW: Esthesioneuroblastoma: The University of Virginia experience 1960–1985. Laryngoscope 96(7):742, 1986

Oberman HA, Rice DH: Olfactory neuroblastoma: A clincopathologic study. Cancer 38:2494, 1976

Rakes SM, Yeatts RP, Campbell RJ: Ophthalmic manifestations of esthesioneuroblastoma. Ophthalmology 92:1749, 1985

Primary Neuroblastoma and Ganglioneuroma

Stout AP: Ganglioneuroma of the sympathetic nervous system. Surg Gynecol Obstet 84:101, 1947

Toppozada HH: Ganglioneuroma of the left maxilla and orbit. J Laryngol 72:733, 1958

PRIMARY ORBITAL MELANOMA

Allen JC, Jaeschle WH: Recurrence of malignant melanoma in the orbit after 28 years. Arch Ophthalmol 76:79, 1966

Coppetto JR, Jaffe R, Gillies CG: Primary orbital melanoma. Arch Ophthalmol 96:2255, 1978

Drews RC: Primary malignant melanoma of the orbit in a Negro. Arch Ophthalmol 93:335, 1975

Dutton JJ, Anderson RL, Schelper RL et al: Orbital malignant melanoma and oculodermal melanocytosis: Report of two cases and review of the literature. Ophthalmology 91:497, 1984

Hagler WS, Brown CC: Malignant melanoma of the orbit arising in a nevus of Ota. Trans Am Acad Ophthalmol Otolaryngol 70:817, 1966

Haim T, Meyer E, Kerner H et al: Oculodermal melanocytosis (nevus of Ota) and orbital malignant melanoma. Ann Ophthalmol December: 1132, 1982

Hidano A: Natural history of nevus of Ota. Arch Dermatol 95:187, 1967

Jakobiec FA, Ellsworth R, Tannenbaum M: Primary orbital melanoma. Am J Ophthalmol 78:24, 1974

Jay B: Malignant melanoma of the orbit in a case of oculodermal melanosis. Br J Ophthalmol 49:359, 1965

Reese AB: Tumors of the Eye, 3rd ed, p 210. Philadelphia, Harper & Row, 1976

Rottino A, Kelly AS: Primary orbital melanoma: Case report with review of the literature. Arch Ophthalmol 27:934, 1942

Shields JA, Augsberger JJ, Donoso LA et al: Hepatic metastasis and orbital recurrence of uveal melanoma after 42 years. Am J Ophthal 100:666, 1985

Wilkes TDI, Uthman EO, Thornton CN et al: Malignant melanoma of the orbit in a black patient with ocular melanocytosis. Arch Ophthalmol 102:904, 1984

Wolter JR, Bryson JM, Blackhurst RT: Primary orbital melanoma. Eye Ear Nose Throat Mon 45 (Aug):64, 1966

RETINAL ANLAGE TUMOR

Blanc WA, Rosenblatt P, Wolff JA: Melanotic progonoma ("retinal anlage" tumor) of the shoulder in an infant. Cancer 11:959, 1958

Borello ED, Gorlin RJ: Melanotic neuroectodermal tumor of infancy: A neoplasm of neural crest origin. Cancer 19:196, 1966

Cutler LS, Chaudhry AP, Topazian R: Melanotic neuroectodermal tumor of infancy: An ultrastructural study, literature review, and reevaluation. Cancer 48:257, 1981

Dehner LP, Sibley RK, Sauk JJ Jr et al: Malignant melanotic neuroectodermal tumor of infancy: A clinical, pathologic, ultrastructural and tissue culture study. Cancer 43:1389, 1979

Hall WC, O'Day DM, Glick AD: Melanotic neuroectodermal tumor of infancy: An ophthalmic appearance. Arch Ophthalmol 97:922, 1979

Halpert B, Patzer R: Maxillary tumor or retinal anlage. Surgery 22:837, 1947

Koudstaal J, Oldhoff, J Panders AK et al: Melanotic neuroectodermal tumor in infancy. Cancer 22:151, 1968

Lamping KA, Albert DM, Lack E et al: Melanotic neuroectodermal tumor of infancy (retinal anlage tumor). Ophthalmology 92:143, 1985

Lurie HI: Congenital melanocarcinoma, melanocytic adamantinoma, retinal anlage tumor, progonoma, and pigmented epulis of infancy: Summary and review of the literature and report of the first case in an adult. Cancer 14:1090, 1961

Lurie HI, Isaacson C: A melanotic progonoma in the scapula. Cancer 14:1088, 1961

Misugi K, Okajima H, Newton WA et al: Mediastinal origin of a melanotic progonoma or retinal anlage tumor: Ultrastructural evidence for neural crest origin. Cancer 18:477, 1965

Navas Palacios JJ: Malignant melanotic neuroectodermal tumor: light and electron microscopic study. Cancer 46:529, 1980

Ricketts RR, Majmudarr B: Epididymal melanotic neuroectodermal tumor of infancy. Hum Pathol 16:416, 1985

Stowens D, Lin TH: Melanotic progonoma of the brain. Hum Pathol 5;105, 1974

Templeton AC: Orbital tumours in African children. Br J Ophthalmol 55:254, 1971

Zimmerman LE: Discussion of melanotic neuroectodermal tumor of infancy (retinal anlage tumor) by Lamping KA, Albert DM, Lack E et al. Ophthalmology 92:143, 1985

ECTOMESENCHYMAL TUMORS

Enzinger FM, Weiss SW: Soft Tissue Tumors, p 639. St Louis, CV Mosby, 1983

Jakobiec FA, Font RL, Tso MOM et al: Mesectodermal leiomyoma of the ciliary body: A tumor of presumed neural crest origin. Cancer 39:2102, 1977

Jakobiec FA, Iwamoto T: Ocular adnexa: Introduction to lids, conjunctiva and orbit. In Jakobiec FA (ed): Ocular Anatomy, Embryology, and Teratology. Philadelphia, Harper & Row, 1982

Karcioglu ZA, Someren A, Mathes SJ: Ectomesenchymoma: A malignant tumor of migratory neural crest (ectomesenchyme) remnants showing gangliotic, schwannian, melanocytic, and rhabdomyoblastic differentiation. Cancer 39:2486, 1977

MESENCHYMAL TUMORS

Barnes L: Surgical Pathology of the Head and Neck, Vol 2, p 883. New York, Marcel Dekker, 1985

Batsakis JG: Tumors of the Head and Neck: Clinical and Pathological Considerations, 2nd ed. Baltimore, Williams & Wilkins, 1979

Blodi FC: Pathology of orbital bones. Am J Ophthalmol 81:8, 1976

Blodi FC, Unusual orbital neoplasms. Am J Ophthalmol 68:407, 1969

Dahlin DC: Bone Tumors: General Aspects and Data on 6,221 Cases, 3rd ed. Springfield, Charles C Thomas, 1978

Enzinger FM, Weiss SW: Soft Tissue Tumors. St Louis, CV Mosby, 1983

Forrest AW: Intraorbital tumors. Arch Ophthalmol 41:198, 1949

Fu YS, Perzin KH: Non-epithelial tumors of the nasal cavity, paranasal sinuses, and nasopharynx: A clinicopathologic study. II: Osseous and fibro-osseous lesions, including osteoma, fibrous dysplasia, ossifying fibroma, osteoblastoma, giant cell tumor and osteosarcoma. Cancer 33:1289, 1974

Jaffe HL: Tumours and Tumorous Conditions of the Bones and Joints. London, Henry Kimpton, 1958

Jakobiec FA, Font RL: Mesenchymal Tumors. In Spencer WH (ed): Ophthalmic Pathology: An Atlas and Textbook, 3rd ed, Vol 3, p 2554. Philadelphia, WB Saunders, 1986

Jakobiec FA, Tannenbaum M: Embryological perspectives on the fine structure of orbital tumors. Int Ophthalmol Clin 15:85, 1975b

Jones I, Jakobiec F: Diseases of the Orbit, p 461. Philadelphia, Harper & Row, 1979

Krohel GB, Stewart WB, Chavis RM: Orbital Disease: A Practical Approach. New York, Grune & Stratton, 1981

Lucas RB: Pathology of Tumours of the Oral Tissues, 4th ed, p 191. Edinburgh, Churchill Livingstone, 1984

Mirra JM: Bone Tumors: Diagnosis and Treatment. Philadelphia, JB Lippincott, 1980

Ni C, Albert DM: Tumors of the Eyelid and Orbit: A Chinese-American Collaborative Study, Vol 22, No. 1, p 183. Boston, Little, Brown, 1982

Ozanics V, Jakobiec FA: Prenatal development of the eye and its adnexa. In Jakobiec FA (ed): Ocular Anatomy, Embryology and Teratology, p 11. Philadelphia, Harper & Row, 1982

Rootman J, Kemp EG, Lapointe JS et al: A review of orbital tumours originating in bone. (Submitted to Br J Ophthalmol)

Spranger JW, Langer LO, Wiedemann HR: Bone Dysplasias: An Atlas of Constitutional Disorders of Skeletal Development, p. 203. Philadelphia, WB Saunders, 1974

RHABDOMYOSARCOMA

Abramson DH, Ellsworth RM, Tretter P et al: The treatment of orbital rhabdomyosarcoma with irradiation and chemotherapy. Ophthalmology 86:1330, 1979

Acquaviva A, Barber L, Bernardini C et al: Medical therapy of orbital rhabdomyosarcoma in children. J Neurosurg Sci 26:45, 1982

Albert DM, Wong VG, Henderson ES: Ocular complications of vincristine therapy. Arch Ophthalmol 78:709, 1967

Ashton N, Morgan G: Embryonal sarcoma and embryonal rhabdomyosarcoma of the orbit. J Clin Pathol 18:699, 1965

Bale PM, Parson RE, Stevens MM: Diagnosis and behavior of juvenile rhabdomyosarcoma. Hum Pathol 14:596, 1983

Calhoun FP Jr. Reese AB: Rhabdomyosarcoma of the orbit. Arch Ophthalmol (ns) 27:558, 1942

Cassady JR, Sagerman RH, Tretter P et al: Radiation therapy for rhabdomyosarcoma. Radiology 91:116, 1968

Chess J, Ni C, Yin FQ et al: Rhabdomyosarcoma. Int Ophthalmol Clin 22:63, 1982

Ellenbogen E, Lasky MA: Rhabdomyosarcoma of the orbit in the newborn. Am J Ophthalmol 80:1024, 1975

Exelby PR: Solid tumors in children: Wilm's tumor, neuroblastoma and soft tissue sarcomas. CA 28:146, 1978

Font RL, Hidayat AA: Fibrous histiocytoma of the orbit: A clinicopathologic study of 150 cases. Hum Pathol 13:199, 1982

Frayer WC, Enterline HT: Embryonal rhabdomyosarcoma of the orbit in children and young adults. Arch Ophthalmol 62:203, 1959

Green DM, Jaffe N: Progress and controversy in the treatment of childhood rhabdomyosarcoma. Cancer Treat Rev 5:7, 1978

Grosfeld JL, Weber TR, Weetman RM et al: Rhabdomyosarcoma in childhood: Analysis of survival in 98 cases. J Pediatr Surg 18:141, 1983

Haik BG, Jereb B, Smith ME et al: Radiation and chemotherapy of parameningeal rhabdomyosarcoma involving the orbit. Ophthalmology 93:1001, 1986

Heyn R, Ragab A, Raney B et al: Late effects of therapy in orbital rhabdomyosarcoma. (Report from Intergroup Rhabdomyosarcoma Study I). Proc Am Soc Clin Oncol (Abst C257) 2:66, 1983

Horn RC, Enterline HT: Rhabdomyosarcoma: A clinicopathological study of 39 cases. Cancer 11:181, 1958

Jones IS, Reese AB, Krout J: Orbital rhabdomyosarcoma: An analysis of 62 cases. Am J Ophthalmol 61:721, 1966

Kahn HF, Yeger H, Kassin O et al: Immunohistochemical and electron microscopic assessment of childhood rhabdomyosarcoma: Increased frequency of diagnosis over routine histologic methods. Cancer 51:1897, 1983

Kassel SH, Copenhauer R, Arean VM: Orbital rhabdomyosarcoma. Am J Ophthalmol 60:811, 1965

Kingston JE, McElwain TJ, Malpas JS: Childhood rhabdomyosarcoma: Experience of the children's solid tumour group. Br J Cancer 48:195, 1983

Kirk RC, Zimmerman LE: Rhabdomyosarcoma of the orbit. Arch Ophthalmol 81:559, 1969

Knowles DM II, Jakobiec FA, Potter GD et al: Ophthalmic striated muscle neoplasms. Surv Ophthalmol 21:219, 1976

Knowles DM II, Jakobiec FA, Potter GD et al: The diagnosis and treatment of rhabdomyosarcoma of the orbit. In Jakobiec FA (ed): Ocular and Adnexal Tumors, Chapter 49. Birmingham, Aesculapius, 1978

Kroll AJ: Fine-structural classification of orbital rhabdomyosarcoma. Invest Ophthalmol 6:531, 1967

Landers PH: X-ray treatment of embryonal rhabdomyosarcoma of orbit: Case report of a 13-year survival without recurrence. Am J Ophthalmol 66:745, 1968

Lederman M: Radiation treatment of primary malignant tumors of the orbit. In Boniuk M (ed): Ocular and Adnexal Tumors: New and Controversial Aspects, p 477. St Louis, CV Mosby, 1964

Leff SR, Henkind P: Rhabdomyosarcoma and late malignant melanoma of the orbit. Ophthalmology 90:1258, 1983

Masson JK, Soule EH: Embryonal rhabdomyosarcoma of the head and neck: Report on eighty-eight cases. Am J Surg 110:585, 1965

Maurer H, Foulkes M, Gehan E: Intergroup Rhabdomyosarcoma Study (IRS) II, preliminary report. Proc Am Soc Clin Oncol (Abst C274) 2:70, 1983

Messmer EP, Font RL: Applications of immunohistochemistry to ophthalmic pathology. Ophthalmology 91:701, 1984

Morales AR, Fine G, Horn RC Jr: Rhabdomyosarcoma: An ultrastructural appraisal. Pathol Annu 7:81, 1972

Palmer NF, Foulkes M: Histopathology and prognosis in the second intergroup rhabdomyosarcoma study (IRS-II). ASCO Abstracts, C897, p 229, 1983

Palmer NF, Sachs N, Foulkes M: Histopathology and prognosis in rhabdomyosarcoma (IRS-I). ASCO Abstracts, C660, p 170, 1982

Polack DM, Kanai A, Hood CI: Light and electron microscopic studies of orbital rhabdomyosarcoma. Am J Ophthalmol 71:75, 1971

Porterfield JT, Zimmerman LE: Rhabdomyosarcoma of the orbit: A clinicopathologic study of 55 cases. Arch Pathol Anat 335:329, 1962

Rootman JR, Dimick J: Rhabdoid tumor of the orbit. (Submitted)

Rubin P, Casarett GW: Clinical Radiation Pathology, Vol 2, p 674, Philadelphia, WB Saunders 1968

Sagerman RH, Cassady JR, Tretter P: Radiation therapy for rhabdomyosarcoma of the orbit. Trans Am Acad Ophthalmol Otolaryngol 72:849, 1968

Sanderson PA, Kuwabara T, Cogan DG: Optic neuropathy presumably caused by vincristine therapy. Am J Ophthalmol 81:146, 1976

Stobbe GD, Dargeon HW: Embryonal rhabdomyosarcoma of the head and neck in children and adolescents. Cancer 3:826, 1950

Stout AP: Rhabdomyosarcoma of the skeletal muscles. Ann Surg 123:447, 1946

Stout AP: Tumors of the soft tissues. In Atlas of Tumor Pathology, Section 2, Fascicle 5, p 89. Washington DC, Armed Forces Institute of Pathology, 1953

Suton WW, Lindberg RD, Gehan EA et al: Report from Intergroup Rhabdomyosarcoma Study: Three year relapse free survival rates in childhood rhabdomyosarcoma of the head and neck. Cancer 49:2217, 1982

Tefft M, Lindberg R, Gehan E (for the Intergroup Rhabdomyosarcoma Study Committee): Radiation of rhabdomyosarcoma in children combined with systemic chemotherapy. Local control in patients enrolled into the Intergroup Rhabdomyosarcoma Study (IRS). Natl Cancer Inst Monogr 56:75, 1981

Tsokos M, Howard R, Costa J: Immunohistochemical study of alveolar and embryonal rhabdomyosarcoma. Lab Invest 48:148, 1983

Weichert KA, Bove KC, Aron BS et al: Rhabdomyosarcoma in children: A clinicopathologic study of 35 patients. Am J Clin Pathol 66:692, 1976

Weichselbaum RR, Cassady JR, Albert DM et al: Multimodality management of orbital rhabdomyosarcoma. Int Ophthalmol Clin 20(2):247, 1980

SMOOTH MUSCLE TUMORS

Folberg R, Cleasby G, Flanagan JA et al: Orbital leiomyosarcoma after radiation therapy for bilateral retinoblastoma. Arch Ophthalmol 101:1562, 1983

Font RL, Jurco S III, Brechner RJ: Postradiation leiomyosarcoma of the orbit complication bilateral retinoblastoma. Arch Ophthalmol 101:1557, 1983

Jakobiec FA, Howard G, Rosen M et al: Leiomyoma and leiomyosarcoma of the orbit. Am J Ophthalmol 80:1028, 1975

Jakobiec FA, Jones IS, Tannenbaum M: Leiomyoma: An unusual tumor of the orbit. Br J Ophthalmol 57:825, 1973

Jakobiec FA, Mitchell JP, Chauhan PM et al: Mesectodermal leiomyosarcoma of the antrum and orbit. Am J Ophthalmol 85:51, 1978

Patton RB, Horn RC Jr: Rhabdomyosarcoma: Clinical and pathological features and comparison with human fetal and embryonal skeletal muscle. Surgery 52:572, 1962

Sanborn GE, Valenzuela RE, Green WR: Leiomyoma of the orbit. Am J Ophthalmol 87:371, 1979

Wojno T, Tenzel RR, Nadji M: Orbital leiomyosarcoma. Arch Ophtalmol 101:1566, 1983

ADIPOSE TUMORS

Lipoma

Bartley GB, Yeatts RP, Garrity JA et al: Spindle cell lipoma of the orbit. Am J Ophthalmol 100:605, 1985

Forrest AW: Intraorbital tumors. Arch Ophthalmol 41:198, 1949

Johnson BL, Linn JG: Spindle cell lipoma of the orbit. Arch Ophthalmol 97:133, 1979

Morris D, Henkind P: Fatty infiltration of orbits and heart. Am J Ophthalmol 69:987, 1970

Moss HM: Expanding lesions of the orbit: A clinical study of 230 consecutive cases. Am J Ophthalmol 54:761, 1962

Reese AB: Tumors of the Eye, 2nd ed. Philadelphia, Harper & Row, 1963

Reese AB: Expanding lesions of the orbit (Bowman lecture). Trans Ophthalmol Soc UK 91:85, 1971

Silva D: Orbital tumors. Am J Ophthalmol 65:318, 1968

Liposarcoma

Abdalla MI, Ghaly AF, Hosni F: Liposarcoma with orbital metastases: Case report. Br J Ophthalmol 50:426, 1966

Blodi FC: Unusual orbital neoplasms. Am J Ophthalmol 68:407, 1969

Enterline HT, Culberson JD, Rochlin DB et al: Liposarcoma: A clinical and pathological study of 53 cases. Cancer 13:932, 1960

Enzinger FM, Weiss SW: Soft Tissue Tumors. St Louis, CV Mosby, 1983

Friedman M, Egan JW: Effect of irradiation on liposarcoma. Acta Radiol 54:225, 1960

Jakobiec FA, Jones IS: Mesenchymal and fibro-osseous tumors. In Duane TD (ed): Clinical Ophthalmology, Vol 2, Chapter 44. Philadelphia, Harper & Row, 1976

Mortada A: Rare primary orbital sarcomas. Am J Ophthalmol 68:919, 1969

Naeser P, Mostrom U: Liposarcoma of the orbit: A clinocopathological case report. Br J Ophthalmol 66:190, 1982

Quere MA, Camain R, Baylet R: Liposarcome orbitaire. Ann Ocul (Paris) 196:994, 1963

Schroeder W, Kastendieck H, von Domarus D: Primares myxoides Liposarkom der Orbita. Ophthalmologica 172:337, 1976

Tong ECK, Rubenfeld S: Cardiac metastasis from myxoid liposarcoma emphasizing its radiosensitivity. Am J Roentgenol 103:792, 1968

FIBROUS TISSUE TUMORS

Fibroma

Case TD, LaPiana FG: Benign fibrous tumor of the orbit. Ann Ophthal 7:813, 1975

Fowler JG, Terplan KL: Fibroma of the Orbit. Arch Ophthalmol (ns) 28:263, 1942

Herschorn BJ, Jakobiec FA, Horblass A et al: Tenonoma: An epibulbar subconjunctival fibroma. Ophthalmology 90:1490, 1983

Mortada A: Fibroma of the orbit. Br J Ophthalmol 55:350, 1971

Nodular Fasciitis

Ferry AP, Sherman SE: Nodular fasciitis of the conjunctiva apparently originating in the fascia bulbi (Tenon's capsule). Am J Ophthalmol 78:514, 1974

Font RL, Zimmerman LE: Nodular fasciitis of the eye and adnexa: A report of ten cases. Arch Ophthalmol 75:475, 1966

Levitt JM, de Veer JA, Oguzhan MC: Orbital nodular fasciitis. Arch Ophthalmol 81:235, 1969

Mackenzie DH: The Differential Diagnosis of Fibroblastic Disorders. Oxford, Blackwell Scientific Publications, 1970

Meacham CT: Pseudosarcomatous fasciitis. Am J Ophthalmol 77:747, 1974

Perry RH, Ramoni PS, McAllister V et al: Nodular fasciitis causing unilateral proptosis. Br J Ophthalmol 59:404, 1975

Tolls RE, Mohr S, Spencer WH: Benign nodular fasciitis originating in Tenon's capsule. Arch Ophthalmol 75:482, 1966

Fibromatoses, Fibrosarcoma, and Myxoma

Abramson DH, Ellsworth RM, Zimmerman LE: Nonocular cancer in retinoblastoma survivors. Trans Am Acad Ophthalmol Otolaryngol 81:OP454, 1976

Abramson DH, Ronner HJ, Ellsworth RM: Second tumors in irradiated bilateral retinoblastoma. Am J Ophthalmol 87:624, 1979

Balsaver AM, Butler JJ, Martin RG: Congenital fibrosarcoma. Cancer 20:1607, 1967

Chung EB, Enzinger FM: Infantile fibrosarcoma. Cancer 38:729, 1976

Eifrig DC, Foos RY: Fibrosarcoma of the orbit. Am J Ophthalmol 67:244, 1969

Enzinger FM, Weiss SW: Soft Tissue Tumors. St Louis, CV Mosby, 1983

Forrest AW: Tumors following radiation about the eye. Int Ophthalmol Clin 2:543, 1962

Gonzales-Crussi F: Ultrastructure of congenital fibrosarcoma. Cancer 26:1289, 1970

Hidayat AA, Font RL: Juvenile fibrosarcomatosis of the periorbital region and eyelid: A clinicopathologic study of six cases. Arch Ophthalmol 98:280, 1980

Jakobiec FA, Tannenbaum M: The ultrastructure of orbital fibrosarcoma. Am J Ophthalmol 77:899, 1974

Mackenzie DH: The Differential Diagnosis of Fibroblastic Disorders. Oxford, Blackwell Scientific Publications, 1970

Mortada A: Rare primary orbital sarcomas. Am J Ophthalmol 68:919, 1969

Nasr AM, Blodi FC, Lindahl S et al: Congenital generalized multicentric myofibromatosis with orbital involvement. Am J Ophthalmol 102:779, 1986

Rootman J, Carvounis EP, Dolman CL et al: Congenital fibrosarcoma metastatic to the choroid. Am J Ophthalmol 87:632, 1979

Sagerman R, Cassady J, Tretter P et al: Radiation-induced neoplasia following external beam therapy for children with retinoblastoma. Am J Roentgenol Radium Ther Nucl Med 105:529, 1966

Schnitka T, Asp D, Horner R: Congenital generalized fibromatoses. Cancer 11:627, 1958

Schutz JS, Rabkin MD, Schutz S: Fibromatous tumor (desmoid type) of the orbit. Arch Ophthalmol 97:703, 1979

Soloway H: Radiation induced neoplasms following curative therapy for retinoblastoma. Cancer 19:1984, 1966

Stout AP: Fibrosarcoma in infants and children. Cancer 15:1028, 1962

Stout AP, Lattes R: Tumors of the soft tissues. In Atlas of Tumor Pathology, 2nd Series, Fascicle 1. Washington, DC, Armed Forces Institute of Pathology, 1967

Strickland P: Fibromyxosarcoma of the orbit: Radiation induced tumor 33 years after treatment of "bilateral ocular glioma." Br J Ophthalmol 50:50, 1966

Weiner JM, Hidayat AA: Juvenile fibrosarcoma of the orbit and eyelid. Arch Ophthalmol 101:253, 1983

Yanoff M, Scheie HG: Fibrosarcoma of the orbit: Report of two patients. Cancer 19:1711, 1966

Myxoma

Blegvad O: Myxoma of the orbit. Acta Ophthalmol (Kbh) 22:131, 1944

Blodi FC: Unusual orbital neoplasms. Am J Ophthalmol 68:407, 1969

Gifford SR: Multiple myxoma of the orbit. Arch Ophthalmol 5:445, 1931

Jakobiec FA, Jones IS: Mesenchymal and fibro-osseous tumors, p 461. In Jones IS, Jakobiec FA (eds): Diseases of the Orbit. Philadelphia, Harper & Row, 1979

Kreuger EG, Polifrone JC, Baum G: Retrobulbar orbital myxoma and its detection by ultrasonography. J Neurosurg 26:87, 1967

Lamb HD: Myxoma of the orbit, with case report and anatomical findings. Arch Ophthalmol 57:425, 1928

FIBROUS HISTIOCYTOMA

Biedner B, Rothkoff L: Orbital fibrous histiocytoma in an infant. Am J Ophthalmol 85:548, 1978

Cabellero LRC, Rodriguez AC, Sopelana AB: Angiomatoid malignant fibrous histiocytoma of the orbit. Am J Ophthalmol 92:13, 1981

Cole SH, Ferry AP: Fibrous histiocytoma (fibrous xanthoma) of the lacrimal sac. Arch Ophthalmol 96:1647, 1978

Enzinger FM: Angiomatoid malignant fibrous histiocytoma: A distinct fibrohistiocytic tumor of children and young adults simulating vascular neoplasm. Cancer 44:2147, 1979

Font RL, Hidayat AA: Fibrous histiocytoma of the orbit: A clinicopathologic study of 150 cases. Hum Pathol 13:199, 1982

Hoffman MA, Dickerson GR: Malignant fibrous histiocytoma: An ultrastructural study of eleven cases. Hum Pathol 14:913, 1983

Iwamoto T, Jakobiec FA, Darrell RW: Fibrous histiocytoma of the corneoscleral limbus: The ultrastructure of a distinctive inclusion. Ophthalmology 88:1260, 1981

Jakobiec FA, DeVoe AG: Fibrous histiocytoma of the tarsus. Am J Ophthalmol 84:794, 1977

Jakobiec FA, Howard G, Jones IS et al: Fibrous histiocytoma of the orbit. Am J Ophthalmol 77:333, 1974

Jakobiec FA, Jones IS: Mesenchymal and fibro-osseous tumors. In Duane TD (ed): Clinical Ophthalmology, Vol 2, Chapter 44. Philadelphia, Harper & Row, 1978

John T, Yanoff M, Scheie HG: Eyelid fibrous histiocytoma. Ophthalmology 88:1193, 1981

Kauffman SL, Stout AP: Histiocytic tumors (fibrous xanthoma and histiocytoma) in children. Cancer 14:469, 1961

Kim JH, Chu FC, Woodward HQ et al: Radiation-induced soft tissue and bone sarcoma. Radiology 129:501, 1978

Lattes R: Tumors of the soft tissues. An Atlas of Tumor Pathology, 2nd Series, Fascicle 1 (revised). Washington, DC, Armed Forces Institute of Pathology, 1982

Marback RL, Kincaid MC, Green WC et al: Fibrous histiocytoma of the lacrimal sac. Am J Ophthalmol 93:511, 1982

O'Brien JE, Stout AO: Malignant fibrous xanthomas. Cancer 17:1445, 1964

Ozzello L, Stout AP, Murray MR: Cultural Characteristics of malignant histiocytomas and fibrous xanthomas. Cancer 16:331, 1963

Rodrigues MM, Furgiuele FP, Weinreb S: Malignant fibrous histiocytoma of the orbit. Arch Ophthalmol 95:2025, 1977

Russman BA: Tumor of the orbit: A 33 year follow up. Am J Ophthalmol 64:273, 1967

Soule E, Enriquez P: Atypical fibrous histiocytoma, malignant fibrous histiocytoma, maligiant histiocytoma, and epithelioid sarcoma. Cancer 30:128, 1972

Stewart WB, Newman NM, Cavender JC et al: Fibrous histiocytoma metastatic to the orbit. Arch Ophthalmol 96:871, 1978

Tewfik HH, Tewfik FA, Latourette HB: Postirradiation malignant fibrous histiocytoma. J Surg Oncol 16:199, 1981

Turner RR, Wood GS, Beckstead JH et al: Histiocytic malignancies: Morphologic, immunologic and enzymatic heterogeneity. Am J Surg Pathol 8:485, 1984

Weiss SW, Enzinger FM: Malignant fibrous histiocytoma. An analysis of 200 cases. Cancer 41:2250, 1978

Zimmerman LE: Changing concepts concerning the malignancy of ocular tumors. Arch Ophthalmol 78:166, 1967

XANTHOGRANULOMA

Gaynes PM, Cohen GS: Juvenile xanthogranuloma of the orbit. Am J Ophthalmol 63:755, 1967

Sanders TE: Infantile xanthogranuloma of the orbit: A report of three cases. Am J Ophthalmol 61:1299, 1966

Zimmerman LE: Ocular lesions of juvenile xanthogranuloma: Nevoxantho-endothelioma. Trans Am Acad Ophthalmol Otolaryngol 69:412, 1965

TUMORS ORIGINATING IN BONE

Blodi FC: Unusual orbital neoplasma. Am J Ophthalmol 68:407, 1969

Blodi FC: Pathology of orbital bones. Am J Ophthalmol 81:1, 1976

Forrest AW: Intraorbital tumors. Arch Ophthalmol 41:198, 1949

Fu YS, Perzin KH: Non-epithelial tumors of the nasal cavity, paranasal sinuses, and nasopharynx: A clinicopathologic study. II: Osseous and fibro-osseous lesions, including osteoma, fibrous dysplasia, ossifying fibroma, osteoblastoma, giant cell tumor and osteosarcoma. Cancer 33:1289, 1974

Ni C, Albert DM: Tumors of the Eyelid and Orbit: A Chinese-American Collaborative Study, vol. 22, no. 1, p. 183. Boston, Little, Brown & Co, 1982

Rootman J, Kemp EG, Lapointe JS, Quenville NF: A review of orbital tumors originating in bone. (submitted)

Fibrous Dysplasia

Dehner LP: Tumors of the mandible and maxilla in children. Cancer 31:364, 1973

Fries JW: The roentgen features of fibrous dysplasia of the skull and facial bones. Am J Radiol 77:71, 1957

Liakos GM, Walker CB, Carruth JAS: Ocular complications in craniofacial fibrous dysplasia. Br J Ophthalmol 63:611, 1979

Moore AT, Buncic JR, Munro IR: Fibrous dysplasia of the orbit in childhood. Clinical features and management. Ophthalmology 92:12, 1985

Moore RT: Fibrous dysplasia of the orbit. Surv Ophthalmol 13:321, 1969

Ronner HJ, Trokel SL, Hilal S: Acute blindness in a patient with fibrous dysplasia. Orbit 1:231, 1982

Sevel D, James HE, Burns R et al: McCune-Albright syndrome (fibrous dysplasia) associated with an orbital tumor. Ann Ophthalmol 16:283, 1984

Shapiro A, Tso MOM, Putterman AM et al: A clinicopathologic study of hematic cysts of the orbit. Am J Ophthalmol 102:237, 1986

Osteoma and Ossifying Fibroma

Khalil MK, Leib ML: Cemento-ossifying fibroma of the orbit. Can J Ophthalmol 14:195, 1979

Lehrer HZ: Ossifying fibroma of the orbital roof: Its distinction from "blistering" or intra-osseous meningioma. Arch Neurol 20:536, 1969

Margo CE, Ragsdale BD, Perman KI et al: Psammomatoid (juvenile) ossifying fibroma of the orbit. Ophthalmology 92:150, 1985

Margo CE, Weiss A, Habal MB: Psammomatoid ossifying fibroma. Arch Ophthalmol 104:1347, 1986

Marks MW, Newman MH: Transcoronal removal of an atypical orbitoethmoid osteoma. Plast Reconstr Surg 72:874, 1983

Miller NR, Gray J, Snip R: Giant mushroom-shaped osteoma of the orbit originating from the maxillary sinus. Am J Ophthalmol 83:587, 1977

Pagani JJ, Bassett LW, Winter J et al: Osteogenic sarcoma after retinoblastoma radiotherapy. Am J Radiol 133:699, 1979

Shields JA, Nelson LB, Brown JF et al: Clinical, computed tomographic, and histopathologic characteristics of juvenile ossifying fibroma with orbital involvement. Am J Ophthalmol 96:650, 1983

Whitson WE, Orcutt JC, Walkinshaw MD: Orbital osteoma in Gardner's syndrome. Am J Ophthalmol 101:236, 1986

Wilkes SR, Trautmann JC, DeSanto LW et al: An unusual cause of amaurosis fugax. Mayo Clin Proc 54:258, 1979

Osteoblastoma

Abdalla MI, Hosni F: Osteoblastoma of the orbit: Case report. Br J Ophthalmol 50:95, 1966

Dahlin DC, Johnson EW Jr: Giant osteoid osteoma. J Bone Joint Surg [Am] 36:559, 1954

Jackson RP: Recurrent osteoblastoma: A review. Clin Orthop 131:229, 1978

Lowder CY, Berlin AJ, Cox WA et al: Benign osteoblastoma of the orbit. Ophthalmology 93:1351, 1986

McLeod RA, Dahlin DC, Beabout JW: The spectrum of osteoblastoma. Am J Roentgenol 126:321, 1976

Ronis ML, Obando M, Bucko MI et al: Benign osteoblastoma of temporal bone. Laryngoscope 84:857, 1974

Shepherd WFI, Maguire CJF, Bailey IC: Abstract: Benign osteoblastoma of the orbit. Ir J Med Sci 146:150, 1977

Williams RN, Boop WC Jr: Benign osteoblastoma of the skull: case report. J Neurosurg 41:769, 1974

Reparative Granuloma

Cook H: Giant-cell granuloma. Br J Oral Surg 3:97, 1965

deMello DE, Archer CR, Blair JD: Ethmoidal fibro-osseous lesion in a child: Diagnostic and therapeutic problems. Am J Surg Pathol 4:595, 1980

Friedberg SA, Eisenstein R, Wallner LJ: Giant cell lesions involving the nasal accessory sinuses. Laryngoscope 69:763, 1969

Hirschl S, Katz A: Giant cell reparative granuloma outside the jaw bone. Hum Pathol 5:171, 1974

Hoopes PC, Anderson RL, Blodi FC: Giant cell (reparative) granuloma of the orbit. Ophthalmology 88:1361, 1981

Sood GC, Malik SR, Gupta DK et al: Reparative granuloma of the orbit causing unilateral proptosis. Am J Ophthalmol 63:524, 1967

Aneurysmal Bone Cyst

Klepach GL, Ho REM, Kelly JK: Aneurysmal bone cyst of the orbit: A case report. J Clin Neuro-Ophthalmol 4:49, 1984

Powell JO, Glaser JS: Aneurysmal bone cyst of the orbit. Arch Ophthalmol 93:340, 1975

Ronner HJ, Jones IS: Aneurysmal bone cyst of the orbit: A review. Ann Ophthalmol 15:626, 1983

Sanerkin NG, Mott MG, Roylance J: An unusual intraosseous lesion with fibroblastic, osteoclastic, osteoblastic, aneurysmal and fibromyxoid elements: Solid variant of aneurysmal bone cyst. Cancer 51:2278, 1983

Yee RD, Cogan DG, Thorp TR et al: Optic nerve compression due to aneurysmal bone cyst. Arch Ophthalmol 95:2176, 1977

Xanthomatous Lesions

Nicholls JV: Cholesterol containing granuloma of the orbital wall. Arch Ophthalmol 41:234, 1956

Parke DW II, Font RL, Boniuk M et al: "Cholesteatoma" of the orbit. Arch Ophthalmol 100:612, 1982

Thacker EA: Epidermoid tumors of the frontal bone, sinus and orbit. Arch Otolaryngology 51:400, 1950

Brown Tumor

Holzer NJ, Croft CB, Walsh JB et al: Brown tumor of the orbit. JAMA 238:1758, 1977

Naiman J, Green WR, D'Heurle D et al: Brown tumor of the orbit associated with primary hyperparathyroidism. Am J Ophthalmol 90:565, 1980

Parrish CM, O'Day DM: Brown tumor of the orbit. Arch Ophthalmol 104:1199, 1986

Som PM, Lawson W, Cohen BA: Giant cell lesions of the facial bones. Radiology 147:129, 1983

Chondroma

Bowen JH, Christensen FH, Klintworth GK et al: A clinicopathologic study of a cartilaginous hamartoma of the orbit. Ophthalmology 88:1356, 1981

Jepson CM, Wetzig PC: Pure chondroma of the trochlea. Surv Ophthalmol 11:656, 1966

Chondrosarcoma

Albert DA, Ni C, Sebag J et al: Rare orbital tumors. Int Ophthalmol Clin 22:183, 1982

Cardenas-Ramirez L, Albores-Saavedra J, De Buen S: Mesenchymal chondrosarcoma of the orbit. Arch Ophthalmol 86:410, 1971

Guccion J, Font RL, Enzinger FM et al: Extraskeletal mesenchymal chondrosarcoma. Arch Pathol 95:336, 1973

Holland MG, Allen JH, Ichinose H: Chondrosarcoma of the orbit. Trans Am Acad Ophthalmol Otolaryngol 65:898, 1961

Rosenthal DI, Schiller AL, Mankin HJ: Chondrosarcoma: Correlation of radiological and histological grade. Radiology 150:21, 1984

Sevel D: Mesenchymal chondrosarcoma of the orbit. Br J Ophthalmol 58:882, 1974

Chordoma

Ferry AP, Haddad HM, Goldman JL: Orbital invasion by an intracranial chordoma. Am J Ophthalmol 92:7, 1981

Osteogenic Sarcoma

Abramson DH, Ellsworth RM, Zimmerman LE: Non-ocular cancer in retinoblastoma survivors. Trans Am Acad Ophthalmol Otolaryngol 81:454, 1976

Abramson DH, Ronner HJ, Ellsworth R: Second tumors in nonirradiated bilateral retinoblastoma. Am J Ophthalmol 87:624, 1979

Bone RC, Biller HF, Harris BL: Osteogenic sarcoma of the frontal sinus. Ann Otolaryngol 82:162, 1973

Rosen G: Pre-operative (neoadjuvant) chemotherapy for osteosarcoma: A ten year experience. Orthopedics 8:659, 1985

Small ML, Green WR, Johnson LC: Lipoma of the frontal bone. Arch Ophthalmol 97:129, 1979

Sundaresan N, Huvos AG, Galicich JH: Combined modality treatment of osteosarcoma of the skull. Neurosurgery 63:563, 1985

Rare Tumors of Orbital Bone

Brackup AH, Haller MD, Danber MM: Hemangioma of the bony orbit. Am J Ophthalmol 90:258, 1980

deSmet MD, Rootman J: Orbital manifestation of plasmacytic lymphoproliferations. (Accepted Ophthalmology 1987)

Friendly DS, Font RL, Milhorat T: Hemangioendothelioma of frontal bone. Am J Ophthalmol 93:482, 1982

Gross JH, Roth AM: Intraosseous humangioma of the orbital roof. Am J Ophthalmol 86:565, 1978

Hayes FA, Thompson EI, Hustu HO et al: The response of Ewing's sarcoma to sequential cyclophosphamide and adriamycin induction therapy. J Clin Oncol 1:45, 1983

Hornblass A, Zaidman GW: Intraosseous orbital cavernous hemangioma. Ophthalmology 88:1351, 1981

Phillips WC, Kattapuram SV, Doseretz DE et al: Primary lymphoma of bone: Relationship of radiographic appearance and prognosis. Radiology 144:285, 1982

Razek A, Perez A, Tefft M et al: Intergroup Ewing's sarcoma study, local control related to radiation dose, volume and site of primary lesion of Ewing's sarcoma. Cancer 46:516, 1980

Rosen G, Capartos B, Nirenberg A et al: Ewing's sarcoma, ten year experience with adjuvant chemotherapy. Cancer 47:2204, 1981

Fibrous Histiocytoma of Bone

Caballero LR, Rodriguez AC, Sopelina AB: Angiomatoid malignant fibrous histiocytoma of the orbit. Am J Ophthalmol 92:12, 1981

Cappana R, Bertoni F, Bacchini P et al: Malignant fibrous histiocytoma of bone. The experience at the Rizzoli Institute: Report of 90 cases. Cancer 54:177, 1984

Font RL, Hidaijal AA: Fibrous histiocytoma of the orbit: A clinicopathologic study of 150 cases. Hum Pathol 13:199, 1982

Paling MR, Hyams DM: Computed tomography in malignant fibrous histiocytoma. J Comput Assist Tomogr 6:785, 1982

Ros PR, Viamonte M Jr, Rywlin AM: Review: Malignant fibrous histiocytoma: Mesenchymal tumor of ubiquitous origin. Am J Radiol 142:753, 1984

LACRIMAL

Ashton N: Epithelial tumors of the lacrimal gland. Mod Probl Ophthalmol 14:306, 1975

Balchunas WR, Quencer RM, Byrne SF: Lacrimal gland and fossa masses: Evaluation by computed tomography and A-Mode echography. Radiology 149:751, 1983

Canavan YM, Logan WC: Benign hemangioendothelioma of the lacrimal gland fossa. Arch Ophthalmol 97:1112, 1979

Cykiert RC, Albert DM, Cornog, JL Jr et al: Suspected multiple primary tumors of the lacrimal and parotid glands. Arch Ophthalmol 94:1530, 1976

Dagher G, Anderson RL, Ossoinig KC et al: Adenoid cystic carcinoma of the lacrimal gland in a child. Arch Ophthalmol 98:1098, 1980

Dardick I, van Hostrand AWP, Phillips MJ: Histogenesis of salivary gland pleomorphic adenoma (mixed tumor) with an evaluation of the role of the myoepithelial cell. Hum Pathol 13:62, 1982

Font RL, Gamel JW: Epithelial tumors of the lacrimal gland: An analysis of 265 cases. In Jakobiec FA (ed): Ocular and Adnexal Tumors, p 787. Birmingham, Aesculapius, 1978

Font RL, Gamel JW: Adenoid cystic carcinoma of the lacrimal gland: A clinicopathologic study of 79 cases. In Nicholson DH (ed): Ocular Pathology Update, p 277. New York, Masson Publishing USA, 1980

Gamel JW, Font RL: Adenoid cystic carcinoma of the lacrimal gland: The clinical significance of a basaloid histologic pattern. Hum Pthol 13:219, 1982

Henderson JW, Farrow GM: Primary malignant mixed tumors of the lacrimal gland. Ophthalmology 87:466, 1980

Henderson JW, Neault RW: En bloc removal of intrinsic neoplasms of the lacrimal gland. Am J Ophthalmol 82:905, 1976

Hesselink JR, Davis KR, Dallow RL et al: Computed tomography of masses in the lacrimal gland region. Radiology 131:143, 1979

Iwamoto T, Jakobiec FA: A comparative ultrastructural study of the normal lacrimal gland and its epithelial tumors. Hum Pathol 13:236, 1982

Iwamoto T, Jakobiec FA: Lacrimal glands. In Jakobiec FA (ed): Ocular Anatomy, Embryology and Teratology, p 761. Philadelphia, Harper & Row, 1982

Jacobs L, Sirkin S, Kinkel W: Ectopic lacrimal gland in the orbit identified by computerized axial transverse tomography. Ann Ophthalmol 9:591, 1977

Jakobiec FA, Yeo JH, Trokel SL et al: Combined clinical and computed tomographic diagnosis of primary lacrimal fossa lesions. Am J Ophthal 94:785, 1982

Janecka I, Housepian E, Trokel S et al: Surgical management of malignant tumors of the lacrimal gland. Am J Surg 148:539, 1984

Lee DA, Campbell RJ, Waller RR et al: A clinicopathologic study of primary adenoid cystic carcinoma of the lacrimal gland. Ophthalmology 92:128, 1985

Lloyd GAS: Lacrimal gland tumours: The role of CT and conventional radiology. Br J Radiol 54:1034, 1981

Ludwig ME, LiVolsi VA, McMahon RT: Malignant mixed tumor of the lacrimal gland. Am J Surg Pathol 3, No. 5: 457, 1979

Marsh JL, Wise DM, Smith M et al: Lacrimal gland adenoid cystic carcinoma: Intracranial and extracranial en bloc resection. Plast Reconstr Surg 68:577, 1981

McPherson SD Jr: Mixed tumor of the lacrimal gland in a seven-year-old boy. Am J Ophthalmol 61:501, 1966

Mindlin A, Lamberts D, Barsky D: Mixed lacrimal gland tumor arising from ectopic lacrimal gland tissue in the orbit. J Pediatr Ophthalmol 14:44, 1977

Mueller EC, Borit A: Aberrant lacrimal gland and pleomorphic adenoma within the muscle cone. Ann Ophthalmol 11:661, 1979

Ossoff RH, Jones JA, Bytell DE: Recurrent benign mixed tumor of lacrimal gland: Report of a case with intracranial extension. Otolaryngol Head Neck Surg 89:599, 1981

Perzin K, Jakobiec FA, LiVolsi V et al: Lacrimal gland mixed tumors. Cancer 45:2593, 1980

Portis JM, Krohel GB, Stewart WB: Calcifications in lesions of the fossa of the lacrimal gland. Ophthalmic Plast Reconstr Surg 1:137, 1985

Riley FC, Henderson JW: Report of a case of malignant transformation in benign mixed tumor of the lacrimal gland. Am J Ophthalmol 70:767, 1970

Sidrys LA, Fritz KJ, Variakojis D: Fast neutron therapy for orbital adenoid cystic carcinoma. Ann Ophthalmol 14:42, 1982

Spiro RH, Huvos G, Strong EW: Malignant mixed tumor of salivary origin. Cancer 39:388, 1977

Stewart WB, Krohel GB, Wright JE: Lacrimal gland and fossa lesions: An approach to diagnosis and management. Ophthalmology 86:886, 1979

Wagoner MD, Chuo N, Gonder JR et al: Nucoepidermoid carcinoma of the lacrimal gland. Ann Ophthalmol 14:383, 1982

Waller RR, Riley FC, Henderson JW: Malignant mixed tumor of the lacrimal gland: Occult source of metastatic carcinoma. Arch Ophthalmol 90:297, 1973

Witschel H, Zimmerman LE: Malignant mixed tumor of the lacrimal gland: A clinicopathologic report of two unusual cases. Graefes Arch Clin Exp Ophthalmol 216:327, 1981

Wright JE: Factors affecting the survival of patients with lacrimal gland tumours. Can J Ophthalmol 17:3, 1982

Wright JE, Stewart WB, Krohel GB: Clinical presentation and management of lacrimal gland tumours. Br J Ophthalmol 63:600, 1979

Zimmerman LE, Sanders TE, Ackerman LV: Epithelial tumors of the lacrimal gland: Prognostic and therapeutic significance of histologic types. Int Ophthalmol Clin 2:337, 1962

Zimmerman LE, Sobin LH: Histological Typing of Tumours of the Eye and Its Adnexa. International Histological Classification of Tumours No. 24. Geneva, World Health Organization, 1980

ORBITAL METASTASES

Abdalla MI, Ghaly AF, Hosni F: Liposarcoma with orbital metastases: Case report. Br J Ophthalmol 50:426, 1966

Albert DM, Rubenstein RA, Scheie HG: Tumor metastasis to the eye. II: Clinical study in infants and children. Am J Ophthalmol 63:727, 1967

Alvarez-Berdecia A, Schut L, Bruce DA: Localized primary intracranial Ewing's sarcoma of the orbital roof: Case report. J Neurosurg 50:811, 1979

Appen RE, DeVenecia G, Selliken JH et al: Meningeal carcinomatosis with blindness. Am J Ophthalmol 86:661, 1978

Ballinger WH Jr, Wesley RE: Seminoma metastatic to the orbit. Ophthalmic Surg 15:120, 1984

Bullock JD, Yanes B: Ophthalmic manifestations of metastatic breast cancer. Ophthalmology 87:961, 1980

Divine RD, Anderson RL: Metastatic small cell carcinoma masquerading as orbital myositis. Ophthalmic Surg 14:483, 1982

Divine RD, Anderson RL, Ossoinig KC: Metastatic carcinoid unresponsive to radiation therapy presenting as a lacrimal fossa mass. Ophthalmology 89:516, 1982

Dresner SC, Kennerdell JS, Dekker A: Fine needle aspiration biopsy of metastatic orbital tumors. Surv Ophthalmol 27:397, 1983

Ferry AP, Font RL: Carcinoma metastatic to the eye and orbit: I. A clinicopathologic study of 227 cases. Arch Ophthalmol 92:276, 1974

Font RL, Ferry AP: Carcinoma metastatic to the eye and orbit: III. A clinicopathologic study of 28 cases metastatic to the orbit. Cancer 38:1326, 1976

Font RL, Naumann G, Zimmerman LE: Primary malignant melanoma of the skin metastatic to the eye and orbit. Am J Ophthalmol 63:738, 1967

Fratkin JD, Purcell JJ, Krachmer JH et al: Wilms' tumor metastatic to the orbit. JAMA 238:1841, 1977

Glassburn JR, Klionsky, M, Brady LW: Radiation therapy for metastatic disease involving the orbit. Am J Clin Oncol 7:145, 1984

Grubb BP, Thant M: Orbital metastasis of prostatic carcinoma. J Ocul Ther Surg 3:273, 1984

Healy JF: Computed tomographic evaluation of metastases to the orbit. Ann Ophthalmol 15:1026, 1983

Henderson JW, Farrow GM: Orbital Tumors, 2nd ed, p 67. New York, Brian C Decker, 1980

Hesselink JR, David KR, Weber AL et al: Radiological evaluation of orbital metastases, with emphasis on computed tomography. Radiology 137:363, 1980

Hood CI, Font RL, Zimmerman LE: Metastatic mammary carcinoma in the eyelid with histiocytoid appearance. Cancer 31:793, 1973

Hou PK, Garg MP: Tumors of the orbit: A report of 193 consecutive cases. In Blodi FC (ed): Current Concepts in Ophthalmology, Vol 2, p 176. St Louis, CV Mosby Co, 1972

Howard GM, Jakobiec FA, Iwamoto T et al: Pulsating metastatic orbital tumor. Am J Ophthalmol 85:767, 1978

Jakobiec FA: Presentation, pathology and management of orbital metastatic disease. Presented at 5th International Symposium on Orbital Disorders. Amsterdam, September 1985

Jakobiec FA, Austin P, Iwamoto T et al: Primary infiltrating signet ring carcinoma of the eyelids. Ophthalmology 90:291, 1983

Jakobiec FA, Font RL: Ocular and orbital tumors. In Johanessen JV (ed): Electron Microscopy in Human Diseases, Vol VI: The Nervous System, Sensory Organs and Respiratory Tract, p 346. New York, McGraw-Hill, 1979

Jakobiec FA, Font RL, Iwamoto T: Diagnostic ultrastructural pathology of ophthalmic tumors. In Jakobiec FA (ed): Ocular and Adnexal Tumors, p 359. Birmingham, Aesculapius, 1978

Jensen OA: Metastatic tumours of the eye and orbit. A histopathological analysis of a Danish series. Acta Pathol Microbiol Scand [Suppl] 212:201, 1970

Kennedy RE: An evaluation of 820 orbital cases. Trans Am Ophthalmol Soc 82:134, 1984

Kraus HR, Slamovits TL, Sibony PA et al: Letter: Orbital metastasis of bladder carcinoma. Am J Ophthalmol 94:265, 1982

Krohel GB, Perry S, Hepler RS: Acute hypertension with orbital carcinoid tumor. Arch Ophthalmol 100:106, 1982

Leyson JF: Mediastinal seminoma associated with exophthalmos and gynecomastia. Urology 3:336, 1974

Mackay B, Ordonez NG: The role of the pathologist in the evaluation of poorly differentiated tumors. Semin Oncol 9:396, 1982

Mann AS: Bilateral exophthalmos and seminoma. J Clin Endocrinol Metab 27:1500, 1967

Mottow-Lippa L, Jakobiec FA, Iwamoto T: Pseudoinflammatory metastatic breast carcinoma of the orbit and lids. Ophthalmology 88:575, 1981

Musarella MA, Chen HSL, DeBoer G et al: Ocular involvement in neuroblastoma: Prognostic implications. Ophthalmology 91:936, 1984

Neumann KH, Nystrom JS: Metastatic cancer of unknown origin: Nonsquamous cell type. Semin Oncol 9:427, 1982

Osher RH, Schatz NJ, Duane TD: Acquired orbital retraction syndrome. Arch Ophthalmol 98:1798, 1980

Reifler DM: Orbital metastasis with enophthalmos: a review of the literature. Henry Ford Hosp Med J 33:171, 1985

Robert NJ, Garnick MB, Frei E III: Cancers of unknown origin: Current approaches and future perspectives. Semin Oncol 9:526, 1982

Rootman J: Orbital metastatic disease. Presented at 5th International Symposium on Orbital Disorders. Amsterdam, September 1985

Rothfus WE, Curtin HD: Extraocular muscle enlargement: A CT review. Radiology 151:677, 1984

Rush JA, Older JJ, Richman AV: Testicular seminoma metastatic to the orbit. Am J Ophthalmol 91:258, 1981

Rush JA, Waller RW, Campbell RJ: Orbital carcinoid tumor metastatic from the colon. Am J Ophthalmol 89:636, 1980

Shields JA, Bakewell B, Augsburger JJ et al: Classification and incidence of space-occupying lesions of the orbit. Arch Ophthalmol 102:1606, 1984

Stewart WB, Newman NM, Cavender JC et al: Fibrous histiocytoma metastatic to the orbit. Arch Ophthalmol 96:871, 1978

Taylor JB, Soloman BH, Levine RE et al: Exophthalmos and seminoma: Regression with steroids and orchiectomy. JAMA 240:860, 1978

Third National Cancer Survey: NCI Monograph 41, 1975

Walker RA: Immunohistochemistry of biological markers of breast carcinoma. In DeLettis RA (ed): Advances in Immunohistochemistry, p 223. Chicago, Year Book Medical Publishers, 1984

Winkler CF, Goodman GH, Eiferman A et al: Orbital metastasis from prostatic carcinoma: Identification by an immunoperoxidase technique. Arch Ophthalmol 99:1406, 1981

Wolter JR, Hendrix RC: Osteoblastic prostate carcinoma metastatic to the orbit. Am J Ophthalmol 91:648, 1981

Yeo JH, Jakobiec FA, Iwamoto T et al: Metastatic carcinoma masquerading as scleritis. Ophthalmol 90:184, 1983

Zimmerman LE, Stangl R, Riddle PJ: Primary carcinoid tumor of the orbit. Arch Ophthalmol 101:1395, 1983

THERAPY FOR ORBITAL METASTASES

Breast Cancer

Bonadonna G: Advances in Antracycline Chemotherapy: Epirubicin. Milano, Masson Italia Editori, 1984

Buchanan RB, Blamey RW, Turrant KR et al: A randomized

comparison of tamoxifen with surgical oophorectomy in premenopausal patients with advanced breast cancer. J Clin Oncol 4:1326, 1986

Canellos GP, De Vita VT, Gold GL et al: Combination chemotherapy for advanced breast cancer: Response and effect on survival. Ann Intern Med 84:389, 1976

Canetta R, Florentine S, Hunter H et al: Magestrol acetate. Cancer Treat Rep 10:141, 1983

De Lena N, Brambilla C, Valagussa P et al: High dose methdroxyprogestrone acetate in breast cancer resistant to endocrine in cytotoxic therapy. Cancer Chemother Pharmacol 2:175, 1979

Dukart G, Posner L, Henry D et al: Comparative cardiotoxicity of mitoxantrone versus doxorubicin. Am Soc Clin Oncol 5:48, 1986

Eder JP, Antman K, Peters W et al: High dose combination alkylating agent chemotherapy with autologous bone marrow support for metastataic breast cancer. J Clin Oncol 4:1592, 1986

Harris AL, Powles TJ, Smith IE: Aminoglutethimide for the treatment of advanced postmenopausal breast cancer. Eur J Cancer 19:11, 1983

Henderson IC, Canellos GP: Medical progress: Cancer of the breast: the past decade. N Engl J Med 302:17; 78, 1980

Hryniuk W, Bush H: The importance of dose intensity in chemotherapy of metastatic breast cancer. J Clin Oncol 2:1281 1984

Luft R, Olivecrona H, Ikkos D et al: Hyphysectomy, the management of metastatic cancer of the breast. In Curry A (ed): Endocrine Aspects of Breast Cancer, p 27. Edinburgh, Livingstone, 1958

Mouridsen H, Palshof T, Patterson J et al: Tamoxifen in advanced breast cancer. Cancer Treat Rep 5:131, 1978

Peto R: Overview of mortality of adjuvant therapy of breast cancer. Presented at Overview meeting of Trialists. Bethesda, Maryland, November, 1985

Santen RJ, Worgul TJ, Samojlik E et al: Randomized trial comparing surgical adrenalectomy with aminoglutethimide plus hydrocrotisone in women with advanced breast cancer. N Engl J Med 305:545, 1981

Carcinoma of the Lung

Abeloff MD, Ettinger DS, Khouri NF, et al: Intensive induction therapy for small cell carcinoma of the lung. Cancer Treat Rep 63:519, 1979

Britell JC, Eagan RT, Ingle JN et al: Cistichlorodiammineplatinum (2) alone followed by adriamycin plus cyclophosphamide as progression versus cistichlorodiammineplatinum (2) adriamycin, and cyclophosamide in combination for adenocarcinoma of the lung. Cancer Treat Rep 62:1207, 1978

Bunnpa PA Jr, Ihde DC: Small cell bronchogenic carcinoma: A review of therapeutic results. In Livingstone RB (ed): Lung Cancer: Advances in Research and Treatment, p 169. The Hague, Martinus Nijhoff, 1981

Cohen MH, Creaven PJ, Fossieck BE et al: Intensive chemotherapy of small cell bronchogenic carcinoma. Cancer Treat Rep 61:349, 1977

Evans WK, Murray N, Feld R et al: Canadian multicenter randomized trial comparing standard and alternating combina-

tion chemotherapy in extensive small cell lung cancer. Proc Am Soc Clin Oncol 5:169, 1986

Goldie JH, Coldman AJ: A mathematical model for relating the drug sensitivity of tumors to their spontaneous mutation rate. Cancer Treat Rep 63:1727, 1979

Goldie JH, Coldman AJ, Gaudauskaus GA: Rationale for the use of alternating noncross resistant chemotherapy. Cancer Treat Rep 66:439, 1982

Higgins GA, Shields TW: Experience of the veterans administration surgical adjuvant group. Prog Cancer Res Ther 11:422, 1979

Idhe DC, Deisseroth AB, Lichter AS et al: Late intensive combined modality therapy followed by autologous bone marrow infusion in extensive stage small cell lung cancer. J Clin Oncol 4:1443, 1986

Linga Berry R: Treatment of small cell carcinoma of the bronchus. Lancet 1:129, 1975

Neuroblastoma

Finklestein JZ, Klemperer MR, Evans A et al: Chemotherapy for metastatic neuroblastoma. Med Pediatr Oncol 6:179, 1979

Green AA, Hayes FA, Hushu HO: Sequential cyclophosphamide and doxorubicin for induction of complete remission in children with disseminate neuroblastoma. Cancer 48(10):2310, 1981

Leikin S, Evans A, Huyn R et al: The impact of chemotherapy on advanced neuroblastoma: Survival of patients diagnosed in 1956, 1962 and 1966–1968 in childrens' cancer study group Am J Pediatr 84:131, 1974

Robinson WA, Mughal T, Thomas MR et al: Treatment of advanced malignant melanoma with subcutaneous recombinant interferon. Proc Am Soc Clin Oncol 5:132, 1986

Carcinoma of the Prostate

Blackard CE, Byar DP, Jordan WP: Orchiectomy for advanced prostatic carcinoma: a re-evaluation. Urology 1:553, 1973

Einhorn L, Donohue JP: Cis-diamminedichloroplastinum vinblastin and bleomycin combination chemotherapy in disseminated testicular cancer. Ann Intern Med 87(3):293, 1977

Einhorn L, Williams ST, Troner M et al: The role of maintenance therapy in disseminated testicular cancer. N Engl J Med 305:727, 1981

Ekman P, Snochowski M, Zetterberg A et al: Steroid receptor content in human prostatic carcinoma in response to endocrine therapy. Cancer 44:1173, 1979

Geller J, Albert J, Yen SSC: Treatment of advanced cancer of prostate with megestrol acetate. Urology 12:537, 1978

Huggins C, Stevens RE, Hodges CV: Studies on prostatic cancer: The effects of castration on advanced carcinoma of the prostate gland. Arch Surg 43:209, 1941

Labrie F, Belanger A, Cusan L et al: Anti-fertility effects of LHRH in the male. J Androl 1:209, 1980

Labrie F, Dupona A, Belanger A et al: New approach in the treatment of prostate cancer: Complete instead of only partial withdrawal of androgens. Prostate 4:579, 1983

Manni A, Santen R, Boucher A et al: Androgen priming and response to chemotherapy in advanced prostate cancer. Proc Am Soc Clin Onc 5:96, 1986

Menon M, Walsh PC: Hormonal therapy for prostatic cancer. In Murphy GP (ed): Prostatic Cancer, p 175. Littleton, MA, PSG Publishing, 1979

Murray N, Coppin C, Murphy K: Mitoxantrone as first line chemotherapy for metastatic prostate cancer: Phase II results. Recent advances in chemotherapy. Proceedings of the 14th International Congress on Chemotherapy, Kyoto, 1985

Peckham MJ, Barrett A, Liew KH et al: The treatment of metastatic germ cell testicular tumors with bleomycin, etoposide and cis-platin (BEP). Br J Cancer 47:613, 1983

Sogani PC, Whitmore WF: Experience with flutamide in previously untreated patients with advanced prostatic cancer. J Urol 122:640, 1979

Torti FM, Carter SK: Chemotherapy of prostate cancer. Ann Intern Med 92:681, 1980

Williams ST, Einhorn LH: Etoposide salvage therapy for refractory germ cell tumors: an update. Cancer Treat Rev [Suppl A] 9:67, 1982

Gastrointestinal Carcinoma

Bitran JT, Desser RK, Kozloff MF et al: Treatment of metastatic pancreatic and gastric adenocarcinomas with 5-fluorouracil, adriamycin and mitomycin C (FAM). Cancer Treat Rep 63:2049, 1979

Chabner D: 5-FU and high dose folinic acid therapy: Biochemical rationale. Presented at the 4th Chemotherapy Foundation Symposium. New York, November, 1986

Clarke JS, Cruze K, El Farra S et al: The natural history and results of surgical therapy for carcinoma of the stomach: An analysis of 250 cases. Am J Surg 102:143, 1961

Douglass H, Lavin PT, Goudsmit A et al: Phase 1–2 evaluation of combinations of methylCCNU, mitomycin C, adriamycin and 5-FU in advanced measurable gastric cancer (est-2277). Proc Am Soc Clin Oncol 2:121, 1983

MacDonald JS, Schein PS, Woolley PV et al: 5-fluorouracil, mitomycin C and adriamycin (FAM): A new combination chemotherapy program for advanced gastric carcinoma. Ann Intern Med 93:533, 1980

Schein PS, Smith FP, Wooley PV et al: Current management of advanced and locally and unresectable gastric carcinoma. Cancer 50:2590, 1982

Shah A, MacDonald W, Gudauskas G, et al: 5-FU infusion in advanced colorectal cancer: A comparison of three dose schedules. Cancer Treat Reports Vol 69, 1985

Renal Cell Carcinoma

Hahn DM, Schimpff SC, Ruckdschel JC et al: Single agent chemotherapy for renal cell carcinoma: CCNU vinblastin, thiotepa or bleomycin. Cancer Treat Rep 61:1585, 1977

Neidhart J, Gagen M, Kisner D et al: Therapy of renal cancer with low (LD) intermediate (ID) and high (HD) dose regimens of human lymphoblastoid interferon (age BLI): Welfaron. Proc Am Soc Clin Oncol 3:60, 1984

Paulson DF, Perez CA, Anderson T: Cancer of the kidney and ureter. In De Vita VT Jr, Hellman S, Rosenberg SA (eds): Cancer: Principles and Practice of Oncology, p 895. Philadelphia, JB Lippincott, 1985

Rosenberg S: Treatment with interleuken II. Presented at the 4th Chemotherapy Foundation Symposium. New York, November, 1986

Rosenberg SA, Lotze AT, Muul LM et al: Alterations on the systemic administration of autologous lymphokine activated killer cells and recombinant interleukin-II to patients with metastatic cancer. N Engl J Med 313:1485, 1985

Melanoma

Robinson WA, Mughal T, Thomas MR et al: Treatment of advanced malignant melanoma with subcutaneous recombinant interferon. Proc Am Soc Clin Oncol 5:132, 1986

Rosenberg S: Treatment with interleuken II. Presented at the 4th Chemotherapy Foundation Symposium. New York, November, 1986

Rosenberg SA, Lotze AT, Muul LM et al: Alterations on the systemic administration of autologous lymphokine activated killer cells and recombinant interleukin-II to patients with metastatic cancer. N Engl J Med 313:1485, 1985

Thyroid Carcinoma

Brennan MF, MacDonald JS: Cancer of the endocrine system. In De Vita VT Jr, Hellman S, Rosenberg SA (eds): Cancer: Principles and Practice of Oncology, p 1179. Philadelphia, JB Lippincott, 1985

Gottlieb JA, Hill CS Jr, Ibanez ML et al: Chemotherapy of thyroid cancer: An evaluation of experience with 37 patients. Cancer 30:848, 1972

Harada T, Nishikawa Y, Suzuki T et al: Bleomycin treatment for cancer of the thyroid. Am J Surg 122:53, 1971

Leight GS, Farrell RE, Wells SA et al: Effect of chemotherapy on calcitonin levels in patients with metastatic medullary thyroid carcinoma. Proc Am Assoc Cancer Res 21:155, 1980

Maxon HR, Thomas SR, Hertzburg VS et al: Relation between effective radiation dose and outcome of radioiodine therapy for thyroid cancer. N Engl J Med 309:937, 1983

Shimaoka K, Schoenfeld DA, Lerner H et al: A randomized trial of adriamycin plus cis-diammine-dichloroplatinum in thyroid carcinoma. Proc Am Soc Clin Oncol 2:168, 1983

Carcinoid

Kelsen DP, Cheng E, Kemeny N: Streptozotocin and adriamycin in the treatment of APUD tumors. Proc Am Assoc Cancer Res 23:433, 1982

Marks C: Carcinoid tumors: A clinical pathological study. Boston, GK Hall, 1979

Mengel CE, Shafer RD: The carcinoid syndrome. In Holland JF, Frei E (eds): Cancer Medicine, p 1584. Philadelphia, Lea & Febiger, 1973

Wick MR, Scott RE, Li CY et al: Carcinoid tumor of the thymus: A clinicopathological report of 7 cases with review of the literature. Mayo Clin Proc 55:246, 1980

Seminoma

Loehrer PJ, Birch R, Williams ST et al: Cis-platin combination chemotherapy in metastatic seminoma: The South Eastern Cancer Study Group Experience. Proc Am Assoc Clin Oncol 5:106, 1986

Sonntag R, Tshopp L, Obrecht P et al: Treatment of metastatic seminoma with chemotherapy. Proc Am Assoc Clin Oncol 4:106, 1985

SINUS AND NASOPHARYNGEAL TUMORS

Batsakis JG: Tumors of the Head and Neck: Clinical and Pathological Considerations, 2nd ed. Baltimore, Williams & Wilkins, 1979

Batsakis JG: Pathology of tumors of the nasal cavity and paranasal sinuses. In Thawley SE, Panje WR (eds): Comprehensive Management of Head and Neck Tumors, Vol 1, p 327. Philadelphia, WB Saunders, 1987

Batsakis JG, Regezi JA, Solomon AR et al: The pathology of head and neck tumors: Mucosal melanomas. Head Neck Surg 4:404, 1982

Batsakis JG, Rice DH, Solomon AR: The pathology of head and neck tumors: Squamous and mucous gland carcinomas of the nasal cavity, paranasal sinuses, and larynx. Head Neck Surg 2:497, 1980

Christensen WN, Smith RRL: Schneiderian papillomas: A clinicopathologic study of 67 cases. Hum Pathol 17:393, 1986

Conley J: Concepts in Head and Neck Surgery, p 55. Grune & Stratton, New York, 1970

Fechner RE, Alford DD: Inverted papilloma and squamous cell carcinoma. Arch Otolaryngol 88:507, 1968

Flores AD, Anderson DW, Doyle PJ et al: Paranasal sinus malignancy: A retrospective analysis of treatment methods. J Otolaryngol 13:141, 1984

Frazell EL, Lewis JS: Cancer of the nasal cavity and accessory sinuses. A report of the management of 416 patients. Cancer 16:1293, 1963

Godtfredsen E, Lederman M: Diagnostic and prognostic roles of ophthalmoneurologic signs and symptoms in malignant nasopharyngeal tumors. Am J Ophthalmol 59:1063, 1965

Henderson JW: Orbital Tumors, 2nd ed. New York, Brian C Decker (Thieme-Stratton), 1980

Johnson LN, Krohel GB, Yeon EB et al: Sinus tumors invading the orbit. Ophthalmology 91:209, 1984

Jones HM: Some orbital complications of nose and throat conditions. J R Soc Medicine 74:409, 1981

Mohan H, Sen DK, Gupta DK: Orbital affection in nasal and paranasal neoplasms. Acta Ophthalmol 47:289, 1969

Moss WT: Radiation therapy for tumors of the nasal cavity and paranasal sinuses. In Thawley SE, Panje WR (eds): Comprehensive Management of Head and Neck Tumors, Vol 1, p 344. Philadelphia, WB Saunders, 1987

Sakai S, Fuchihata H, Hamasaki Y: Treatment policy for maxillary sinus carcinoma. ACTA Otolaryngol 83:171, 1976

Smith JL, Wheliss JA: Ocular manifestations of nasopharyngeal tumors. Trans Am Acad Ophthalmol Otolaryngol 66:659, 1962

Spiro RH, Huvos AG, Strong EW: Adenoid cystic carcinoma of salivary origin: A clinicopathologic study of 242 cases. Am J Surg 128:512, 1974

Spiro RH, Huvos AG, Strong EW: Adenoid cystic carcinoma: Factors influencing survival. Am J Surg 138:579, 1979

Weber AL, Stanton AC: Malignant tumors of the paranasal sinuses: Radiologic, clinical and histopathologic evaluation of 200 cases. Head Neck Surg 6:761, 1984

Weiss JS, Bressler SB, Jacobs EF Jr et al: Maxillary ameloblastoma with orbital invasion: A clinicopathologic study. Ophthalmology 92:710, 1985

LID TUMORS

Basal Cell Carcinoma

Bertelsen K, Gadeberg C: Carcinoma of the eyelid. Acta Radiol [Oncol] 17:58, 1978

Daly NJ, de Lafontan B, Combes PF: Results of the treatment of 165 lid carcinomas by iridium wire implant. Int J Radiat Oncol Biol Phys 10:455, 1984

De Silva SP, Dellon AL: Recurrence rate of positive margin basal cell carcinoma: Results of a five-year prospective study. J Surg Oncol 28:72, 1985

Fitzpatrick PJ, Thompson GA, Easterbrook WM et al: Basal and squamous cell carcinoma of the eyelids and their treatment by radiotherapy. Int J Radiat Oncol Biol Phys 10:449, 1984

Gladstein AH: Efficacy, simplicity, and safety of x-ray therapy of basal-cell carcinomas on periocular skin. J Dermatol Surg Oncol 4:586, 1978

Jakobiec FA, Rootman J, Jones IS: Secondary and metastatic tumors of the orbit. In Jones IS, Jakobiec FA (eds): Disease of the Orbit. Philadelphia, Harper & Row, 1979

Luxemberg M, Guthrie T Jr: Chemotherapy of eyelid and periorbital tumors. Trans Am Ophthalmol Soc 83:162, 1985

McDougall AL, Chaplin AJ, Jones RL: Infiltration of the supraorbital nerve by basal cell carcinoma. Am J Dermatopathol 5:381, 1983

McGregor JC: A study of basal cell carcinoma of the inner canthus, 1967–72. Br J Surg 66:522, 1979

Mehta H: Surgical management of carcinoma of eyelids and periorbital skin. Br J Ophthalmol 63:578, 1979

Mohs FE: Chemosurgery for the microscopically controlled excision of cutaneous cancer. Head Neck Surg Nov/Dec:150, 1978

Nordman EM, Nordman LEO: Treatment of basal cell carcinoma of the eyelid. Acta Ophthalmol 56:349, 1978

Weimar VM, Ceilley RI: Basal-cell carcinoma of a medial canthus with invasion of supraorbital and supratrochlear nerves: Report of a case treated by Mohs' technique. J Dermatol Surg Oncol 5:279, 1979

Squamous Cell Carcinoma

Duke-Elder S, MacFaul PA: The ocular adnexa. In Duke-Elder S (ed): System of Ophthalmology, Vol 8, p 420. London, Henry Kimpton, 1974

Henderson JW: Orbital Tumors, 2nd ed, p 425. New York, Thieme-Stratton, 1980

Reifler DM, Hornblass A: Squamous cell carcinoma of the eyelid. Surv Ophthalmol 30:349, 1986

Trobe JD, Hood CI, Parsons JT et al: Intracranial spread of squamous cell carcinoma along the trigeminal nerve. Arch Ophthalmol 100:608, 1982

Malignant Melanoma of Skin

Clark WH et al: The histogenesis and biologic behavior of primary human malignant melanomas of the skin. Cancer Res 29:705, 1969

Clark WH et al: The developmental biology of malignant melanomas. Semin Oncol 2:83, 1975

Clark WH et al: Current concepts of the biology of human cutaneous malignant melanoma. Adv Cancer Res 24:267, 1977

Clark WH et al: Origin of familial malignant melanomas from heritable melanocytic lesions. Arch Dermatol 114:732, 1978

Elder DE et al: Dysplastic nevus syndrome. Cancer 46:1787, 1980

Elwood JM, Gallagher RP, Hill GB et al: Pigmentation and skin reaction to sun as risk factors for cutanenous melanoma: The Western Canada Melanoma Study. Br Med J 288:99, 1984

Font RL: Eyelids and lacrimal drainage system. In Spencer W: Ophthalmic Pathology, Vol 3, p 2189. Philadelphia, WB Saunders, 1986

Kopf AW et al: Malignant melanoma: A review. J Dermatol Surg Oncol 3:1, 1977

Mihm MC, Lopansri S: A review of the classification of malignant melanoma. J Dermatol 6:131, 1979

Robbins SL, Cotran RS, Kumar V: Pathologic Basis of Disease 3rd ed, p 1279. Philadelphia, WB Saunders, 1984

Sebaceous Carcinoma of the Ocular Adnexa

Aurora A, Blodi F: Lesions of the eyelids: A clinicopathologic study. Surv Ophthalmol 15:94, 1970

Boniuk M, Zimmerman LE: Sebaceous carcinoma of the eyelid, eyebrow, caruncle, and orbit. Trans Am Acad Ophthalmol Otolaryngol 72:619, 1968

Brownstein S, Codere F, Jackson WB: Masquerade syndrome. Ophthalmology 87:259, 1980

Cavanagh HD, Green WR, Goldberg HK: Multicentric sebaceous adenocarcinoma of the meibomian gland. Am J Ophthalmol 77:326, 1974

Doxanas MT, Green WR: Sebaceous gland carcinoma: Review of 40 cases. Arch Ophthalmol 102:245, 1984

Ginsberg J: Present status of meibomian gland carcinoma. Arch Ophthalmol 73:271, 1965

Hendley RL, Rieser JC, Cavanagh HD et al: Primary radiation therapy for meibomian gland carcinoma. Am J Ophthalmol 87:206, 1979

Ni C, Searl SS, Kuo PK et al: Sebaceous cell carcinomas of the ocular adnexa. In Ni C, Albert DM (eds): Tumors of the Eyelid and Orbit: A Chinese-American Collaborative Study, Vol 22, p 23. Boston, Little Brown & Co, 1982

Rao NA, Hidayat AA, McLean IW et al: Sebaceous carcinomas of the ocular adnexa: A clinicopathologic study of 104 cases, with five-year follow-up data. Hum Pathol 13:113, 1982

Rao NA, McLean IW, Zimmerman LE: Sebaceous carcinoma of the eyelids and caruncle: Correlation of clinicopathologic features with prognosis. In Jakobiec FA (ed): Ocular and Adnexal Tumors, p 461. Birmingham, Aesculapius, 1978

Rulon DB, Helwig EB: Cutaneous sebaceous neoplasms. Cancer 33:82, 1974

Shields JA, Bakewell B, Augsburger JJ et al: Classification and incidence of space-occupying lesions of the orbit: A survey of 645 biopsies. Arch Ophthalmol 102:1606, 1984

Tenzel RR, Stewart WB, Boynton JR et al: Sebaceous adenocarcinoma of the eyelid: Definition of surgical margins. Arch Ophthalmol 95:2203, 1977

Wagoner MD, Beyer CK, Gonder JR et al: Common presentations of sebaceous gland carcinoma of the eyelid. Ann Ophthalmol 14:159, 1982

Other Adnexal Carcinomas

Font RA: Eyelids and lacrimal drainage system. In Spencer WH: Ophthalmic Pathology, Vol 3, p 2214. Philadelphia, WB Saunders, 1986

Khalil M, Brownstein S, Codere F et al: Eccrine sweat gland carcinoma of the eyelid with orbital involvement. Arch Ophthalmol 98:2210, 1980

Ni C, Kuo PK, Dryja TP et al: Sweat gland tumors in the eyelids: A clinicopathological analysis of 55 cases. In Ni C, Albert DM (eds): Tumors of the Eyelid and Orbit: A Chinese-American Collaborative Study. Boston, Little, Brown & Co, 1982

SQUAMOUS CARCINOMA OF THE CONJUNCTIVA

Blodi FC: Squamous cell carcinoma of the conjunctiva. Doc Ophthalmol 34:93, 1973

Brownstein S: Mucoepidermoid carcinoma of the conjunctiva with intraocular invasion. Ophthalmology 8:1126, 1981

Cohen BH, Green R, Iliff NT et al: Spindle cell carcinoma of the conjunctiva. Arch Ophthalmol 98:1809, 1980

Gamel JW, Eiferman RA, Guibor P: Mucoepidermoid carcinoma of the conjunctiva. Arch Ophthalmol 102:730, 1984

Gelender H, Forster Rk: Papanicolaou cytology in the diagnosis and management of external ocular tumors. Arch Ophthalmol 98:909, 1980

Illif WJ, Marback R, Green W: Invasive squamous cell carcinoma of the conjunctiva. Arch Ophthalmol 93:119, 1975

Li WW, Pettit TA, Zakka KA: Intraocular invasion by papillary squamous cell carcinoma of the conjunctiva. Am J Ophthalmol 90:697, 1980

Milik MOA, Sheikh EH el: Tumors of the eye and adnexa in the Sudan. Cancer 44:293, 1979

Nicholson DH, Herschler J: Intraocular extension of squamous cell carcinoma of the conjunctiva. Arch Ophthalmol 95:845, 1977

Patipa M, Hull DS: Chronic unilateral conjunctivitis: Consider malignancy. Am Fam Physician 22(i):69, 1980

Pizzarello LD, Jakobiec FA: Bowen's disease of the conjunctiva a misnomer. In Jakobiec FA (ed): Ocular and Adnexal Tumors. Birmingham, Aesculapius, 1981

Rao NA, Font RL: Mucoepidermoid carcinoma of the conjunctiva. Cancer 38:1699, 1976

Rasteiro A, Cunha-Vaz JG: Squamous cell carcinoma of the limbus with intraocular invasion. Ophthalmologica 173:332, 1976

Rootman J, Roth A, Crawford JB et al: Extensive squamous cell carcinoma of the conjunctiva presenting as orbital cellulitis. Can J Ophthalmol (accepted for publication, 1987)

Searl SS, Krigstein JH, Albert DM et al: Invasive squamous cell carcinoma with intraocular mucoepidermoid features: Conjunctiva carcinoma with intraocular invasion and diphasic morphology. Arch Ophthalmol 100:109, 1982

Zimmerman LE: Squamous cell carcinoma and related lesions of the bulbar conjunctiva. In Boniuk M: Ocular and Adnexal

Tumors: New and Controversial Aspects, p 49. St Louis, CV Mosby, 1964

Zimmerman LE: The cancerous, precancerous and pseudocancerous lesions of the lid and conjunctiva. In Rycroft PV (ed): Plastic Surgery: Proceedings of the Second International Corneo-Plastic Conference, p 54. England, Pergamon Press, 1969

MALIGNANT MELANOMA OF THE CONJUNCTIVA

Bernardina VB, Naidoff M, Clark WH: Melanomas of the conjunctiva. Am J Ophthalmol 82:383, 1976

Crawford JB: Conjunctiva melanomas: Prognostic factors. A review and analysis of a series. Trans Am Ophthalmol Soc 78:476, 1980

Folberg R, McLean WI, Zimmerman LE: Malignant melanoma of the conjunctiva. Hum Pathol 16:136, 1985

Folberg R, McLean IW, Zimmerman LE: Primary acquired melanosis of the conjunctiva. Hum Pathol 16:129, 1985

Jakobiec FA: Conjunctival melanoma: Unfinished business. Arch Ophthalmol 98:1378, 1980

Jakobiec FA, Brownstein S, Albert W et al: The role of cryotherapy in the management of conjunctival melanoma. Ophthalmology 89:502, 1982

Jakobiec FA, Rootman J, Jones IS: Secondary and metastatic tumors of the orbit. In Duane TD: Clinical Ophthalmology, Vol 2, p 15. Philadelphia, Harper & Row, 1976

Jay B: Naevi and melanomata of the conjunctiva. Br J Ophthalmol 49:169, 1964

Lederman M, Wybar K, Busby E: Malignant epibulbar melanoma: Natural history and treatment by radiotherapy. Br J Ophthalmol 68:605, 1984

Lewis PM, Zimmerman LE: Delayed recurrence of malignant melanomas of the bulbar conjunctiva. Am J Ophthalmol 45:536, 1958

Liesegang TJ, Campbell J: Mayo Clinic experience with conjunctival melanomas. Arch Ophthalmol 98:1385, 1980

Manschot WA: Melanotic lesions of the conjunctiva. Mod Prob Ophthalmol 14:344, 1975

Reese AB: Precancerous melanoma and diffuse malignant melanoma of the conjunctiva. Arch Ophthalmol 19:354, 1938

Rodriguez-Sains RS: Ocular findings in patients with dysplastic nevus syndrome. Ophthalmology 93:661, 1986

Shields JA, Shields CL, Augsburger JJ: Current options in the management of conjunctival melanomas. Orbit 6:25, 1986

Spencer WH, Zimmerman LE: Conjunctiva. In Spencer WH: Ophthalmic Pathology: An Atlas and Textbook, 3rd ed, Vol 1, p 109. Philadelphia, WB Saunders, 1985

Zimmerman LE: The histogenesis of conjunctiva melanomas. In Jakobiec FA (ed): Ocular and Adnexal Tumors, p 572. Birmingham, Aesculapius, 1978

EXTRASCLERAL AND ORBITAL EXTENSION OF UVEAL MELANOMA

Affeldt JC, Minckler DS, Azen SP et al: Prognosis in uveal melanoma with extrascleral extension. Arch Ophthalmol 98:1975, 1980

Callender GR, Wilder HC, Ash JE: Five hundred melanomas of the choroid and ciliary body followed five years or longer. Am J Ophthalmol 25:962, 1942

Chisholm JF Jr: A long term follow-up on malignant melanomas of the choroid based on the Terry and Johns series. Am J Ophthalmol 36:61, 1953

Dunphy EB, Forrest AW, Leopold IH et al: The diagnosis and management of intraocular melanomas: A symposium. Trans Am Acad Ophthalmol Otolaryngol 62:517, 1958

Henderson JW: Orbital Tumors, p 335. Philadelphia, WB Saunders, 1973

Jensen OA: Malignant melanomas of the uvea in Denmark 1943–1952: A clinical, histopathological and prognostic study. Acta Ophthalmol, Suppl 75, 1963

Kersten RC, Blodi FC: Prognosis of choroidal melanomas. Ophthalmic Forum 1:21, 1983

Kersten RC, Tse DT, Anderson RL et al: The role of orbital exenteration in choroidal melanoma with extrascleral extension. Ophthalmology 92:436, 1985

McLean IW, Foster WD, Zimmerman LE: Prognostic factors in small malignant melanomas of choroid and ciliary body. Arch Ophthalmol 95:48, 1977

Paul EV, Parnell BL, Fraker M: Prognosis of malignant melanomas of the choroid and ciliary body. Int Ophthalmol Clin 2:387, 1962

Raivio I: Uveal melanoma in Finland: An epidemiological, clinical, histological and prognostic study. Acta Ophthalmol [Suppl] 133:40, 1977

Rendahl I: Does exenteratio orbitae improve the prognosis in orbital tumor? Acta Ophthalmol 32:431, 1954

Shammas HF, Blodi FC: Orbital extension of choroidal and ciliary body melanomas. Arch Ophthalmol 95:2002, 1975

Shammas HF, Blodi FC: Prognostic factors in choroidal and ciliary body melanomas. Arch Ophthalmol 95:63, 1977

Shields JA: Approaches to the management of choroidal melanoma. In Jakobiec FA (ed): Ocular and Adnexal Tumors, p 4. Birmingham, Aesculapius, 1978

Shields JA, Augsburger JJ, Corwin S et al: The management of uveal melanomas with extrascleral extension. Orbit 5:31, 1986

Shields JA, Augsburger JJ, Donoso LA et al: Hepatic metastasis and orbital recurrence of uveal melanoma after 42 years. Am J Ophthalmol 100:666, 1985

Starr HJ, Zimmerman LE: Extrascleral extension and orbital recurrence of malignant melanomas of the choroid and ciliary body. Int Ophthalmol Clin 2:369, 1962

Warren RM: Prognosis of malignant melanomas of the choroid and ciliary body. In Blodi FC (ed): Current Concepts in Ophthalmology, Vol 4, p 158. St Louis, CV Mosby, 1974

ORBITAL EXTENSION OF RETINOBLASTOMA

Brown DH: The clinicopathology of retinoblastoma. Am J Ophthalmol 61:508, 1966

Carbajal UM: Metastasis in retinoblastoma. Am J Ophthalmol 48:47, 1959

Devesa SS: The incidence of retinoblastoma. Am J Ophthalmol 80:263, 1975

Duke-Elder S: Diseases of the Retina, Vol X. System of Ophthalmology, p 672. London, Henry Kimpton, 1967

Ellsworth RM: The practical management of retinoblastoma. Trans Am Ophthalmol Soc 67:462, 1969

Ellsworth R: Orbital retinoblastoma. Trans Am Ophthalmol Soc 72:79, 1974

Francois J, Matton-van Leuwen MT: Recent data on the heredity of retinoblastoma. In Boniuk M: Ocular and Adnexal Tumours, New and Controversial Aspects, p 123. St Louis, CV Mosby, 1964

Fraser GR, Friedman AI: The causes of blindness in children. Baltimore, John Hopkins Press, 1967

Goldberg L: Management of retinoblastoma in patients presenting with orbital involvement. 2nd International Symposium on Retinoblastoma, 1982

Kodilinye HC: Retinoblastoma in Nigeria: Problems of treatment. Am J Ophthalmol 63:469, 1967

Merriam GR: Retinoblastoma. Analysis of seventeen autopsies. Arch Ophthalmol 44:71, 1950

Miller RW: Fifty-two forms of childhood cancer: US mortality experience 1960–66. J Pediatr 75:685, 1969

Perez C et al: Phase II sequential chemotherapy treatment in advanced retinoblastoma. 2nd International Symposium on Retinoblastoma, 1982

Redler LD, Ellsworth RM: Prognostic importance of choroidal invasion in retinoblastoma. Arch Ophthalmol 90:294, 1973

Reed M, Culham J: Skeletal metastases from retinoblastoma. J Cancer Assoc Radiol 26:249, 1975

Reese AB: Extension of retinoblastoma in the optic nerve. Arch Ophthalmol 5:269, 1931

Reese AB: Invasion of the optic nerve by retinoblastoma. Arch Ophthalmol 40:553, 1948

Reese AB: Tumors of the Eye, 3rd ed, p 89. New York, Harper & Row, 1976

Rootman J, Carruthers JDA, Miller RR: Retinoblastoma: An overview. Perspect Pediatr Pathol Vol 10, 1986

Rootman J, Ellsworth R, Hofbauer J et al: Orbital extension of retinoblastoma: A clinicopathologic study. Can J Ophthalmol 13:72, 1978

Rootman J, Hofbauer J, Ellsworth R: Invasion of the optic nerve by retinoblastoma. Can J Ophthalmol 11:106, 1976

Stannard C, Lipper S, Sealy R et al: Retinoblastoma correlation of invasion of the optic nerve and choroid with prognosis and metastasis. Br J Ophthalmol 63:560, 1979

Stannard CE, Sealy R, Sevel D et al: Treatment of malignant meningitis in retinoblastoma. Br J Ophthalmol 59:362, 1969

Tarkkanen A, Tuovinen E: Retinoblastoma in Finland, 1912–64. Acta Ophthalmol 49:293, 1971

Zimmerman LE: The registry of ophthalmic pathology: Past, present and future. Trans Ophthalmol Otolaryngol 65:88, 1961

NEUROEPITHELIAL TUMORS OF THE CILIARY BODY

Apple DJ, Rabb MF: Ocular Pathology: Clinical Applications and Self-Assessment, 3rd ed. St Louis, CV Mosby, 1985

Broughton WL, Zimmerman LE: A clinicopathologic study of 56 cases of intraocular medulloepitheliomas. Am J Ophthalmol 85:407, 1978

Green WR: Retina. In Spencer WH: Ophthalmic Pathology: An Atlas and Textbook, 3rd ed, Vol 2, p 589. Philadelphia, WB Saunders, 1985

Henderson JW: Orbital Tumors, 2nd ed. New York, Brian C Decker, 1980

Jakobiec FA, Jones IS: Diseases of the Orbit. Philadelphia, Harper & Row, 1979

Zimmerman LE: Verhoeff's "terato-neuroma": A critical reappraisal in light of new observations and current concepts of embryonic tumors. Am J Ophthalmol 72:1039, 1971

EXTENSION FROM THE LACRIMAL SAC

Ashton N, Choyce DP, Fison LG: Carcinoma of lacrimal sac. Br J Ophthalmol 35:366, 1951

Flanagan JC, Stokes DDP: Lacrimal sac tumors. Ophthalmology 85:1282, 1978

Font R: Lacrimal drainage system. In Spencer WH: Ophthalmic Pathology: An Atlas and Textbook, p 2317. Philadelphia, WB Saunders, 1985

Harry J, Ashton N: The pathology of tumours of the lacrimal sac. Trans Ophthalmol Soc UK 88:19, 1968

Hornblass A, Jakobiec FA, Bosniak S et al: The diagnosis and management of epithelial tumors of the lacrimal sac. Ophthalmology 87:476, 1980

Jones IS: Tumors of the lacrimal sac. Am J Ophthalmol 42:561, 1956

Jones IS, Jakobiec FA, Rootman J: Secondary and metastatic tumors of the orbit. In Jones IS, Jakobiec FA: Diseases of the Orbit, p 503. Philadelphia, Harper & Row, 1979

Lloyd WC III, Leone CR Jr: Malignant melanoma of the lacrimal sac. Arch Ophthalmol 102:104, 1984

Milder B, Smiith ME: Carcinoma of lacrimal sac. Am J Ophthalmol 65:782, 1968

Ryan SJ, Font RL: Primary epithelial neoplasms of the lacrimal sac. Am J Ophthalmol 76:73, 1973

CHAPTER 13

Structural Lesions

Jack Rootman and Jocelyn S. Lapointe

■ CONGENITAL LESIONS

Cystic

DERMOID CYSTS

Dermoid cysts of the orbital and periorbital region present in a variety of ways depending upon the suture of origin, size, and rate of growth. They are developmental choristomas composing 3% to 9% of all orbital masses with an average of 4.7% in pooled series. Our series included 27 dermoids (15 superficial and 12 deep) constituting about 6% of orbital tumors and 2% of all orbital conditions. In the head and neck region, they are thought to arise from ectodermal rests pinched off at suture lines. About 10% of head and neck dermoids are orbital and in most series the upper outer quadrant dominates, but they may occur virtually anywhere within and adjacent to the orbit. They typically exert mass effect by expanding slowly and displacing adjacent structures without infiltration.

Clinically, dermoids can be divided into two groups as suggested by Grove: superficial (simple) and deep (complicated). The presentation, progression, complications, and management are related to the type of dermoid.

Superficial Dermoids

Superficial dermoids usually present in infancy as localized rounded periorbital masses, often situated temporally and less frequently medially (Fig. 13-1). In our series the site of origin was frontozygomatic suture in nine, frontolacrimal suture in four, and the deep temporalis fossa in two. They are characteristically painless, firm, and immobile and cause little ocular or lid displacement. On palpation, the posterior edge does not extend around the bony margin into the deep orbit. They are generally 1 to 2 cm in size and nonfluctuant.

On CT scan they are rounded, clearly defined masses frequently containing a lucent center suggestive of fat

(Fig. 13-2). They are usually not associated with significant bony defect other than a focal minor indentation. They are easily managed by direct excision (Fig. 13-3) of the intact dermoid including its base. In our experience these have been histologically typical dermoid cysts, usually with intact walls lined by keratinized squamous epithelium (Fig. 13-4). Occasionally, however, focal areas of granulomatous inflammation line the wall of the cyst at sites of previous rupture. We usually remove superficial dermoids between the first and fifth years of life to avoid traumatic rupture.

Deep Dermoids

Deep or complicated orbital dermoids present as slow-growing masses later in life, frequently noted in retrospect to have been present for many years. They can arise from virtually any suture site medially, laterally, or even from the apical portion of the orbit. The suture of origin in the deep dermoids seen in our clinic was frontozygomatic in five, ethmoid in three, adjacent to the superior orbital fissure in two, and undetermined in two extensive ones. The palpable portion, when present, typically consists of a rounded anterior margin with extension of the mass deep into the orbit. Unless they have been previously incised, they rarely cause entrapment of adjacent structures, and thus are dominated clinically by mass effect alone. We had one patient with a dumbbell dermoid of the frontozygomatic suture presenting as a chronic, draining, focally inflamed fistula secondary to partial excision (Fig. 13-5). In our experience with patients referred to our clinic, the extent and complexity of deeper dermoids were frequently underestimated, especially when the anterior margin was palpable superficially (Fig. 13-6). When large, they may cause visual or oculomotor disturbances.

Careful investigation is important to distinguish deep from superficial lesions, because deep dermoids may extend beyond the orbit into the temporalis fossa or even intracranially. On CT scan, deep orbital dermoids have a constellation of findings that together may permit a spe-

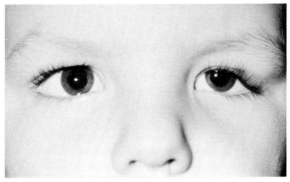

A

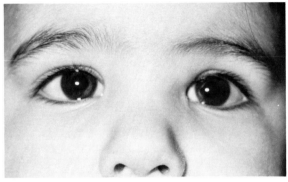

B

FIGURE 13-1. *(A)* A 2½-year-old boy with a left superotemporal superficial dermoid arising from the frontozygomatic suture. *(B)* A 14-month-old boy with a firm, rounded, superficial dermoid in the superomedial lid which was attached to a frontolacrimal suture line. (Sherman RP, Rootman J, Lapointe JS: Orbital dermoids: Clinical presentation and management. Br J Ophthalmol 68:642, 1981)

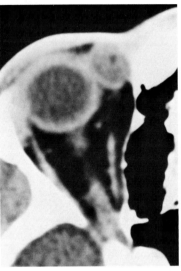

FIGURE 13-2. An axial CT scan of an anterior medial superficial dermoid showing a well-defined capsule and contents of lower density. Note the small area of fat density in the center of the lesion.

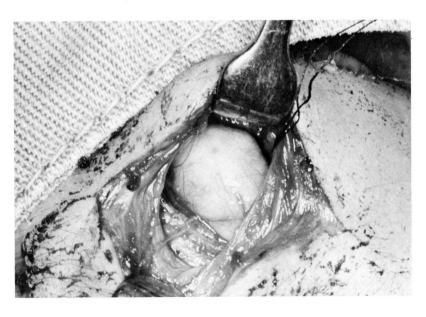

FIGURE 13-3. Surgical appearance of the dermoid shown in Figure 13-1A. Note the smooth contour and pale color. (Sherman RP, Rootman J, Lapointe JS: Orbital dermoids: Clinical presentation and management. Br J Ophthalmol 68:642, 1981)

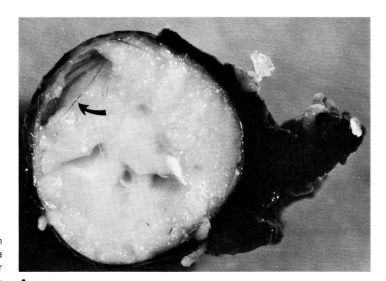

A

FIGURE 13-4. *(A)* Gross photograph of the dermoid in Figure 13-3 showing a thin wall, keratin and lipid debris, and hair *(arrow)*. *(B)* Cyst wall showing keratinized lining, abortive sebaceous structures, and hair (H&E, original magnification × 10). (Sherman RP, Rootman J, Lapointe JS: Orbital dermoids: Clinical presentation and management. Br J Ophthalmol 68:642, 1981)

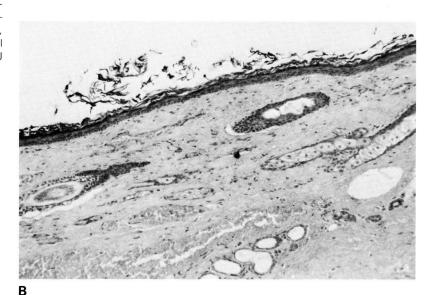

B

cific diagnosis. Characteristically, dermoids have relatively well-defined margins. The central portion of most lesions is intermediate in density between fat and muscle (Fig. 13-7). Variation in density may occur within the lesion (Fig. 13-8), but actually only a minority of lesions contain low-density areas that give CT attenuation values equivalent to pure fat. When present, however, this finding is virtually pathognomonic. A few lesions have the same density as muscle, in which case the appearance is much less specific. Calcification, particularly in the rim of the lesion, is frequent in the giant dermoids. This is a useful sign, because most soft tissue masses of the orbit

(other than some mucoceles) do not have rim calcification (Fig. 13-9). The most useful CT finding is that of bony change. Focal or generalized enlargement of the orbit with erosion into the sinuses or the cranial cavity may occur. Almost invariably there is evidence of a break or full-thickness defect of the orbital bony wall, which most characteristically has irregular or notched borders (Fig. 13-10).

Lateral dermoids arising from the frontozygomatic suture may be difficult to differentiate from solid, malignant, and erosive lacrimal gland lesions. An important distinguishing feature is that bony change tends to in-

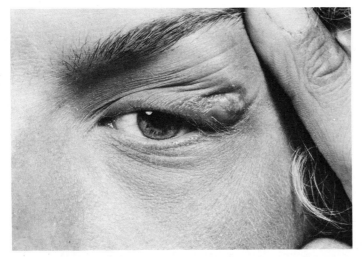

A

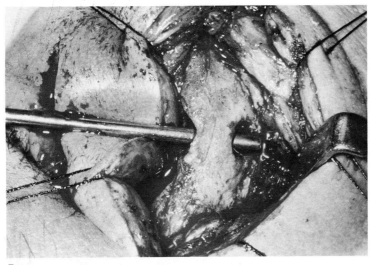

B

FIGURE 13-5. *(A)* Left eye of a 21-year-old patient showing a mass and a draining fistula in the superolateral aspect of the lid. *(B)* Photograph taken at surgery of the same patient. Suction tip extends through a defect in the frontozygomatic suture into the temporalis fossa where the outer portion of a dumbbell dermoid lay. (Sherman RP, Rootman J, Lapointe JS: Orbital dermoids: Clinical presentation and management. Br J Ophthalmol 68:642, 1981)

clude or extend only to the frontozygomatic suture in dermoids, whereas lacrimal tumors will produce bony changes extending beyond the suture (Fig. 13-11). In addition, the rounded, well-defined margins and relatively lucent, central areas typical of dermoids are not seen with malignant lacrimal masses. Ultrasonography may identify dermoids as cystic, but when they contain much debris (including keratin and fat) they may have internal echoes suggestive of a solid tumor. In addition, deeper orbital lesions may be more difficult to characterize with ultrasonography.

The location, relationship to bone, and cystic nature help to diagnose dermoids. The differential diagnosis depends on the location of the mass. In the lacrimal fossa, primary and secondary lacrimal tumors should be considered, especially if there is evidence of bony erosion or calcification. Medially, retention cysts or mucoceles can be distinguished by their relationship to the sinuses, evidence of focal destruction of bones, and the associated opacification and expansion of the affected sinuses. We have encountered two cases of orbitofrontal dermoids and two mucoceles in this location that had similar radiographic features. The clue to the diagnosis of the mucoceles was the presence of an old fracture site in the lateral portion of the frontal sinus that led to obstruction and formation of the mucocele, which ultimately eroded into

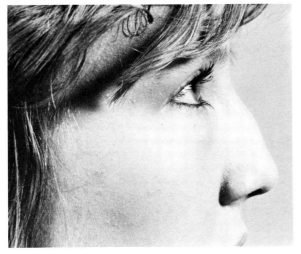

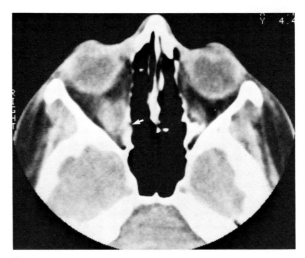

A   **B**

FIGURE 13-6. *(A)* This 17-year-old girl presented with a thickened right lower lid and elevated globe due to an inferior deep orbital dermoid that had been excised, but had recurred repeatedly prior to referral. *(B)* CT scan of the same patient showing the posterior aspect of the orbital mass, which was immediately inferior to the optic nerve and abutting the medial orbital wall. Note dehiscence in the posterior medial wall *(arrow)*. This was the site of origin noted at the time of excision of the dermoid cyst. (Sherman RP, Rootman J, Lapointe JS: Orbital dermoids: Clinical presentation and management. Br J Ophthalmol 68:642, 1981)

FIGURE 13-7. A massive, deep orbital dermoid in a 72-year-old man. It had been partially excised 35 years earlier. Note the central lucency due to fat within the lesion. At surgery, it was found to be attached to the bone adjacent to the superior orbital fissure.

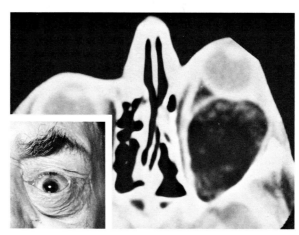

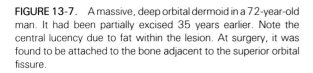

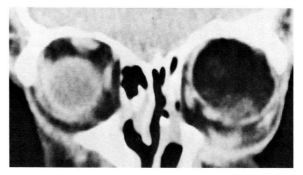

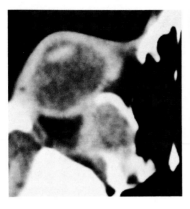
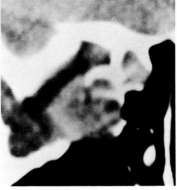

FIGURE 13-8. Axial and coronal CT scans of a patient who was referred with a recurrent incompletely excised deep orbital dermoid attached to the medial wall. Note variable density and calcific exostoses.

the orbit. An encephalocele may occur medially, in which case a focal defect continuous with the cranial cavity may be noted, generally at the base of the nose; however, it may be difficult to distinguish between encephalocele and dermoid in some cases. Injection of a nonionic water-soluble contrast medium into the lesion, or withdrawal and analysis for evidence of cerebrospinal fluid may help distinguish an encephalocele from other cystic lesions involving the orbit, sinuses, and intracranial cavity. Any of the solid tumors of the orbit should be included in the differential diagnosis, especially if there is a focal bony defect.

The treatment of deep dermoids can be complicated owing to size, location, and involvement of orbital structures, and should not be undertaken by the inexperienced orbital surgeon. They operative approach should be based on thorough preoperative assessment of size, location, extent, and relationship to adjacent structures. In principle, the base of the dermoid is believed to be the active growth center, but total removal of the lining is mandatory to prevent recurrence or fistulization. We attempt to dissect completely the orbital side of the lesion

while it is firm before evacuating it, because the dissection planes are more clearly defined when it is intact. Because of the large size of these lesions, evacuation followed by microdissection of the remaining lining is frequently necessary. The deep lesions may extend intracranially and require anterior, lateral, or combined orbitotomy for total extirpation. As long as the complete lining and contents of the dermoid are removed, intraoperative rupture does not appear to lead to early or late postoperative morbidity. Once the lining of the cyst is removed, the adjacent bone can be smoothed out using a diamond drill to remove any crevices or exostoses, which are common in dermoids. Rarely, lesions extending apically to the intracranial cavity may be impossible to remove completely because of the potential to produce serious functional deficits. Some practitioners have advocated marsupialization in these circumstances, but this may be dangerous because of the potential for infection. We would not recommend it. In one such case, the incomplete removal with total evacuation has allowed considerable intervals between procedures (20 years) with preservation of ocular function. The best management

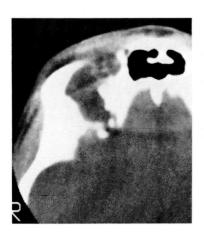
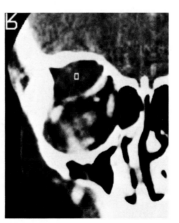

FIGURE 13-9. Axial and coronal CT scans of a deep dermoid in the orbital roof showing irregular excavation of bone, a lucent center, and rim calcification of the capsule (right).

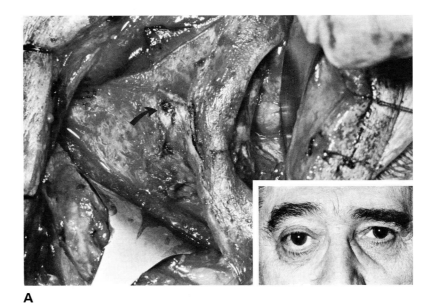

A

FIGURE 13-10. *(A)* A 56-year-old man with a long-standing history of progressive proptosis and downward displacement of his right eye due to an extensive deep orbital dermoid. The surgical photograph shows the dermoid in the lateral orbit eroding through the bony wall *(arrow)*. *(B)* Axial and coronal views of the dermoid show erosion of the superior, lateral, and posterolateral walls of the orbit. Note low-density areas due to the presence of fat as well as irregular calcification and exostosis associated with the dermoid.

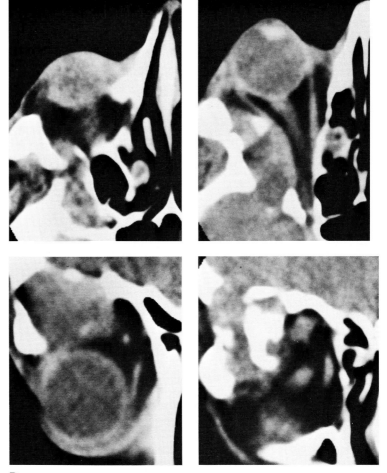

B

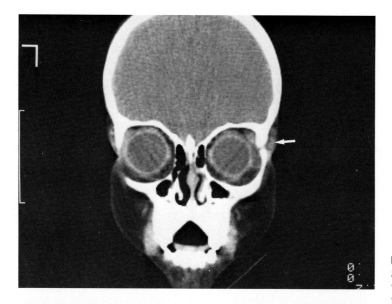

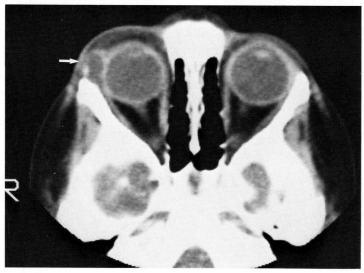

FIGURE 13-11. Coronal *(top)* and axial *(bottom)* CT scans of a dermoid extending through the frontozygomatic suture into the temporalis fossa *(top, arrow)*. Note the low-density central area due to fat as well as focal calcification of the capsule *(bottom, arrow)*.

remains total removal, and all attempts should be directed to achieve it. Ruptured dermoid cysts that erode adjacent bone produce a characteristic yellowish discoloration of the bone.

Pathologically, giant dermoids almost universally have evidence of rupture with a granulomatous foreign body reaction. In fact, the entire lining of the cyst may be a granulomatous infiltrate with evidence of retained fat, cholesterol clefts, old hemorrhage, and hairs. (Fig. 13-12). Calcification may also be noted within the large dermoid cysts. (Fig. 13-13). Elsewhere, the lining may consist of typical keratinizing squamous epithelium with adnexal structures, which are sometimes extensive (Fig. 13-14). It is of interest that in spite of histologic evidence

of previous rupture, very few of our patients presented with a history of acute orbital inflammatory signs and symptoms. The single patient with a fistula had a chronic, low-grade, localized inflammatory reaction.

LACRIMAL CYSTS

Cysts of the lacrimal gland may occur rarely as a congenital anomaly. More usually they are seen as a lesion of the adult. When seen in the infant, they arise within the orbital lobe and can attain significant size, in contrast to acquired ductal cysts, which are usually smaller and in the palpebral lobe. The more common acquired lacrimal cyst will be discussed later in the chapter.

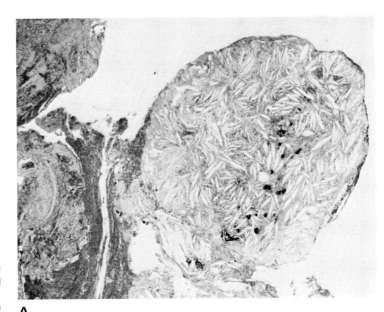

FIGURE 13-12. *(A)* A nodule of tissue from the wall of a deep dermoid containing cholesterol clefts surrounded by foreign body reaction (H&E, original magnification × 2.5). *(B)* Histology of the wall of a deep dermoid showing hair *(arrow)* surrounded by scar and inflammatory reaction (H&E, original magnification × 10). (Sherman RP, Rootman J, Lapointe JS: Orbital dermoids: Clinical presentation and management. Br J Ophthalmol 68:642, 1981)

A

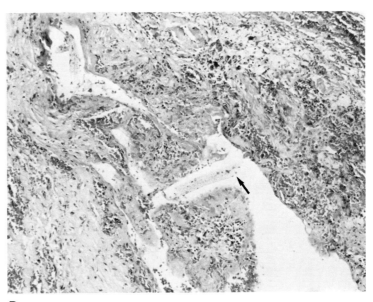

B

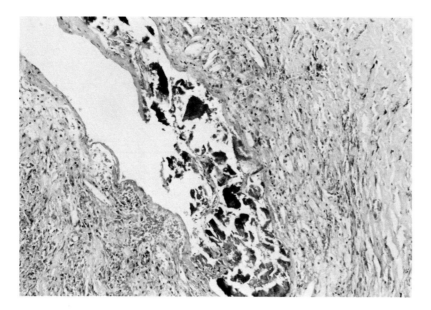

FIGURE 13-13. Histology of part of the wall of a deep dermoid cyst showing calcification surrounded by scar and many lipid-laden macrophages (H&E, original magnification × 10). (Sherman RP, Rootman J, Lapointe JS: Orbital dermoids: Clinical presentation and management. Br J Ophthalmol 68:642, 1981)

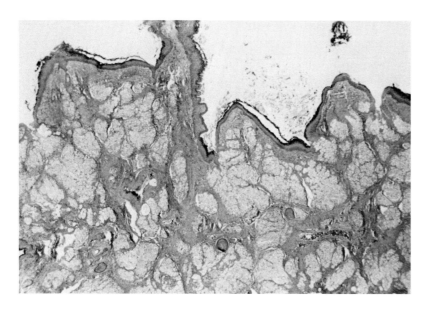

FIGURE 13-14. Wall of a giant dermoid cyst showing many sebaceous adnexal structures and keratinized epithelium (H&E, original magnification × 2.5). (Sherman RP, Rootman J, Lapointe JS: Orbital dermoids: Clinical presentation and management. Br J Ophthalmol 68:642, 1981)

MICROPHTHALMOS WITH CYST AND CONGENITAL CYSTIC EYE

Failure of the fetal fissure to close and proliferation of the neuroepithelium through the opening may lead to formation of an orbital cyst. The size of the resultant cyst varies from a minor histologic finding to massive involvement of the orbit. Large cysts extend inferiorly to involve the lower lid and orbit. They appear as blue-gray, transilluminating lesions (Fig. 13-15). Typically, the associated eye is deformed, microphthalmic, and displaced upward appearing as a small nubbin of tissue on the surface of the cyst. Microphthalmos with cyst may occur bilaterally.

Microphthalmos with cyst occurs at the fourth week of embryonic life. In contrast, congenital cystic eye develops earlier because of arrested development of the primary optic vesicle. This cyst may also be large but usually involves the upper rather than the lower lid. It has no visible associated ocular structures, instead, the orbit is filled with cystic and solid tissue consisting of abnormal, dysplastic neuroepithelium. We have seen a severe case of microphthalmos with cyst in which the eye was completely disrupted and the orbit filled with a large, partially cystic structure that appeared as a massive swelling of the upper lid. It was associated with a severe developmental anomaly of the ipsilateral brain (Fig. 13-16).

These congenital cystic lesions of the orbit should be differentiated from teratomas, which are usually more rapid in development, associated with a normal appearing but protruding eye, and of a denser hue. In addition, they should be distinguished from orbital cephalocele. Management of large lesions is surgical excision of the cyst, globe, and abnormal neuroepithelial structures.

ORBITAL CEPHALOCELE

Cranial orbital cephaloceles are rare, and result from failure of separation of the surface ectoderm and neuroectoderm leading to a dehiscence in bone and protrusion of either a dural (meningocele) or an encephalic (encephalocele, meningoencephalocele) cyst. They usually present as congenital lesions but, particularly when in the deep orbit, may appear later in life. They are frequently associated with other congenital facial anomalies. Characteristically, the midline structures are involved. Those that occur anteriorly usually affect the base of the nose, causing hypertelorism and a superomedial mass that either displaces the globe downward and outward or extends anteriorly toward the brow. Deeper orbital cephaloceles may be occult and result in proptosis with or without ocular dysfunction. Those that are visible may be fluctuant, transilluminate, pulsate, and change in size with Valsalva maneuver.

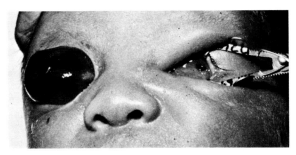

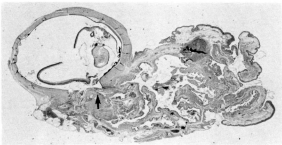

FIGURE 13-15. *(Top)* An infant born with a massive cyst on the right and a microphthalmic eye on the left. *(Bottom)* Low-power histologic view of the right microphthalmic eye attached to the extensive neuroepithelial-lined cyst. Note coloboma in the deformed globe inferiorly *(arrow)*.

The importance of recognizing these cysts is to plan appropriate management rather than have an accidental surgical encounter. On investigation, there may be evidence of a variable sized bony dehiscence suggesting the presence of a cephalocele. If an undiagnosed cyst is encountered at surgery, and a cephalocele suspected, aspiration of the contents will yield CSF. Management, when the defect is small, consists of excision, closure, and ligation of the base with patching of the bony defect from the orbital side. When large, a transfrontal craniotomy with excision, patching, and closure is necessary.

RETENTION AND ADNEXAL CYSTS

Cysts originating from accessory lacrimal, adnexal, and epithelial structures may occur in the anterior orbit. More usually they arise from scarring and implantation secondary to trauma or inflammation. They can, however, appear independent of predisposing cause and are presumably ectopias in this situation. We have encountered two of these in the deep lid, and both were lined by double layers of epithelium and filled with a serous fluid. They also occur deep to the conjunctiva and extend into the orbit and may be lined by ductal, sweat gland, sebaceous, or conjunctival epithelium. Usually they are mo-

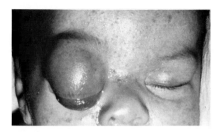

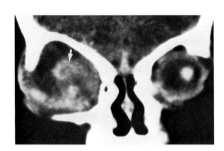

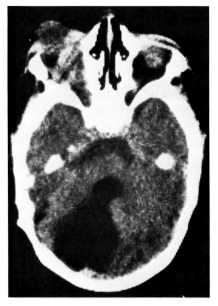

FIGURE 13-16. An infant born with a large multilocular cystic and solid lesion of the orbit and upper lid. It was associated with a partial absence of the right cerebral hemisphere. (Wilson RD, Traverse L, Hall JG et al: Oculocerebrocutaneous syndrome. Published with permission from The American Journal of Ophthalmology 99: 142–148, copyright 1985 by The Ophthalmic Publishing Company)

bile, and transilluminate; they may or may not be fluctuant. Management consists of microdissection and excision or marsupialization.

RATHKE POUCH CYST

We have seen a single unusual case of massive cystic destruction of the base of the skull, including the maxillary sinus, which presented with upward and axial displacement of the globe (Fig. 13-17A). On CT scan there was a large, apparently destructive, lesion, which led to a presumptive clinical and radiologic diagnosis of a sarcoma (Fig. 13-17B). At the time of planned biopsy through the nose, a huge gush of fluid was obtained with decompression of the orbit (Fig. 13-17C). The lining of the cyst was histologically consistent with a Rathke pouch cyst, accounting for the lesion at the base of the skull. Following drainage there has been no recurrence with a 5-year follow up.

ISOLATED MUSCLE CYST

Another unusual cystic lesion we have seen involved the lateral rectus muscle. It appeared clinically as a bluish discoloration of the lateral conjunctiva associated with proptosis and inward displacement of the globe. The clinical diagnosis was consistent with a cyst or a lateral orbital varix in spite of the fact that the patient did not show evidence of expansion during a Valsalva maneuver and venography was negative. The cyst had been present

for many years, and was progressively enlarging. Therefore, it was explored. A large, clear, thin cystic lesion was found within the lateral rectus muscle and was resected (Fig. 13-18A and B). Histologically and on electron microscopy, it consisted of a single layer of cells of probable epithelial origin (Fig. 13-18C).

Bony Anomalies

ORBITAL ASYMMETRY

Minor degrees of facial and orbital asymmetry were the most common causes of pseudoproptosis in our orbital clinic (Fig. 13-19). We have seen a total of 30 patients (2.3% of orbital cases) referred for evaluation of proptosis that were essentially related to varying degrees of bony asymmetry. In almost all instances the asymmetry is identifiable clinically by an associated facial asymmetry. A simple clue to picking this up is to observe the patient from behind while he faces a mirror. The reversal of the images makes facial asymmetry particularly noticeable. For the most part these patients had minor degrees of asymmetry involving all of the hemifacial structures. However, in a few instances the asymmetry was related to maxillary hypoplasia resulting in a relatively retroplaced orbit on the affected side (Fig. 13-20). In several cases familial asymmetry was evident when examining the siblings or parents. Retrospective photographic review is useful to demonstrate how long the patient has had this anomaly.

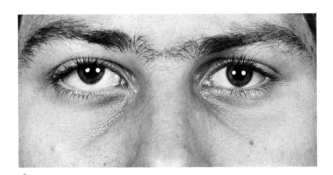

A

FIGURE 13-17. *(A)* A 17-year-old boy who presented with upward displacement and mild proptosis of the right globe and diplopia in downgaze. *(B)* Axial CT scan of the same patient showing a large, apparently destructive, lesion of the base of the skull. *(C)* Axial CT scan after intranasal drainage of the cyst at biopsy. It was diagnosed as a Rathke's pouch cyst. Note air and fluid within the cyst cavity, which extends into the middle cranial fossa.

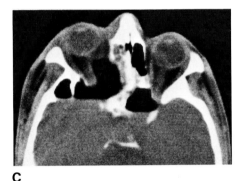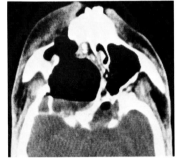

B

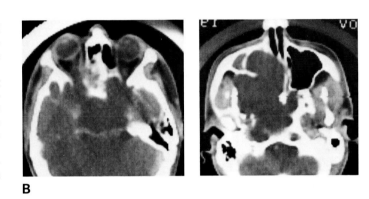

C

CRANIOFACIAL DYSOSTOSIS AND DEVELOPMENTAL ANOMALIES OF THE SKULL

Craniofacial dysostosis and developmental anomalies may result in profound orbital abnormalities. The most common orbital abnormality associated with craniofacial dysostosis is extreme shallowing as the result of arrested growth of the affected cranial bones. The flattening of the face and the shallowing of the orbits may produce profound and threatening exophthalmos. In Crouzon's disease there may also be an associated developmental hypoplasia of the superior rectus muscles leading to marked exodeviations, particularly in upgaze. Narrowing

of the optical canal may lead to optic atrophy. The cosmetic and functional disturbances related to the dysostosis, hypertelorism, and exorbitism are the domain of a multidisciplinary craniofacial team, which should include an ophthalmologist. Their definition and management is beyond the scope of this book and constitute a separate medical discipline.

MESODERMAL DEFECTS

Part of the abnormality associated with von Recklinghausen's disease (multiple neurofibromatosis) may be a developmental anomaly of the cranial bones, in particu-

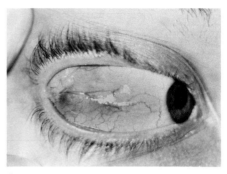
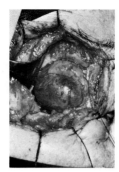

A

FIGURE 13-18. *(A)* A bluish discoloration and swelling of the lateral subconjunctiva. It was due to a large cyst found within the lateral rectus muscle. *(B)* Axial and coronal CT scans show a large cyst, which had caused smooth erosion of the lateral orbital wall.

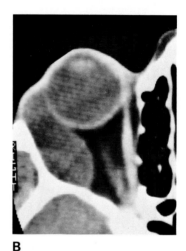
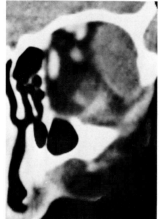

B

lar, absence of the sphenoid wing (Fig. 13-21.) This may lead to pulsatile exophthalmos or rarely enophthalmos because of the adjacency of the dura and periorbita.

Tumors and Ectopias

DERMOLIPOMAS

Dermolipomas are not usually lesions of the orbit and are properly described as conjunctival tumors. They are included here because of the frequent clinical confusion with true orbital dermoids. Dermolipomas are an ectopia of skin to conjunctiva probably related to sequestration at the time of embryonic development of the lids. They typically occur on the superolateral epibulbar surface and are usually asymptomatic (Fig. 13-22). Histologically, the surface consists of keratinizing squamous epithelium with adnexal structures, including hair, which may be sufficient to cause constant irritation that requires treat-

ment. If asymptomatic, excision is not necessary. Because of their intimate association with the lacrimal duct structures, it is important to avoid damage to the ducts at the time of excision. We usually remove them under the microscope, identify the abnormal epithelium with hairs on it, and excise that portion of the surface as an ellipse, identifying and avoiding the lacrimal ducts. The underlying dermis usually contains fat and connective tissue septae and can be debulked with ease, again avoiding the lacrimal ducts and the underlying lateral rectus muscle. Deep excision is unnecessary because the offending feature consists of the superficial ectopic skin. Aggressive orbital dissection should be avoided.

LACRIMAL ECTOPIA

Although not infrequent in conjunctiva, caruncle, and epibulbar sites, ectopic lacrimal tissue is rare in the deep orbit. When it occurs here, it is isolated from ductal

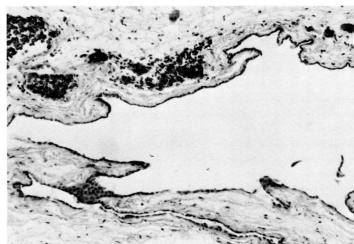

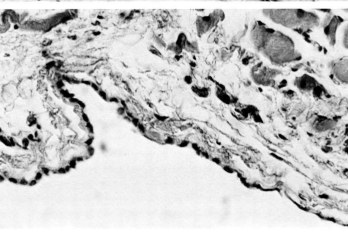

FIGURE 13-18. *(Continued).* *(C)* Histopathology of the intramuscular cyst. It was lined by a single layer of epithelium (H&E, original magnification *top* × 2.5; *bottom* × 25).

C

structures and accumulated secretions are said to incite a local cicatricial inflammatory response. Depending on the location, there may be evidence of both mass and infiltrative effect with reduction in extraocular movements, proptosis, and visual deterioration. Diagnosis requires reliable evidence of lacrimal tissue obtained from a site remote from the lacrimal gland. Many of the cases described have been characterized by progressive chronic inflammatory infiltration of the orbit. Suggested management has been surgical excision. We have seen one such case with massive infiltration of the orbit; the patient responded dramatically to orbital irradiation with regression of the inflammatory component.

ORBITAL TERATOMA

The broadest definition of teratoma is a tumor made of tissues derived from more than one germ layer and usually from all three. They are believed to arise from pluripotential embryonic tissue. Overall, teratomas are said to account for 6.6% of childhood tumors, most commonly occurring in the testes, ovaries, and retroperitoneum. The orbit is a rare site of teratoma, particularly if they are defined as tumors that contain components of elements from all three germ layers. Only 58 such cases have been described in the literature.

Characteristically, they present as a rapidly developing unilateral tumor of the infant orbit. In older age groups, they are generally smaller and develop more slowly. The common clinical feature is extreme unilateral proptosis, with marked stretching of the lids by a solid or more frequently cystic mass. The eye is usually of normal size but may be degenerated secondary to protrusion and exposure. The orbit is increased in size. Although massive intracranial teratomas with orbital extension have been described, the vast majority are primary lesions of the orbit.

Histologically, the totipotential cells differentiate along ectodermal, neuroectodermal, mesodermal, and

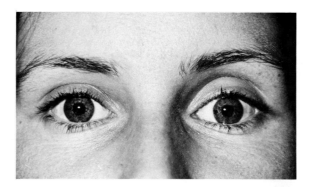

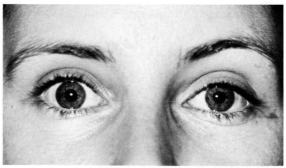

FIGURE 13-19. *(Top)* A 36-year-old patient with orbital asymmetry and left enophthalmos. (Note deepened superior sulcus.) *(Bottom)* The same patient following augmentation of the orbit with a bone graft in the floor.

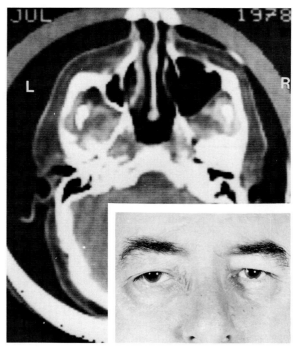

FIGURE 13-20. This 57-year-old man had a history of long-standing prominence of the right eye. Note, however, left enophthalmos and flattening of the premaxillary area. The CT scan shows left maxillary hypoplasia, which was associated with enophthalmos. (Cline RA, Rootman J: Enophthalmos: A clinical review. Ophthalmology 91:229, 1984)

endodermal lines. The presence of gastrointestinal, glandular, and secretory choroid plexus accounts for the frequently cystic and rapidly developing features of these tumors. Although malignant teratomas are not uncommon elsewhere, only one documented case has been described in the orbit.

The importance of this tumor lies in the differential diagnosis of a rapidly growing orbital tumor of infancy. This includes benign (orbital hemangioma and lymphangioma) and malignant tumors (rhabdomyosarcoma and metastatic tumor, particularly neuroblastoma and leukemia). In addition, congenital anomalies such as microphthalmos with cyst, congenital cystic eyeball, unilateral congenital glaucoma, cephaloceles, and plexiform neurofibromas should be ruled out. Inflammatory lesions in this age group rarely mimic tumors.

The majority of these in the past have been treated by exenteration. However, with improvements in preoperative diagnostic imaging and surgical technology, excision of the tumor alone is possible. This is particularly true if the tumor is smaller and there is evidence of preservation of ocular function.

■ ACQUIRED LESIONS

Cystic

MUCOCELE

Jack Rootman and Larry Allen

Pathogenesis and Development

Mucoceles are cystic, slowly expanding lesions originating from the sinuses. Their etiology is related to obstruction of the normal sinus ostea and entrapment of the secretory epithelium, which continues to secrete mucous, filling the normally aerated space and exerting pressure on the surrounding bony structures. This leads to effacement of the normal septae, expansion of the sinus, thinning of the bony walls, and ultimately extension through the wall into the adjacent orbit, nasopharynx, or cranial cavity. The respiratory epithelium lining the sinus may undergo atrophy with loss of the normal cilia and goblet cells and replacement by a fibrous capsule

(Fig. 13-23). The majority of mucoceles, therefore, contain a clear to slightly yellowish mucoid material. Rarely a pyocele filled with purulent material may be formed when the contents are infected. In the antibiotic era, this is increasingly infrequent. Thus, cyst contents vary from mucoid or viscous to purulent with the majority containing a clear sterile fluid.

It has been suggested that the usual cause of osteal obstruction is inflammation with secondary scarring, but other contributing factors include fractures (see Fig. 13-23), osteomas, polyps, nasal septal deviation, mucous retention cysts, and congenital narrowing of the ostea. Hemorrhage within a mucocele is rare, and associated with brown fluid and cholesterol crystals. A review of the history of patients in our own series revealed that 40% had fractures, 35% had a history of chronic sinusitis and sinus surgery, and the remaining 25% had no antecedent history.

Incidence and Distribution

Of the structural lesions in our clinic, mucoceles constituted 13% while overall they represented 1.7% of orbital patients seen. The incidence varies, depending on the series studied, from 2% to 15% but the estimated frequency is about 3% or 4% of orbital patients. Most mucoceles involve the frontal or ethmoid sinuses, or both, and occur at any age in both sexes. The majority, however, are seen between the fourth and seventh decades. In our own series, the average age was 46.3 years. Rare mucoceles of infancy and childhood may suggest an underlying cystic fibrosis. They develop slowly with an average duration of symptoms of 10 months.

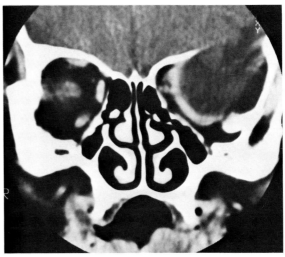

FIGURE 13-21. Coronal CT scan of a patient with absence of the left sphenoid wing and pulsating exophthalmos due to neurofibromatosis. The temporal lobe has herniated into the orbit through the bony defect.

Clinical Features

The clinical features are an expansive, noninfiltrating mass effect dominated by the site of bony erosion or expansion. Thus, mucoceles of the frontal sinus lead to downward and outward displacement of the globe with minimal proptosis, particularly when they occur anteriorly. Posterior extension from the sinus may lead to more downward displacement and proptosis. Psychophysical

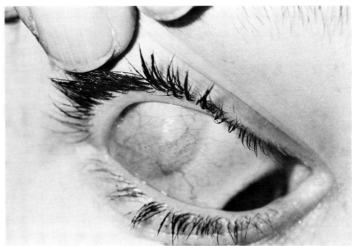

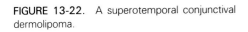
FIGURE 13-22. A superotemporal conjunctival dermolipoma.

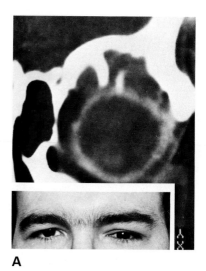
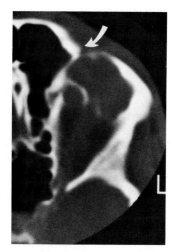

A

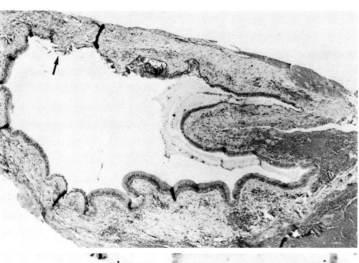

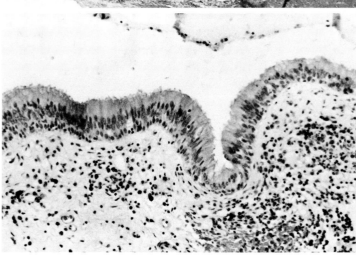

FIGURE 13-23. *(A)* This 34-year-old man presented with downward displacement of the left eye. He had also noted diplopia in upgaze. The axial and coronal CT scans show a mucocele arising lateral to a fracture site *(arrow)* in the frontal sinus and extending inferiorly into the orbit. Note the smooth, scalloped edges and focal calcification. *(B)* Histopathology of the mucocele shows pseudostratified respiratory epithelium, areas of thinning and loss of epithelium *(top, arrow),* mucin debris, and surrounding inflammation (H&E, original magnification *top* × 2.5; *bottom* × 25).

B

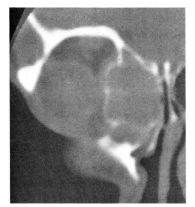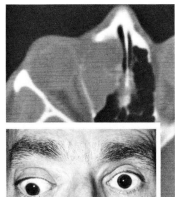

FIGURE 13-24. This 48-year-old man had downward and outward displacement of his right globe due to a fronto-ethmoid mucocele, which is shown on axial and coronal CT scan. Note characteristic expansion of the ethmoid sinus with smooth, scalloped margins and bone formation in the periorbita.

or oculomotor dysfunction is rare and usually a reflection of an extremely large lesion.

Frontoethmoid mucoceles cause outward and downward displacement, and are often associated with a fullness in the superonasal and medial canthal region with flattening of the nasion and a palpable mass (Fig. 13-24). Rarely they may be bilateral, leading to a hyperteloric appearance (Fig. 13-25). In our experience ethmoid mucoceles tended to be smaller and characterized by lateral displacement of the globe with minimal exophthalmos. Mucoceles arising from the frontoethmoid complex, when associated with a palpable mass, can be felt above the medial canthal ligament in contrast to lesions of the lacrimal sac, which are generally felt below the ligament. When they penetrate bone, the periosteal tissues may develop metaplastic bone formation, producing a shell and palpable exostosis at the margin of the lesion (see Figs. 13-23 and 13-24). Mucoceles of the frontoethmoid complex, particularly in the young, must be differentiated from cephaloceles. In children. cephaloceles may vary with a Valsalva maneuver, may be pulsatile, and are usually associated with hypertelorism. On investigation the bony dehiscence from the cranial cavity should be obvious. Nevertheless, the bone dehiscence may be very tiny, particularly in an adult, and differentiation may be difficult. Fluid withdrawal would help to differentiate between CSF and mucus content.

Mucoceles originating in the sphenoid and posterior ethmoid sinus, because of their intimate relationship to the optic nerve, cavernous sinus, and orbital apex, tend to present with functional abnormalities related to these structures rather than globe displacement and soft tissue changes (Fig. 13-26). Characteristically, the patients have visual symptoms, retrobulbar pain, or nerve palsies, and about half of them have nasal symptoms. Encroachment on the optic canal may cause optic atrophy. Apical orbital

and cavernous sinus involvement lead to extraocular muscle palsies in 50% of the patients (usually third nerve). Sensory nerve compression leads to intermittent apical orbital pain, which may be confused with migraine. The location and ophthalmic manifestations of our series of mucoceles are summarized in Tables 13-1 and 13-2.

An unusual presentation is that of enophthalmos secondary to erosion of the floor of the orbit caused by a maxillary sinus mucocele (Fig. 13-27). Mucoceles of the maxillary sinus are rare and usually lead to upward displacement of the globe; however, erosion of the floor may cause the eye to sink into the expanded orbit. We have seen two such patients; both had intermittent facial pain with deepening of the superior sulcus and downward displacement of the globe. One was aware of a filling of the sulcus on awakening in the morning brought about by her recumbent position during the night. Both had x-ray evidence of chronic opacification of the maxillary sinus with destruction of the orbital floor.

When present for prolonged periods of time, sinus polyposis may cause proptosis by expansion of the sinuses and erosion of the bone. Polyposis usually occurs within the context of very long-standing allergic rhinitis. The polypoid tissue may erode the wall focally, in multiple sites, or may cause diffuse expansion of the sinuses. In addition, polyposis may contribute to the development of mucocele (Fig. 13-28).

Another unusual manifestation of mucocele was exemplified by a patient who developed intermittent exophthalmos and downward displacement of the globe related to a pyocele that had caused a fistula, which extended through the orbit and the upper lid. Intermittent drainage led to resolution of his symptoms. Finally, we have seen two patients with chronic sinusitis and pyocele extending into the orbit, causing intermittent and recurrent episodes of orbital cellulitis.

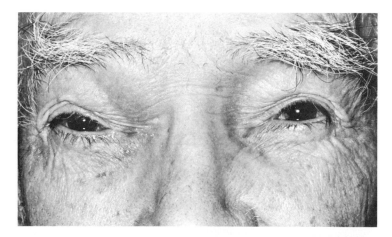

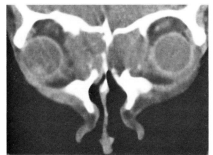

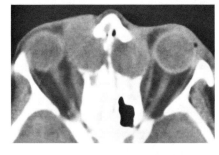

FIGURE 13-25. This 80-year-old man had progressive hypertelorism due to extensive bilateral muco-celes involving the fronto-ethmoid and maxillary sinuses.

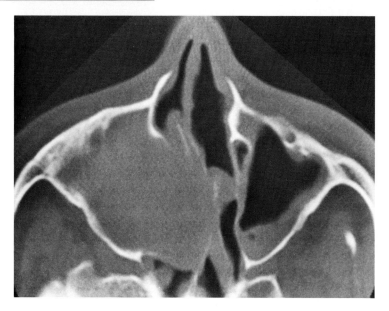

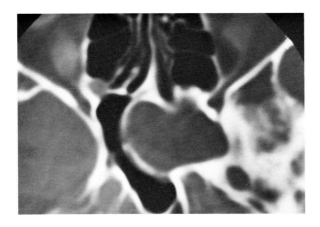

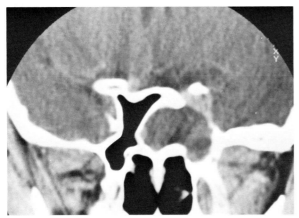

FIGURE 13-26. Axial *(top)* and coronal *(bottom)* CT scans of a sphenoid sinus mucocele that led to a mild left optic neuropathy due to pressure on the optic nerve.

acteristic of fluid-filled lesions. Those that contain debris may show some internal echoes and be confused with solid lesions.

Management

Management is directed to complete removal of the cyst lining, reestablishment of normal drainage, or obliteration of the sinus. This is usually the domain of the otorhinolaryngologist, but ophthalmologic expertise may be necessary for management of the orbital portion. Recurrence has been frequently noted in the past and attributed to incomplete excision of the lining or restenosis of the new osteum.

When the mucocele is clearly isolated, we usually completely excise the lining and smooth the bone with a drill to remove any crevices that may be lined by epithelium. When large and involving the frontoethmoid complex, either a silastic tube or a nasal flap is placed in the opening to reestablish and maintain it. It is useful to complete the orbital dissection prior to collapse of the cyst, because the definition of the margin of the mucocele is much easier while the mass is tense, facilitating dissection from the periorbita. Usually this margin is dissected free with ease, but in instances of recurrent inflammation careful and meticulous sharp dissection may be necessary because of fibrosis.

Investigations

Radiologically, mucoceles expand the sinus cavity while thinning the sinus walls and destroying the normal internal septae (see Figs. 13-23, 13-24, and 13-25). The margin of the mucocele on CT or polytomography may be a thin shell of bone (see Figs. 13-23, 13-24). On CT scan the sinus is homogeneously opacified by material of soft tissue density. The leading margin in the orbit is usually well defined, rarely enhances, and is smooth in contour. An associated old, healed bony fracture may be noted at the margin of the mucocele (see Fig. 13-23). Findings on polytomography are similar, although frequently less clearly demonstrated than by CT. On ultrasonography mucoceles are usually smooth in outline, rounded, and clearly defined from surrounding orbital structures. In addition, they have few internal echoes, good sound transmission, and good definition of the deep wall, char-

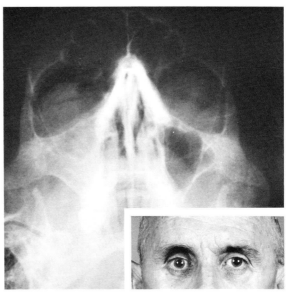

FIGURE 13-27. A 59-year-old man with a right maxillary mucocele that had caused progressive right enophthalmos and globe ptosis. Note the deepened right superior sulcus. (Cline RA, Rootman J: Enophthalmos: A clinical review. Ophthalmology 91:229, 1984)

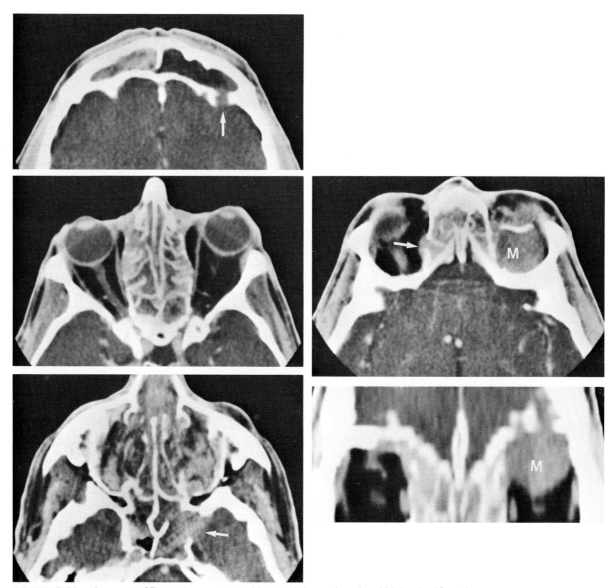

FIGURE 13-28. Composite CT scan demonstrates widespread sinus polyposis, which involved frontal, ethmoid, sphenoid, and maxillary sinuses. It was associated with multiple focal areas of erosion *(arrows)* due to polypoid tissue and the development of a large mucocele *(M)* in the roof of the left orbit.

TABLE 13-1.
MUCOCELE LOCATION, UNIVERSITY OF BRITISH COLUMBIA ORBITAL CLINIC, 1976–1984

Sinus	Right	Left	Bilateral	Total
Frontal	4	2		6
Ethmoid	2	5		7
Fronto-ethmoid	1	2		3
Maxillary	1	1		2
Sphenoid	2			2
Fronto-ethmoid-maxillary			1	1
			Total	21

TABLE 13-2.
MUCOCELE OF THE ORBIT: OPHTHALMIC MANIFESTATIONS, UNIVERSITY OF BRITISH COLUMBIA ORBITAL CLINIC, 1976–1984

Clinical Findings	Sinus Involved						Total
	F	E	M	S	F-E	F-E-M	
Loss of vision	2			2			4
Afferent pupil	1			2			3
Proptosis > 2 mm	5	5	1				11
Diplopia	2		1				3
Lid edema	3	3	1	1	1		9
Headache	2	1				1	4
Displacement							
Up			1				1
Down	2	1					3
Horizontal					1	1	2
Down and horizontal	4	3					7

F, Frontal; E, Ethmoid; M, Maxillary; S, Sphenoid

LACRIMAL DUCTAL CYSTS

Lacrimal ductal cysts are a rare, but important consideration in the differential diagnosis of mass lesions of the anterior orbit, especially those in the region of the lacrimal gland. They have been known for hundreds of years. Schmidt coined the term *dacryops* for this condition in 1803. Classically they are said to be symptomless swellings, usually nontender, mobile, tense, and fluctuant. However, in our experience (nine cases) two thirds of the cases seen had some degree of irritation or tenderness. In the majority of instances, eversion of the upper lid causes protrusion of the cysts into the conjunctival cul-de-sac where they appear as somewhat bluish lesions that transilluminate (Figs. 13-29 and 13-30). They tend to expand slowly and, on occasion, may vary in size due to intermittent discharge. We had several patients who noted swelling of the cyst when crying and one who experienced swelling and pain when deep sea diving. Rarely, a lacrimal duct cyst may present as a sudden expansion due either to inflammation within the cyst or hemorrhage. Infection with the development of fistulous discharge has been described.

Two types of lacrimal ductal cysts were seen: unilateral or bilateral (multiple). Bilateral cysts may be associated with blepharochalasis. Usually the cysts are relatively small and isolated, but they may be sufficiently large to cause displacement of the globe, and they may be multilocular (Fig. 13-30).

Histologically these cysts are lined by a double layer of epithelium; the inner lining is cuboidal and the outer myoepithelial (Fig. 13-31). The intervening stroma is frequently fibrotic and contains an inflammatory cell infiltrate (see Fig. 13-31). In occasional instances intense inflammation and granulation tissue may be seen. The pathogenesis is probably related to trauma or inflammation that weakens the ductal walls, destroying their neuromuscular contractility, allowing dilatation with

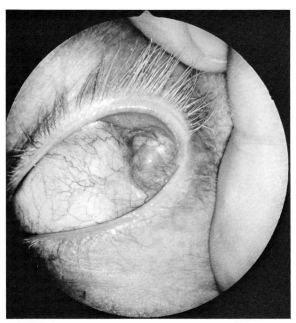

FIGURE 13-29. The left superotemporal fornix of a 44-year-old man who presented with painful, tender swelling of the upper lid due to a lacrimal cyst. (Smith S, Rootman J: Lacrimal ductal cysts: Presentation and management. Surv Ophthalmol 30:245, 1986)

blockage even at low secretory pressures. The clinical diagnosis is usually obvious on the basis of the visible cystic lesion. In large lesions ultrasonography and CT scan may demonstrate the cystic structure. Cysts of the lacrimal ducts must be differentiated from other cystic and noncystic lesions of the lids and lacrimal fossa with which they may be confused. We found the following potentially confusing cystic lesions in this region: dermoid cysts (particularly those that are superficial), laterally located frontal mucoceles, implantation cysts, aneurysmal bone cysts, and a muscle cyst in the lateral rectus. In addition to those seen in our series, the literature cites parasitic cysts and cysts of the lid adnexal structures in the differential diagnosis. The latter are most commonly seen in association with cicatrizing conditions such as pemphigoid and trachoma. Solid tumors of the lacrimal gland may be mistaken for ductal cysts, but are for the most part recognizable on clinical and laboratory studies as solid lesions.

If symptomatic or cosmetically bothersome, lacrimal duct cysts may be treated by complete excision or marsupialization; the latter technique is preferred for patients with decreased tear production on the affected side as shown on Schirmer's testing, which should be done in all cases. In several instances we have noted that the ductal cysts are multiple, a feature visible only at the time of excision. Simple lancing, incomplete excision, or aspiration alone usually results in a recurrence of the cyst.

IMPLANTATION CYSTS

Orbital implantation cysts are usually the result of previous trauma or surgery. We have encountered a number of cysts that developed following muscle surgery. These can reach significant size and extend deep into the orbit (Fig. 13-32). Management is by excision of the cyst under the microscope, avoiding damage to the usually scarred and partially incorporated muscle. Rarely, implantation cysts may result from penetrating trauma to the orbit.

Trauma

Jack Rootman and Janet Neigel

CLINICAL PRESENTATION AND EXAMINATION

Orbital injury may be isolated, but is often seen in association with damage to local structures including the globe, paranasal sinuses, nasolacrimal system, nose, and brain. In addition, the injury may be complicated by shock, inebriation, or loss of consciousness. The first priority is establishment of an airway, control of bleeding, and restoration of circulation. Once the patient is stabilized, attention can be directed to the local structures. The globe should be promptly examined before the onset of soft tissue swelling. The minimum requirement is to obtain a visual acuity with the least amount of trauma to the potentially damaged ocular structures. Tightly swollen lids can be gently separated by Desmarres retractors; if they are unavailable, a retractor can be fashioned from paper clips. If there is no significant orbital tension, blepharospasm, or obvious ocular injury, a speculum may be gently inserted. When necessary, a lid block can be given to reduce blepharospasm to perform an adequate ocular examination. In children or restless and pugnacious patients, examination aided either by sedation or anesthesia may be necessary. Major ocular injuries indicated by a soft globe, prolapsing tissue, rupture, hemorrhage, and loss of the red reflex should be ruled out promptly and dealt with in the operating room.

A careful, thorough history is not always possible, but should include circumstances of injury, exact nature of the offending object, distance and direction that it travelled, time of occurrence, any previous ocular disorder, history of surgery, allergies, systemic medical problems, or current medications. Pretrauma photographs may be useful.

Once the globe has been assessed, an orbital examination can be done. Gross external inspection of the facial structures is helpful in defining major facial fractures. Horizontal, vertical, and axial displacement of the globe and orbit should be documented. The lids should be checked for abnormality of height, width, inclination,

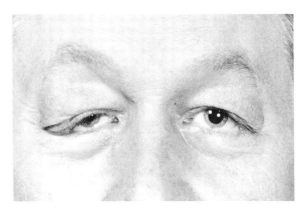

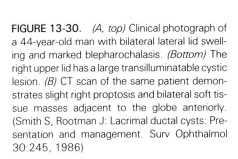

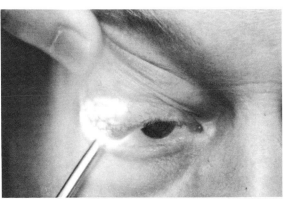

FIGURE 13-30. *(A, top)* Clinical photograph of a 44-year-old man with bilateral lateral lid swelling and marked blepharochalasis. *(Bottom)* The right upper lid has a large transilluminatable cystic lesion. *(B)* CT scan of the same patient demonstrates slight right proptosis and bilateral soft tissue masses adjacent to the globe anteriorly. (Smith S, Rootman J: Lacrimal ductal cysts: Presentation and management. Surv Ophthalmol 30:245, 1986)

A

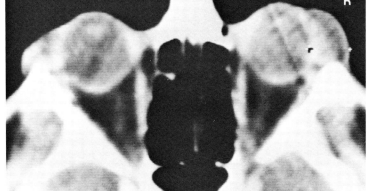

B

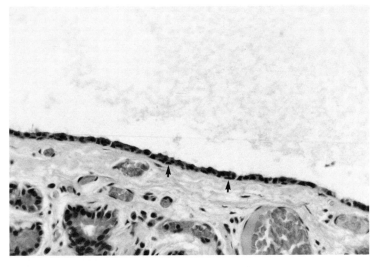

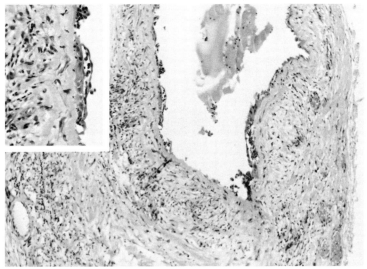

FIGURE 13-31. *(Top)* Photomicrograph of a portion of the cyst wall obtained from the patient shown in Figure 13-29. Note inner cuboidal layer and outer myoepithelial cells *(arrow)*. The lumen contains inspissated secretions, and the wall of the cyst is somewhat fibrotic. Note also lacrimal structures (H&E, original magnification × 25). *(Bottom)* Another portion of the cyst wall from the same patient shows degeneration of the epithelial surface associated with more marked inflammation and fibrosis (H&E, original magnification × 10). *(Inset)* High power of the same specimen (× 25). (Smith S, Rootman J: Lacrimal ductal cysts: Presentation and management. Surv Ophthalmol 30:245, 1986)

and interpalpebral distance. The mobility of the lids (levator function), ptosis, and pseudoptosis should be evaluated. The assessment of ptosis may be particularly difficult in the presence of significant lid swelling. The medial and lateral canthal ligaments should be checked for any alteration in level and increase in intercanthal distance (telecanthus). The position of the globe may be altered due to avulsion of the suspensory ligaments or fractures of adjacent sites. Malar flattening with or without globe ptosis, downward displacement of the lateral canthus, and lower lid retraction may be evidence of a displaced trimalar fracture of the zygoma. In contrast, lower lid retraction without flattening may be seen with a simple orbital rim fracture. Telecanthus, especially when associated with depression of the nasal bridge, can be seen with a midline fracture (Fig. 13-33). Enophthalmos may be due to increased orbital volume secondary to herniation of tissues into adjacent sinuses, disturbances in the periorbital fat, or an absolute deficiency of fat when it is altered by liquefaction or subsequent fibrosis (Fig. 13-34). Traumatic exophthalmos is relatively rare, but may result from reduction in orbital volume due to inward displacement of orbital walls, hemorrhage, and emphysema. A pseudoproptotic appearance may result from a complete third nerve palsy. Pulsating exophthalmos may indicate an orbital roof fracture with secondary herniation of the anterior cranial fossa contents or a carotid cavernous fistula. Another cause of pseudoptosis may be a deepened superior sulcus related to enophthalmos or downward displacement of the globe.

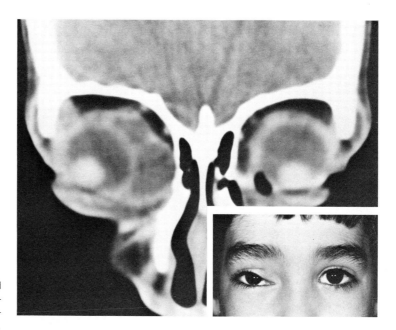

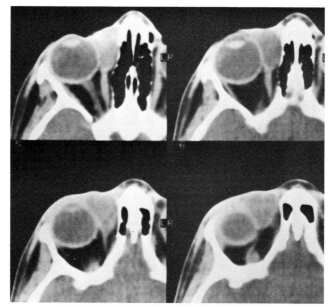

FIGURE 13-32. An 8-year-old boy presented with a history of progressive swelling of the superior lid and medial canthal region following extraocular muscle surgery done 8 months after birth. The axial and coronal CT scans demonstrate a large epithelial cyst that is attached to the medial rectus muscle posteriorly.

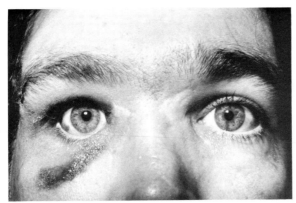

FIGURE 13-33. Clinical photograph of a patient who had a midfacial fracture resulting in flattening of the base of the nose and hypertelorism.

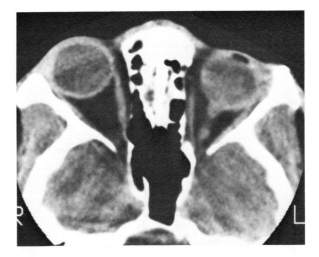

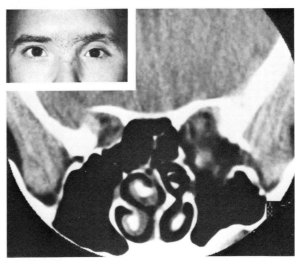

FIGURE 13-34. Clinical features and axial and coronal CT scans of a blow-out fracture of the orbit, with left enophthalmos and downward displacement of the inferior orbital structures. Note globe ptosis, enophthalmos, and deepened superior sulcus.

Extraocular movements and diplopia should be documented in all fields of gaze, to assess acute motor status and progressive change. If there is any reduction in eye movements, forced duction testing should be performed to distinguish entrapment and muscle contusion from paresis (Fig. 13-35). Topical proparacaine or cocaine is instilled in the eye, and a cotton-tipped applicator or pledget saturated with anesthetic is placed over the insertion of the muscle for 5 minutes. The muscle is then grasped with a forcep and the eye rotated in the affected direction of gaze.

Palpation of the orbital rim may reveal local tenderness, displacement, and degree of comminution of the fracture site. Tissue emphysema and crepitus may suggest a paranasal sinus fracture (Figs. 13-36 and 13-37). A bruit may be present when a traumatic arteriovenous shunt has occurred.

Sensation should be tested, particularly in the distribution of the infraorbital, frontal, zygomatico-facial, and zygomatico-temporal nerves. CSF rhinorrhea may occur, especially with a significant naso-orbital or roof fracture. Anosmia may be an indication of a dural tear in the roof of the ethmoid sinus or cribriform plate.

Lacerations should be explored to evaluate the integrity of the orbital septum and the major anterior orbital structures, especially the levator muscle and lacrimal structures. In addition, a careful assessment for retained foreign bodies should be made. If possible, photographs or sketches of the injury should be obtained.

SOFT TISSUE INJURY AND ORBITAL HEMORRHAGE

Blunt or penetrating trauma may result in soft tissue injuries with damage to vital orbital structures. The optic nerve, extraocular muscles, or neurovascular structures may be affected either directly or indirectly by shearing forces. The signs and symptoms of soft tissue injury include ecchymosis, lid swelling, proptosis, and ophthalmoplegia. Orbital hemorrhage can be classified according to the site of accumulated blood, as shown in the following list.

1. Hemorrhage in the eyelid anterior to the orbital septum
2. Hemorrhage posterior to the orbital septum, including subconjunctival hemorrhage
3. Hemorrhage within the muscle cone
4. Subperiosteal hematoma

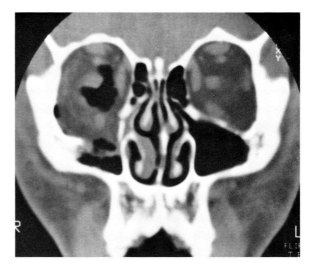

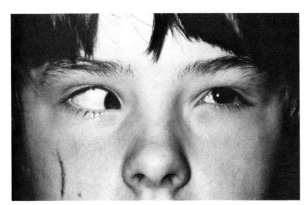

FIGURE 13-35. Clinical photograph of a patient with a medial wall blow-out fracture, which led to limitation of abduction on the left side.

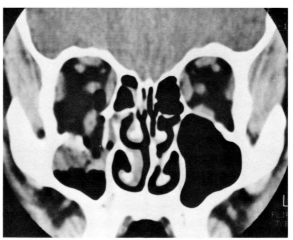

FIGURE 13-37. Coronal CT scans of a patient with a blow-out fracture of the orbit demonstrate orbital emphysema and downward displacement of the inferior orbital structures. The patient was supine for these direct coronal images, causing fluid in the right maxillary antrum to layer in the superior, dependent portion of the sinus.

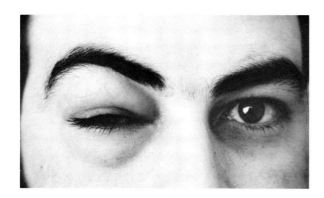

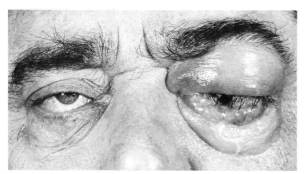

FIGURE 13-36. Clinical photographs showing orbital emphysema following trauma. *(Top)* The soft tissues of the lid are primarily involved. This occurred 1 day after orbital trauma, when he blew his nose. *(Bottom)* Massive orbital emphysema following a blow-out fracture of the orbit.

5. Intracranial hemorrhage that spreads to the orbit by means of the medial portion of the superior orbital fissure or by means of the space between the dura mater and the optic nerve in the optic canal.

Abrasions and avulsion of tissue usually produce superficial defects. Simple closed injuries lead to contusions with tenderness, swelling, and ecchymosis, which present as limited or localized ecchymosis, edema, and subconjunctival hemorrhage (the "black eye"). The blood typically accumulates in the preseptal tissues or the superficial conjunctiva. In contrast, subconjunctival hemorrhages secondary to orbital trauma accumulate in the retrobulbar, intraconal, and extraconal spaces and track anteriorly or posteriorly. In such situations visible ecchymosis may not appear for a few days, and when present, can be seen in the fornix extending beneath both the bulbar and tarsal conjunctivae. Deeper and intracranial hemorrhages may also take a few days to present either by tracking from the subgaleal space or into the intraconal space through the superior orbital fissure extending extraconally as it tracks forward. Intracranial bleeding may also pass directly into the extraconal space through the medial aspect of the superior orbital fissure.

By and large, management of soft tissue hemorrhage that does not threaten vision is usually conservative and consists of thorough inspection, cleansing and repair of wounds, and cold compresses in the early phase followed by warm compresses. Hematomas, on the other hand, may appear as swollen fluctuant areas, which may be drained or aspirated. In the later stages, hematomas become organized, and if they cause significant orbital pressure need to be surgically evacuated.

Soft tissue injuries often result in trauma to vital structures in the orbit. The optic nerve, extraocular muscles, or neurovascular structures may be affected either directly or indirectly.

OPTIC NERVE TRAUMA

Injuries to the optic nerve are rare and can result from simple contusion, avulsion, fractures of the optic canal, compression secondary to intracanalicular hematoma, and optic nerve edema within the canal. In addition, the nerve may be damaged intracranially due to sudden deceleration. Types of optic nerve injury are summarized in the following list.

A. Direct Orbital Trauma
1. Penetrating: pencils, antenna, ice picks, etc. Occasionally with minimal soft tissue trauma; rule out cranial penetration or carotid injury
2. Missiles: removal seldom improves vision
3. Avulsion
4. Strangulation

B. Indirect Damage to Optic Nerve
1. Sudden deceleration of head
2. Usually supraorbital blow; rarely occipital or parietal
3. Immediate loss of vision; prognosis poor
4. Recovery within a few days, if at all
5. Altitudinal or arcuate visual field defects or central scotoma
6. Work up: pupils, orbital CT scan
7. Treatment: Surgery only if secondary visual loss; no surgery on unconscious patient; high-dose steroids (questionable)

C. Traumatic Chiasmal Syndrome
1. Severe head trauma: vertex, upper forehead
2. AP distortion of skull: deceleration
3. Usually one eye blind; temporal defect in other eye
4. Occasionally pure bitemporal defect
5. Associated findings: cranial nerve palsies; diabetes insipidus, pituitary insufficiency; anosmia; CSF rhinorrhea, meningitis; carotid-cavernous fistula

D. Herniation
1. Third nerve compression
2. Posterior cerebral artery compression
3. Optic nerve compression (gyrus rectus syndrome, frontal lobe herniation)

It is important to monitor visual loss and pupillary reactions. The time of onset in relation to the trauma may point to a secondary optic nerve compression from an enlarging hematoma or vascular compromise. Visual loss when immediate is usually complete and irreversible, reflecting laceration, avulsion, or severe contusion with ischemic necrosis. Decompression is not useful for this type of injury.

Usually the site of injury is the intracanalicular portion of the nerve because it is here that the nerve is surrounded by, and partially adherent to, the bony canal (Fig. 13-38). The intraorbital segment is encased in orbital fat. Here the nerve is loose and has some give, and may stretch with retrobulbar hemorrhage. Hemorrhage apically, however, may affect the nerve rapidly by confining it in the tight space (Fig. 13-39). The intracranial portion is surrounded by brain and skull and is well isolated from all but extreme trauma.

Secondary lesions are circulatory events subsequent to the initial injury and may be due to edematous swelling of the nerve following contusion or hypoxia, necrosis from local compression, or vascular obstruction (thrombosis or arterial spasm). A fracture is not necessary for nerve damage to occur but is a reflection of the severity of the traumatic insult to the optic canal and nerve.

Damage to the nerve may also be caused by remote or contrecoup injury. Clinically, a patient with indirect optic nerve injury presents with a history of blunt trauma to the brow or orbital rim. There is a gradual visual deteri-

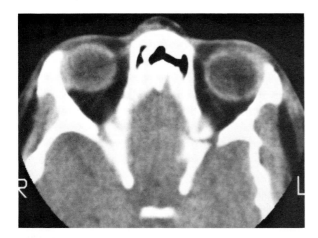

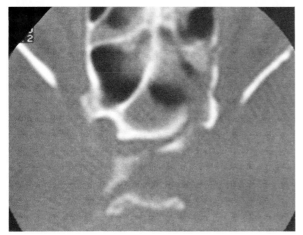

FIGURE 13-38. Axial CT scans of the apex of the orbit and the optic canal region demonstrate a fracture involving the orbital roof and the tuberculum sellae adjacent to the optic canal. This was associated with a left optic neuropathy.

oration with a sluggish or absent ipsilateral pupillary reflex and normal consensual reaction. The fundus is also normal. Associated findings may include epistaxis and concussion. A visual field defect inferiorly suggests a down fracture of the superior bony canal. Optic nerve sheath hemorrhages may present with proptosis along with the visual loss.

Delayed or progressive visual loss carries a better prognosis and is potentially reversible. Aggressive management should be undertaken if the history suggests some vision immediately following the injury, or in the case of an unconscious patient if there is a deterioration in the pupillary light response and no evidence of intracranial injury. Medically, such patients may be treated with megadose steroids in the range of 120 mg of prednisone daily to reduce circulatory spasm, edema, and cell

necrosis. Failure to respond within 1 week would indicate permanent damage, and the steroids should be discontinued. Optic nerve decompression may be indicated in some patients, although the visual results have been inconclusive.

A superior orbital fissure syndrome may be seen in isolation without optic nerve injury secondary to medial displacement of the greater wing of the sphenoid bone. This is a rare complication of orbital fractures and is probably best treated by observation and monitoring of optic nerve function.

FRACTURES OF THE ORBIT

Fractures of the orbit may be suggested by a variety of clinical signs and symptoms but usually cannot be clearly defined without x-ray studies, because most of these signs and symptoms can be produced by orbital edema and hemorrhage alone. Fractures of the roof may be associated with hemorrhage into the upper lid and lateral subconjunctiva. Occasionally CSF rhinorrhea may also be seen. Lateral wall fractures are more likely to be associated with avulsion of the optic nerve. Orbital emphysema may be produced by medial wall or floor fractures.

The etiology of orbital fractures may be divided into direct (orbital rim) fractures that occur when the force is applied to the bone or group of bones, and indirect (blow-out or blow-in) when the force is transmitted through the oribital soft tissues. Fractures in and around

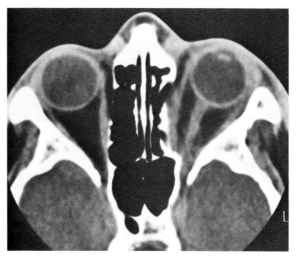

FIGURE 13-39. CT scan shows a medial blow-out fracture of the orbit and hemorrhage into the orbital apex. The latter accounted for the sudden onset of an optic neuropathy following the trauma.

the orbit tend to follow the line of least resistance. Site and extent are dependent on the degree and direction of impact.

Plain x-rays, including Waters, Caldwell, and lateral views, may demonstrate blowout and orbital rim fractures as well as those of other facial bones (Fig. 13-40). Opacification of the maxillary antrum is suggestive of floor fracture. Tissue emphysema may also be noted following sinus fracture.

CT scanning can demonstrate soft tissue injuries and entrapped extraocular muscles. Management decisions when dealing with fractures must be individualized because no two injuries are alike.

Fifty-three para-orbital fractures were referred to the University of British Columbia Orbital Clinic. Of these, 42 were male and 11 female; 19 were right sided and 34 were left sided. The high incidence of trauma on the left side reflects the major cause and right-handedness of the assailant.

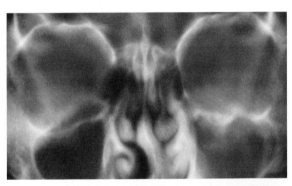

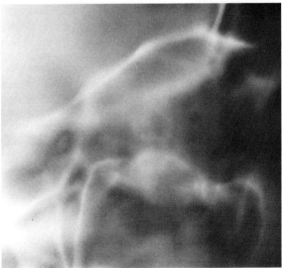

FIGURE 13-40. Coronal and lateral tomograms of the orbit demonstrate a left orbital blow-out fracture with opacification of the maxillary sinus. The orbital floor is disrupted.

Blow-Out Fractures

Blow-out fractures result from compression of soft tissue and sudden increase in orbital hydraulic pressure. The force is transmitted to the walls and fractures occur in the areas of least resistance. They are usually caused by a blunt, rounded object greater than 5 cm in diameter, such as a fist, knee, elbow, hockey puck, tennis ball, or dashboard edge.

The site of least resistance is in the orbital floor medial to the infraorbital groove, immediately in front of the inferior orbital fissure (see Figs. 13-34 and 13-37). It is here that the inferior rectus and inferior oblique muscles and their fat and fascial attachments may become entrapped. The nerve to the inferior oblique, because of its course along the lateral border of the rectus, may be injured without actual entrapment of the muscle. The medial wall and uncommonly the roof of the orbit may be involved in a blow-out type fracture (Fig. 13-41).

Physical findings suggestive of a blow-out fracture include orbital rim tenderness, infraorbital hypesthesia, motility disturbances with a positive forced duction, enophthalmos, and pseudoptosis. There is usually extensive edema and ecchymosis and there may be crepitus.

Infraorbital hypesthesia, when present, suggests a fracture of the central portion of the floor of the orbit. A defect medial or lateral to the infraorbital canal may leave sensation intact. Anesthesia in the distribution of the zygomatic nerve may be associated with a lateral fracture.

True muscle incarceration is usually not found at the time of surgery. Most cases of acute movement disturbances are caused by orbital septal disruption or injury to muscles, including laceration, avulsion, hemorrhage, and peripheral nerve injury. The great majority of orbital blow-out fractures lead to impairment of movement in all fields of up and down gaze, reflecting both inferior oblique and inferior rectus involvement (Fig. 13-42). The disruption of the connective tissue septae not only involves the system of the inferior orbit, but can have tractional effects on the medial and lateral rectus muscles, which explains some of the bizarre motility patterns seen following blow-out fractures.

Acute enophthalmos may occur due to prolapse and escape of fat and orbital contents into a sinus or due to increased orbital volume. Initial enophthalmos may be masked by edema or hematoma. Enophthalmos may be associated with a pseudoptosis of the upper eyelid, a deepening of the supratarsal sulcus, and a decrease in the interpalpebral fissure. Late enophthalmos can develop as the result of fat atrophy and necrosis and the globe may be retracted by short, fibrotic entrapped muscles.

Facial x-rays may show the tear-drop sign due to soft tissue protrusion into the superior portion of the maxillary antrum through the fracture site. A coronal CT scan can be very helpful to determine soft tissue injuries and

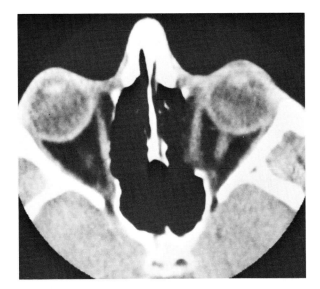

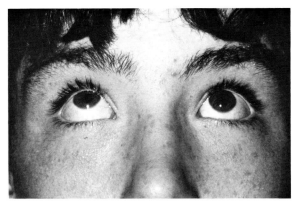

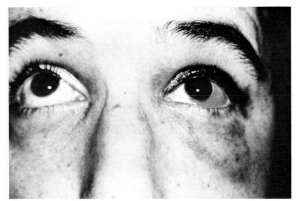

FIGURE 13-42. Features of limitation of supraduction associated with blow-out fractures of the orbit.

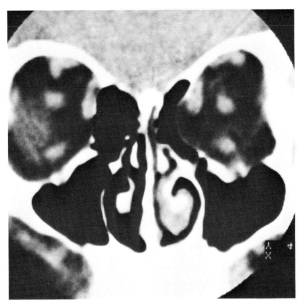

FIGURE 13-41. Axial and coronal CT scans of a medial orbital blow-out fracture with entrapment of the left medial rectus muscle. Note medial displacement of the posterior portion of the muscle with adherence to the bone at the posterior end of the fracture.

recognize entrapped extraocular muscles. In some cases, tethering of the muscles by connective tissue strands may be seen, along with alterations of the normal rectangular or elliptical contour of the muscle in cross section.

As a general guideline, a blow-out fracture need not necessarily be considered an emergency unless the globe is in the maxillary sinus. Thus, there is time for contemplative assessment of the patient. In patients who are initially asymptomatic the incidence of late complications following untreated blow-out fractures is extremely low. Indications for surgery include unresolved diplopia over a 10-day to 2-week period with a persistent positive forced duction or cosmetically unacceptable enophthalmos, or both. With the introduction of careful coronal, axial, and sagittal CT scanning, significant muscle displacement and tethering may be identified earlier and could lead to the development of criteria for direct intervention. Infraorbital hypesthesia alone is not an indication for acute repair. A number of authors have described long-term hypesthesia relieved by surgically disimpacting the nerve within the infraorbital canal. During the early assessment period, the patient should be warned not to blow his nose or sneeze because of the risk of orbital emphysema. There should be careful follow up for evidence of infection (rare). Early motility exercises may improve ocular excursion and might stimulate the formation of a functional connective tissue system around the muscles.

Operative repair is directed toward freeing the entrapped orbital tissue and restoring the integrity of the orbital floor. The approach may be percutaneous, through the maxillary sinus, or by a combination of the two. There are four percutaneous routes. One may enter the orbit through the conjunctival cul-de-sac, which avoids a visible scar but provides limited access to the floor. Usually a lateral canthotomy must be added to this to obtain adequate exposure of the fracture site. The subciliary incision is our preference, although there is an increased risk of ectropion and it does take a bit longer to expose the fracture site. A lower eyelid incision can be made in a skin crease approximately half the distance between the lash margin and the orbital rim. The orbicularis muscle should be split horizontally a few millimeters lower than the skin lesion to obtain a better cosmetic result. An orbital rim incision is quicker but results in more noticeable scarring, greater risk of ectropion, and implant extrusion. A fracture of the orbital floor may also be approached through the maxillary sinus. A traction suture should be placed through the inferior rectus muscles to aid in identification of entrapped tissues.

After the incarcerated tissues are released from the fracture site an implant is placed over the defect. Frequently if the repair is done some time after the injury, there is adherence of the orbital soft tissues to the margin of the fracture, requiring sharp dissection for release. Alloplastic implants (Teflon, Supramid, Sialastic, and Cranioplast) and autogeneous implants (bone or cartilage from iliac crest, ribs, or walls of maxillary or ethmoid sinuses) have all been successful. It is important to avoid using too large an implant, which may lead to damage of the optic nerve and other posterior orbital structures. Small defects may be covered by absorbable gelatin film. Throughout and at the end of the procedure a forced duction test should be performed. A Frost suture may be used to apply traction to the lower lid to prevent lid retraction postoperatively.

Treatment of late enophthalmos depends upon the cosmetic results desired and is often difficult. One should wait 4 to 6 months until the enophthalmos stabilizes. To test the likelihood of successful repair, the forward traction test has been advocated. One applies a forceps to the medial and lateral rectus muscle and exerts forward traction. If the globe comes forward prognosis for repair is better than if the globe cannot be advanced. Globe ptosis and enophthalmos can be repaired by placement of an implant in the floor. This implant should have a greater volume posteriorly in order to increase orbital volume, and advance and elevate the globe. However, if the cosmetic deformity consists of a narrow palpebral fissure or ptosis, one could correct this with appropriate lid surgery. For a deepened superior sulcus one could remove the skin and some orbital fat from the contralateral eye and elevate the crease to provide symmetry.

Of the 53 cases of orbital fracture seen at the University of British Columbia Orbital Clinic, 33 were blow-out fractures. The most common presenting symptom was diplopia in 25 patients. Thirteen of these demonstrated restricted extraocular excursions. Ten patients presented with infraorbital hypesthesia. Enophthalmos of more than 2 mm was present initially in six patients, and subsequently in three others. Two patients presented with proptosis, three with ptosis, and another three with orbital emphysema. Surgery was necessary in 13 cases with the following indications: enophthalmos in six cases, strabismus with enophthalmos in three, and one case each of orbital hemorrhage, decreased visual acuity, removal of bony spurs, and a large defect in the floor. Eight patients showed definite improvement following surgery whereas two others did not. Complications in 13 cases operated on included one case of muscle imbalance following repair with Sialastic implant and one case of implant extrusion. Of the 20 cases managed conservatively, six had improvement of initial symptoms. Two patients had worsened enophthalmos, and 12 did not return for follow up after initial improvement.

Zygomatic Fractures

Zygomatic fractures (Fig. 13-43) usually result from a lateral blow on the cheek. They are also referred to as tripod or tripartite fractures because of dislocation of the zygoma from the frontal bone above, the arch laterally, and the maxilla medially. The fracture usually extends posteriorly into the floor of the orbit and may result in symptoms of a blow-out. The incidence of blow-out fractures with zygomatic injuries is between 33% and 41%. If the zygoma is displaced posteriorly, a step-like deformity and tenderness of the inferior orbital rim may be noted. There may be edema and depression of the normal convexity of the cheek with ecchymosis, unilateral epistaxis, and emphysema. If there is rotation of the fracture, the level of the globe or lateral canthus, or both, will be altered.

Five trimalar fractures were evaluated at the University of British Columbia Orbital clinic. The etiology in two was direct fist injury, in one a fall, in one a hockey puck, and in the fifth a direct blow with a hammer.

Initial presenting signs included malar flattening in two, a step deformity in a third, and swelling and ecchymosis around the orbit in the remaining two. Two of these patients had decreased visual acuity to less than 20/100, secondary to a ruptured globe in one and a macular hole in the other. Surgical repair was necessary in four of the five cases.

Indications for surgical treatment are trismus (inability to open the mouth) and unacceptable facial asymmetry. Undisplaced fractures require no treatment.

Le Fort Fractures

Fractures involving the maxilla have been divided into three groups (Fig. 13-44):

- Le Fort I is a low transverse maxillary fracture above the teeth with no orbital involvement.
- Le Fort II has a pyramidal configuration including nasal, lacrimal, and maxillary bones. These involve the medial orbital floors (which also may be blown out).
- Le Fort III involves craniofacial dysjunction in which the entire facial skeleton is detached from the base of the skull and suspended only by soft tissues. They involve the medial and lateral orbital walls and orbital floor.

Thus, fractures of the central third of the facial skeleton (Le Fort II and III types) may involve the orbit. They are often asymmetric.

Six patients presented with fractures involving more than one orbital wall, including two Le Fort III fractures. Three of these were caused by motor vehicle accidents, one by an industrial accident, one by a fall, and one by a blow to the face. All six required surgical intervention.

Midfacial Fractures

Comminuted naso-orbital-ethmoidal fractures are one of the most common patterns affecting the facial skeleton. A force that fractures the nasal bones usually fractures the medial orbital walls, ethmoid sinuses, and cribriform plate (which may result in CSF rhinorrhea) (Fig. 13-45). The most common etiology is a dashboard injury. In minor injuries only the nasal bones and frontal processes of the maxillae are displaced posteriorly and impacted into the interorbital space, collapsing and spreading internally (Fig. 13-46). In more severe trauma the lacrimal and ethmoid bones crumble and telescope, leading to hypertelorism and associated displacement of the medial canthal ligaments with telecanthus (see Fig. 13-33). Severe epistaxis may result from laceration or avulsion of the anterior ethmoid artery. A rare late complication of nasal fracture is incarceration of mucosa with failure of union, which leads to recurrent hemorrhage into the adjacent soft tissues leading to ecchymosis and hemosiderin deposition (Fig. 13-47).

Clinically, the patient usually presents with a flattened bridge of the nose and swollen medial canthal areas. Dacryostenosis is a common complication.

Treatment of these injuries should be done at one time and consists of correction of the epicanthal folds, restoration of bony contour, repair of the lacrimal system, and medial canthoplasty.

Orbital Apex Fractures

Orbital apex fractures occur alone or in combination with other facial fractures. Injury to the optic nerve with loss of vision, CSF leaks, and carotid cavernous fistulas *(Text continues on p. 518.)*

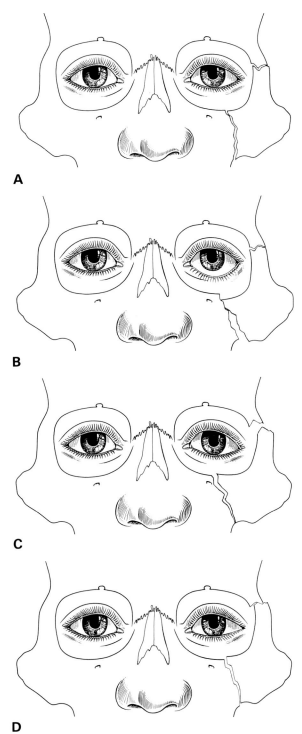

A

B

C

D

FIGURE 13-43. Schematic demonstrates the ocular features of trimalar fractures. *(A)* An undisplaced fracture does not change the lid or eye position. *(B)* Rotation of the inferolateral orbital margin causes inferior lateral scleral show. *(C)* A downward displacement of the fragment pulls the lateral canthus down. *(D)* Upward displacement causes elevation of the canthus and stretching and flattening of the lateral lid.

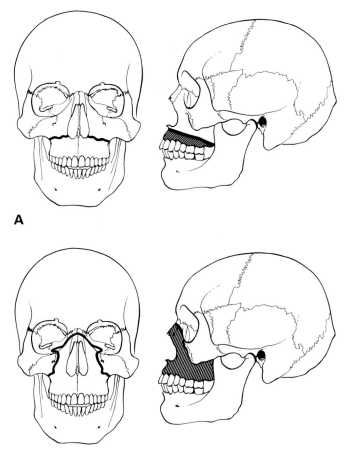

A

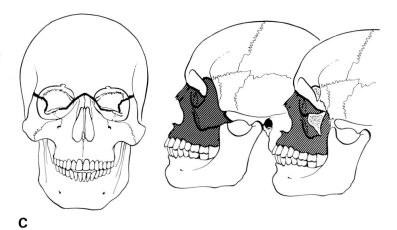

B

C

FIGURE 13-44. Le Fort fractures: *(A)* Le Fort I; *(B)* Le Fort II; *(C)* Le Fort III.

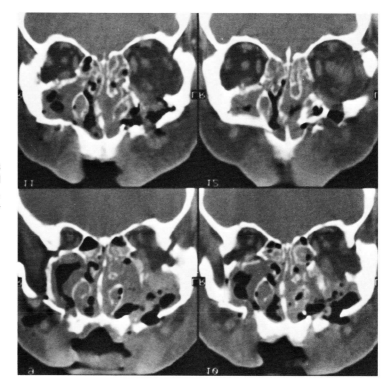

FIGURE 13-45. Composite coronal CT scans demonstrate a midfacial fracture with bilateral disruption of the ethmoid and maxillary sinuses, nasal structures, and orbital floors. Note the lateral zygomatic fracture on the left side.

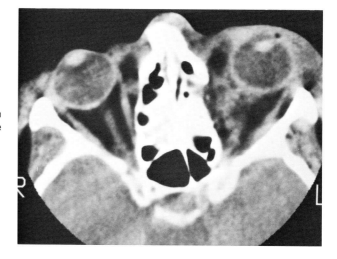

FIGURE 13-46. Axial CT scan of a midfacial smash, with collapse of the ethmoid sinuses and hemorrhage into the medial half of the left orbit.

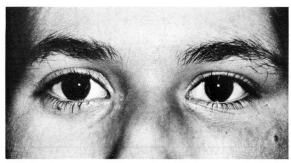

FIGURE 13-47. Clinical photograph of a patient who presented with recurrent bilateral lid and nasal ecchymosis with brownish discoloration of the nose. This was due to recurrent subcuticular hemorrhage from incarcerated nasal mucosa in the fracture site.

are possible associated complications. The diagnosis of a fracture of the optic canal is facilitated by CT scan. Conventional views will also show a linear fracture of the frontal or temporal bones or of the lesser wing of the sphenoid, which has extended into this region.

Orbital Roof Fractures

Orbital roof fractures may also involve the brain, cribriform plate, and the frontal sinuses. They are usually caused by missiles or blunt trauma. Orbital roof fractures may be divided into three types. The first involves the medial third of the rim, the anterior wall of the frontal sinus, and the subjacent area of the orbital roof (Fig. 13-48). Extension through the posterior wall of the frontal sinus into the anterior cranial fossa may occur. The second type involves the lateral third of the rim, which is weakened by the lacrimal fossa. The last type involves the central third and may be associated with a fracture of the frontal bone.

These fractures are dangerous because of potential complications including intracranial hemorrhage, infection, CSF rhinorrhea, pulsating exophthalmos, ptosis, pneumocephalus, and injuries to the optic nerve and lacrimal gland. If the trochlea is involved diplopia may ensue. The patients may also experience painful limitation of upgaze due to downward displaced bone fragments.

The brain often sustains a concussion injury and may even be lacerated if there is a comminuted fracture. The supraorbital rim may be depressed with a step-like deformity and may demonstrate point tenderness. Delayed onset of eyelid ecchymosis may follow a roof fracture. Persons with large frontal sinuses are more susceptible. Management of these fractures should use a team approach with a neurosurgeon and ophthalmologist. Four cases of orbital roof fracture were referred to the University of British Columbia Orbital Clinic. One of the four

required open reduction, whereas the other three were treated conservatively and recovered uneventfully.

ORBITAL FOREIGN BODIES

Foreign bodies may enter the orbit either by traversing between the globe and the orbital wall or by double perforation of the globe, as occurs in 7% of intraocular foreign bodies. It should always be kept in mind that there may be more than one foreign body present. Any laceration or puncture site should be explored for a foreign body.

Orbital foreign bodies are usually dormant and well tolerated. Exceptions to this are copper and organic matter. Copper can incite a purulent inflammatory response even after variable periods of quiescence. Organic foreign bodies such as wood or vegetable matter cannot be seen on conventional x-rays, and CT scan may be helpful in localizing them. If left in the orbit, they can produce cellulitis, granuloma, fistula to the skin or conjunctiva, abscess, osteomyelitis, or periostitis. Organic foreign bodies may also present with serious late complications, such as brain abscess.

A careful history must be obtained because often the initial incident is forgotten. Management depends on the composition, size, and shape of the foreign body and accurate localization by use of plain orbital x-rays, bone free film, or CT scans, or all three (Figs. 13-49 and 13-50). Ultrasonography is of limited value because it may be difficult to differentiate some foreign bodies from traumatized orbital fat. If there is a fistula, a foreign body may sometimes be located surgically by following the fistu-

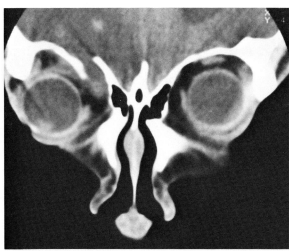

FIGURE 13-48. Coronal CT scan of an orbital roof fracture with a traumatic encephalocele.

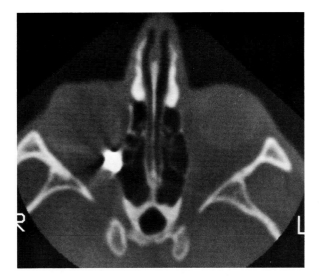

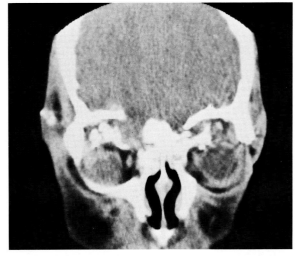

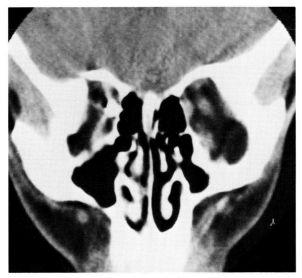

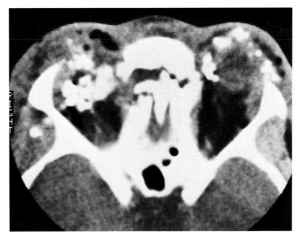

FIGURE 13-50. Coronal and axial CT scans of multiple foreign bodies in the orbit associated with a gunshot injury.

FIGURE 13-49. Axial and coronal CT scans show a metallic foreign body in the orbit following an air gun injury. It caused pressure on the optic nerve. The foreign body was removed surgically, and visual field returned to normal.

lous tract posteriorly. It should be noted in passing that magnetic resonance imaging cannot be used in the presence of a suspected magnetic foreign body, because magnetic fragments may move in the magnetic field and damage critical structures. Once the extent of ocular and orbital damage is assessed, a decision must be made whether or not to remove it. Because there is a good prognosis and removal can be difficult, treatment should be conservative unless there is a severe inflammatory reaction or a compressive effect on a vital orbital structure. Objects located in the orbit posterior to the equator

should be left alone to prevent iatrogenic damage. Inert, smooth-edged objects should also be observed. Generally, foreign bodies should be removed if superficial and anterior in location, if they have sharp edges (that threaten adjacent structures), or if they are composed of organic matter or copper. Removal should be as atraumatic as possible to prevent further damage and fragmentation of the object. It is important to explore the complete extent of injury, and cultures should be obtained.

It must be remembered that a foreign body may enter the orbit and penetrate to the paranasal sinuses, nose, or intracranial cavity (by means of the superior orbital fissure or roof). There is an increased risk of direct penetration of a foreign body into the anterior fossa in children due to the absence of a frontal sinus. This can lead to

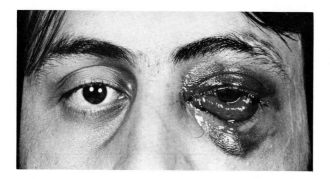

FIGURE 13-51.   Massive orbital tension with chemosis, ecchymosis, and marked proptosis following blunt trauma to the orbit. The patient had raised intraocular pressure, a pulsating central retinal artery, and fixation of the globe with decreasing vision. Treatment by urgent lateral canthotomy restored vision and intraocular pressure immediately.

further damage and serious sequelae. There may not be a fracture evident on x-ray. In a series of 42 transorbital cranial wounds, Webster and co-workers reported a 12% mortality rate. Immediate and delayed neurological complications should always be anticipated.

MANAGEMENT OF CATASTROPHIC DECREASE OF VISION FOLLOWING TRAUMA

Orbital hemorrhage is often associated with an underlying fracture or contusion injury and is divided into five types, as noted in the discussion of Soft Tissue Injury and Orbital Hemorrhage. Hemorrhage in the eyelid anterior to the orbital septum spreads easily, may cause considerable swelling, and extend across the bridge of the nose to the other side. Deep orbital hemorrhage may produce a limitation of extraocular movement or, if diffuse and in the muscle cone, a frozen globe. It may present with sudden pain, loss of vision, and explosive proptosis, with a dramatic increase in intraocular pressure and orbital tension (Fig. 13-51). The optic nerve head may show arterial pulsation, which can antecede an arterial occlusion. There may be loss of the direct light response with preservation of the consensual reflex.

If the periorbita is damaged, the blood may extravasate to appear superficially in the lid or conjunctiva in contrast to subperiosteal or a contained hematoma, which typically present with the abrupt onset of unilateral proptosis and globe displacement or slowly progressive proptosis. Clinically, one may see choroidal striae on fundoscopy and forced ductions may be negative. CT scan may show a mass with a central nonenhancing area of low density surrounded by a thin, isodense soft tissue rim that enhances. Ultrasonography demonstrates an extraconal well-demarcated lesion in the peripheral orbit. Depending on its location, it may interfere with neural structures in the superior orbital fissure or the optic nerve. It is usually of limited size due to the firm adher-

ence of the periorbita at bony suture lines. Significant orbital tension as a result of a subperiosteal hematoma may require urgent evacuation.

Penetrating trauma may result in laceration or avulsion of muscles or damage to nerve supply or both. Avulsion of rectus muscles may decrease the blood supply to the anterior segment and result in ischemic necrosis. An avulsed muscle may be difficult to find because it contracts towards the orbital apex. In searching for a lost muscle, one may note dimpling of Tenon's capsule when the dissected conjunctiva is stretched forward. Injecting Tenon's capsule with epinephrine may help to reduce vascularity and identify the contrasting red muscle.

Serious injury is more common with penetration of the medial upper lid than at other sites. Blunt objects need a greater force to enter the orbit, creating entry wounds larger than the size of the object. Sharp objects enter with minimal force and often the globe shifts away, preventing direct damage. High-speed missiles frequently perforate the globe before penetrating the orbit. A pointed object may even pass through the superior orbital fissure and pierce the internal carotid artery within the cavernous sinus, leading to a carotid-cavernous fistula.

Management of acute retrobulbar hemorrhage includes an emergent lateral canthotomy, antiglaucomatous agents, intermittent digital massage, and, if hemorrhage is severe, paracentesis of the anterior chamber. If there is a rapid accumulation of blood, an 18-gauge needle may be inserted through the lid to aspirate the blood. This may be done with ultrasound guidance. The use of retrobulbar hyaluronidase has been described, but runs a serious risk of increasing orbital tension acutely. An emergent surgical exploration or decompression of the orbit rarely becomes necessary. If there is no visual compromise, drainage is not necessary. Severe orbital swelling after trauma may lead to progressive proptosis, chemosis, and prolapse of conjunctiva. This requires careful monitoring of visual function and symptomatic therapy for prolapsed conjunctiva (with a moisture chamber).

Bibliography

DERMOID CYSTS

Cullen JF: Orbital diploic dermoids. Br J Ophthalmol 58:105, 1974

Grove AS, Jr: Orbital disorders: Diagnosis and management. In McCord CD, Jr (ed): Oculoplastic Surgery, p 274. New York, Raven Press, 1981

Grove AS, Jr: Giant dermoid cysts of the orbit. Ophthalmology 86:1513, 1979

Jones IS, Jakobiec FA, Nolan BT: Patient examination and introduction to orbital disease. In Duane TD (ed): Clinical Ophthalmology II: The Orbit, p 1. Philadelphia, Harper & Row, 1976

Kennedy RE: Marsupialization of inoperable orbital dermoids. Trans Am Opthalmol Soc 68:146, 1970

Moss HM: Expanding lesions of the orbit: A clinical study of 230 consecutive cases. Am J Ophthalmol 54:761, 1962

Pfeiffer RL, Nicholl RJ: Dermoid and epidermoid tumours of the orbit. Arch Ophthalmol 40:639, 1948

Pollard ZF, Calhoun MD. Deep orbital dermoid with draining sinus. Am J Ophthalmol 79:310, 1975

Sherman RP, Rootman J, LaPointe JS: Orbital dermoids: Clinical presentation and management. Br J Ophthalmol 68:642, 1984

MICROPHTHALMOS WITH CYST

Bonner J, Ide CH: Astrocytoma of the optic nerve and chiasm associated with microphthalmos and orbital cyst. Br J Ophthalmol 58:828, 1974

Dollfus MA, Marx P, Langlois J et al: Congenital cystic eyeball. Am J Ophthalmol 66:504, 1968

Ehlers N: Cryptophthalmos with orbito-palpebral cyst and microphthalmos: Report of a bilateral case. Acta Ophthalmol 44:84, 1966

Jensen OA: Microphthalmia with associated pseudogliomatosis of the retina and pseudogliomatous orbital cyst. Acta Ophthalmol 43:240, 1965

Kok-van Alphen CC, Manschot WA, Frederiks E et al: Microphthalmus and orbital cyst. Ophthalmologica 167:389, 1973

Makley TA, Jr, Battles M: Microphthalmos with cyst: Report of two cases in the same family. Surv Ophthalmol 13:200, 1969

Morada A, Eleinein GA, Elshiwy T: Formation of orbital cyst with microphthalmos. Bull Ophthalmol Soc Egypt 62:227, 1969

Waring GO, Roth AM, Rodrigues MM: Clinicopathologic correlation of microphthalmos with cyst. Am J Ophthalmol 82:714, 1976

CONGENITAL CYSTIC EYE

Baghdassarian SA, Tabbara KF, Matta CS: Congenital cystic eye. Am J Ophthalmol 76:269, 1973

Dollfus MA: Congenital cystic eyeball. Am J Ophthalmol 66:504, 1968

Helveston EM, Malone E, Jr, Lashmet MH: Congenital cystic eye. Arch Ophthalmol 84:622, 1970

Wilson RD, Traverse L, Hall JG et al: Oculocerebrocutaneous syndrome. Am J Ophthalmol 99:142, 1985

CEPHALOCELE

Clements DB, Kaushal K: A study of the ocular complications of hydrocephalus and meningomyelocele. Trans Ophthalmol Soc UK 90:383, 1970

Consul BN, Kulshrestha OP: Orbital meningocele. Br J Ophthalmol 49:374, 1965

Dvorak-Theobald G, Middleton WH: Congenital cyst of the optic nerve with encephalocele. Trans Am Acad Ophthalmol Otolaryngol 55:277, 1951

Leone CR, Jr, Marlowe JF: Orbital presentation of an ethmoidal encephalocele. Arch Ophthalmol 83:445, 1970

Mortada A: Pulsating frontocele and exophthalmos. Am J Ophthalmol 65:425, 1968

Pollock JA, Newton TH, Hoyt WF: Transsphenoidal and transethmoidal encephaloceles: A review of clinical and roentgen features in 8 cases. Radiology 90:442, 1968

Rothstein TB, Romano P, Shoch D: Meningomyelocoele-associated ocular abnormalities. Trans Am Ophthalmol Soc 71:287, 1973

Strandberg B: Cephalocele of posterior part of orbit. Arch Ophthalmol 42:254, 1949

LACRIMAL ECTOPIA

Baldridge M: Aberrant lacrimal gland in the orbit. Arch Ophthalmol 84:748, 1970

Green W, Zimmerman L: Ectopic lacrimal gland tissue: Report of eight cases with orbital involvement. Arch Ophthalmol 78:318, 1967

ORBITAL TERATOMA

Alkmade PP: Congenital teratoma of the orbit. Ophthalmologica 173:274, 1976

Appalanarasayya K, Devi O: Teratoma of the orbit. Int Surg 54:301, 1970

Ashley D: Origin of teratomas. Cancer 32:390, 1973

Barber JC, Barber LF, Guerry D, III et al: Congenital orbital teratoma. Arch Ophthalmol 91:45, 1974

Barishak YR, Mashiah M: Congenital teratoma of the orbit. J Pediatr Ophthalmol 14:217, 1977

Chang DF, Dallow RL, Walton DS: Congenital orbital teratoma: Report of a case with visual preservation. J Pediatr Ophthalmol Strabismus 17:88, 1980

Duke-Elder S: System of Ophthalmology, Normal and Abnormal Development, Congenital Deformities. St Louis, CV Mosby 3, No. 2:967, 1963

Ede EH, Davis WE, Block SPW: Orbital teratoma. Arch Ophthalmol 96:1093, 1978

Ferry AP: Teratoma of the orbit: A report of two cases. Surv Ophthalmol 10:434, 1965

Howard GM: Congenital teratoma of the orbit. Arch Ophthalmol 73:350, 1965

Hoyt WF, Joe S: Congenital teratoid cyst of the orbit: A case report and review of the literature. Arch Ophthalmol 68:196, 1962

Jensen OA: Teratoma of the orbit. Acta Ophthalmol 47:317, 1969

Levin ML, Leone CR, Kinkaid MC: Congenital orbital teratomas. AJO 102:476, 1986

Mamalis N, Garland PE, Argyle JC et al: Congenital orbital teratoma: A review and report of two cases. Surv Ophthalmol 30, No. 1:41, 1985

Mortada A: Orbital teratoma. Br J Ophthalmol 55:639, 1971

Saradarian AU: Malignant teratoma of the orbit: Six and one half years' observation. Arch Ophthalmol 37:253, 1947

Simonsen AH, Sogaard H: Teratoma orbitae: Report of a case. Acta Ophthalmol [Copenh] 59:308, 1981

Sinniah D, Prathop K, Somasundram K: Teratoma in infancy and childhood. Cancer 46:630, 1980

MUCOCELE

Alberti PW, Marshall HF, Black JI: Fronto-ethmoidal mucocele as a cause of unilateral proptosis. Br J Ophthalmol 52:833, 1968

Coleman D, Jack R, Franzen L: B-scan ultrasonography of orbital mucocoeles. Eye Ear Nose Throat Mon 51:207, 1972

Guerry R, Smith J: Paranasal sinus carcinoma causing orbital mucocele. Am J Ophthalmol 80:943, 1975

Iliff CE: Mucoceles in the orbit. Arch Ophthalmol 89:392, 1973

Johnson LN, Heplen RS, Yee RD et al: Sphenoid sinus mucocele (anterior clinoid variant) mimicking diabetic ophthalmoplegia and retrobulbar neuritis. AJO 102:111, 1986

Jones HM: Some orbital complications of nose and throat conditions. JR Med Soc 74:409, 1981

Leone CR, Marlowe JF: Orbital presentation of an ethmoidal encephalocele. Arch Ophthalmol 83:445, 1970

Mohan H, Sen KD, Gupta DK: Orbital affection in nasal and paranasal neoplasms. Acta Ophthalmol 47:289, 1969

Montogomery WW: Mucocele of the maxillary sinus causing enophthalmos. Eye Ear Nose Throat Mon 43:41, 1964

Mortada A: Exophthalmos and posterior frontocele with fibrous wall on orbital side. Am J Ophthalmol 72:701, 1971

Pollock J, Newton T, Hoyt W: Trans-sphenoidal and transethmoidal encephaloceles. Radiology 90:442, 1968

Reese AB: Expanding lesions of the orbit. Trans Ophthalmol Soc UK 63:85, 1971

Robertson DM, Henderson JW: Unilateral proptosis secondary to orbital mucocele in infancy. Am J Ophthalmol 68:845, 1969

Silva D: Orbital tumors. Am J Ophthalmol 65:318, 1968

Stanton MB: Sphenoid sinus mucocele. Am J Ophthalmol 70:991, 1970

Stool S, Kertesz E, Sibinga M et al: Exophthalmos due to pyocele of the sinus in children with cystic fibrosis. Trans Am Acad Ophthalmol Otolaryngol 70:811, 1966

Tenzel RR, Gross J: Anterior ethmoidal mucocele presenting in the orbit. Am J Ophthalmol 62:160, 1966

Valvassori GE, Putterman AM: Ophthalmological and radiological findings in sphenoidal mucoceles. Arch Ophthalmol 90:456, 1973

Von Leden H: Orbital mucoceles. Can J Ophthalmol 1:36, 1966

Zizmor J, Fasano CV, Smith B et al: Roentgenographic diagnosis of unilateral exophthalmos. JAMA 197:343, 1966

LACRIMAL DUCTAL CYSTS

Duke-Elder S, MacFaul PA: The ocular adnexa. In Duke-Elder S (ed): System of Ophthalmology, Vol 13, p. 638. St. Louis, CV Mosby, 1974

Duran JA, Cuevas J: Cyst of accessory lacrimal gland. Br. J Ophthalmol 67:485, 1983

Green WR, Zimmerman LE: Ectopic lacrimal gland tissue. Arch Ophthalmol 78:318, 1967

Harris: GJ; Marsupialization of a lacrimal gland cyst. Ophthalmic Surg 14:75, 1983

Rush A, Leone CR, Jr: Ectopic lacrimal gland cyst of the orbit. Am J Ophthalmol 92:198, 1981

Sen KD, Thomas A: Simple dacryops. Am J Ophthalmol 63:161, 1967

Smith S, Rootman J: Lacrimal ductal cysts: Presentation and management. Surv Ophthalmol 30:245, 1986

TRAUMA

Anderson DP, Ford RM: Visual abnormalities after severe head injuries. Can J Surg 23:163, 1980

Anderson RL, Panje WR, Gross CE: Optic nerve blindness following blunt forehead trauma. Ophthalmology 89:445, 1982

Berkowitz RA, Putterman AM, Patel DB: Prolapse of the globe into the maxillary sinus after orbital floor fracture. Am J Ophthalmol 91:253, 1981

Brock L, Tanenbaum HL: Retention of wooden foreign bodies in the orbit. Can J Qphthalmol 15:70, 1980

Cabbabe EB, Shively RE, Malik P: Cranioplasty for traumatic deformities of the frontoorbital area. Ann Plast Surg 13:175, 1984

Callahan M, Callahan A: Ophthalmic Plastic and Orbital Surgery. Birmingham, Aesculapius, 1979

Converse JM, Smith B et al: Orbital blowout fractures: A ten-year survey. Plast Reconstr Surg 39:20, 1967

Emery JM, von Noorden GK, Schlernitzauer DA: Orbital floor fractures: Long-term follow-up of cases with and without surgical repair. Trans Am Acad Ophthalmol Otolaryngol 75:802, 1971

Finkle Dr, Ringler SL et al: Comparison of the diagnostic methods used in maxillofacial trauma. Plast Reconstr Surg 75:32, 1985

Flanagan JC, McLachlan DL, Shannon GM: Orbital roof fractures. Ophthalmology 87:325, 1980

Gilbard SM, Mafee MF et al: Orbital blowout fractures. Ophthalmology 92:1523, 1985

Godoy J, Mathog RH: Malar fractures associated with exophthalmos. Arch Otolaryngol 111:174, 1985

Greenwald HS, Keeney AR, Shannon GM: A review of 128 patients with orbital fractures. Am J Ophthalmol 78:655, 1974

Grove AS, Jr: New diagnostic techniques for the evaluation of orbital trauma. Trans Am Acad Ophthalmol Otolaryngol 83:626, 1977

Grove AS, Jr, Tadmor R et al: Orbital fracture evaluation by coronal computed tomography. Am J Ophthalmol 85:679, 1978

Hoffman JR, Neuhaus RW, Baylis HI: Penetrating orbital trauma. Am J Emergen Med 1:22, 1983

Holtmann, B, Wray RC, Little AG: A randomized comparison of four incisions for orbital fractures. Plast Reconstr Surg 67:731, 1981

Klingele TG, Gado MH, Burde RM et al: Compression of the anterior visual system by the gyrus rectus. J Neurosurg 55:272, 1981

Koornneef L: Current concepts on the management of orbital blow-out fractures Ann Plast Surg 9:185, 1982

Miller GR, Tenzel RR: Ocular complications of midfacial fractures. Plast Reconst Surg 39:37, 1967

Mustarde JR: Repair and Reconstruction in the Orbital Region. Baltimore, Williams & Wilkins, 1966

Paton D, Goldberg MF: Management of Ocular Injuries. Philadelphia, WB Saunders, 1985

Pope-Pegram LD, Hamill MB: Post-traumatic subgaleal hematoma with subperiosteal orbital extension. Surv Ophthalmol 30:258, 1986

Putterman AM: Blow-out fractures of the orbital floor: Interview. Ophthalmic Plast Reconstr Surg 1:33, 1985

Putterman AM: Late management of blow-out fractures of the orbital floor. Trans Am Acad Ophthalmol Otolaryngol 83:OP650, 1977

Putterman AM, Stevens T, Urist MJ: Nonsurgical management of blow-out fractures of the orbital floor. Am J Ophthalmol 77:232, 1974

Seiff SR, Berger MS et al: Computed tomographic evaluation of the optic canal in sudden traumatic blindness. Am J Ophthalmol 98:751, 1984

Sheffield RW: Facial fractures I. Selected Readings Plast Surg 3:1, 1985

Smith B, Grove AS, Jr, Guibor P: Fractures of the orbit. In Duane TD (ed): Clinical Ophthalmology, Chap 48. Philadelphia, Harper & Row, 1976

Smith B, Regan WF: Blow-out fracture of the orbit. Am J Ophthalmol 44:733, 1957

Stewart DJ, Polomeno RC: Total transient visual loss and orbital foreign bodies. Can J Ophthalmol 14:95, 1979

Stewart W (ed): Ophthalmic Plastic and Reconstructive Surgery. San Francisco, American Academy of Ophthalmology, 1984

Wessberg GA, Wolford LM et al: Ophthalmologic considerations in maxillofacial trauma. Int J Oral Surg 10:236, 1981

Wilkins RB, Havins, WE: Current treatment of blow-out fractures. Ophthalmology 89:464, 1982

Zbylski JR: Reconstruction of the war-damaged orbital region. Clin Plast Surg 2:523, 1975

CHAPTER 14

Vascular Lesions

Jack Rootman and Douglas A. Graeb

Vascular lesions of the orbit produce distinct clinical, radiologic, and histopathologic findings that reflect their relationship to, or origin from, the vascular system. The group encompasses a broad range of entities originating from the vascular anlage including tumors, shunts, anomalies, aneurysms, and obstructive lesions.

The pathophysiology, and hence the clinical presentation, are largely determined by the hemodynamic alterations. Although some overlap exists, most of these lesions can be understood in terms of the abnormal hemodynamics unique to each.

Most lesions present with mass effect, which may be positive (proptosis or displacement of the globe), negative (enophthalmos), or intermittent (the pulsatile exophthalmos of posttraumatic carotid-cavernous fistulas, or the proptosis seen with the Valsalva maneuver in some venous malformations).

The specific symptoms tend to reflect the underlying hemodynamics. Lesions associated with a rapid shunt of blood from the arterial to the venous system are characterized by pulsatile bruit, visible and palpable orbital pulsations, and the effects of increased orbital venous pressure (dilatation of episcleral veins, elevation of intraocular pressure, chemosis, orbital tissue swelling, and engorgement of the retinal circulation).

Lesions in which the arteriovenous shunt is less vigorous generally present with milder symptoms and signs. Exophthalmos may be present but is generally nonpulsatile; bruit is frequently absent, and elevation of intraocular pressure is less severe. However, these low-flow shunts are prone to the development of episodes of venous thrombosis, which may either alleviate or aggravate the symptoms depending upon the alteration in hemodynamics produced by such an event.

Of the venous anomalies, some will distend markedly with elevation in venous pressure produced by dependence or the Valsalva maneuver. Others appear to lack significant venous connections and do not respond to changes in venous pressure. These lesions are more often characterized by spontaneous hemorrhage with episodic swelling and features of tissue extravasation.

In summary, the clinical features that lead one to suspect a lesion of vascular origin are individual features or combinations of tumefaction, vascular engorgement (due either to arteriovenous shunting or venous thrombosis), spontaneous hemorrhage (with or without history of an antecedent anomaly), orbital pulsation, and intermittent exophthalmos.

■ TUMORS

We have divided the vascular tumors into hamartomas and neoplasms. All are characterized by development of mass effect, which is modified by their hemodynamic characteristics. Tumors may have high flow (infantile hemangiomas), low flow (cavernous hemangiomas), or reflect little or no flow (lymphangiomas and some solid neoplasms). Malignant lesions may be complicated by local infiltrative features in addition to the mass and hemodynamic effect.

Hamartomas

Although nosologic argument exists, we have classified hemangiomas and lymphangiomas as hamartomas rather than neoplasms. Infantile hemangiomas have a history of rapid onset and a rich blood supply with or without dermal and/or systemic features. On the other hand, cavernous hemangiomas are generally seen in adults and tend to present as slow-growing masses with clinical and radiologic features of a minimal blood supply. In our experience, lymphangiomas appear to lack systemic vascular connections and are characterized by bouts of recurrent hemorrhage with or without associated dermal or mucosal lesions.

HEMANGIOMAS

Infantile Capillary Hemangioma

Infantile capillary hemangiomas represent an abnormal growth of blood vessels dominated by varying degrees of endothelial proliferation. The more endotheliomatous lesions generally demonstrate more rapid growth and re-

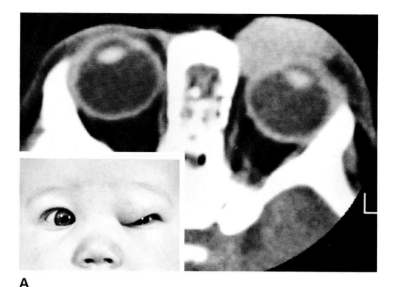

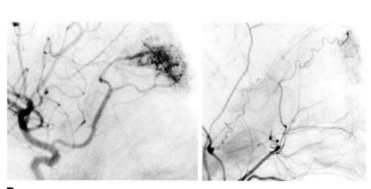

A

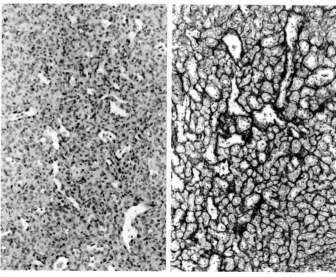

B

C

FIGURE 14-1. *(A)* This 11-month-old infant had a history of a left upper lid mass, noted at 10 weeks of age. The size of the mass increased rapidly over 6 weeks. It was a rubbery, slightly violaceous tumor of the upper lid and anterior orbit behind the septum. It was associated with 4 D of astigmatism, and the child acted amblyopic. Contrast-enhanced CT scan demonstrates a uniformly enhancing, smooth, contoured mass displacing the globe posteriorly. Failure to respond to corticosteroids and the child's significant astigmatism led to excision of the mass under hypotensive anesthesia. *(B)* Preoperative angiography of the mass demonstrates rapid filling of a fine vascular network primarily supplied by the internal carotid system *(left)* with minor external carotid supply *(right)*. *(C, left)* Photomicrograph of lesions shown in *A* and *B* demonstrates a dense hypercellular net of fine endothelially lined vascular channels (hematoxylin-eosin, original magnification × 10). *(Right)* Reticulin stain demonstrates the organization of the capillary channels characteristic of infantile hemangiomas (reticulin, original magnification × 10).

gression. The endothelial cells are organized into a network of basement membrane-lined vascular channels of varying density and size (Fig. 14-1C)

These lesions have a female predominance and usually present within the first months of life, starting as small flat foci that undergo rapid expansion over weeks to months and then typically involute. The involution may take months to years depending upon the size and histopathology (on average, three quarters of cases are involuted by age 7). Lesions undergoing involution are characterized histologically by fewer endothelial cells, larger and less numerous vascular channels, increasing collagen deposition, intralesional fat, and in some instances, inflammatory cell infiltrates (Fig. 14-2C). Many of these are associated with dermal hemangiomas in the head and neck and throughout the body, or with deep visceral capillary tumors. When visceral lesions are of great size, they may lead to sequestration of thrombocytes and red blood cells with attendant thrombocytopenia and bleeding diathesis (the Kasbach-Merritt syndrome).

Our series consisted of 23 infantile capillary hemangiomas, which were divided clinically into three subgroups on the basis of anatomic location and extent, including deep, superficial, and combined hemangiomas (Table 14-1). The superficial infantile capillary hemangioma affects the lid or conjunctival surface alone; deep lesions affect the orbit behind the septum; combined lesions involve both superficial and deep components (Fig. 14-3).

Deep Infantile Hemangioma

The deep infantile hemangiomas are defined as lying posterior to the orbital septum, and may therefore lie in the deep tissues of the lid and anterior orbit or may occur solely within the deep orbit (Figs. 14-1, 14-2, and 14-4). The main clinical features of proptosis or displacement of the globe are caused by their mass effect. Because of their rich blood supply, some will exhibit subtle pulsation if one examines carefully for this feature. They may also enlarge with crying or the Valsalva maneuver. Obvious dilatation of the overlying lid or facial vessels and a blue-violet discoloration of the lids or conjunctiva may be noted. When palpable through the lid, they have a rubbery consistency and a smooth contour. The size and location of these lesions often produce distortion or obstruction of the visual axis with subsequent amblyopia and strabismus. The associated refractive abnormalities have been astigmatism and myopia, and may be of sufficient degree to lead to significant risk of amblyopia if not recognized and treated.

On CT scan, the margins of these lesions vary from moderately well-defined to infiltrating. They may occur in any compartment and frequently cross boundaries, being both intraconal and extraconal, postseptal and pre-septal. Those with a significant deep component cause displacement and occasionally indentation of the globe. The enhancement seen with intravenous contrast varies from moderate to intense, and may be homogeneous or inhomogeneous (see Figs. 14-1 and 14-2). This variable enhancement pattern presumably reflects the changing histology of these lesions as they involute, with the less intense, more inhomogeneous pattern being seen in lesions undergoing involution. We have not seen calcification in these lesions.

B-scan ultrasonography demonstrates either a smooth lobular or irregular contour and high echogenicity. A-scan reveals some irregularity, due to vascular spaces and septae with low to medium internal reflectivity and high spikes produced by the septae. Blood flow is frequently fast and may be demonstrated on Doppler echography.

At angiography, these lesions frequently have multiple feeding vessels from both the ophthalmic artery and external carotid branches (see Fig. 14-1). The feeding vessels are frequently enlarged and early draining veins are often demonstrated, reflecting a hemodynamically rapid circulation through the tumor (see Fig. 14-2). The tumor mass generally opacifies densely, although less vascular areas may be seen, presumably due to involution (see Fig. 14-2B).

Management. The vast majority of deep infantile hemangiomas regress; therefore, this outcome can usually be awaited without surgical intervention. However, larger lesions with considerable proptosis or with associated astigmatism or visual axis obstruction may require more aggressive treatment. A number of modalities have been tried, including radiotherapy (radon seed implantation or external beam therapy), systemic and local corticosteroids (see Fig. 14-2), and surgery. In the presence of very large platelet-consuming lesions associated with the Kasabach-Merrit syndrome, systemic antifibrinolytic agents are used, including aminocaproic acid or tranexamic acid. Both the systemic corticosteroids and antifibrinolytic agents should be monitored under the care of a pediatrician familiar with their use. We use systemic and locally injected corticosteroids in the case of large nonresectable lesions or to shrink resectable lesions. The systemic dosage used is 1.5 mg/kg to 2.5 mg/kg prednisone daily over a few weeks with titration downward depending on response. Local injection is also used in doses of 40 mg to 80 mg triamcinolone with 25 mg methylprednisolone (Solu-Medrol) directly into the lesion. This produces local tension in the lesion, which rapidly dissipates and is usually followed by reduction in the size of the mass. In our experience, corticosteroids are effective in a high percentage of cases, but recurrence and regrowth with diminution of the steroid dose is not infrequent (a rebound phenomenon).

We have performed surgical resection in selected cir-

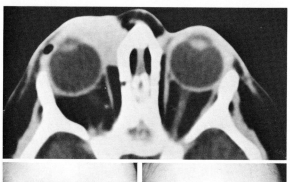
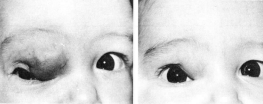
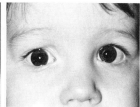

A

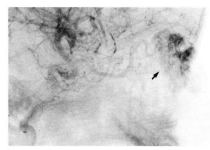
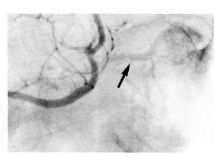

B

FIGURE 14-2. *(A)* Clinical photograph of an 11-month-old child demonstrates an anterior postseptal hemangioma *(left)*. It responded to corticosteroids *(center),* but rebounded and was associated with 5 D of astigmatism. Postoperative results of anterior resection *(right)* with return to emmetropia. CT scan shows a mass with distinct margins causing lateral and posterior displacement of the globe. *(B)* Angiography of the lesion shown in *A* demonstrates hyperdynamic blood flow through an enlarged ophthalmic artery, with rapid shunting into the superior ophthalmic vein *(right, large arrow)*. Note patchy (inhomogeneous) filling of the posterior portion reflecting regressive features *(left, small arrow)*. *(C)* Photomicrographs of the lesion shown in *A* and *B*. Evidence of maturation is demonstrated by larger channels, increased collagen, and intralesional fat deposition (hematoxylin-eosin, original magnification × 10).

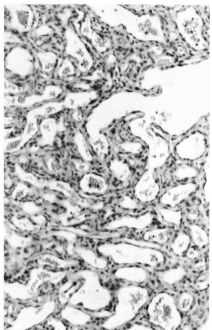
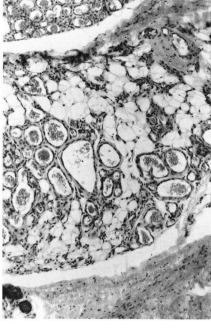

C

TABLE 14-1.
INFANTILE CAPILLARY HEMANGIOMAS, UNIVERSITY OF BRITISH COLUMBIA ORBITAL CLINIC, 1976–1985

Type	No.	Management	Follow-up
Deep	9	5 resected (3 primary and 2 following steroid failures)	Resolved
		4 observed	Partial resolution over 4–5 years
Superficial	7	Observed	Resolved over 2–3 years
Combined	7	Observed for resolution, then cosmetic surgery	Partial resolution over 4–5 years, followed by cosmetic surgery

cumstances (*i.e.*, significant threat to vision with failure to respond to corticosteroids, rebound on steroid withdrawal, and severe steroidal side-effects) or if the lesion is clearly isolated and well-defined with functional deficits. Operative removal requires detailed preoperative investigation (including systemic survey, CT, and angiography), hypotensive anesthesia, and meticulous surgical technique. In these circumstances, a controlled resection can be performed with constant hemostasis. At surgery, these tumors may have fine pseudopodal extensions, which can be cauterized or followed, depending upon the surrounding structures. These extensions frequently insinuated themselves between structures and required microdissection. Surgery has produced rapid resolution and gratifying results in these selected cases (see Fig. 14-2).

We have avoided the use of radiation because of the risk of long-term side-effects; however, several other institutions favor judicious use of either radon seed implantation or external beam therapy, and report clinical resolution.

Superficial Infantile Hemangioma

Superficial capillary hemangiomas are the so-called strawberry nevi and are confined to the dermis. They may be single or multiple, can occur anywhere on the body, and undergo the same pattern of growth and resolution described earlier. An important clinical feature that indicates resolution is the appearance in a previously vascular strawberrylike lesion of fine stellate areas of pale scarring (herald spot). It is very reassuring to point out this feature to the parents of affected children. These lesions are best treated with benign neglect when no functional abnormalities are associated. Larger hemangiomas may need therapy if they bleed frequently or lead to visual obstruction. Therapy may include steroids, dermal laser, cryotherapy, or radiotherapy.

Combined Infantile Hemangiomas

Combined hemangiomas have both dermal and deep components. Clinically, the dermal component is associated with a palpable deeper mass or displacement of the globe. When massive, these lesions are the most startling

and tragic of the infantile hemangiomas. The widespread involvement produces marked deformity of both the skin and the orbit, and they are frequently associated with amblyopia (Fig. 14-5). Management is again governed by the potential visual functional risks, and involves corticosteroids, systemic antifibrinolytic agents, selective angiographic embolization, or perhaps radiotherapy with adjunctive local measures. Cosmetic surgery for skin redundancy and persistent deformities should await resolution of the primary lesion. We have had seven cases of this type with long-term follow up, all of which were treated with cosmetic surgery following spontaneous resolution with reasonable cosmetic results (Fig. 14-6). (*Text continues on p. 532.*)

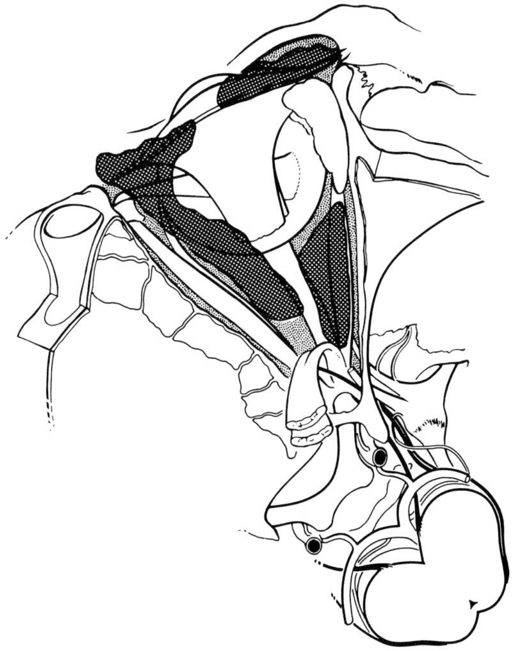

FIGURE 14-3. Schematic of orbit demonstrates major anatomic subtypes of vascular tumors, including superficial (cutaneous, preseptal, conjunctival); deep (behind the septum or intraconal); and combined with superficial and deep components.

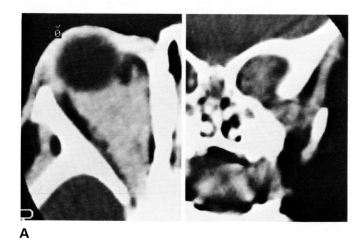

A

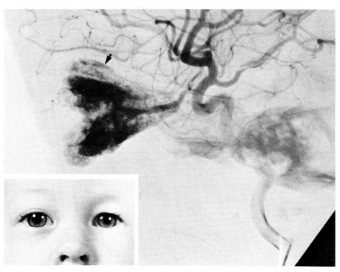

B

FIGURE 14-4. *(A)* Contrast-enhanced CT scan of a 5-month-old infant demonstrates right pulsatile proptosis due to the diffuse enhancing deep intraconal infantile hemangioma *(left)*. Coronal scan *(right)* demonstrates mass in the pterygopalatine fossa. *(B)* Internal carotid angiogram of the same patient demonstrates early dense opacification of a diffuse retrobulbar mass via an enlarged ophthalmic artery. The negative shadow is created by the superior muscle mass *(arrow)*. *(C)* The mass in the pterygopalatine fossa has a supply separate from the internal maxillary artery.

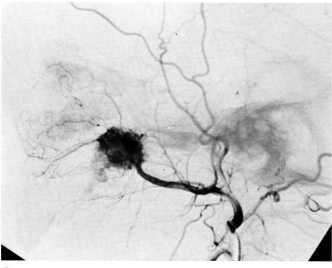

C

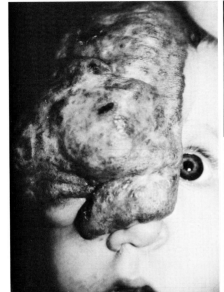
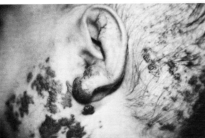
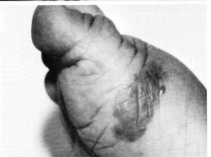

FIGURE 14-5. *(Left)* Clinical photographs demonstrate massive facial and orbital infantile capillary hemangioma. Note patchy stellate areas of pale scarring (herald spots) on the surface. *(Right)* Multiple capillary hemangioma involving the foot, head, and neck.

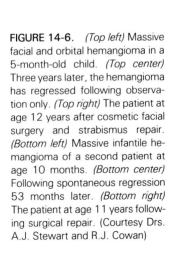
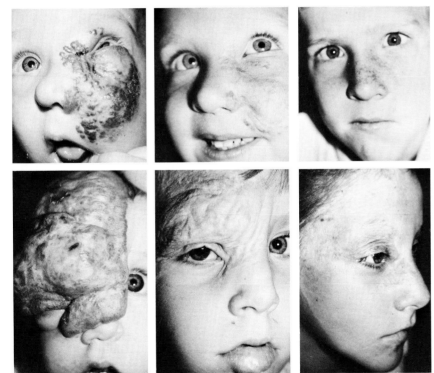

FIGURE 14-6. *(Top left)* Massive facial and orbital hemangioma in a 5-month-old child. *(Top center)* Three years later, the hemangioma has regressed following observation only. *(Top right)* The patient at age 12 years after cosmetic facial surgery and strabismus repair. *(Bottom left)* Massive infantile hemangioma of a second patient at age 10 months. *(Bottom center)* Following spontaneous regression 53 months later. *(Bottom right)* The patient at age 11 years following surgical repair. (Courtesy Drs. A.J. Stewart and R.J. Cowan)

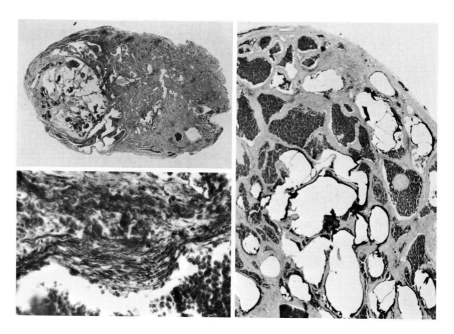

FIGURE 14-7. Photomicrographic series demonstrates the major histopathologic features of cavernous hemangioma: a fine capsule, large endothelially lined vascular channels with smooth muscle in the walls *(bottom left),* and variable density of stromal components *(top left).* Not all channels have filled with a radio-opaque contrast (dark rim) injected after removal of the tumor shown in Figure 14-9 *(top left:* hematoxylin-eosin, original magnification × 1; *bottom left:* phosphotungstic acid–hematoxylin demonstrating dark, smooth muscle fibers, original magnification × 40). *(Right)* After injection of radio-opaque dye, seen as dark rims in some of the vascular channels (hematoxylin-eosin, original magnification × 2.5).

Functional amblyopia was unfortunately present in all cases as a result of the profound alteration of visual axis associated with them. More radical therapy early in the course of this tumor has been advocated, but in our opinion may not produce better functional results and may be more disfiguring. No uniformly successful medical or surgical treatment exists for these massive lesions. Combined hemangiomas have a high attendant risk of amblyopia; therefore, intervention should be based on getting the best cosmetic result with the least risk to the child.

Cavernous Hemangiomas

Cavernous hemangiomas are benign noninfiltrative lesions that exert a slowly progressive mass effect. Histopathology reveals a fine capsule that surrounds a tumor consisting of large endothelially lined channels with abundant, loosely distributed smooth muscle in the vascular walls and stroma (Fig. 14-7).

Although they may undergo evolution with time, only a few in our series were noted to have evidence of scarring, hemosiderin deposition, or significant inflammatory infiltrates. Thus, sudden change reflecting either clinical evidence of inflammation or hemorrhage is the exception and not the rule; rather, the history is one of progressive slow mass effect.

We have seen 12 cavernous hemangiomas, all occurring in adults between the ages of 34 years and 70 years. These tumors are typically intraconal and cause little dysfunction other than that produced by mass effect (*i.e.,* proptosis, posterior pole indentation, and choroidal striae; Fig. 14-8). Because they grow very slowly, the patient is frequently unaware of the duration of the disease, but examination of old photographs often reveals prop-

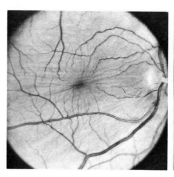

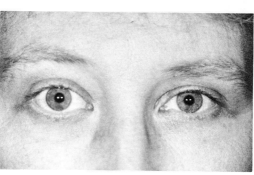

FIGURE 14-8. Left intraconal hemangioma caused posterior indentation and choroidal striae in a 39-year-old patient who had 4 mm of proptosis noted for 6 months and associated with a 2-D induced hyperopia.

tosis of many years' duration. Very large cavernous hemangiomas or those located within the orbital apex may, however, produce optic nerve compression, diplopia, or orbital pain (Fig. 14-9). Two of our patients had the unusual feature of transient amauroses in extremes of gaze due to optic nerve compression induced in this position.

CT scan typically shows a very well-defined oval or rounded intraconal mass with smooth margins, which enhances with intravenous contrast (Fig. 14-10). Occasionally, a small portion of the lesion extends to the extraconal compartment, but the greatest bulk of the tumor is almost always intraconal. The majority of lesions arise laterally and cause medial displacement of the optic nerve; proptosis is generally present and the posterior pole of the globe is frequently indented by the rounded anterior margin of the tumor. About one half of these lesions will show subtle outward bowing of the lateral orbital wall, consistent with a long-standing, slowly growing mass lesion (see Fig. 14-10A).

The enhancement pattern may be homogeneous or somewhat inhomogeneous with approximately equal frequency. The position of the nonenhancing optic nerve can be seen on good quality scans in the majority of cases; the nerve is typically displaced rather than surrounded by the tumor. Small areas of calcification are occasionally seen.

B-scan ultrasonography shows rounded, intraconal, well-circumscribed masses with well-delineated posterior surfaces (see Fig. 14-9C). The acoustic texture is echogenic and the adjacent extraocular muscles may be accentuated. A-scan shows medium reflectivity between regular highly reflective spikes and medium sound attenuation. The borders are usually well defined with a posterior high reflective spike marking the capsule.

Internal carotid angiography typically reveals a few small intratumoral collections or puddles of contrast, which appear late in the arterial phase and persist well into the venous phase (see Fig. 14-9C). The main tumor mass does not opacify. The ophthalmic artery and its branches may be displaced or stretched, but they are not enlarged and supply from external carotid branches is infrequent. Although this appearance is virtually pathognomonic for a cavernous hemangioma, angiography is rarely necessary for investigation. In occasional instances, however, puddling of contrast is not seen and the angiogram may be entirely normal or show only vascular displacement. A rare variant of this tumor has been described in the periorbital bones.

The clinical and angiographic features of cavernous hemangiomas confirm that they are low-flow lesions, in sharp contrast with the features of infantile capillary hemangiomas. Histopathologic confirmation of their low flow character is also seen by the presence of menisci in some vascular spaces, and evidence of decomposed blood. Because of their low flow character, cavernous hemangiomas may be punctured with impunity during surgery after careful exposure and isolation. In fact, this technique leads to exsanguination and shrinkage of the tumor, which facilitates its removal (Fig. 14-11).

Management. The cavernous hemangioma is a classic surgical lesion, and few orbital tumors are removed with greater ease and satisfaction. When exposed, the tumor is a plump, nodular, plum-colored mass with vascular channels on its well-defined surface. It can be removed by blunt dissection of the surface to free it of adjacent orbital structures. Any connecting vascular strands can then be easily identified and cauterized. There is frequently an apical vascular tag, which is best left to the final stage of the procedure because rupture earlier may cause more bleeding and obscure the field (see Fig. 14-11). When these vessels are transected, preferably at the end of removal, there may be a gush of blood, which can be controlled with simple gentle tamponade or can be avoided by identifying the vessels and using bipolar cautery.

LYMPHANGIOMAS

Lymphangiomas are hemodynamically isolated vascular hamartomas. The concept of this lesion in the orbit seems incongruous, because evidence suggests that the postseptal or deeper portions of the orbit do not normally have lymphatic channels. In spite of this, lymphangiomas have been consistently described in the orbit and have been the center of considerable controversy. In particular, separation of lymphangiomas from orbital varices has been a source of confusion. However, we believe the fundamental differentiation should be made on the basis of clinical, hemodynamic, and histopathologic criteria. The distinguishing characteristic of this group of lesions consists of relative hemodynamic isolation, which produces clinical features based on extent and location. Three patterns of occurrence have been noted based on location as superficial, deep, and combined (see Fig. 14-3). The location governs differences in clinical presentation, complications, and management. Histopathologically, lymphangiomas are better understood as a spectrum of vascular hamartomas with similar fundamental components and a relative hemodynamic isolation. The histopathologic features include diaphanous, serous-filled vascular channels, collagenous stromal network, features of recurrent and old hemorrhage, lymphorrhages (accumulations of lymphocytes), dysplastic vessels, and randomly occurring bundles of smooth muscle. For the most part, the endothelially lined channels contain serous fluid but may also contain an admixture of blood and blood products. The interstices generally consist of loose collagen, but include dense lymphorrhages and some randomly arranged smooth muscle as well (Fig.

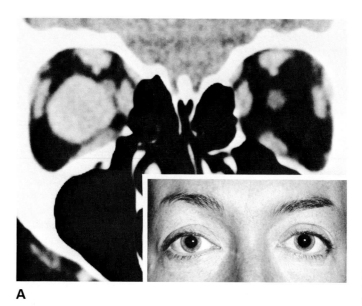

A

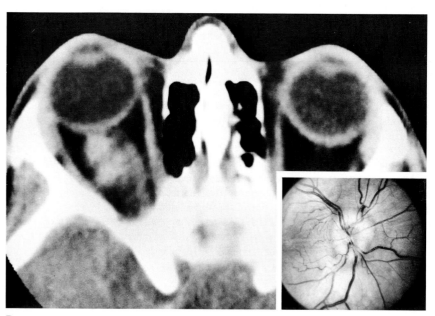

B

FIGURE 14-9. *(A)* Right orbital mass noted for 6 months proved on CT scan to consist of a well-defined intraconal enhancing lesion immediately behind the globe. *(A, B)* Note displacement of the optic nerve leading to disc swelling *(B, inset)* and obscured vision on right lateral gaze.

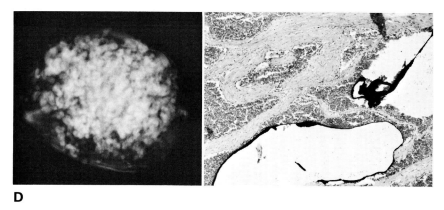

FIGURE 14-9 *(Continued).* *(C)* Venous phase of angiogram demonstrates the characteristic small "puddles" of contrast *(arrow)*. Ultrasonograms *(C, insets)* demonstrate a well-circumscribed echogenic mass on B-scan *(top)* with high and medium internal reflectivity and well-defined highly reflective borders on A-scan. *(D)* Specimen from the same patient injected with radio-opaque contrast after excision. Note interconnected vascular network not all of which has filled, as shown on the right and in Figure 14-7. This suggests multiple sources of blood supply (hematoxylin-eosin, original magnification × 10).

14-12*B*; also see Fig. 14-16). Ultrastructurally, a mixture of abnormal vessels is found, with characteristics of both blood and lymph vessels (see Fig. 14-17).

Superficial Lesions

Superficial lymphangiomas typically consist of a visible lesion of the conjunctiva or lid alone. They consist of multiple clear cystic structures or may contain an admixture of xanthochromic or partially blood-filled cysts. On the other hand, they may simply consist of a transilluminatable bluish cyst just beneath the skin. If cosmetically unacceptable they can be removed with relative ease because of their limited location and small size.

Deep Lesions

The deep lymphangiomas typically present with sudden proptosis due to spontaneous hemorrhage into what was a previously unrecognized lesion (see Fig. 14-12; Fig. 14-13). The majority in our experience occurred in childhood, and in all cases the clinical picture was similar. None demonstrated significant clinical features of either arterial or venous connection (*i.e.,* no change was noted on Valsalva maneuver or alteration of head position, nor was there a bruit or pulsation). Although the majority (five out of six) of those in this category presented with spontaneous hemorrhage, one of our cases developed gradually increasing proptosis and ptosis over several weeks. Half of our cases had significant compressive

(Text continues on p. 538.)

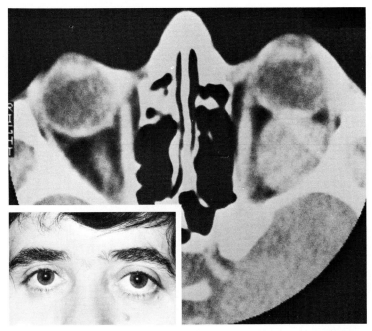

A

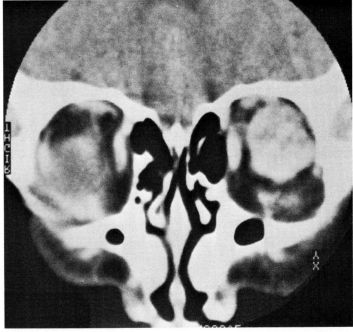

B

FIGURE 14-10. *(A)* Axial and *(B)* coronal CT scans following contrast injection show mottled enhancement of a well-defined left orbital cavernous hemangioma. It had been present in a 38-year-old woman for many years, and is demonstrated by the lateral bowing of the orbit *(A, inset)*.

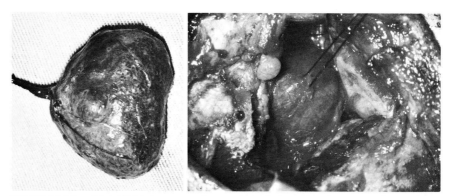

FIGURE 14-11. *(Right)* Orbital cavernous hemangioma during extirpative surgery. Suture allows for traction and, because of the low flow character of these tumors, leads to exsanguination of the mass, which facilitates removal. *(Left)* The gross specimen demonstrates an apical vascular tag.

FIGURE 14-12. *(A)* CT scan after contrast injection shows a right-sided deep lymphangioma presenting as a low-density cystlike mass with rim enhancement. *(Inset)* Ultrasonogram demonstrates a lobular mass with few internal echoes, causing flattening of the globe. The patient presented with a 6-week history of rapid onset of orbital mass effect, which was exacerbated by a needle aspiration several days before referral. *(B)* Orbital venogram of this patient demonstrates only slight stretching and displacement of the superior ophthalmic vein with no connection to the lesion. Histology of the margin shows large, thinwalled, endothelially lined vascular channels with a loose collagenous stroma and little intraluminal blood. The central cavity contained decomposed blood products. (Rootman J, Hay E, Graeb D et al: Orbital–adnexal lymphangiomas. Ophthalmology 93:1558, 1986)

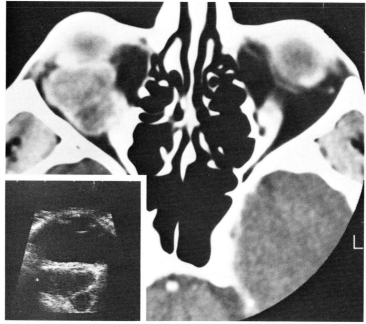
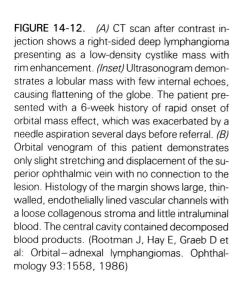

A

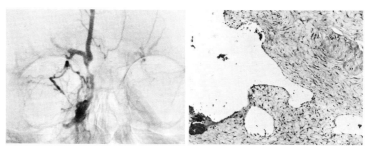

B

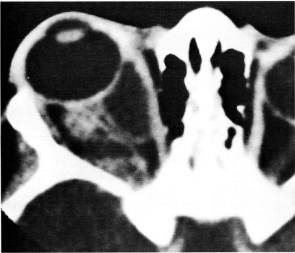
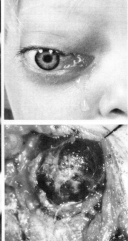

FIGURE 14-13. Deep lymphangioma. Clinical photograph demonstrates massive proptosis progressing over a 2-week period and leading to papilloedema with choroidal folds. CT scan after injection of contrast demonstrates a large medial cystlike area with posterior rim enhancement and a mottled lateral irregularly enhancing component. *Bottom inset* demonstrates the hemorrhagic cystic component at surgery. (Rootman J, Hay E, Graeb D et al: Orbital–adnexal lymphangiomas. Ophthalmology 93:1558, 1986)

symptoms with decreased visual acuity, papilloedema, and conduction defects.

The CT scans of patients in the deep category show low-density cystlike masses behind the orbital septum in the intraconal and extraconal spaces. With contrast injection, a thin rim of enhancement may be noted, which corresponds histologically to abnormal endothelially lined channels (see Figs. 14-12, 14-13). In addition, some of the patients may show focal enhancing areas outside the cystlike region and enlargement of the bony orbit. On ultrasonography, retrobulbar cystic masses are noted. Both angiography and orbital venography fail to demonstrate a vascular component, showing only displacement of normal vessels (see Fig. 14-12).

The acute orbital hemorrhage may cause optic nerve compression and require urgent surgical management. They can be successfully treated by careful dissection, evacuation of hematic cysts, and resection of the offending vascular anomaly (see Fig. 14-13). The contrast CT scan can give some guidance to the area of vascular anomaly, because it appears as either rim or irregular focal enhancement. Nevertheless, the surrounding orbital tissues are not infrequently densely scarred and differentiation of normal and abnormal tissues at the time of surgery may be very difficult, making safe total excision complicated. Postoperative drainage is recommended to avert any sequestration of blood following surgery. Five of our cases underwent surgery: three for compressive optic neuropathy and two for progressive proptosis. One had slow (several months) spontaneous resorption. Two of our cases have required repeat intervention for recurrent hemorrhage on a second occasion, a reflection of the indistinct margins and difficulty of complete excision.

Combined Lesions

Combined lymphangiomas are usually recognized within the first year of life and enlarge slowly over many years. They may have spontaneous hemorrhages. Hemorrhages into the deep portion can cause optic nerve dysfunction; those into the superficial component cause recurrent subconjunctival hemorrhages, periorbital ecchymosis, and swelling. However, unlike the deep type, the diagnosis of lymphangioma is made obvious by the superficial component (Fig. 14-14A). The superficial portion consists of multiple conjunctival and lid cysts. Some of the cysts are filled with clear or xanthochromic fluid and others with blood or menisci. In addition, in a number of these cases (two of six in our series) similar cystic lesions of the mucous membranes of the mouth may be noted (see Fig. 14-14B). The combined lesions are frequently massive in size, involving the intraconal, extraconal, preseptal, and postseptal spaces. The very large lesions produce significant cosmetic disfigurement and frequently decreased vision from either optic atrophy (as a result of spontaneous hemorrhages in the orbit) or amblyopia. Two of our cases have had cerebral hemorrhages due to an isolated intracranial vascular anomaly.

CT scanning demonstrates large soft tissue masses that cross boundaries of both preseptal and postseptal spaces as well as intraconal and extraconal compartments. The lesions are frequently poorly defined at their margins and on contrast injection show inhomogeneous enhancement with some rounded cystlike nonenhancing areas within the tumor mass (see Fig. 14-14C). Enlargement of the orbit is frequent. No connection to the arterial or venous system can be demonstrated clinically or by

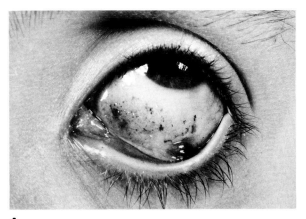

A

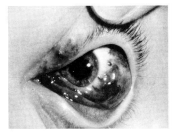
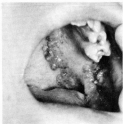

B

FIGURE 14-14. *(A)* Combined lymphangioma. Clinical photograph of a patient shows multiple characteristic conjunctival cysts present since birth, some of which contain clear or xanthochromic fluid and others blood. A deep component was noted behind the globe on CT scan. Biopsy showed a series of fine, endothelially lined vascular channels with only connective tissue stroma. *(B, left)* Epibulbar surface and *(right)* mouth of a patient who had a histologically confirmed combined lymphangioma (vascular hamartoma). Note typical multicystic oral lesions, some with blood and others with clear or xanthochromic fluid. *(C)* Axial CT scan of combined lymphangioma shows a spectrum of findings. Uniform dense enhancement is seen in the medial and lateral subconjunctiva, whereas the retrobulbar region has areas of patchy inhomogeneous enhancement medially, and low-density cystlike areas with rim enhancement laterally. (Rootman J, Hay E, Graeb D et al: Orbital–adnexal lymphangiomas. Ophthalmology 93:1558, 1986)

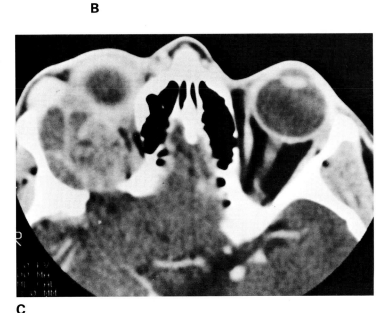

C

contrast studies (intralesional, venous, and arterial; Fig. 14-15).

Combined lesions require surgery either on an urgent basis when there is an acute retrobulbar hemorrhage with optic nerve compression, or on an elective basis to deal with cosmetic disfigurement. Because of the large size and widespread involvement of the orbit, the prognosis for successful management is more guarded than for superficial lesions. Carbon dioxide laser surgery may aid in the management of these lesions.

In summary, lymphangiomas present a spectrum of vascular hamartomas with histopathologic features that identify them as a grouping that parallels the histology of similar lesions elsewhere in the head and neck (Figs. 14-16 and 14-17). This includes the presence of diaphanous, serous-filled vascular channels, a loose connective tissue stroma, lymphorrhages, features of old hemorrhage, randomly distributed smooth muscle bundles, and dysplastic vessels. There is no clinical evidence of active hemodynamic connection (*i.e.*, no bruit or change on Valsalva maneuver), and there is no direct arterial or venous connection on radiographic contrast injection studies. The relative hemodynamic isolation of these thin-walled vascular channels explains the pathophysiology of this lesion. Bleeding may result from sludging, minimal trauma with rupture of a component vessel, or possibly spontaneous hemorrhage from fragile neovascular tufts. In addition, the intermittent and slow expansion of the mass may be related to an osmotic process with imbibed tissue fluids. Overall, the constellation of clinical and investigative features is sufficiently distinctive to warrant a separation of these lesions into a category of

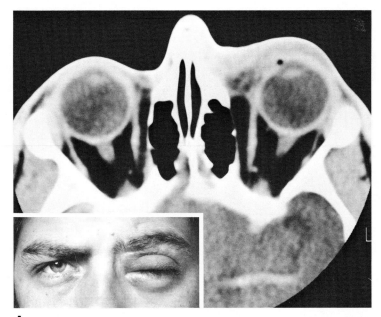

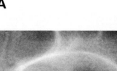

A

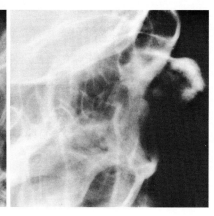

B

FIGURE 14-15. *(A)* Combined lymphangioma. A 19-year-old man had a history of a mass lesion of the lid, conjunctiva, and anterior orbit present since infancy and leading to amblyopia and esotropia. The conjunctival portion had typical cystic elements. He had multiple lid procedures. CT scan with contrast demonstrates a variably enhancing mass in the anterior orbit, lid, and conjunctiva. *(B)* Preoperative intralesional injection of contrast demonstrated multiple fine vascular channels with no dispersement or connection to the venous system demonstrated on either early or late films (done at 30 minutes). (Rootman J, Hay E, Graeb D et al: Orbital–adnexal lymphangiomas. Ophthalmology 93: 1558, 1986)

their own that can be divided into superficial, combined, and deep types. The clinical manifestations, prognosis, and management directly correlate with the pathophysiology described and location of the lesions.

Neoplasia

HEMANGIOPERICYTOMA

Hemangiopericytomas are uncommon tumors that originate from the pericyte and are characterized by infrequent occurrence in the head and neck and an incidence largely in the adult population. They are the source of considerable difficulty in predicting biological behavior on the basis of histopathology. Because the pericyte is a spindle-shaped cell with a moderate amount of cytoplasm and an indistinct border, routine histopathologic differentiation from endothelial cells, histiocytes, and fibroblasts may be difficult. Distinction on a cellular basis may be best achieved by electron microscopy. Since the identification of this entity by Stout, the tumor has been well delineated throughout the body, where it tends to occur in the retroperitoneum and lower limbs. Orbital occurrences have been repeatedly described in multiple case reports; the largest series is that of Croxatto and Font. Generally speaking, the behavior and morphology of this tumor in the orbit is similar to those noted in other sites within the body.

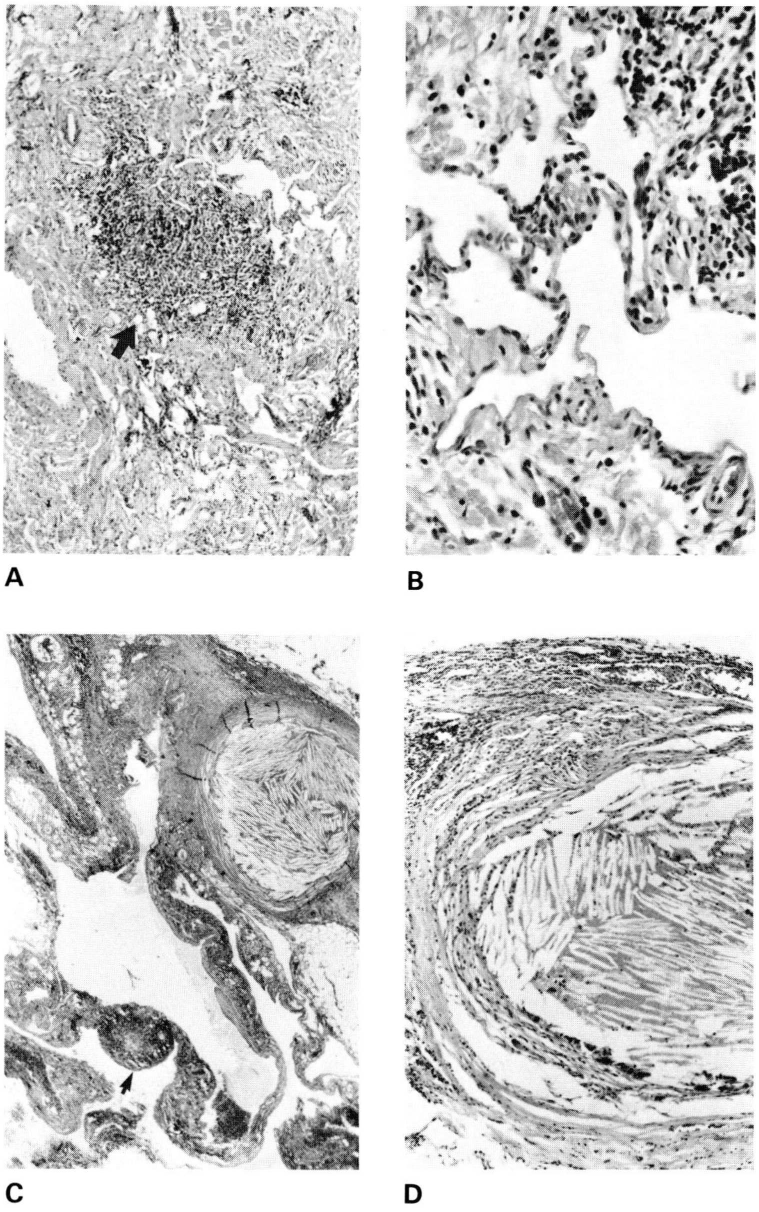

FIGURE 14-16. Histopathologic and electron microscopic spectrum of lymphangiomas, showing large, diaphanous, endothelially lined vascular channels *(B, C)* with stromal connective tissue and lymphorrhages *(A, C: arrows)*. Note evidence of old bleeding with formation of cholesterol clefts *(C, D)* (hematoxylin-eosin, original magnifications: *A*, ×10; *B*, ×25; *C*, ×2.5; *D*, ×10). (Rootman J, Hay E, Graeb D et al: Orbital–adnexal lymphangiomas. Ophthalmology 93:1558, 1986)

The median age of occurrence is in the fourth decade, but hemangiopericytomas have been noted from 20 months of age to 87 years. The major clinical features are proptosis and mass effect, predominantly in the superior part of the orbit, unassociated with pain or features of infiltration or entrapment (Fig. 14-18A). Hemodynamically, they have been shown to have a rapid circulation with a significant amount of shunting of blood. Angiography shows dilated feeding arteries, an early tumor blush, and a rapid venous outflow (see Fig. 14-18B). In spite of this, clinical evidence of active hemodynamics is rare and can be demonstrated only by angiography. Patients will usually have symptoms for less than 1 year on presentation. However, there is wide variation from 1 month to 26 years. On CT scan, these tumors tend to present as well-defined masses with homogeneous enhancement and show a blush on angiography (see Fig. 14-18A and B).

At the time of surgery, most of these tumors appear to be reasonably well circumscribed, pinkish or violaceous masses, and they may have large draining telangiectatic vessels. We have seen only three such tumors. In two

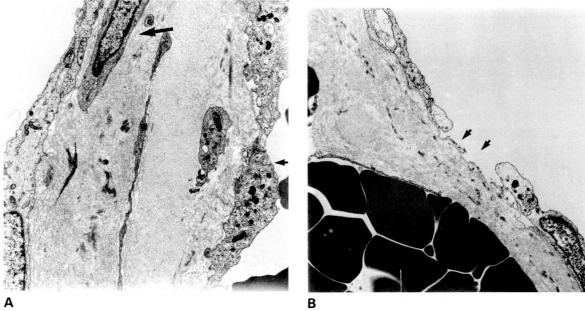

A   **B**

FIGURE 14-17. Electron micrographs of tissue obtained from combined lymphangioma (vascular hamartoma) shown in Figure 14-14C. *(A)* Stroma between two ectatic lumina of a blood vessel-like capillary. Note tight endothelial apposition *(short arrows)* and pericytes *(long arrows)*. *(B)* Lymphatic-like space next to a red cell-containing vascular channel. Note absence of pericytes, and endothelial gap typical of a lymphatic vessel *(short arrows)* adjacent to fluid-containing lumen (original magnifications: *A*, ×7280; *B*, ×5600). (Rootman J, Hay E, Graeb D et al: Orbital–adnexal lymphangiomas. Ophthalmology 93:1558, 1986)

instances, the mass itself appeared to be quite friable; however, the majority have been described at surgery as having circumscribed borders with rare grossly infiltrative lesions noted. In the literature, the majority have been about 3 cm in size, but range all the way from 1.7 cm to 5.5 cm.

The fundamental histopathology of this lesion consists of a uniformly cellular tumor with a sinusoidal vascular component often forming branching (staghorn) channels. The reticulin pattern forms a dense network or mesh around individual cells in contrast to that of capillary hemangiomas (see Fig. 14-18C, *right*). Additional features noted in hemangiopericytomas include myxoid, cellular, storiform, and cystic components. In addition, giant cells may be noted as well as areas of necrosis, hemorrhage, and hyalinization. Three basic patterns have been described, including sinusoidal, solid, and mixed types. Hemangiopericytomas can be divided into benign, intermediate, and malignant tumors on the basis of histopathologic criteria. The benign pattern demonstrates minimal atypia with few mitotic figures, whereas borderline and malignant patterns demonstrate increasing mitosis, compression of vascular spaces, pleomorphism, necrosis, hemorrhage, and infiltrative margins. In spite of these distinctions, it remains difficult to reliably predict the biology on the basis of histopathologic criteria.

The major differential diagnosis in the orbit, besides infantile capillary hemangiomas, includes fibrous histiocytoma and mesenchymal chondrosarcomas. Fibrous histiocytomas are dominated by a storiform highly cellular pattern without a significant vascular component, and mesenchymal chondrosarcomas contain areas of chondroid or cartilaginous tissue. Ultrastructurally, the pericyte has a number of distinct characteristics including frequent pinocytotic vesicles, poorly developed and rare desmosomes, and a striking, frequently multilayered, basal lamina.

About one third of hemangiopericytomas of the orbit will recur, and 10% to 15% overall may develop metastases. Local recurrence correlates most closely with incomplete or piecemeal excision. In addition, there is an increased incidence of recurrence in the malignant and borderline groups. Nevertheless, histologically benign tumors may also recur or metastasize. Because local recurrence and metastatic disease are significant risk in these tumors and may occur after many years, long-term follow up (at least 10 years) is necessary to assure complete cure. Because these tumors usually have a pseudocapsule, careful and complete local excision is the recommended form of therapy. Elsewhere in the body, high-dose radiotherapy has been used in treatment of these tumors when recurrent or aggressive in behavior, but carries attendant morbidity in the orbit. Aggressive local behavior may require exenteration. Systemic chemotherapy has been used in too small a number of cases to comment on its efficacy.

In summary, orbital hemangiopericytomas are unusual vascular tumors that tend to present as well-circumscribed noninfiltrative superior masses. They have an unpredictable pattern of behavior and are best handled by careful local excision, unless they demonstrate biologically aggressive behavior.

MALIGNANT HEMANGIOENDOTHELIOMA: ANGIOSARCOMA

Malignant endothelially derived vascular tumors are extremely rare, representing 1% of all sarcomas. Typically, they occur in the skin, with a predilection for the head and neck of males in later life. They may be multiple and aggressive both locally and systemically. The structural spectrum is diverse, which in part accounts for a lack of standardized nomenclature. The fundamental histologic features are the presence of irregular lumina (frequently containing blood) lined by atypical endothelial cells, which may be papillary in configuration. A wide spectrum of differentiation of these tumors may be noted, from well-defined vascular groupings of atypical endothelial cells with a vascular reticulin pattern, to poorly differentiated (epithelioid) cells that are difficult to distinguish from carcinomas. Ultrastructurally, the morphologic spectrum reflects this diversity, but fundamental endothelial features (a basal lamina, luminal pinocytotic vesicles, tight junctions, cytofilaments, and Weibel-Palade bodies) may be noted. Factor VIII-related antigen, an endothelial marker, may be noted.

About a dozen cases in the orbit have been reported. The dominant presentation has been the development of mass effect over a relatively short period (2 to 3 months). No sex predilection has been noted, and the median age was 24 years. One quarter of the reported cases had local sensory or motor neurologic signs and symptoms. Overall, these tumors have been typically locally aggressive, and wide surgical excision is recommended to prevent recurrence or metastases.

KAPOSI'S SARCOMA

Multifocal hemorrhagic sarcoma was first described in 1872 by Kaposi. Three related clinical syndromes appear to exist, varying with demography, genetic factors, and immune status. The classic syndrome consists of development of discrete violaceous lesions on the extremities (especially the lower) of elderly males (seventh decade) and immune-compromised patients. It typically occurs in patients of eastern European or Mediterranean origin. Progression is characterized by increasing numbers of lesions, nodularity, hemorrhage, and gastrointestinal, genitourinary, lymph node, and visceral involvement. Mortality in this form is between 10% and 20%, typically with a long clinical course over 8 years to 10 years. Second malignancies, especially those of reticuloendothelial origin, are frequent, with 25% of patients succumbing.

A second, more aggressive, syndrome is seen in Central Africa, typically in the fourth decade. Visceral, lymph node, and internal mucosal involvement is more frequent early in the course of the disease, and progression is therefore more rapid. Finally, a particularly aggressive form frequently develops in persons afflicted by the acquired immune deficiency syndrome (AIDS).

Clinically, the disease can be staged into nodular, locally aggressive, and generalized, correlating with the prognosis. Ocular involvement is usually of the skin of the lids or conjunctiva. The African form has been noted to occur in the lacrimal gland.

Histologically, this tumor is believed to arise from a primitive perithelial cell giving rise to a spectrum of findings. Earlier, less aggressive lesions may be dominated by inflammatory cells and resemble pyogenic granuloma with a background of malignant spindle cells. With evolution of the lesion, increasing numbers of spindle cells are noted with increasing atypia and a reduction in the inflammatory cell background. In addition, features of recurrent hemorrhage and slit-like vascular channels are noted.

Treatment depends on staging. Local lesions may be resected or treated with injectable chemotherapeutic agents. Multifocal disease or visceral involvement is treated by systemic chemotherapy and extended field radiation.

ANGIOLYMPHOID HYPERPLASIA

Angiolymphoid hyperplasia (Kimura's disease) is a benign disorder characterized by the development of inflammatory angiomas of the skin, chiefly of the head and neck. It is believed to be a reactive inflammatory disorder that may be associated with systemic eosinophilia, regional adenopathy, focal itching nodules, occasional spontaneous resolution, and inflammatory infiltrates. All of these features support the concept of an inflammatory pathogenesis.

Histologically, the striking feature is a well-circumscribed lesion consisting of a mixture of vascular channels with plump vacuolated endothelial cells and zonal polymorphic inflammatory infiltrate with many eosinophils. Lymphoid follicles and disrupted inflamed larger vessels may be noted.

(Text continues on p. 546.)

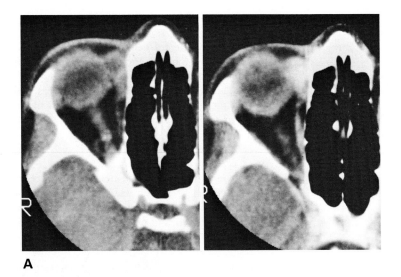

A

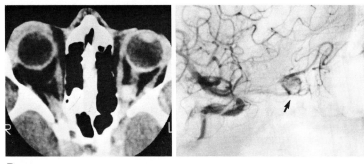

B

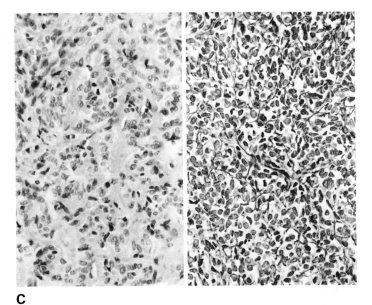

C

FIGURE 14-18. *(A)* Hemangiopericytoma. Axial CT scan without *(left)* and with *(right)* contrast injection. Note well-defined homogeneously enhancing anterior orbital mass. *(B)* Contrast-enhancing apical orbital mass that displaced the optic nerve and led to optic neuropathy. Angiogram on the *right* demonstrates an early uniform fine mesh of enhancing vessels *(arrow)*. *(C)* Histopathology of a solid hemangiopericytoma shown in *B*. This demonstrates a spindle cell population (*left:* hematoxylin-eosin, original magnification ×25) and dense reticulin pattern surrounding individual cells (*right:* reticulin, original magnification ×25).

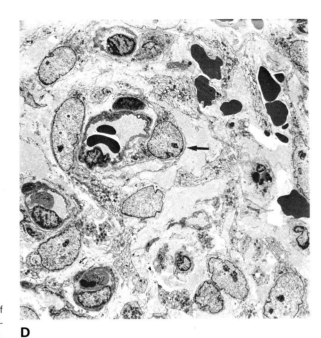

D

FIGURE 14-18 *(Continued).* *(D, E)* Ultrastructural features of hemangiopericytoma from patient shown in *A*. Note characteristic wrapping of pericytes around a vascular channel *(D, arrow)*. Additional features consistent with pericytes include the presence of basement membrane, few intracytoplasmic filaments, and pinocytotic vesicles (original magnifications: *D*, ×2000; *E*, ×9400).

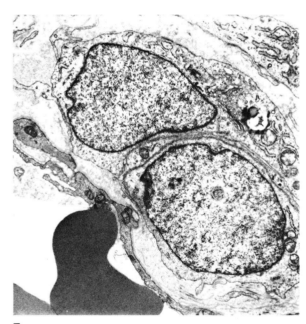

E

TABLE 14-2.
MAJOR PATHOPHYSIOLOGIC AND CLINICAL FEATURES OF ARTERIOVENOUS SHUNTS AND VENOUS ANOMALIES

Lesion	Site of Shunt	Principal Orbital Hemodynamic Pathology	Principal Symptoms
Arteriovenous Shunts			
AVM (arteriovenous malformation)	Intraorbital	Hyperdynamic antegrade shunt with mass effect	Proptosis, faint orbital pulsations, bruit
	Extraorbital	Collateral flow to extraorbital shunt	Epibulbar vascular congestion
Posttraumatic carotid cavernous fistulas	Cavernous sinus	High-flow shunt with pulsatile retrograde flow into orbital veins	Bruit, prominent orbital pulsation, orbital congestion with elevated venous pressure
Dural arteriovenous fistulas of cavernous sinus	Cavernous sinus	Low-flow shunt with faintly pulsatile or nonpulsatile retrograde flow in orbital veins	Same as above but to a lesser degree
Venous Anomalies			
Nondistensible	No shunt	Spontaneous hemorrhage	Episodic hemorrhages with frequent spontaneous resolution
Distensible	No shunt	Enlargement with elevation of systemic venous pressure	Intermittent proptosis

Orbital involvement has been described, and consists chiefly of well-defined soft tissue masses of the anterior orbit, canthus, or lids. This lesion, which is essentially a benign disorder, is included because of the vascular component, necessitating a differentiation of this from a number of important orbital lesions. The differential diagnosis includes angiosarcomas, epithelioid hemangioendotheliomas, nonspecific orbital inflammations, insect bite, pyogenic granuloma, eosinophilic granuloma, angiomatous lymphoid hamartoma, and granuloma faciale.

Because it is a benign, well-defined mass lesion, the treatment of choice is local incision alone. For lesions that are incompletely excised or recurrent, radiotherapy has also been advocated.

VASCULAR LEIOMYOMA (ANGIOMYOMA)

Vascular leiomyoma is a rare, usually subcuticular, tumor that arises from smooth muscle of blood vessels. The few cases described in the orbit have been slow growing, encapsulated masses occurring chiefly in the fourth and fifth decades of life. Although the dominant clinical feature is mass effect, pain and change on Valsalva maneuver may be noted. Histologically, they are characterized by the presence of fascicular interwoven bundles of spindle cells with a significant vascular pattern. Myxoid areas may be noted. Densely vascular lesions may be confused with hemangiopericytoma. The diagnosis is substantiated by identification of smooth muscle origin by

means of histochemistry or electron microscopy. Because they are well encapsulated and benign, the treatment of choice is complete excision. Incomplete removal may lead to recurrence locally.

■ ARTERIOVENOUS SHUNTS AND VENOUS ANOMALIES

Congenital and Acquired Arteriovenous Shunts

The orbital vessels may be involved in arteriovenous shunts to varying degrees and by different mechanisms (Table 14-2). The effect they have on orbital structures is directly related to the site and degree of shunting and is proportional to the volume of flow. Increased arteriovenous flow and pressure leads to venous dilatation, fluid transudation, and vascular turbulence, which may result in sludging and thrombosis. Higher-flow shunts have a greater effect, resulting in orbital swelling, chemosis, increased episcleral venous pressure (therefore, increased intraocular pressure), retinal vascular dilatation, pulsatile exophthalmos, and bruit. In contrast, low-flow shunts tend to manifest lesser signs and symptoms, consisting of edema and vascular dilatation with or without increased intraocular pressure (Fig. 14-19). Primary orbital shunts (defined as those in which the arteriovenous shunt is situated within the orbit) are quite rare, and consist mainly of congenital arteriovenous malformations (Fig. 14-20).

FIGURE 14-19. Clinical manifestations of low-flow arteriovenous shunts. *(Top)* Vascular dilatation and tortuousness in the left posterior pole (versus normal right posterior pole). This was associated clinically with epibulbar vascular dilatation *(bottom left)* and 3 mm of proptosis, which occurred spontaneously in a 72-year-old woman. *(Bottom right)* Epibulbar vascular dilatation and tortuousness in a 74-year-old woman who presented with a mild sixth nerve palsy, raised intraocular pressure (34 mm Hg), and 2 mm of proptosis due to a low-flow shunt (shown in Figure 14-27).

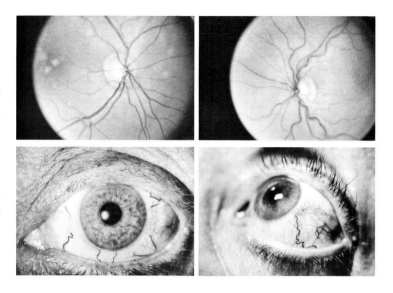

FIGURE 14-20. *(A)* A primary orbital arteriovenous malformation in a 17-year-old girl with a 3-year history of proptosis. Close clinical observation demonstrated orbital pulsation synchronous with the pulse. CT scan shows calcification within a poorly defined enhancing mass and marked enlargement of the superior ophthalmic vein. *(B)* Arteriography of this patient demonstrates enlarged ophthalmic artery *(center)* and external carotid branches *(left)* supplying a tangle of anomalous vessels, with early drainage to the markedly enlarged superior ophthalmic vein *(right)*.

A

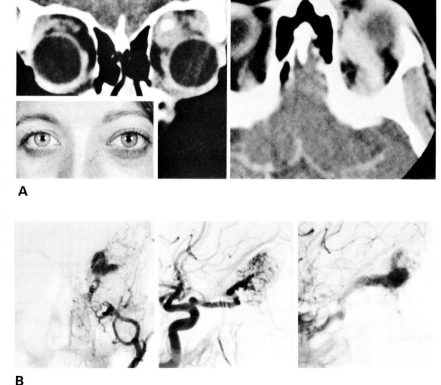

B

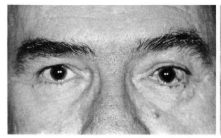
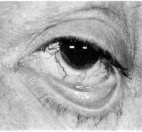

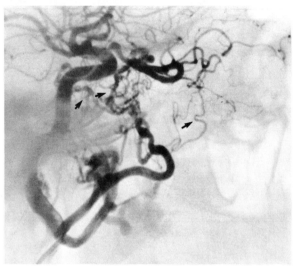

FIGURE 14-21. *(Top)* This patient demonstrates lid and epibulbar arterial dilatation. It was related to participation of these vessels in supplying a large post-traumatic arteriovenous fistula of the face, shown on angiography *(below)*. Multiple enlarged anastomotic vessels *(arrows)* from the ophthalmic and internal carotid arteries reconstitute the previously ligated internal maxillary artery.

These may occur alone or as part of congenital syndromes such as the Wyburn-Mason and Osler-Weber-Rendu syndromes (see Fig. 14-35). Although arteriovenous malformations can be high-flow shunts, the venous drainage is antegrade in the orbital veins; thus, signs and symptoms are generally less profound than in fistulas, wherein the flow is retrograde due to distal obstruction and shunting. (The congenital arteriovenous malformations are discussed in a later section of this chapter.)

Much more frequently, the orbital veins participate secondarily in an arteriovenous shunt that is located outside the orbit, most commonly, in or near the cavernous sinus. These lesions drain to the orbit, producing retrograde flow in the orbital veins and thus increasing the venous pressure. These shunts may be high flow or low flow, with the associated symptoms described previously. They may be of spontaneous onset or follow obvious severe head trauma.

Rarely, the orbital arteries may participate in the arterial supply of an arteriovenous shunt that occurs outside the orbit. In these cases, the main feature is arterial engorgement (Fig. 14-21).

Venous thrombosis in the cavernous sinus is probably the initiating factor in the arteriovenous shunts of spontaneous onset (see below), but may also play an important role in the subsequent clinical course. Thrombosis of the superior ophthalmic vein will lead to eventual resolution of the orbital symptoms (Fig. 14-22). On the other hand, thrombosis of the other venous exit routes of the cavernous sinus may increase the flow of blood to the superior ophthalmic vein and aggravate the symptoms.

Posttraumatic carotid-cavernous fistulas result from a tear within the cavernous portion of the internal carotid artery itself (Fig. 14-23). The tear is the result of major head trauma, often associated with basal skull fracture. Occasionally, fistulas may follow a penetrating injury that passes through the orbit and superior orbital fissure to perforate the internal carotid artery. In either instance, a sizable hole is usually produced in the intracavernous portion of the artery. Because this portion of the artery is encased within a plexus of veins, an arteriovenous fistula results, which transmits increased blood flow and elevated pressure to the cavernous sinus and its tributaries, including retrograde drainage to the ophthalmic veins. The large arteriovenous shunt that results produces the signs and symptoms of a high-flow vascular lesion. The patient is usually aware of a pulsatile bruit from the time of the injury. Pulsatile exophthalmos is frequent and is associated with chemosis, orbital swelling, episcleral venous congestion, and elevation of intraocular pressure.

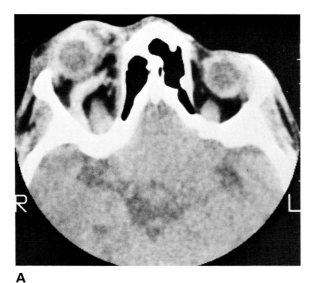

A

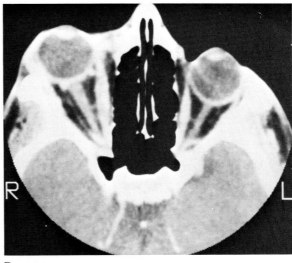

B

FIGURE 14-22. Contrast CT scan and angiographic features of a low-flow spontaneous arteriovenous shunt that demonstrates dilated superior ophthalmic (A) and vortex veins (B). Note moderate enlargement of extraocular muscles and proptosis (B). (C) Contrast-enhanced CT scan taken 1 month later. At this time, the patient demonstrated partial resolution of symptoms 2 days after angiography. Note intraluminal nonenhancing area consistent with a spontaneous thrombus (arrow). (D, E) Angiographic features of the carotid cavernous shunt of the same patient. Note initial filling of the posterior cavernous sinus (D) with delayed retrograde opacification of the anterior cavernous sinus and the enlarged superior ophthalmic vein (E).

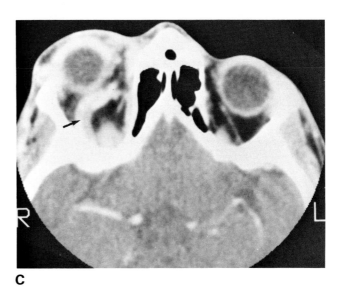

C

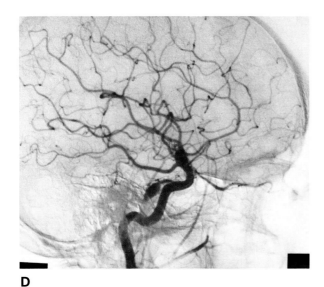

D

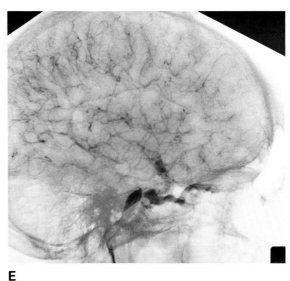

E

549

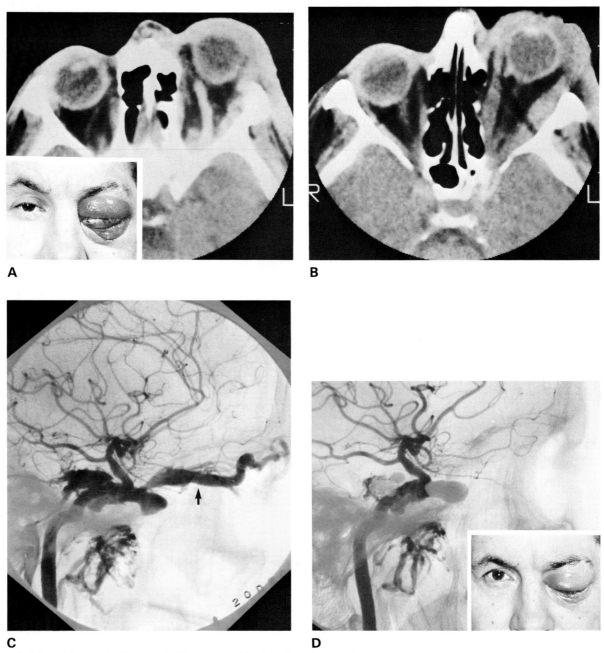

FIGURE 14-23. *(A, B)* CT and clinical features of a high-flow shunt following head trauma with marked orbital engorgement both clinically and on CT scan. Note enlarged superior ophthalmic vein, marked proptosis with tethering of the globe, and markedly enlarged extraocular muscles. *(C)* Arteriogram of the same patient shows a post-traumatic carotid-cavernous fistula, with high-flow shunt into the cavernous sinus and retrograde drainage into the superior ophthalmic vein *(arrow)*. *(D)* Angiogram following detachable balloon embolization of two separate fistulas with occlusion of the shunt to the superior ophthalmic vein. *(Inset)* Early resolution 1 week after embolization.

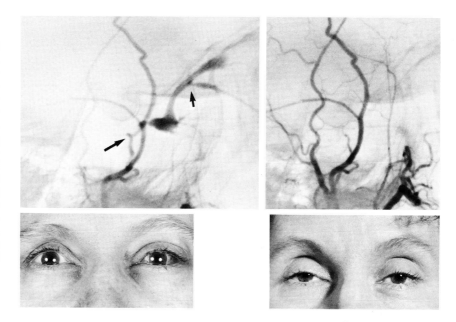

FIGURE 14-24. Angiography of a low-flow arteriovenous shunt. The 54-year-old patient had a history of left lid swelling, mild proptosis, chemosis, decreased abduction, slightly raised intraocular pressure (22 mm Hg), and epibulbar injection *(left)*. Note slow filling of cavernous sinus from the accessory meningeal artery *(long arrow)* and retrograde drainage to a mildly dilated superior ophthalmic vein *(short arrow)*. *(Right)* The same patient is shown 6 months later following embolization of the shunt; with absence of flow in the superior ophthalmic vein. Note resolution of ocular signs.

Cranial nerve palsies (usually third or sixth, or both) may result from pressure on the distended cavernous sinus, but may also occur as the direct effect of trauma. Symptoms are frequently bilateral but are milder in the contralateral eye. Occasionally, if the hole in the internal carotid artery is quite small, posttraumatic carotid-cavernous fistulas may present as a low-flow shunt.

The etiology of spontaneous arteriovenous shunts in the region of the cavernous sinus is still somewhat speculative. However, most of these lesions appear identical angiographically to dural arteriovenous malformations that have been described in relation to the dural sinuses elsewhere within the cranium. These lesions have been shown to be acquired, and probably develop following thrombosis of the venous sinuses. It is postulated that as the thrombosed sinus (in this case, the cavernous sinus) becomes recanalized, preexisting microscopic arteries in the wall of the dural sinus become enlarged sufficiently to constitute a significant hemodynamic shunt. These lesions occur most frequently in postmenopausal females. The lesions are prone to a chronic fluctuating course with occasional exacerbations. Spontaneous resolution also occurs and is as frequent as 40% in some series (see Fig. 14-22). Angiographically, they are characterized by a network of fine meningeal vessels that may arise from the internal or the external carotid arteries and shunt blood directly into the cavernous sinus (Fig. 14-24). The arterial supply to these lesions is frequently bilateral, and in most the shunt is relatively small. Bruit may be absent in as many as 50% of patients, and the orbital symptoms are correspondingly mild. Evidence of thrombosis within the cavernous sinus or its tributary veins is usually found.

This ongoing thrombosis is responsible for the periodic exacerbations and remissions, and for the spontaneous resolution that occurs in this entity. Thrombosis of the cavernous sinus itself is curative. Thrombosis of the superior ophthalmic vein will protect the orbit from the hemodynamic effects of the lesion and lead to resolution of the orbital symptoms (see Fig. 14-22). On the other hand, if the other drainage routes of the cavernous sinus (such as the superior and inferior petrosal sinuses and the pterygoid plexus) become thrombosed, the entire shunt may be directed by retrograde flow to the superior and inferior ophthalmic veins, producing an acute exacerbation.

A less frequent group of "spontaneous" arteriovenous shunts in the cavernous sinus region may result directly from minor trauma. In these lesions, rather than a network of arteries, one sees only a single meningeal feeding artery with a small shunt into the cavernous sinus. It has been postulated that minor trauma, hypertension, or straining may result in rupture of normal meningeal arteries to cause this variety of "spontaneous" arteriovenous shunt (see Fig. 14-24).

Shunts in other portions of the intracranial dural sinus network may occasionally cause orbital symptoms if the elevated pressure is transferred to the superior ophthalmic vein. Very rarely, the rapid venous drainage from intracerebral arteriovenous malformations may cause similar orbital symptoms.

In summary, arteriovenous shunts, whether congenital or acquired, are hemodynamically either high flow or low flow. The high-flow lesions are usually posttraumatic carotid cavernous fistulas or arteriovenous malformations. The low-flow shunts are dural arteriovenous fis-

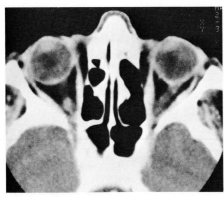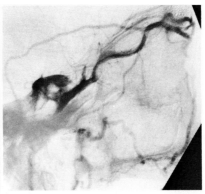

FIGURE 14-25. CT and angiographic features of a spontaneously occurring low-flow arteriovenous shunt in a 59-year-old woman. Note mild extraocular muscle enlargement on CT scan, and a shunt from the external carotid branches to the cavernous sinus with retrograde drainage into a relatively normal-size superior ophthalmic vein on angiography. This was associated with 3 mm of proptosis, normal intraocular pressure, slightly dilated retinal veins, and episcleral venous dilatation.

tulas of the cavernous sinus region and are usually spontaneous or, less often, posttraumatic (see Table 14-2).

We have seen 15 arteriovenous shunts affecting the orbit. Five of these were high-flow shunts associated with pulsatile exophthalmos and bruit. The remaining 10 were low-flow lesions with venous dilatation in all, but chemosis in only three. Intraocular pressure was elevated in eight of the low-flow lesions but to a lesser degree than that noted in the high-flow shunts. In addition, we have seen two other patients with raised episcleral venous pressure and dilatation associated with raised intraocular pressure in the absence of arteriovenous shunting. This is a well-described syndrome not associated with any identifiable shunt. Thus, patients with raised episcleral venous pressure and diltation should be investigated angiographically. Four of our five patients with high-flow shunts had evidence of preexisting trauma. Two were congenital malformations (one high flow, one low flow), and the remainder were spontaneous in onset and occurred in women between the ages of 24 years and 74 years (average age 56 years).

CT scanning will demonstrate proptosis with enlargement of the superior ophthalmic vein and frequent enlargement of the extraocular muscles proportional to the degree of shunting (see Figs. 14-22 and 14-23; Fig. 14-25). There may be CT evidence of venous thrombosis in the form of a nonenhancing defect in the lumen of the superior ophthalmic vein or cavernous sinus (see Fig. 14-22). Ultrasonography may demonstrate similar changes and Doppler echography may reveal a bruit due to the blood flow (Fig. 14-26). Orbital venography will demonstrate failure to fill the orbital veins on the affected side. However, the definitive diagnostic procedure in arteriovenous

shunts is angiography, which shows retrograde opacification of the cavernous sinus and the orbital venous system (Fig. 14-27). Angiography confirms the clinical diagnosis and aids in planning definitive therapy. In spontaneous shunts, bilateral internal and external carotid injections with subtraction are required. Superselective studies of the external carotid branches that are likely to be involved (middle meningeal, accessory meningeal, and ascending pharyngeal arteries, and the artery of the foramen ovale) may be necessary. Several case reports in the literature document closure of spontaneous shunts following angiography.

Management. Treatment is almost always indicated in the posttraumatic high-flow carotid-cavernous fistulas, because the ultimate rate of visual loss without treatment is as high as 40% to 50%. Until recently, neurosurgical techniques have attempted to isolate the fistula by various trapping procedures involving ligation of the internal carotid artery both extracranially and intracranially. Of various newly developed alternate techniques, detachable balloon embolization has now become the treatment of choice because it offers the prospect of safe occlusion of the fistula while preserving flow in the internal carotid artery in the majority of cases (Table 14-3; see Figs. 14-23 and 14-24).

Because of the tendency toward resolution in the spontaneous arteriovenous shunts, treatment is not required except in the presence of impending visual loss, significant elevation of intraocular pressure, marked chemosis and tissue swelling with exposure, or severe pain or bruit. In these cases, intravascular embolization is the treatment of choice, using either particles or liquid tissue adhesives but the success rate in these lesions is not as

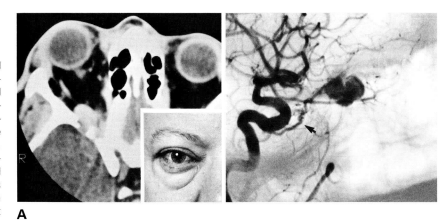

FIGURE 14-26. *(A)* CT scan and clinical photograph of a 53-year-old woman with an apical orbital venous aneurysm due to an arteriovenous shunt causing edema, chemosis, raised intraocular pressure (24 mm Hg versus 10 mm Hg), 7 mm of proptosis, and a reduction of vision. An audible temporal bruit was present. CT scan shows venous aneurysm associated with a bony defect due to enlargement of the canal of Hyrtl. Angiogram shows internal carotid supply to the shunt *(arrow)* and straightening of the ophthalmic artery due to proptosis. *(B)* Right-selective middle meningeal angiogram also demonstrates supply to the venous aneurysm. *(Inset)* Ultrasonogram shows dilated superior ophthalmic vein. *(Right)* Angiogram after surgical closure of the middle meningeal supply and clipping of the orbital aneurysm, which led to resolution of symptoms.

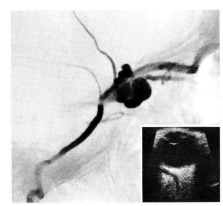

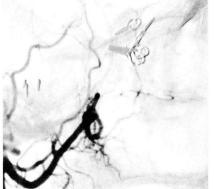

high as in the posttraumatic variety. Surgical intervention with clipping of all feeding vessels may be necessary for lesions that are not easily accessible to catheterization or embolization (see Fig. 14-26).

Venous Anomalies

The venous anomalies consist of either segmental irregular dilatations of the venous outflow system or a tangled mass of abnormal venous channels. They appear to be associated with two different clinical syndromes, which can be explained on the basis of the size of functioning connections to the systemic venous system. Lesions with large connections to the systemic venous system respond to changes in venous pressure and are readily distensible. These patients may describe proptosis and pain that increases with such activities as straining, forward bending, or the Valsalva maneuver. Lesions with little or small functioning systemic venous connections are nondistensible and do not respond obviously to changes in systemic

venous pressure. These lesions are characterized by stagnant blood flow, which leads to thrombosis or hemorrhage, or both. We have encountered five distensible venous anomalies and nine nondistensible venous anomalies.

NONDISTENSIBLE VENOUS ANOMALIES

Varix

Varix presents near the end of the first decade or early in the second decade of life with two clinical syndromes depending upon whether the site of involvement is superficial or deep. Both syndromes are characterized by episodes of acute exacerbation and remission, which are related to hemorrhage or thrombosis within the lesion. Hemorrhage or thrombosis within deeper lesions leads to sudden proptosis and pain with increased pressure in the orbital tissues. There may be mechanical restriction of ocular movement or visual deficit (Fig. 14-28). We have rarely noted subconjunctival extension of the ecchy-

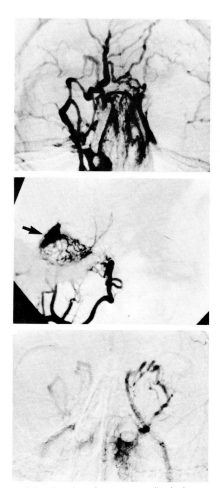

FIGURE 14-27. A series of contrast studies in the same patient demonstrates the hemodynamics of an arteriovenous dural shunt. *(Top)* A venogram with failure to opacify the left orbital veins due to raised venous pressure. *(Center)* Arteriography of the dural shunt in lateral view with early opacification of the posterior cavernous sinus *(arrow)*. *(Bottom)* AP view demonstrates subsequent retrograde filling of both superior ophthalmic veins.

mosis following deep orbital hemorrhage within varix. Patients with a superficial component will also have swelling and disfigurement of the lids and conjunctiva, which may extend into the deep orbit (Fig. 14-29).

In some respects, the distinction between nondistensible varices and lymphangiomas is difficult on clinical grounds, but in our opinion, there are a number of differing features. The superficial component of lymphangiomas is generally more striking with evidence of varying types of tortuous vascular channels, some of which contain blood, menisci, or clear fluid, compared with the larger, blood-filled channels of a varix (compare Fig. 14-14 with Fig. 14-30). In addition, lymphangiomas may be associated with expansion during intercurrent illness,

and similar lesions may be seen elsewhere in the skin and mucous membranes of the head and neck. The histopathological distinction between these two lesions may also be difficult; however, the varix is clearly a venous lesion in character with well-defined venous channels, whereas the lymphangioma is composed of thin-walled endothelially lined vessels, stromal lymphorrhages, and serous or blood-filled channels (some of which may be dysplastic) with the less uniform presence of smooth muscle. It is not surprising that the clinical syndromes are similar when the varix is nondistensible, because both lesions have either very slow or no flow and are probably of similar embryologic origin. However, the varix can frequently be demonstrated to have venous connections on direct injection or injection of tributary veins (orbital or internal jugular venography). In contrast, the findings on direct injection of lymphangiomas fail to reveal any connection to either the arterial or the venous system, in our experience. B-scan ultrasonography and CT scan may show abnormally dilated irregular veins or, when there has been hemorrhage, multilobular lesions. A-scan ultrasonography shows well-delineated regular structures with low internal reflectivity and minimal attenuation due to the congested pools of blood in the dilated veins. In our experience, the described appearance on CT scan and ultrasonography is not pathognomonic.

Management. There are two indications for intervention in the case of orbital varices: one is extreme orbital pressure with functional deficit, and the other is cosmetic disfigurement. Profound orbital hemorrhage leading to visual deterioration and severe pain may necessitate surgical intervention, but in our experience this is rare and in most instances the hemorrhages resolve. Surgical management consists of deep orbital exposure with evacuation of clotted blood and excision of the associated varix. In contrast to the lymphangiomas, we have noted clotted blood in a few spaces and a mixture of spaces filled with fresh, nonclotted old blood at the time of surgery. However, it may be impossible to find the originating varix, in which case only evacuation and decompression can be performed. The more superficial

TABLE 14-3.
MANAGEMENT OF ARTERIOVENOUS SHUNTS, UNIVERSITY OF BRITISH COLUMBIA ORBITAL CLINIC, 1976–1985

Management	Result	
	No Effect	Closure
Observation	5	2
Ocular treatment only	1	
Particle embolization	2	2
Balloon embolization		2
Surgical	1	2

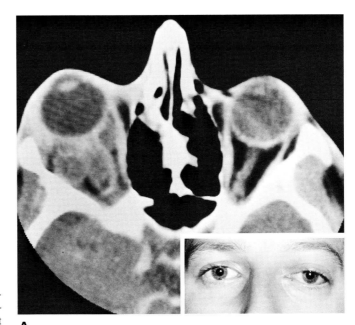

FIGURE 14-28. *(A)* CT scan and clinical photograph of a deep orbital varix in a 16-year-old patient. The varix was associated with an abrupt onset of proptosis due to retrobulbar hemorrhage. The lesion resolved over a 1-month period. *(B)* Ultrasonogram of the same patient demonstrates echo-poor area consistent with retrobulbar hemorrhage.

A

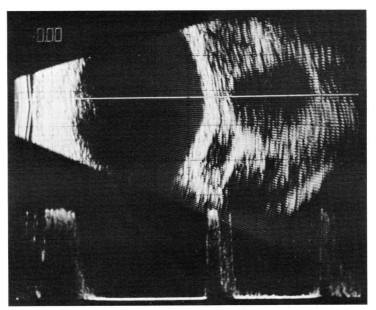

B

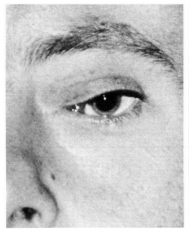
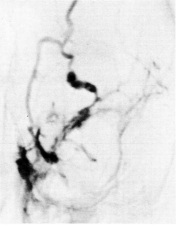

FIGURE 14-29. Lid swelling was associated with a deep orbital varix shown on venography *(right)* to involve the second and third segments of the superior ophthalmic vein.

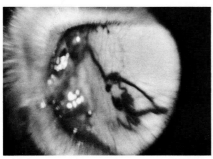
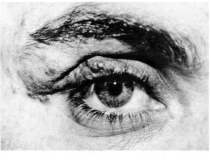

A

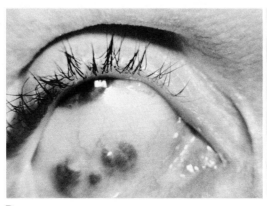
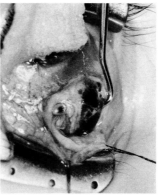

B

FIGURE 14-30. *(A)* Clinical photograph of conjunctival *(left)* and lid *(right)* varix. Note tortuous blood-filled aneurysmal venous network. *(B, left)* Epibulbar component of a deep orbital varix. *(Right)* Surgical photograph of a superficial varix demonstrates involvement of the inferior anterior orbit.

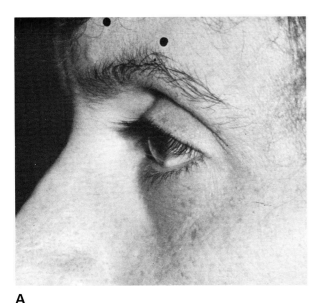 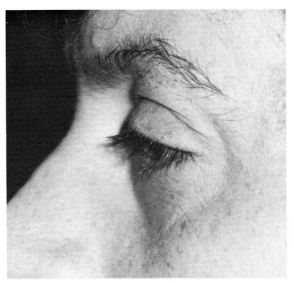

A
B

FIGURE 14-31.   Clinical photographs of a normally enophthalmic patient with a distensible orbital varix before *(A)* and after *(B)* Valsalva maneuver leading to proptosis and fullness of the lid. This patient was 33 years old and had noted the intermittent proptosis since childhood. (Cline RA, Rootman J: Enophthalmos: A clinical review. Ophthalmology 91:229, 1984)

components can be handled by a subcutaneous or anterior orbital dissection with frequent use of bipolar cauterization. The recent development of high-powered surgical carbon dioxide and YAG lasers may facilitate removal of these superficial and subcutaneous varices.

DISTENSIBLE VENOUS ANOMALIES

Of our five patients with distensible venous anomalies, all had evidence of the lesion within the first decade of life. The primary feature is extreme variation based on changes in jugular venous pressure (Figs. 14-31 and 14-32). Three patients had deep lesions, and at rest the affected eye was enophthalmic due to enlarged orbits and perhaps some fat atrophy. Increased jugular venous pressure produced extreme proptosis in all three cases. One lesion was confined to the superficial lid and temporalis fossa, but was also characterized by extreme distention on elevation of jugular venous pressure. One lesion affected the lid and anterior orbital structures alone (see Fig. 14-32). None of these patients had episodes of persistent orbital swelling due to hemorrhage or thrombosis, although this has been rarely described in the distensible variety. In three patients, we have demonstrated changes in the size of the lesion on CT scanning when done with and without elevation of the jugular venous pressure (Fig. 14-33). One of our cases was familial and multifocal with varices also present in the neck and shoulder. B-scan ul-

trasonography may also show increased size of the echo-free spaces with a Valsalva maneuver, and flow may be noted on Doppler echography.

During episodes of extreme engorgement, pain may be noted, especially in younger patients. Only one of our patients has requested intervention because of an active physical life, which produced intermittent pain in the lesion. In this patient, we successfully identified and resected the vessels under hypotension with intermittent display of the varix by increasing intrathoracic pressure intraoperatively.

■ CONGENITAL VASCULAR ANOMALIES

Of the four congenital vascular anomalies discussed in this section, one (Sturge-Weber syndrome) is a phakomatosis as originally and classically described. (The other conditions are tuberous sclerosis, neurofibromatosis, and von Hippel-Lindau disease.) The phakomatoses are characterized by the presence of cutaneous or mucosal nevi, hamartomas, or neoplastic growths. The central nervous system and eyes are most prominently involved, but abnormalities are frequently seen in other organ systems as well.

The term *phakomatosis* is purely morphologic and descriptive and does not imply any pathogenetic link among these disorders. More recently, many new syndromes, including the three other conditions discussed in

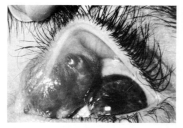
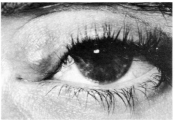
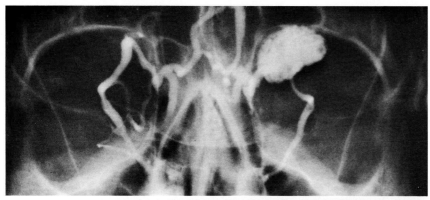

A

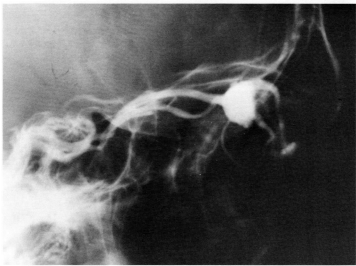

B

FIGURE 14-32. *(A)* Clinical photograph demonstrating the anterior component of a varix with *(left)* and without distention *(right)*. *(B)* Venogram demonstrates the posterior component of the varix on AP and lateral view.

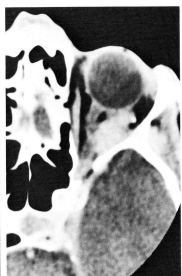

FIGURE 14-33. The CT scan of a distensible orbital varix before *(left)* and after *(right)* distention brought about by increased venous pressure. Note phlebolith.

this section (hereditary hemorrhagic telangiectasia, Wyburn-Mason syndrome, and Klippel-Trenaunay syndrome) have been added to the phakomatoses, and the term *neurocutaneous syndromes* applied to all of them.

These conditions are all rare. Sturge-Weber syndrome is the most common, followed by hereditary hemorrhagic telangiectasia, Klippel-Trenaunay syndrome, and Wyburn-Mason syndrome. In all of them, ophthalmologic involvement is more frequent and integral to the diagnosis than is orbital involvement.

Sturge-Weber Syndrome

A multitude of descriptive terms exist for Sturge-Weber syndrome, the most widely accepted being *encephalofacial angiomatosis.* However, it is the mesodermal coverings of the brain, meninges, and cranial bone that are involved by the angiomatous malformation, rather than the brain itself. The term *meningofacial angiomatosis* would more accurately describe this syndrome.

The minimum criteria for the diagnosis consist of a port wine nevus (nevus flammeus) of the face with ipsilateral leptomeningeal angiomatosis. The angiomatosis is responsible for the highly characteristic intracranial calcification and also very frequently results in focal seizures and contralateral hemiparesis. Ipsilateral glaucoma and buphthalmos are very common. Although incomplete forms have been reported in families, the heredity of this syndrome is uncertain.

The facial nevus is present at birth. It is usually flat, reddish-violet, and blanches on pressure. There are no case reports of the Sturge-Weber syndrome in which the

nevus did not involve at least the upper eyelid or the supraorbital face and scalp. This anomaly is usually unilateral, but frequently the medial boundary does not conform strictly to the midline. Occasionally, it may cross the midline or be present to a more or less equal extent bilaterally (Fig. 14-34A). Similar dermal lesions are frequently found in the oropharynx, trunk, and limbs. Pathologically, they consist of dilated endothelially lined vessels situated in the mid-dermis and deep dermis.

The leptomeningeal angiomatosis is almost always unilateral and most commonly in the occipital or parieto-occipital region, although infrequently the entire hemisphere may be involved. The thickened meninges contain a dense tangle of malformed vessels several layers thick. Frequent areas of hyalinized connective tissue are seen in their walls. Hypervascularity of the underlying cerebral cortex and subcortical white matter is frequently found, without frank vascular malformations. The cortex underlying the malformation is generally atrophic, with microscopic evidence of nerve cell loss, degeneration, and gliosis. Associated cerebral malformations are invariable, including microgyria, agyria, polygyria, heterotopias, and ectopias. Capsular hypertrophy and ectopia of the ipsilatral gasserian ganglion have also been described, implying a topographic coordination between the meningofacial malformation and the trigeminal sensory root ganglion. Meningeal hypervascularity has also been described in the spinal cord along with ectopic dorsal root ganglion cells and glial proliferation. Capillary angiomas may also be found in the kidneys, spleen, ovaries, intestine, adrenals, thyroid, pancreas, and lung.

Microscopically, two kinds of calcification are noted, consisting of fine granular deposition in the walls of small

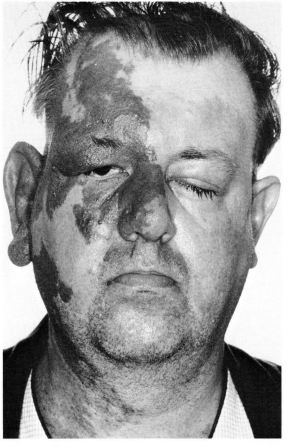
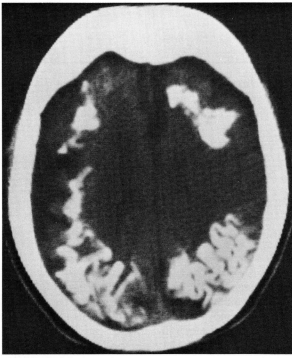

A   B

FIGURE 14-34. *(A)* Clinical photograph of a patient with Sturge-Weber syndrome (meningofacial angiomatosis). Note that facial nevus flammeus does not conform to the midline. The patient had ipsilateral glaucoma. The left eye is closed secondary to recent radioactive plaque surgery for an unrelated uveal melanoma. *(B)* CT scan demonstrates characteristic serpiginous calcifications conforming to the sulcal convolutions.

vessels and large coarse calcifications that are free within the cortex, predominantly in layers two and three (the molecular and pyramidal layers). These calcifications are seldom radiologically apparent before the age of 2 years, but become almost universal by adolescence. The finding of paired parallel serpiginous calcifications conforming to the sulcal convolutions on either plain films or CT is diagnostic (see Fig. 14-34*B*). The calcifications are believed to be secondary to vascular stasis and tissue hypoxia.

Nevi confined to the forehead tend to be associated with angiomatosis overlying the occipital lobe, whereas nevi involving the maxillary area are associated with parietal angiomatosis. This is explained by the close anatomic relationship of these areas during early fetal life when the primitive circulation to the brain and its coverings is being differentiated. A congenital lack of vasomotor innervation has been thought to be a contributing factor in the secondary vascular abnormalities, leading to hyperplasia and dilatation of the abnormal vessels. It has been postulated that the deficiency is in the parasympathetic supply, which is distributed by means of sensory branches of the trigeminal nerve.

At angiography, the leptomeningeal angiomatosis does not opacify or is opacified only faintly, presumably due to very slow flow. A decreased number of superficial cortical veins has been described in the region of the angiomatosis, with a corresponding increase in the deep venous system, which serves as a collateral route of drainage.

Homonymous hemianopia can be seen because of involvement of the visual cortex by leptomeningeal angiomatosis, although this sign may be difficult to elicit in many of these patients owing to intellectual abnormalities.

Seizures, both focal and generalized, usually begin in infancy and ultimately affect 90% of patients. Subnormal mentality is also present in about 50%. Hemiparesis and intellectual impairment may progress with uncontrolled seizures, and early lobectomy has been recommended by some for controlling seizures and preventing progressive neurologic and intellectual deficit.

From the ophthalmologic point of view, lid involvement, buphthalmos, and/or glaucoma are the most common abnormalies, found in about 30% of patients. Although not entirely agreed upon the cause is thought to be related to both elevated episcleral venous pressure secondary to episcleral hemangiomas and angle cleavage anomalies. If the patient develops retinal detachment for a long period of time, neovascular glaucoma may ensue.

Choroidal angiomas are also frequently found and recognized fundoscopically as an elevation that may be gray, yellow, or dark red. They are usually situated at the posterior pole near the optic disk. Microscopically, these are cavernous hemangiomas consisting of large, dilated, endothelially lined channels separated by scanty connective tissue. Atrophy and cystic degeneration of the overlying retina are frequently present. Accumulation of serous subretinal exudate may lead to retinal detachment. The angiomas may calcify, occasionally sufficiently to be seen radiographically. Angiomas may also be seen in the conjunctiva or episclera. Glial proliferation of the optic nerve and generalized hypervascularity of the globe and nerve may also be found.

Hereditary Hemorrhagic Telangiectasia (Osler-Weber-Rendu Syndrome)

Hereditary hemorrhagic telangiectasia is a rare autosomal dominant disorder that is characterized by the presence of numerous telangiectasias of skin and mucous membranes associated with repeated episodes of hemorrhage. The telangiectasias range in size from pinpoint lesions to spider nevi several millimeters in diameter; they are usually flat but may occasionally be nodular. Varying in color from bright red to purple or violet, they are seldom seen before the second or third decade, and increase in size and number thereafter. In addition to the skin, frequent sites of involvement include the nasal, oral, and gastrointestinal mucosa. Repeated episodes of epistaxis and gastrointestinal hemorrhage are common.

Widespread visceral involvement is also frequent, with pulmonary arteriovenous fistulas and malformations being the most important clinically. These are often multiple, predominate in the lower lobes, and are respon-

sible for polycythemia, paradoxic embolism, and brain abscess. Hemoptysis is also seen and may rarely be associated with air embolism. About 15% of patients with hereditary hemorrhagic telangiectasia have demonstrable pulmonary arteriovenus fistulas; 40% to 60% of patients with pulmonary arteriovenous fistulas or malformations have hereditary hemorrhagic telangiectasia.

Involvement of the liver is associated with a process resembling cirrhosis and rarely with portosystemic encephalopathy. The spleen, pancreas, and genitourinary tract may also be involved.

In the central nervous system, a wide range of vascular abnormalities may be seen. The most frequent are small punctate telangiectatic lesions; they may be single or multiple, in any part of the brain, and are almost always asymptomatic. Arteriovenous malformations, aneurysms, dural arteriovenous fistulas, and cavernous angiomas have all been described.

Orbital involvement in the disease is uncommon. Scattered case reports describe conjunctival telangiectasia, varix-like ectatic formations of the retinal veins, telangiectasia of the optic nerve, and orbital arteriovenous malformations (Fig. 14-35). A proliferative vascular retinopathy has also been described.

The telangiectatic lesion has a similar pathology in all organs studied and consists of proliferation and dilatation of small venules. Electron microscopic studies have shown defective overlapping of terminal villi of the endothelial cells, with many endothelial gaps plugged with thrombi. These small venules lack perivascular support due to an absence of pericytes, smooth muscles, and elastic fibers, thus increasing their tendency to hemorrhage. Local hyperfibrinolysis has also been described in these lesions.

Wyburn-Mason Syndrome

The rare Weber-Mason syndrome consists of the association of retinal arteriovenous communications with deep-seated ipsilateral cerebral arteriovenous malformations (AVM) involving the visual pathway. AVM may also be found in the facial soft tissues, mandible, or maxilla. Facial nevi are the least constant element in this syndrome, and are usually ipsilateral within the trigeminal nerve distribution. They most commonly consist of a faint reddish blush with scattered punctate red spots, but typical portwine pigmented nevi may also be found.

The retinal lesion consists of a direct communication between a retinal artery and vein, usually without any intervening vascular network. Retinal arteriovenous communications may also rarely occur as an isolated abnormality. There is a broad spectrum of abnormality, ranging from barely visible single communications to

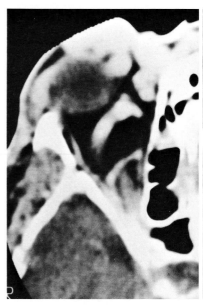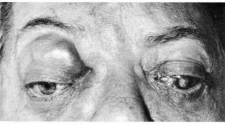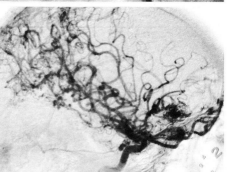

FIGURE 14-35. Clinical CT scan and angiographic features of a case of Rendu-Osler-Weber syndrome. Clinical photograph shows a massively enlarged pulsatile vein in the right upper lid. CT scan shows enlarged superior ophthalmic and lid veins. Arteriogram demonstrates multiple arteriovenous malformations, aneurysms, and fistulas including an arteriovenous malformation in the orbit.

multiple complex communications with strikingly prominent findings. The more complex lesions are the ones that tend to be associated with the Wyburn-Mason syndrome (Fig. 14-36, *insert*).

The involved arteries and draining veins are enlarged and tortuous, sometimes reaching 500 μm to 600 μm in diameter, and it may be difficult to distinguish arteries from veins on fundoscopy. Fluorescein angiography demonstrates rapid flow through the feeding artery. The site of arteriovenous communication is usually evident as an abrupt increase in vessel caliber when the dye reaches the venous side. Laminar flow is usually seen in the draining vein, with rapidly flowing shunted blood occupying the central portion of the blood vessel column.

The larger, more complex communications are associated with visual impairment or total visual loss, retinal edema and exudates, and cystic retinal degeneration. Retinal hemorrhages also occur and may be related to thrombosis of a draining vein.

The cerebral arteriovenous malformation may occupy part or all of the ipsilateral visual pathway from the optic nerve to the visual cortex. There is frequent extension into the dorsal midbrain, pons, cerebellum, and thalamus.

The clinical findings are related to the amount and site of involvement. There is usually some impairment of visual acuity with the large malformations seen in the Wyburn-Mason syndrome, although the smaller isolated arteriovenous communications are frequently incidental. The patient frequently presents in childhood with unilat-

eral amblyopia, esotropia, or both. Later in life visual failure may develop, either suddenly or gradually. Involvement of the optic nerve and orbital soft tissues by an arteriovenous malformation may be associated with pulsatile proptosis. Hemianopia is frequent owing to involvement of the optic chiasm or post-chiasmatic visual pathway. The cerebral AVM may lead to hemiparesis, hemiplegia, seizures, or subarachnoid hemorrhage.

Plain orbital radiographs and CT scans will show enlargement of the optic canal and occasionally of the bony orbit due to involvement of the optic nerve and orbital structures with AVM. The arteriovenous malformation itself will be seen on CT scan as a poorly defined enhancing mass. Contrast-enhanced CT scanning of the head and orbits followed by confirmatory angiography should be performed in all patients with retinal arteriovenous communications to diagnose the full extent of the abnormality (see Fig. 14-36).

Klippel-Trenaunay Syndrome

Klippel-Trenaunay syndrome consists of the association of cutaneous hemangiomas and venous varicosities, usually confined to a single limb, with bony and soft tissue hypertrophy of that limb. There are rare reports of associated orbital vascular anomalies, which include varices, conjunctival telangiectasia, retinal varicosities, and angiomas of the conjunctiva, sclera, and choroid.

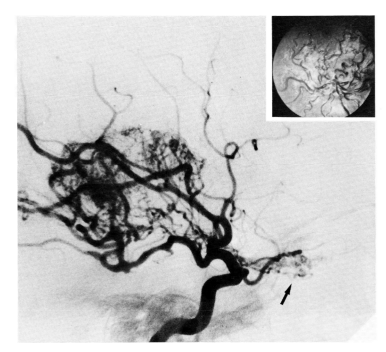

FIGURE 14-36. Angiogram demonstrates deep-seated cerebral and orbital *(arrow)* arteriovenous malformations associated with Wyburn-Mason syndrome. *Inset* demonstrates the complicated arteriovenous communication of the retinal vessels in this disorder.

■ ANEURYSMS

Arterial aneurysms within the vascular network of the orbit may be noted as incidental findings on angiography done for other reasons. Rarely do aneurysms in the orbit cause functional deficits. However, we have encountered one orbital venous aneurysm (demonstrated in Fig. 14-26) that occurred as a complication of an arteriovenous shunt and led to a tumefaction in the apex of the orbit. This mass effect caused some associated pressure on the apical structures and ultimately led to the development of an optic neuropathy.

■ OBSTRUCTIVE LESIONS

Many of the foregoing lesions, including arteriovenous fistulas, orbital varices, and some of the tumors, have obstructive elements either on the arterial or venous side. On the other hand, arterial and venous obstructive processes can be complications of other systemic and local diseases, as demonstrated in a patient with sudden chemosis, edema, and retinal venous dilatation due to orbital vein thrombosis secondary to sphenoid sinusitis (Fig. 14-37). Rarely, orbital vein thrombosis has been described as a spontaneous phenomenon presenting as a sudden hemorrhage, chemosis, edema, and retinal

venous dilatation due to a superior orbital vein obstruction. With recanalization, the signs and symptoms abate spontaneously. We have encountered such a history once in an elderly male presenting with sudden development of chemosis, venous dilatation, raised episcleral venous pressure, and proptosis. This failed to evidence any abnormalities on CT scan, other than dilatation of the superior ophthalmic vein. Signs and symptoms resolved spontaneously over a 4-week period. Although the CT scan was negative, the patient refused angiography and one could not rule out a spontaneous thrombosis of the superior ophthalmic vein owing to a minor arteriovenous shunting process. In addition, we have experienced a case of superior ophthalmic vein thrombosis following marked orbital inflammation subsequent to repeated ocular surgery.

■ UNCLASSIFIED SPONTANEOUS AND POSTTRAUMATIC ORBITAL HEMORRHAGES

Orbital hemorrhage may be a feature of trauma and may be of sufficient degree to lead to functional visual sensory or motor threat. Management in the acute situation may require emergency canthotomy, CT- or ultrasound-guided aspiration, or even decompression. In our experi-

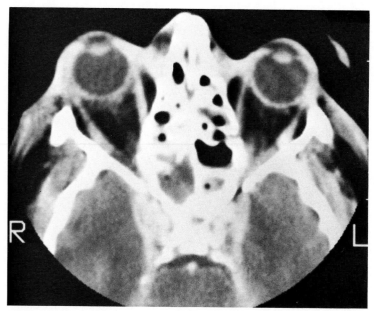

A

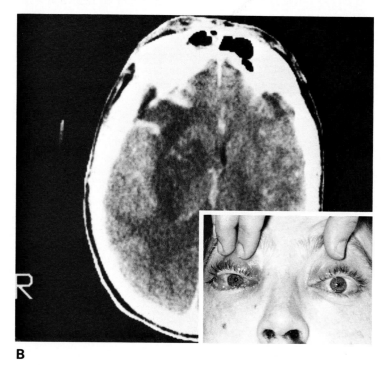

B

FIGURE 14-37. *(A)* CT scan of a patient with sphenoid sinusitis that caused cavernous sinus thrombosis associated with proptosis, chemosis, and cerebral infarction *(B)*. Note low-density areas within the cavernous sinus, indicating thrombosis *(A)*.

ence, spontaneous orbital hemorrhage of an idiopathic variety has not been noted although it is frequently described in the literature. All of the cases of spontaneous hemorrhage we have encountered have been related to underlying vascular, hemodynamic, and hematologic abnormalities.

An important but rare cause of spontaneous orbital hemorrhage is the postoperative hemorrhage that occurs approximately 3 to 4 days following orbital surgery. The hemorrhage may be due to dissolution of intravascular clots. In part it could be related to postoperative inflammation or the release of proteolytic enzymes that result from damage to the orbital fat.

Bibliography

GENERAL

Duke-Elder S, MacFaul PA: The ocular adnexa: II. Lacrimal, orbital and para-orbital diseases. In Duke-Elder S (ed): System of Ophthalmology, Vol 13, p 1086. St. Louis, CV Mosby, 1974

Enzinger FM, Weiss SW: Soft Tissue Tumors, p 379. St. Louis, CV Mosby, 1983

Henderson JW: Orbital Tumors, 2nd ed, p 128. New York, BC Decker, 1980

Jones IS, Jakobiec FA: Diseases of the Orbit, p 269. Philadelphia, Harper & Row, 1979

Reese AB: Tumors of the Eye, 3rd ed. Philadelphia, Harper & Row, 1976

CAPILLARY HEMANGIOMA

Haik BG, Jakobiec FA, Ellsworth RM et al: Capillary hemangioma of the lids and orbit: An analysis of the clinical features and therapeutic results in 101 cases. Trans Am Acad Ophthalmol 86:760, 1979

Henriksson P, Nilsson IM, Bergentz SE et al: Giant hemangioma with a disorder of coagulation. Acta Paediatr Scand 60:227, 1971.

Isacson S: Effect of prednisolone on the coagulation and fibrinolytic systems. Scand J Haematol 7:212, 1970

Kasaback HH, Merritt KK: Capillary hemangioma with extensive purpura. Am J Dis Child 59:1063, 1940

Kennedy RE: Arterial embolization of orbital hemangiomas. Tr Am Ophthalmol Soc 76:266, 1978

Kushner BJ: Intralesional corticosteroid injection for infantile adnexal hemangioma. Am J Ophthalmol 93:496, 1982

Lang PE, Dubin HV: Hemangioma-thrombocytopenia syndrome. Arch Dermatol 111:105, 1975

Neidhart JA, Roach R: Successful treatment of skeletal hemangioma and Kasabach-Merritt syndrome with aminocaproic acid. Am J Med 73:434, 1982

Pasyk KA, Dingman RO, Argenta LC et al: The management of hemangiomas of the eyelid and orbit. Head Neck Surg 6, No. 4:851, 1984

Pearce RL, Summers L, Hermann RP: The management of patients with the Kasabach-Merritt syndrome. Br J Oral Surg 13:188, 1975

Plesner-Rasmussen H, Marushak D, Goldschmidt E: Capillary hemangiomas of the eyelids and orbit. Acta Ophthalmol 61:645, 1983

Steahly LP, Almquist HT: Steroid treatment of an orbital or periocular hemangioma. J Pediatr Ophthalmol 14, No. 1:35, 1977

Stigmar G, Crawford JS, Ward CM et al: Ophthalmic sequelae of infantile hemangiomas of the eyelids and orbit. Am J Ophthalmol 85:806, 1978

Wisnick JL: Hemangiomas and vascular malformations. Ann Plast Surg 12:1, 1984

CAVERNOUS HEMANGIOMA

Coleman DJ, Jack RL, Franzen LA: High resolution B-scan ultrasonography of the orbit. II. Hemangiomas of the orbit. Arch Ophthalmol 88:368, 1972

Dilenge D: Arteriography in angiomas of the orbit. Radiology 113:355, 1974

Flanagan JC: Vascular problems of the orbit. Ophthalmology 86:896, 1979

Forbes GS, Sheedy PF, Waller RR: Orbital tumors evaluated by computer tomography. Radiology 136:101, 1980

Harris GJ, Jakobiec FA: Cavernous hemangiomas of the orbit. J Neurosurg 51:219, 1979

Harris GJ, Jakobiec FA: Cavernous hemangioma of the orbit: A clinicopathologic analysis of sixty-six cases. In Jakobiec FA (ed): Ocular and Adnexal Tumors, p 741. Birmingham, Alabama, Aesculapius, 1978

Kopelow SM, Foos RY, Straatsma BR et al: Cavernous hemangioma of the orbit. Int Ophthalmol Clin 11, No. 3:113, 1971

Krayenbuhl H: The value of orbital angiography for diagnosis of unilateral exophthalmos. J Neurosurg 19:289, 1962

Reese AB: Expanding lesions of the orbit. Trans Ophthalmol Soc UK 91:85, 1971

Vignaud T, Clay C, Bilaniuc LT: Venography of the orbit: An analytical report of 413 cases. Radiology 110:373, 1974

Wende S, Kazner E, Grumme T: The diagnostic value of computed tomography and orbital diseases: A cooperative study of 520 cases. Neurosurg Rev 3:43, 1980

Wright JE: Orbital vascular anomalies. Trans Am Ophthalmol Soc 78:606, 1980

LYMPHANGIOMAS

Batsakis JG: Tumors of the Head and Neck, p 301. Baltimore, Williams & Wilkins, 1979

Cline RA, Rootman J: Enophthalmos: A clinical review. Ophthalmology 91, No. 3:229, 1984

Engzinger FM, Weiss SW: Soft Tissue Tumors, p 482. St Louis, CV Mosby, 1983

Iliff WJ, Green WR: Orbital lymphangiomas. Symposium on Orbital Diseases 86:914, 1979

Jakobiec FA, Jones IS: Vascular tumors, malformations and degenerations. In Jones IS, Jakobiec FA (eds): Diseases of the Orbit, p 269. Philadelphia, Harper & Row, 1979

Jones IS: Lymphangiomas of the ocular adnexa: Analysis of 62 cases. Trans Am Ophthalmol Soc 57:602, 1959

Pang P, Jakobiec FA, Iwamoto T et al: Small lymphangiomas of the eyelids. Ophthalmology 91:1278, 1984

Rootman J, Hay E, Graeb D et al: Orbital-adnexal lymphangiomas: A spectrum of hemodynamically isolated vascular hamartomas. Ophthalmology 93:1558, 1986

Waldo ED, Vuletin JC, Kaye GI: The ultrastructure of vascular tumors: Additional observations and a review of the literature (part 2). Pathol Annu 12:279, 1977

Williams BH: Hemangiomas and lymphangiomas. Adv Surg 15:337, 1981

HEMANGIOPERICYTOMA

Angervall L, Kindnblom LG, Nielson JM et al: Hemangiopericytoma: A clinicopathologic, angiographic and microangiographic study. Cancer 42:2412, 1978

Brown DN, MacCarty CS, Soule EH: Orbital hemangiopericytoma: Review of the literature and report of four cases. J Neurosurg 22:354, 1965

Croxatto JO, Font RL: Hemangiopericytoma of the orbit. Hum Pathol 13:210, 1982

Enzinger FM, Smith BH: Hemangiopericytoma: An analysis of 106 cases. Hum Pathol 7:61, 1976

Fox SA: Hemangiopericytoma of the orbit. Am J Ophthalmol 40:786, 1955

Francois J, Hassens M: Hemangiopericytome de l'orbite. Ann Oculist 446:873, 1963

Genslen S, Caplan LH, Laufman H: Giant benign hemangiopericytoma functioning as an arteriovenous shunt. JAMA 198:203, 1966

Goodman SA: Hemangiopericytoma of the orbit. Am J Ophthalmol 40:237, 1955

Haney RF: Hemangiopericytoma of the orbit. Arch Ophthalmol 71:206, 1964

Henderson JW, Farrow GM: Primary orbital hemangiopericytoma: An aggressive and potentially malignant neoplasm. Arch Ophthalmol 96:666, 1978

Jakobiec FA, Howard GM, Jones IS et al: Hemangiopericytoma of the orbit. Am J Ophthalmol 78:816, 1974

Kauffman SL, Stout AP: Hemangiopericytomas in children. Cancer 13:695, 1960

Macoul KL: Hemangiopericytoma of the lid and orbit. Am J Ophthalmol 66:731, 1968

McMaster MJ, Soule EH, Ivins JC: Hemangiopericytoma: A clinicopathologic study and long-term follow-up of 60 patients. Cancer 36:2232, 1975

Russman BA: Tumor of the orbit: A 33-year follow-up. Am J Ophthalmol 64:273, 1967

Spaeth EB, Valdes-Dapena A: Hemangiopericytoma. Arch Ophthalmol 60:1070, 1958

Stout AP: Hemangiopericytoma: A study of twenty-five new cases. Cancer 2:1027, 1949

Stout AP, Murray MR: Hemangiopericytoma: A vascular tumor featuring Zimmermann's pericytes. Ann Surg 116:26, 1942

Sugar HS, Fishman GR, Kobernick S et al: Orbital hemangiopericytoma or vascular meningioma? Am J Ophthalmol 70:103, 1970

MALIGNANT HEMANGIOENDOTHELIOMA: ANGIOSARCOMA

Bankaci M, Myers EN, Barnes L et al: Angiosarcoma of the maxillary sinus: Literature review and case report. Head Neck Surg 1:274, 1979

Carelli PV, Cangelosi JP: Angiosarcoma of the orbit. Am J Ophthalmol 31:453, 1948

Forrest AW: Intraorbital tumors. Arch Ophthalmol 41:198, 1949

Maddox JC, Evans HL: Angiosarcoma of skin and soft tissue: A study of forty-four cases. Cancer 48:1907, 1981

Messmer EP, Font RL, McCrang JA et al: Epithelioid angiosarcoma of the orbit presenting as Tolosa-Hauf syndrome. Ophthalmology 90:1414, 1983

Nath K, Gogi R, Khan AA et al: Vascular hamartoma and vascular tumours of orbit. Indian J Ophthalmol 25:18, 1977

Sekimoto T, Nakaseko H, Kondo K et al: A case of malignant hemangioendothelioma in the orbit. Folio Ophthalmol Jpn 22:535, 1971

Stout AP: Hemangio-endothelioma: A tumor of blood vessels featuring vascular endothelial cells. Ann Surg 118:445, 1943

Treheux A, Reny A, Picard JL et al: Tumeur rare de l'orbite chez l'enfant. J Radiol Electrol Med Nucl 56:279, 1975

Tsuda N, Takaku I: A case report of malignant vascular tumor of the orbit in a newborn. Folio Ophthalmol Jpn 21:728, 1970

KAPOSI'S SARCOMA

Dayan AD, Lewis PD: Origin of Kaposi's sarcoma from the reticuloendothelial system. Nature 213:889, 1967

Giraldo G, Beth E, Coeur P et al: Kaposi's sarcoma: A new model in the search for viruses associated with human malignancies. J Natl Cancer Inst 49:1495, 1972

Giraldo G, Beth E, Huang ES: Kaposi's sarcoma and its relationship to cytomegalovirus (CMV), III, CMV, DNA and CMV early antigens in Kaposi's sarcoma. Int J Cancer 26:23, 1980

Holland GN, Gottlieb MS, Yee RD et al: Ocular disorders associated with a new severe acquired cellular immunodeficiency syndrome. Am J Ophthalmol 93:393, 1982

Holecek MJ, Harwood AR: Radiotherapy of Kaposi's sarcoma. Cancer 41:1733, 1978

Howard G, Jakobiec F, DeVoe A: Kaposi's sarcoma: The subconjunctival hemorrhage that never clears. Am J Ophthalmol 79:420, 1975

Kalinske M, Leone C: Kaposi's sarcoma involving eyelid and conjunctiva. Ann Ophthalmol 14, No. 5:497, 1982

Lanzotti VJ, Campos LT, Sinkouris JG et al: Chemotherapy for advanced Kaposi's sarcoma. Arch Dermatol 111:1331, 1975

Macher A, Palestine A et al: Multicentric Kaposi's sarcoma of the conjunctiva in male homosexuals with the acquired immunodeficiency syndrome. Ophthalmology 90:879, 1983

O'Brien PH, Brasfield RD: Kaposi's sarcoma. Cancer 19:1497, 1966

Odom R, Goett D: Treatment of cutaneous Kaposi's sarcoma with intralesional vincristine. Arch Dermatol 114:1693, 1978

Rothman S: Some clinical aspects of Kaposi's sarcoma in the European and North American population. Acta Un Int Cancer 18:364, 1962

Safai B, Mike V, Giraldo G et al: Association of Kaposi's sarcoma with second primary malignancies: Possible etiopathogenic implications. Cancer 45:1472, 1980

Sezer N, Ercikan C: Kaposi's sarcoma with ocular manifestations. Br J Ophthalmol 48:223, 1964

Templeton AC, Bhanna D: Prognosis in Kaposi's sarcoma. J Natl Cancer Inst 55:1361, 1975

ANGIOLYMPHOID HYPERPLASIA

Castro C, Winkelman RK: Angiolymphoid hyperplasia with eosinophilia in the skin. Cancer 34:1696, 1974

Gardener JH, Amonette RA, Chesney TM: Angiolymphoid hyperplasia with eosinophilia. J Dermatol Surg Oncol 7:414, 1981

Hisayat AA, Cameron DJ, Font RL et al: Angiolymphoid hyperplasia with eosinophilia (Kinura's disease) of the orbit and ocular adnexa. Am J Ophthalmol 96:176, 1983

Jones EW, Bleehen SS: Inflammatory angiomatous nodules with abnormal blood vessels occurring about the ears and scalp (pseudo or atypical pyogenic granuloma). Br J Dermatol 81:804, 1969

Mehregan AH, Shapiro L: Angiolymphoid hyperplasia with eosinophilia. Arch Dermatol 103:50, 1971

Moesner J, Pallesen R, Sorensen B: Angiolymphoid hyperplasia with eosinophilia (Kimura's disease). Arch Dermatol 117:650, 1981

Reed RJ, Tarazakis N: Subcutaneous angioblastic lymphoid hyperplasia with eosinophilia (Kimura's disease). Cancer 29:489, 1972

Rosai J, Gold J, Landy R: The histiocytoid hemangiomas: A unifying concept embracing several previously described entities of the skin, soft tissue, large vessels, bone, and heart. Hum Pathol 10:707, 1979

Takenaka T, Okuda M, Usami A et al: Histochemical and immunological studies on eosinophilic granuloma of soft tissue, so called Kimura's disease. Clin Allergy 6:27, 1976

Wells, GC, Whimster, IW: Subcutaneous angiolymphoid hyperplasia with eosinophilia. Br J Dermatol 81:1, 1969

VASCULAR LEIOMYOMA

Duhig JJ, Ayer JP: Vascular leiomyoma: A study of 61 cases. Arch Pathol 68:424, 1959

Henderson JW, Harrison EG, Jr: Vascular leiomyoma of the orbit: Report of a case. Trans Am Acad Ophthalmol Otolaryngol 74:970, 1970

Jakobiec FA, Howard GM, Rosen M et al: Leiomyomas and leiomyosarcoma of the orbit. Am J Ophthalmol 80:1028, 1975

Jakobiec FA, Jones IS, Tannenbaum M: Leiomyoma: An unusual tumor of the orbit. Br J Ophthalmol 57:825, 1973

Nath K, Shukla BR: Orbital leiomyoma and its origin. Br J Ophthalmol 47:369, 1963

Sanborn GE, Valenzuela RE, Green RW: Leiomyoma of the orbit. Am J Ophthalmol 87:371, 1979

Wolter JR: Hemangio-leiomyoma of the orbit. Eye Ear Nose Throat Mon 44:42, 1965

ARTERIOVENOUS SHUNTS AND VENOUS ANOMALIES

Brismar G, Brismar J: Spontaneous carotid-cavernous fistulas: Phlebographic appearance and relation to thrombosis. Acta Radiologic Diagnosis 17, Fasc. 2, March 1976

Chaudhary MY, Sachdev VP, Soo HC et al: Dural arteriovenous malformation of the major venous sinuses: an acquired lesion. AJNR 3:13, 1982

Grove AS, Jr: The dural shunt syndrome: Pathophysiology and clinical course. Ophthalmology 91:31, 1984

Houser OW, Campbell JK, Campbell RJ et al: Arteriovenous malformation affecting the transverse dural venous sinus: An acquired lesion. Mayo Clin Proc 54:651, 1979

Newton TH, Hoyt WF: Dural arteriovenous shunts in the region of the cavernous sinus. Neuroradiology 1:71, 1970

Seeger JF, Gabrielsen TO, Giannotta SL et al: Carotid-cavernous sinus fistulas and venous thrombosis. AJNR 1:141, 1980

Talusan ED, Fishbein SL, Schwartz B: Increased pressure of dilated episceral veins with open-angle glaucoma without exophthalmos. Ophthalmology 90:257, 1983

Wright JE: Orbital vascular anomalies. Trans Am Acad Ophthalmol 78:OPH-606, 1974

CONGENITAL VASCULAR ANOMALIES

Ritch R, Shields MB: The secondary Glaucomas. St Louis, CV Mosby, 1982

Vinken PJ, Bruyn GW (eds): Handbook of Clinical Neurology, Vol 14, The Phakomatoses. New York: American Elsevier, 1972

STURGE-WEBER SYNDROME

Haberland C: The phakomatoses. In Vinken PJ, Bruyu GW (eds): Handbook of Clinical Neurology, Vol 31, p 18. New York, American Elsevier, 1977

Nellhaus G, Haberland C, Hill BJ: Sturge-Weber disease with bilateral intracranial calcifications at birth and unusual pathologic findings. Acta Neurol Scand 43:314, 1967

Phelps CD: The Pathogenesis of glaucoma in Sturge-Weber syndrome: Ophthalmology 85:276, 1978

Wohlwill FJ, Yakovlev PI: Histopathology of meningo-facial angiomatosis (Sturge-Weber's disease). J Neuropathol Exp Neurol 16:341, 1957

HEREDITARY HEMORRHAGIC TELANGIECTASIA

Davis DG, Lawton Smith J: Retinal involvement in hereditary hemorrhagic telangiectasia. Arch Ophthalmol 85:618, 1971

Hashimoto K, Pritzker MS: Hereditary hemorrhagic telangiectasia. Oral Surg 34:751, 1972

Hieshima GB, Cahan LD, Berlin MS et al: Calvarial, orbital and dural vascular anomalies in hereditary hemorrhagic telangiectasia. Surg Neurol 8:263, 1977

Hodgson CH, Burchell HB, Allen GC et al: Hereditary hemorrhagic telangiectasia and pulmonary arteriovenous fistula. N Engl J Med 261:625, 1959

Roman G, Fisher M, Perl DP et al: Neurological manifestations of hereditary hemorrhagic telangiectasia (Rendu-Osler-Weber disease): Report of 2 cases and review of the literature. Ann Neurol 4:130, 1978

WYBURN-MASON SYNDROME

Archer DB, Ernest JT, Krill AE: Arteriovenous communications of the retina. Ophthalmol 75:224, 1973

Theron J, Newton TH, Hoyt WF: Unilateral retinocephalic vascular malformations. Neuroradiology 7:185, 1974

Wyburn-Mason R: Arteriovenous aneurysm of mid-brain and retina, facial naevi and mental changes. Brain 66, part 3:12, 1943

KLIPPEL-TRENAUNAY SYNDROME

Limaye SR, Doyle HA, Tang RA: Retinal varicosity in Klippel-Trenaunay syndrome. J Pediatr Ophthalmol Strabismus 16:371, 1979

Rathbun JE, Hoyt WF, Beard C: Surgical management of orbitofrontal varix in Klippel-Trenaunay-Weber syndrome. Am J Ophthalmol 72:109, 1970

CHAPTER 15

Degenerations and Depositions

Jack Rootman

The category of disease involving degenerations and depositions constitutes the smallest group of patients (2%) encountered in our orbital practice. It includes a range of atrophies and abiotrophies that lead to degenerative change of the orbit or of the orbital contents. Patients may present in an orbital practice on the basis of pseudoproptosis (myopia, buphthalmus; Fig. 15-1), enophthalmos (fat atrophies), ocular motor abnormalities (progressive external ophthalmoplegia, amyloid deposition), or mass effect (amyloid deposition, orbital fat prolapse).

Myopia was the most common cause of pseudoproptosis in our orbital practice. Other causes include failure of recognition of facial asymmetry, unilateral bony hypoplasia, ptosis, buphthalmus, and staphyloma.

Orbital atrophy may occur secondary to fatty degeneration following severe orbital trauma, hemorrhage, inflammation, or radiotherapy. Orbital radiotherapy (particularly when delivered in childhood) causes fat atrophy and enophthalmos; unfortunately, this is a common consequence of retinoblastoma treatment with external beam radiotherapy (Fig. 15-2). In addition, it may be seen as part of localized disorders such as scleroderma (as illustrated previously; see Chapter 4), as an idiopathic syndrome in the elderly (Fig. 15-3), or as part of hemifacial atrophy. The cicatrizing process associated with scleroderma appears to involve and restrict the extraocular muscles as well as those of the lid. The primary orbital fat atrophies do not affect muscle balance. Another commonly seen degenerative condition is in the patient who presents with a mass, usually in the region of the lacrimal gland, due to a prolapse of fat through the degenerating Tenon's capsule. This, of course, is a disease of the elderly. It is easily diagnosable on the basis of the ease of retropulsion of the orbital fat prolapse, evidence of the fat seen through Tenon's capsule on slit-lamp examination, and normal ocular motor and orbital findings. On CT scan this has a dramatic appearance of a focal area of radiolucency adjacent to the sclera anteriorly (Fig. 15-4).

Orbital Amyloidosis

Jack Rootman and Peter Dolman

Given what is known about pathogenesis, it could be argued that amyloid belongs in the category of inflammatory or lymphoproliferative disease processes. However, we have included it here as a deposition because of the varied and overlapping distribution, changing nomenclature, and uncertain classification (Table 15-1). Amyloid deposits are not chemically distinct entities, but are a group of diseases that have in common the deposition of several types of abnormal fibrillar proteins with similar physical chemical properties. The symptoms associated with deposition depend on the site, distribution, and magnitude of amyloid, with renal involvement being the most serious. The diagnosis is by biopsy evidence of amyloid in the system involved.

These proteins appear as an amorphous, eosinophilic, hyaline material on light microscopy with routine hematoxylin-eosin stains. A pathognomonic feature is positive congophilia (Congo red stain) with blue-green birefringence (dichroism) on polarizing microscopy. In addition, these deposits may be defined histochemically by metachromasia with crystal or methyl violet and fluorescence in ultraviolet light following thioflavin T or thioflavin S staining. Ultrastructurally, amyloid consists of parallel rows of fibers 75 nm to 100 nm in diameter that show a cross beta-pleated sheet structure on x-ray diffraction.

Chemically, amyloid is made up of 90% fibrils and 10% P component, which is a glycoprotein similar to C reactive protein. The fibrils are derived from polypeptide fragments of normal serum proteins and vary depending on the clinical setting. Amyloidosis can be divided on the basis of distribution into systemic and localized disease, and the systemic type can be divided into immunocyte related (systemic) and secondary (related to inflammatory

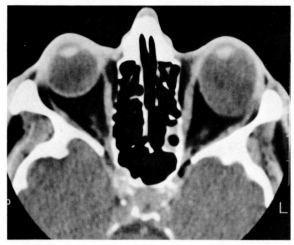

FIGURE 15-1. Axial CT scan demonstrates a buphthalmic left eye in a 67-year-old man who presented with a history of childhood amblyopia and strabismus, and a recent awareness of increasing prominence of the left eye. On physical examination the left globe was 2 mm more prominent than the right, and displaced downward 3 mm with an 18-D right hypertropia. On fundus examination there was left peripapillary atrophy and old chorioretinal scars. The CT scan supports a diagnosis of a large globe causing the appearance of proptosis.

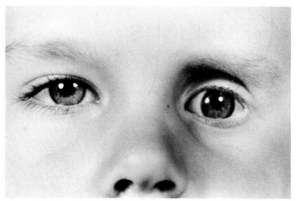

FIGURE 15-2. This child with bilateral retinoblastoma had been treated several years earlier with left orbital radiotherapy and local therapy on the right side. The radiotherapy has led to obvious orbital shrinkage. (Cline RA, Rootman J: Enophthalmos: A clinical review. Ophthalmology 91:229, 1984)

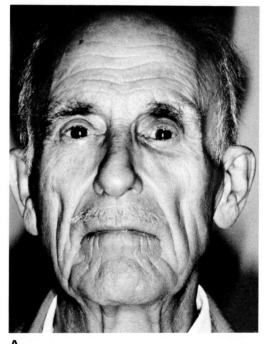

A

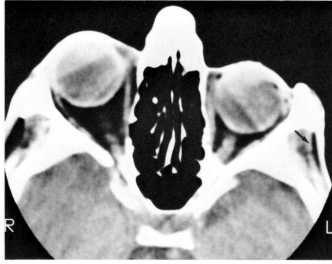

B

FIGURE 15-3. *(A)* This 78-year-old man seen in 1986 had noted ''sinking'' of the left eye for 1 to 2 years. He was otherwise healthy, had no known sinus problems, and had no other ocular symptoms. Vision was normal, as were extraocular movements. There was a markedly deepened left superior sulcus and temporalis fossa. From a clinical point of view, he appeared to have some orbital fat atrophy and similar atrophy in the temporalis fossa. Photographic review revealed that since 1983 this atrophy had been progressive. *(B)* The CT scan showed left enophthalmos with reduced orbital fat and a diminution of fat in the temporalis fossa *(arrow)* when compared to the right side. A diagnosis of senile fat atrophy was made.

disease). In the immunocyte-related amyloidosis (*i.e.*, primary systemic amyloidosis without underlying disease) and lymphoma-related amyloidosis, the fibrils are composed of fragments from a variable region of immunoglobulin light chains and are termed *AL amyloid*. They are typically deposited around blood vessels, in skin, nerve and muscle of the tongue, heart, and gastrointestinal tract. Skin is a characteristic site in so-called primary amyloidosis, where amyloid deposits as yellow plaques associated with frequent ecchymosis due to rupture of the fragile vessels.

Secondary amyloidosis occurs in conjunction with a variety of inflammatory conditions including rheumatoid arthritis (14% to 26% of patients with arthritis), dermatomyositis, scleroderma, inflammatory bowel disease, osteomyelitis, lung abscess, and leprosy. The protein fibrils in secondary amyloidosis *(AA amyloid)* are derived from an acute-phase reactant, serum amyloid A protein. This is thought to be due to proteolytic cleavage of the precursor acute-phase reactant in response to sustained activation of macrophages. Both overproduction and defective degradation of precursor proteins are involved in the pathogenesis of fibril deposition in both types of systemic amyloidosis. The organs commonly affected in secondary amyloidosis are liver, spleen, kidneys, and adrenals. The heredofamilial systemic amyloidosis syndromes are rare. They are usually described on the basis of geographic origin of the cases, and can be divided into neuropathies (Portuguese), nephropathies (familial Mediterranean fever), cardiopathies, and miscellaneous (including lattice corneal dystrophy, medullary tumor of the thyroid, and cerebral amyloidosis). The neuropathies have AF amyloid derived from pre-albumin.

The various forms of localized amyloidosis can be divided into primary or secondary. The primary type is unassociated with any known local disorder, and the secondary types may be associated with local inflammatory disease, degeneration, or focal lymphoproliferative processes.

The eye and periocular tissues are variably involved by any of the amyloid syndromes. Immunocyte-related systemic amyloidosis (primary and lymphoma related) commonly form subcutaneous, waxy yellow eyelid nodules, but may also infiltrate cranial nerves or extraocular muscles and rarely involve the vitreous, retina, choroid, and sclera. Secondary systemic amyloidosis rarely affects the orbit but may involve the periorbital skin.

A primary localized amyloid has been frequently reported in the cornea and conjunctiva. Less commonly, it extends into the orbit. When in the orbit alone, it may appear as a mass in any site including the lacrimal gland, where it may develop as a slowly expanding mass lesion. When it affects the extraocular muscles, it characteristically causes a nodular enlargement of the muscle notable

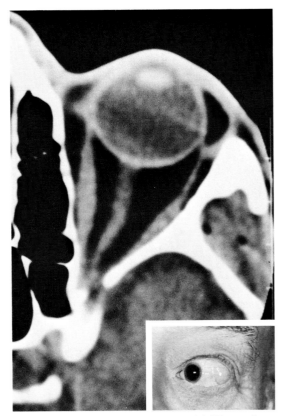

FIGURE 15-4. Clinical photograph and axial CT scan demonstrate lateral prolapse of orbital fat through Tenon's capsule, a clinical syndrome that often presents as an apparent anterior orbital mass.

on CT scan. Immunamyloidosis may be due to a production of amyloidogenic light-chain immunoglobulin protein by a proliferating clone of plasma cells, which may be localized or disseminated in distribution. The benign localized form of this disease has been found in various organs, particularly the bronchopulmonary tree and ocular sites such as orbit, eyelid, and conjunctiva. We have reported an example of localized ocular immunamyloidosis involving the caruncle due to a single clone of plasma cells. Marsh and co-workers have also reported a case of localized conjunctival amyloidosis in a patient who subsequently (within 1 year) developed a diffuse mixed small and large cell lymphoma of the scapula with amyloid in the stroma. Localized amyloid secondary to chronic inflammation or infections of the conjunctiva or cornea usually is subclinical and is identified only at the time of microscopy, and does not involve the orbit.

In short, orbital infiltration by amyloid is most often primary and localized, although it may be part of a sys- *(Text continues on p. 575.)*

TABLE 15-1.
AMYLOIDOSIS: GENERAL, OCULAR, AND ORBITAL FEATURES

Type	General Features	Ocular Features	Orbital Features	Physical Chemistry	Management and Outcome
I. Systemic A. Immunocyte related 1. Primary	Heart—especially in the elderly Skin 55% Tongue GI Peripheral nerves Lower respiratory 30% Liver—90% on biopsy Spleen Majority have monoclonal immunoglobulin in serum or urine		Yellow—ecchymotic skin plaques seen more frequently than in secondary amycoidosis Orbital infiltrate may occur	AL—denatured by formalin Does not lose congophilia after incubation with potassium permanganate	Colchicine and DMSO Death generally 14 months to 10 years Local management of masses

2. Lymphoma related
(a) myeloma—seen in 5%–15% of patients with myeloma
(b) lymphoma
  Waldenstrom's macroglobulinemia
  Heavy chain disease
  Solitary plasmacytoma
  Nodular lymphoma
	Skin 42%
	Tongue
	Arthropathy
	Lower respiratory 30%
	Liver 100% on biopsy
	Kidney most serious
	Spleen
	Adrenal
	Heart—rare
	Monoclonal peak
			May involve skin and orbit	AL—from circulating light chains	Majority are dead in 6 months if myeloma related

B. Familial 1. Neuropathy (a) Lower limb (Portuguese) (b) Upper limb		Scalloped pupils Cornea—vitreous		AFp—pre-albumin	
2. Nephropathy Familial Mediterranean fever, etc.	Autosomal recessive Fever and inflamed pleura, synovium, peritoneam Systemic distribution of amyloid Skin 100%			AA—from SAA	Colchicine and DMSO

572

Classification	Distribution / Notes	Ocular tissue	Biochemistry / Findings	Treatment

3. Cardiopathy
  Progressive heart failure
  Persistent atrial standstill
	Autosomal dominant		ASc—pre-albumin	

4. Miscellaneous (a) Medullary tumor of thyroid	Local amyloid in tumor		AE—prohormone for thyrocalcitonen	
(b) Lattice corneal dystrophy	Autosomal dominant	Cornea		May rarely regress after treatment of the primary disorder
(c) Cerebral hemorrhage				

C. Secondary
 1. Chronic inflammatory disease
  Rheumatoid arthritis
  14%–26% of patients with rheumatoid arthritis
  Dermatomyositis
  Scleroderma
  Inflammatory bowel disease
  Regional enteritis
  Ulcerative colitis
	Seem to be the most severe systemic involvement
	Kidney
	Liver
	Spleen
	Lymph nodes
	Adrenal
	Thyroid
		Less frequently involves the orbit than primary localized	AA—related to SAA
			Loss of congophilia after incubation with potassium permangate not denatured by formalin	

2. Chronic infection
  TB
  Bronchiectasis
  Chronic osteomyelitis				

3. In association with tumors
  Hodgkin's
  Renal cell carcinoma				

II. Localized A. Primary idiopathic	Lung Bladder Tongue Orbit—masses or on microscopy alone	Conjunctiva	Some have been shown to have AL with localized inflammatory cells	Local resection if possible and symptomatic
B. Secondary 1. Lymphoproliferative (local immunocyte related)	Masses or microscopic		Occasionally have demonstrated local monoclonal immunoglobulins	Local resection
2. Inflammatory	Chronic conjunctival inflammatory disease vernal conjunctivitis trachoma	Conjunctiva especially Histologic finding		Local treatment

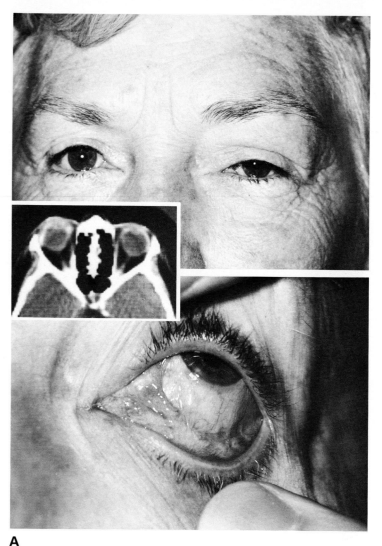

FIGURE 15-5. *(A)* This 62-year-old woman had left orbital aching and drooping of the lid present for 18 months. In addition, she was aware of inferior conjunctival thickening and injection. On physical examination the lower lid and orbit had a doughy consistency. The tissues of the semilunar fold and both inferior and superior conjunctival fornices were thickened by a firm, yellowish, subconjunctival infiltrate *(bottom)*. There was reduced corneal sensation, full extraocular movement, normal exophthalmometry, and normal fundus examination. The CT scan shows an increased density of the left upper lid and thickening of the anterior portion of the sclera and orbit. *(B)* Visual fields demonstrate a general constriction on the left side, which progressed over the next year. The anterior orbital and subconjunctival amyloid mass was debulked.

A

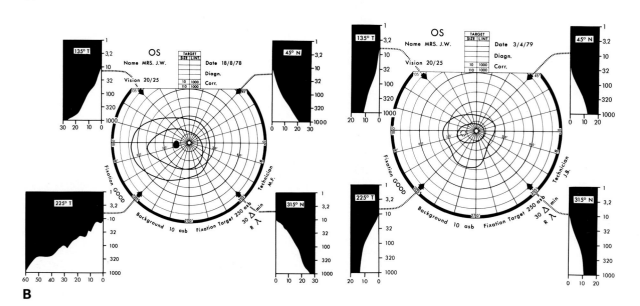

B

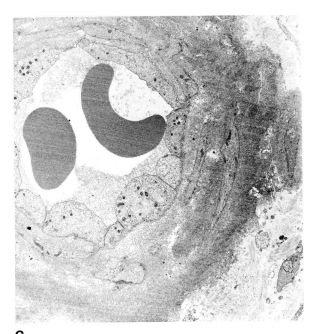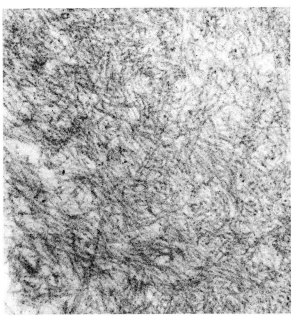

C

FIGURE 15-5 *(Continued).* *(C, top)* Electron microscopy of the orbital specimen demonstrates extracellular amyloid filaments in close relation to endothelial and smooth muscle cells. The amyloid encases perivascular cells (original magnification × 5600). *(Bottom)* Higher power electron micrograph demonstrates extracellular amyloid filaments forming a dense meshwork (original magnification × 94,000). We postulated that peripheral amyloid deposition had affected the pial vessels, leading to the extremely steep profile of the constricted isopters demonstrated on static perimetry in *B*.

temic syndrome wherein there is usually lid involvement as well. Deposits of primary amyloid often initially occur in the conjunctiva and later extend to involve more posterior tissues. This may cause proptosis or infiltrate the extraocular muscles to produce motility disturbances or ptosis. In the late stages, complete fixation of the globe can occasionally occur. Lacrimal gland involvement can lead to expansion of the lacrimal fossa and tumefaction with associated keratoconjunctivitis indistinguishable from a slow-growing tumor of the lacrimal gland. We have encountered a case of orbital amyloidosis that led to visual field contraction (Fig. 15-5), and others have described orbital pain secondary to nerve infiltration. In addition, recurrent orbital hemorrhages and eyelid purpura from perivascular deposits have been noted. At the time of surgery, because of the vascular involvement and stromal amyloid deposits, these lesions are frequently hemorrhagic and rather friable.

Infiltrates usually develop so insidiously, the diagnosis is often late. Biopsy and histopathologic examination with special stains (including immunohistochemistry) are mandatory. Evaluation for systemic involvement includes a thorough physical examination, blood and urine protein immunoelectrophoresis, 24-hour urine assessment for Bence Jones proteins (immunoglobulin light chain fragments), and bone marrow aspirate in cases of suspected multiple myeloma. Rectal and abdominal fat biopsies may help rule out the presence of systemic disease.

Definitive treatment for localized amyloidosis is surgical excision and reconstruction where possible. Damage is restricted to the involved tissue, because localized amyloidosis apparently never sytematizes. Therefore, the prognosis is favorable for most orbital cases. However, the systemic variety follows a gloomier course. In some cases of secondary amyloidosis, elimination of chronic infection or removal of the inciting neoplasm may result in resorption of the deposits. However, most primary and secondary systemic cases progress inexorably to cause major organ failure with a mean survival following diagnosis of between 1 and 4 years. Death is on the average within 14 months, but may occur any time between that period and 10 years. Patients with myeloma and amyloidosis are usually dead within 6 months. There have been recent attempts to treat familial Mediterranean fever and primary systemic amyloidosis with colchicine and dimethylsulfoxide (DMSO).

Bibliography

Borodic GE, Beyer-Machule CK, Millin J et al: Immunoglobulin deposition in localized conjunctival amyloidosis. Am J Ophthalmol 98:617, 1984

Campos EC, Melato M, Manconi R et al: Pathology of ocular tissues in amyloidosis. Ophthalmologica 181:31, 1980

Cline RA, Rootman J: Enophthalmos: A clinical review. Ophthalmology 91:229, 1984

Cohen AS: Amyloidosis. In Petersdorf RG, Adams RD, Braunwald E et al (eds): Harrison's Principles of Internal Medicine, 10th ed, p 368. New York, McGraw-Hill, 1983

Cohen AS et al: Editorial: Amyloid proteins, precursors, mediator, and enhancer. Lab Invest 48:1, 1983

Cooper JH, Ramsey M, Rootman J: Extramedullary plasmacytoma (amyloid tumor) of the caruncle. Submitted for publication, 1987

Da Costa P, Corrin B: Amyloidosis localized to the lower respiratory tract: Probable immunamyloid nature of the tracheobronchial and nodular pulmonary forms. Histopathology 9:703, 1985

Doughman DJ: Ocular amyloidosis. Surv Ophthalmol 13:133, 1968

Duane T: Amyloidosis. In Clinical Ophthalmology, Vol 2, Chap. 35, p 42. Philadelphia, Harper & Row, 1984

Finlay KR, Rootman J, Dimmick J: Optic neuropathy in primary orbital amyloidosis. Can J Ophthalmol 15:189, 1980

Glenner GG: Amyloid deposits and amyloidosis: The Beta fibrilloses. N Engl J Med 302:1283, 1333, 1980

Goodman TF Jr, Abele DC, West CS Jr: Electron microscopy in the diagnosis of amyloidosis. Arch Dermatol 106:393, 1972

Howard G: Amyloid tumours of the orbit. Br J Ophthalmol 50:421, 1966

Hui AN, Koss MN, Hochholzer L et al: Amyloidosis presenting in the lower respiratory tract. Arch Pathol Lab Med 110:212, 1986

Kaiser-Kupfer MI, McAdam KPWJ, Kuwabara T: Localized amyloidosis of the orbit and upper respiratory tract. Am J Ophthalmol 84:721, 1977

Khalil MK, Huang S, Viloria J et al: Extramedullary plasmacytoma of the orbit: Case report with results of immunocytochemical studies. Can J Ophthalmol 16:39, 1981

Kisilevsky R: Amyloidosis: A familiar problem in the light of current pathogenetic developments. Lab Invest 49:381, 1983

Knowles D, Jakobiec F, Rosen M et al: Amyloidosis of the orbit and adnexae. Surv Ophthalmol 19:367, 1975

Kyle RA, Greipp PR: Amyloidosis (AL): Clinical and laboratory features in 229 cases. Mayo Clin Proc 58:665, 1983

Levine MR, Buckman G: Primary localized orbital amyloidosis. Ann Ophthalmol 18:165, 1986

Lucas DR, Knox F, Davies S: Apparent monoclonal origin of lymphocytes and plasma cells infiltrating ocular adnexal amyloid deposits: Report of two cases. Br J Ophthalmol 66:600, 1982

Marsh WM, Streeten BW, Hoepner JA et al: Localized conjunctival amyloidosis associated with extranodal lymphoma. Ophthalmology 94:61, 1987

Nehen J: Primary localized orbital amyloidosis. Acta Ophthalmol (Copenh) 57:287, 1975

Radnot M, Lapis K, Feher J: Amyloid tumor in the lacrimal gland. Ann Ophthalmol 3:727, 1971

Raflo G, Farrell T, Sioussat R: Complete ophthalmoplegia secondary to amyloidosis associated with multiple myeloma. Am J Ophthalmol 92:221, 1981

Robbins SL, Cotran RS: Amyloidosis. In Pathologic Basis of Disease, 3rd ed, p 195. Philadelphia, WB Saunders, 1984

Schaldenbrand JD, Keren DF: IgD amyloid in IgD-lambda monoclonal conjunctival amyloidosis. Arch Pathol Lab Med 107:626, 1983

Simpson GT, Skinner M, Strong MS et al: Localized amyloidosis of the head and neck and upper aerodigestive and lower respiratory tracts. Ann Otol Rhinol Laryngol 93:374, 1984

PART IV

Management of Diseases
of the Orbit

CHAPTER 16

Orbital Surgery

Jack Rootman

In the last 20 years advances in investigative techniques, anesthesia, and surgery have vastly improved the operative potential for diseases within the orbit. Preoperative localization and characterization by computed tomography, ultrasonography, and special radiographic procedures allow ophthalmic surgeons to be more certain of the nature of orbital pathology. The surrounding tissues are more clearly defined and the approach can be better planned. For major orbital procedures, in the absence of systemic contraindications, the use of hypotensive anesthesia facilitates more deliberate, contemplative, bloodless surgery. Operative microscopy, fiberoptic illumination, and special instrumentation enhances the field of view and allows meticulous dissection of orbital lesions.

The orbital contents are within 30 cc of space surrounded by bone, nasal sinuses, and the intracranial contents. The complex of neurosensory, motor, and secretory structures are tightly confined and any insensitive mechanical insult could have disastrous effects on ocular function. Surgery in this space is properly the domain of the experienced ophthalmic surgeon or multidisciplinary team familiar with the anatomy and physiology of the orbit and the periorbital structures. Careful preoperative planning, meticulous operative technique, and fastidious postoperative care are fundamental to successful management. There is nothing more frustrating or humiliating than choosing the wrong approach or the wrong instruments for the wrong lesion.

■ INDICATIONS

The timing and approach of surgical intervention are based on the nature of the orbital disease process defined by clinical and laboratory study. The basic indications for surgery of the orbit are biopsy, excision of a cyst or mass, repair and reconstruction, drainage of an abscess, decompression, and exenteration.

Orbital Mass Lesions

The need for surgical intervention for orbital mass lesions can be broadly separated into two categories:

1. Well-defined, slow-growing, or nonprogressive lesions (cystic, neoplastic, and structural) without functional deficit can be observed. Intervention is based on size, location, rate of progression, or extension. Surgery is usually extirpative in these cases. The specific surgical approach is established by knowing the location, contours, and effect of the mass based on preoperative studies.
2. Progressive, infiltrative lesions causing entrapment or functional damage to neurosensory and motor structures generally require incisional biopsy prior to definitive management.

Biopsy is the single most demanding and underestimated orbital procedure. Meticulous care directed to hemostasis and exposure is mandatory, because many orbital lesions may present only subtle alterations in color, texture, and contour that differentiate them from surrounding normal tissues. Occasionally differences may be so subtle that a frozen section biopsy might be required to be sure that the appropriate pathology has been identified. It is important to identify adjacent landmarks carefully and to correlate them with preoperative imaging before either incisional or excisional biopsy. Preoperative or intraoperative evaluation prior to biopsy should include consultation with the pathologist, because the material obtained from this critical site may require special fixation and handling to maximize its diagnostic value. In addition to obtaining guidance as to disposition of tissue, it may be worthwhile to ascertain in advance the size of biopsy necessary for appropriate histopathologic study.

Orbital Foreign Bodies

Orbital foreign bodies that disturb function, are potentially toxic, or result in infection should be removed. In particular, vegetable matter requires removal to prevent infection or fistula formation. On the other hand, metallic foreign bodies lying within fat are rarely of major concern and should not be aggressively sought after unless they are potentially reactive or cause direct damage to orbital structures.

Trauma

Orbital and periorbital trauma that interferes with function or causes significant structural defects requires exploration and repair. Acute soft tissue injuries to the orbit may cause extensive hemorrhage or swelling, which threatens ocular and orbital structures, and may require urgent decompression. Bony fragments associated with complicated fractures need to be carefully removed and realigned when necessary. Because of the frequently complicated nature of facial trauma, reconstruction and repair may be done by a team consisting of ophthalmologist, otorhinolaryngologist, neurosurgeon, or reconstructive facial surgeon.

Drainage

Management of abscesses trapped within the orbit or periorbital spaces requires appropriate drainage, culture, and antibiotic administration. Drainage should be by the correct route depending upon the origin of the infection and the localization within the orbit. When suppurative infections originating from superficial wounds or pyemic sources loculate, they should be drained by the most direct route. On the other hand, sinus infections are a frequent source of orbital cellulitis that may form abscesses. Treatment should include antibiotics aimed at the likely organisms depending on age group, culture, and local epidemiology and may involve drainage of the abscess and sinus cavity. Prompt, frequent, and adequate monitoring of ocular functions is vital in management of these problems because functional deterioration can be rapid, even catastrophic.

Decompression

Graves' orbitopathy, sudden severe hemorrhage, or massive orbital swelling may jeopardize visual, sensory, and motor function, necessitating decompression. In a reversible, short-lived disorder such as a hemorrhage, a simple lateral canthotomy or aspiration may suffice to deal with the immediate threat to vision or ocular function. Failing this, a full exploration and decompression may be necessary.

In Graves' orbitopathy, progressive exophthalmos with severe exposure keratopathy, compressive optic neuropathy and marked cosmetic disfigurement are indications for decompression. Decompression can be lateral, inferior, medial, or by combined approach, but must breach the periorbita to be effective. The periorbital tissues represent a relatively inelastic plane, and unless they are incised at the time of decompression minimal effect will result. The nature of the decompression should be individualized according to the experience of the surgeon and the need of the patient. In my opinion, the superior or intracranial approach is rarely, if ever, necessary and produces much less satisfying decompression when compared to other routes. In the case of optic neuropathy the pathogenesis is apical orbital crowding; thus, surgery should be aimed at adequate apical decompression. In this situation I prefer direct anterior routes (ethmoidal and inferior, with or without lateral) for decompression. Through the incision for an ethmoidal decompression, the periorbital tissues may also be elevated inferiorly and the medial floor of the orbit removed, allowing extension of the medial decompression. On the other hand, medial decompression can be augmented by direct orbital floor fracture through the lid or by a lateral decompression if necessary. A combined medial, floor, and lateral decompression may be achieved with a medial and lateral approach. The Caldwell-Luc approach through the maxillary sinus is another means to remove the floor and ethmoid sinuses.

Exenteration and Superexenteration

Total removal of the orbital contents (exenteration) is indicated when malignant disease processes originate within the orbit and threaten to extend beyond it. The operation usually consists of removal of the orbit and periorbital contents. The exenteration can be either total when the anterior orbital contents or lids are involved, or subtotal when only the anterior orbit is involved without the lids. Subtotal exenteration consists of splitting the lids, removing the orbital contents, and using the remaining lid and subcuticular tissue for lining the cavity or for closure over an orbital implant. Superexenteration involves the en bloc excision of the orbital contents within bone or with surrounding structures. In the case of malignant epithelial tumors of the lacrimal gland, or of bony invasion, en bloc resection of the orbital contents and surrounding bone may be necessary. Malignant epithelial neoplasia originating in the sinuses and nasopharynx may also require en bloc orbital resection along with excision of the nasopharyngeal and sinus structures.

■ SURGICAL APPROACHES TO THE ORBIT

Three routes are used in orbitotomy: anterior, lateral, and superior. The orbit may be approached by any one route or by a combination of these. The position within the surgical spaces and the character of the lesion determine the specific choice. A team approach with a neurosurgeon, otorhinolaryngologist, or reconstructive surgeon may be necessary for lesions contiguous to or extending from the intracranial or sinus cavities.

Anterior

The majority of orbital procedures can be carried out through an anterior incision in skin or conjunctiva. This approach is useful for biopsy of lesions anywhere in the orbit or to remove well-defined anteriorly located tumors. Access can be through conjunctiva or skin. When approached through skin, the dissection may be either extraperiosteal or more directly through the orbital septum. The main incision sites are superior, inferior, in the quadrants, medial, lateral, or directly over a palpable lesion.

Lateral

Lateral orbitotomy with removal of the wall allows clear access to the orbital contents. The amount of bony excision can be customized to include more of the superolateral orbital rim, and even the zygomatic arch when necessary, depending on the size and location of various lesions. Most retrobulbar and parabulbar lesions can be handled by an anterior or lateral orbitotomy alone or in combination.

Superior

The superior approach to the orbit is either by transfrontal or temporofrontal (panoramic) incision. These approaches are necessarily the domain of the combined ophthalmologic and neurosurgical team. When operating on the apex of the orbit, we prefer a panoramic bony excision. A superior or coronal incision can also be used to do an orbital exploration without necessarily including a frontal craniotomy. This is a particularly useful approach when one wishes to avoid any facial scarring. The combined superior approaches are necessitated in compound trauma of the orbit and intracranial cavity, de-compression of the optic canal, or for removal of apical or combined apical intracranial lesions.

Variations and Combinations

All of the approaches defined above can be used in combinations or with variations to obtain access to any of the surgical spaces of the orbit. Widening bony incisions and even removing part or all of sinus structures to expand the surgical space may rarely be necessary. In complex lesions of the floor of the orbit, a combined inferior sinus approach with an orbital floor dissection may be necessary.

■ OPERATIVE PRINCIPLES

There are five major operative principles governing orbital technique:

1. Maintenance of a bloodless field;
2. Adequate exposure and visualization;
3. Safe atraumatic manipulation of tissue;
4. Entering through nonpathologically involved planes;
5. Adequate postoperative drainage.

Bloodless Field

A bloodless operative field is necessary in orbital surgery where the identification of subtle differences in coloration and texture of normal and pathological tissue may be difficult. In addition the operative space may be very small and any amount of bleeding will obscure visualization. We maintain hemostasis by a combination of hypotensive anesthesia, patient positioning, and meticulous local control. For major orbital procedures where no systemic contraindication exists, hypotensive anesthesia delivered by an experienced anesthetist is recommended. Hypotension is obtained by a combination of alpha blocking agents, halothane, curare, and a microdrip of nitroprusside or nitroglycerine. This allows a minute-to-minute control of blood pressure, which is monitored on a continual basis by intra-arterial catheterization. The blood pressure is maintained at a systolic mean of 60 mm Hg to 80 mm Hg. The patient is placed in a reverse Trendelenburg position to reduce both arterial flow and venous backpressure of the orbit (Fig. 16-1). Local hemostasis is obtained with fine bipolar coagulators (with and without fluid modes), microvascular clips, bone wax, vacuum suction, neurosurgical paddies, and chemical coagulators.

Adequate Exposure and Visualization

Adequate exposure and visualization involves careful retraction, periosteal elevation, excellent lighting, the use of multiple incisions when necessary, wide bony cuts, and the introduction of operative magnification. We have developed a surgical stage that can be attached to the face of the patient using temporary surgical glue. The stage can then act as a platform for attaching retraction sutures and devices (Fig. 16-2). Kennerdell and Maroon have also designed a fixed retraction system for orbital surgery.

Safe Atraumatic Manipulation of Tissue

Safe atraumatic manipulation of tissue, particularly in the hypotensive situation, requires gentle intermittent pressure and the use of delicate forceps. In principle, the removal of a mass demands minimal trauma to the surrounding complex and delicate neurosensory and motor structures. Thus, the established plane of dissection in the removal of benign lesions should be close to the tumor or cyst. In effect, the surgeon manipulates the mass and distracts it away from the surrounding tissues rather than dissecting these structures directly. For removal of malignant lesions or benign mixed tumors of the lacrimal gland, a safe margin of normal tissue is necessary.

Entering Through Nonpathologically Involved Planes

To establish the appropriate planes of dissection or to identify differences between surrounding normal tissues and disease, definition of the plane of entry is extremely important. Again, in principle, it is necessary to be familiar preoperatively with the location and nature of the lesion to plan surgery accordingly. In addition, the dissection should avoid direct entry into the lesion. Rather, one should enter by distracting the more easily dissected and pliable normal adjacent tissues to identify the exact level of involvement of the lesion, unless, of course, the mass or infiltration is extremely accessible and a more direct approach is possible. Regardless, the zone between normal and abnormal tissue is vital to the careful identification, biopsy, and extirpation of lesions.

Adequate Postoperative Draining

One of the problems of orbital surgery is operating in a small space that is confined by rigid structures; any excessive postoperative swelling could cause serious damage to surrounding orbital structures. Both postoperative or in-

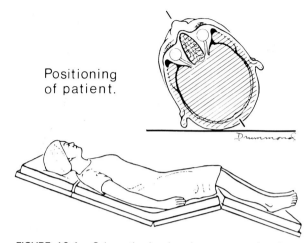

Positioning of patient.

FIGURE 16-1. Schematic drawing demonstrates the placement of a patient for orbital surgery in a reverse Trendelenburg position to reduce venous backflow. Upper drawing shows head position for right lateral orbitotomy.

traoperative closure of the lids should be condemned for this reason. Excessive postoperative pressure applied through the closed lids could be dangerous. The use of early postoperative drains helps to prevent excessive tissue swelling, especially following significant operative manipulation of tissues. When required following an anterior orbitotomy, an ordinary Penrose drain is adequate. However, for major orbital procedures vacuum drains are inserted and extended out through fresh ab externo incisions. The amount of postoperative edema is greatly reduced by providing external drainage for the first 24 to 48 hours.

■ INSTRUMENTATION

Properly organized and specific instrumentation facilitates surgery within the orbit. For this reason, we have designed and organized special instruments (manufactured by Downs Surgical Limited) that address specific functions and needs of the orbital discipline, both on macroscopic and microscopic levels. In addition, many of the microsurgical, neurosurgical, and otohinolaryngologic instruments can be used or adapted for orbital surgery.

Retractors

Gentle, convenient, and appropriate retraction of surrounding structures demands instruments of varying sizes and shapes. We use a series of straight and curved ribbon as well as angled retractors designed to facilitate the nu-

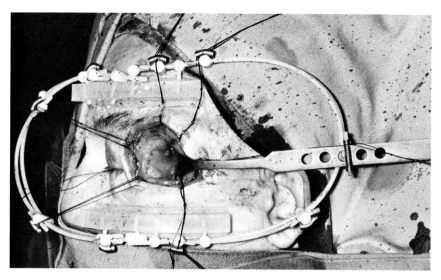

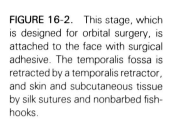

FIGURE 16-2. This stage, which is designed for orbital surgery, is attached to the face with surgical adhesive. The temporalis fossa is retracted by a temporalis retractor, and skin and subcutaneous tissue by silk sutures and nonbarbed fishhooks.

merous stages of dissection (Fig. 16-3). A special triangular temporalis retractor improves orbital access after dissection of the temporalis muscle from its fossa (Fig. 16-4). Additional retraction of skin or fascial layers can be accomplished with silk sutures, nonbarbed fish hooks (Fig. 16-4 B), and special skin retractors (Fig. 16-5). Figure 16-6 illustrates a vascular retractor that allows exposure of a vessel for clipping or cautery. The vessel is placed in the gap and the flat prongs retract the surrounding tissue.

Periosteal Elevators

Elevation of the periosteum is best accomplished with a variety of instruments that address the specific sizes and contours within and surrounding the orbit. The periosteal elevators have 5-mm, 7-mm, and 11-mm squared and 7.5-mm rounded ends (Fig. 16-7). In addition, for special purposes, elevators with right- and left-curved ends have been made.

Forceps

For manipulation of orbital masses, curved ovarian-style forceps and fine tissue forceps allow firm control with minimal trauma to solid masses.

Microdissectors

In principle, operations within the orbit are best achieved with wide exposure and meticulous blunt dissection allowing for careful identification of diseased and normal tissues. Blunt dissection of orbital masses or cysts is vastly improved by the use of fine microdissecting instruments. The ones shown in Figure 16-8 have rounded ends measuring 1.5 mm, 3 mm, 4 mm, and 5 mm, in both straight and curved modes designed for the orbit. They are based on longer dissectors used in neurosurgery (Fig. 16-8 A). In addition, sharp and blunt right-angled manipulators may provide a means of tissue traction (Fig. 16-8 B).

Magnification

For most orbital procedures, two- to five-power loupes provide all the magnification necessary. However, for surgery on the optic nerve, on the lacrimal gland, and in the orbital apex the operative microscope may be necessary. For example, removal of benign mixed tumors of the lacrimal gland requires a large bony incision and a very careful periosteal elevation by an extraperiosteal approach. The entire lacrimal gland must be removed. Therefore, the extension of the palpebral lobe through the levator aponeurosis must be identified with magnification prior to extirpation of the gland.

Bone-Cutting Instruments

Modern air-driven microsurgical bone-cutting instruments are more convenient and less cumbersome than old-fashioned saws. There are three types of instruments: sagittal saws, reciprocating saws, and air-driven drills. We use a microsurgical saw that is small, light, easily manipulated, and can be controlled by a foot pedal to facilitate firm hand control.

(Text continues on p. 587.)

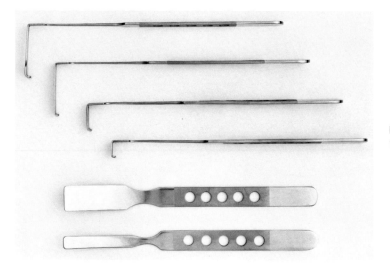

FIGURE 16-3. Straight and angled orbital retractors.

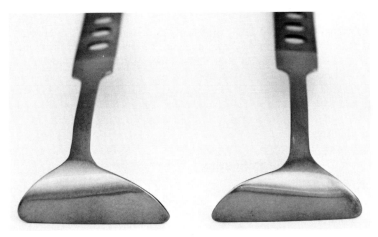

A

FIGURE 16-4. (A) Right and left temporalis retractors. (B) Use of the angled and the temporalis retractors in orbital surgery.

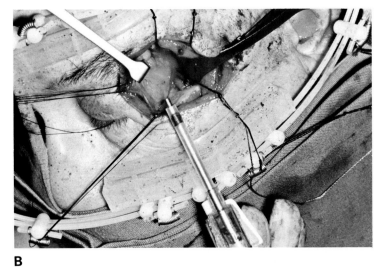

B

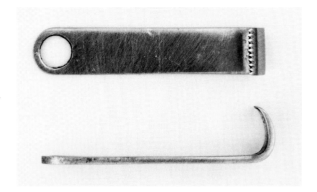

FIGURE 16-5. Skin retractors.

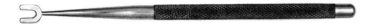

FIGURE 16-6. Vascular retractor.

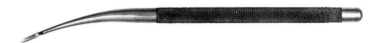

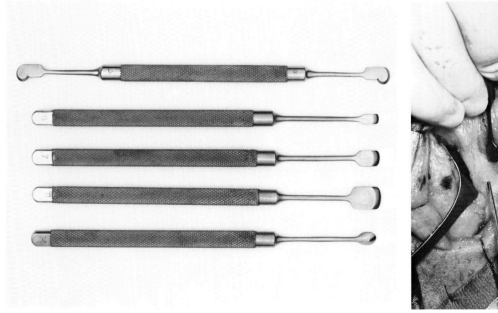

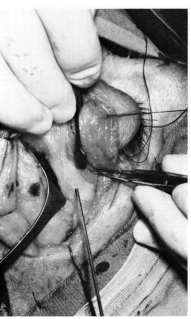

A   **B**

FIGURE 16-7. *(A)* A variety of periosteal elevators with right and left curved ends and 5-mm, 7-mm, and 11-mm squared ends and a 7.5-mm rounded end. *(B)* This demonstrates the use of the periosteal elevator in dissecting the lateral periorbita.

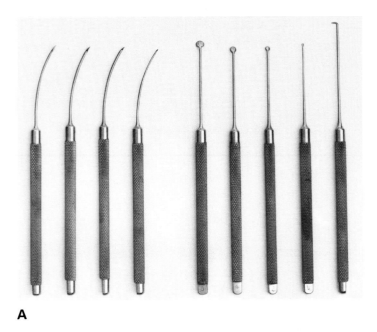

A

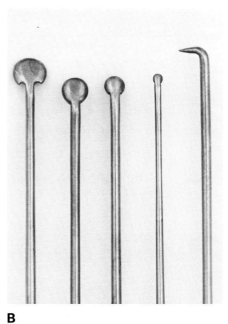

B

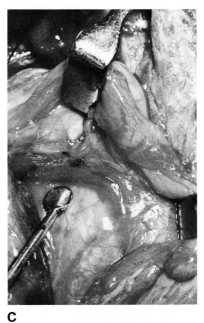

C

FIGURE 16-8.   *(A,B)* Straight and curved microdissectors. The ends of the dissectors are 1.5 mm, 3 mm, 4 mm, and 5 mm in diameter. The right-angled end is used for distracting tissue. *(C)* Clinical photograph demonstrates a 4-mm round dissector being used in orbital surgery.

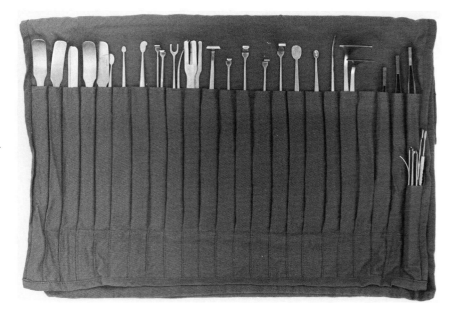

FIGURE 16-9. A method of organizing orbital instruments.

Coagulators

For hemostasis, extraorbital bleeding can be controlled by unipolar cautery. In certain situations chemical coagulators are necessary to avoid potential damage induced by cautery. The bipolar coagulators with and without fluid modes allow precise control of the bleeding sites, particularly for fine vessels, and can be tailored to specific needs and stages of surgery.

Organization of Instruments

Instruments should be organized according to function and well displayed. This will facilitate an efficient operative interchange between the surgeon and assistants (Fig. 16-9).

■ SPECIFIC OPERATIVE PROCEDURES

Anterior Orbitotomy

There are three anterior orbital approaches: transconjunctival, extraperiosteal, and trans-septal. The trans-septal approach can be accessed through the relaxation lines around the eye (Fig. 16-10).

TRANSCONJUNCTIVAL APPROACH

Some anterior periocular and intraconal lesions can be approached by direct conjunctival incision and dissection (Fig. 16-11). A rectus muscle may be disinserted to enter the intraconal space and retractors placed between the muscle and the globe. In addition, the optic nerve may be accessed by this route where it can be operated upon following disinsertion of the medial rectus muscle, and lateral rotation and anterior distraction of the globe. This is a particularly useful approach to optic nerve sheath decompression for chronic papilledema.

EXTRAPERIOSTEAL APPROACH

The anterior extraperiosteal approach is most useful for lesions occurring in the peripheral orbital space adjacent to periosteum or arising from and involving bone (Fig. 16-12). In particular, lesions such as dermoid cysts are readily accessible by this approach. The skin incision is usually made just at the orbital rim and carried down to the level of the periosteum, which can then be incised and elevated. The extraperiosteal space can then be safely and extensively explored. An alternative route of access inferiorly can be by means of subciliary incision through skin and orbicularis with dissection along the plane of the orbital septum and incision of the periosteum at the orbital margin. The entire floor of the orbit can then be easily explored.

For the most part anterior orbitotomies do not require bony resection, but we have noted that some large superior orbital lesions can be more readily accessed by temporary removal of the superior orbital margin (Fig. 16-12 *B*). A clearer view of the entire superior orbital space can be gained this way. It is not necessary to tran-

(Text continues on p. 590.)

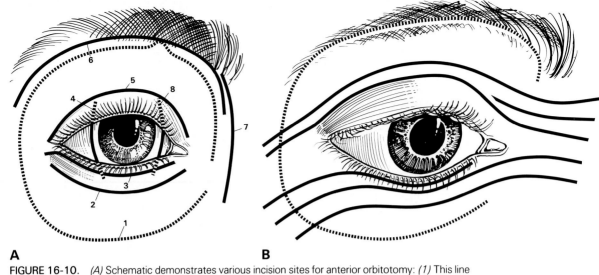

A   **B**

FIGURE 16-10. *(A)* Schematic demonstrates various incision sites for anterior orbitotomy: *(1)* This line defines the position of the orbital margin; *(2)* lower lid; *(3)* subciliary; *(4)* lateral conjunctival; *(5)* lid crease; *(6)* supraorbital; *(7)* medial (Lynch); and *(8)* medial conjunctival. *(B)* The relaxation lines around the eyes are useful sites for line of incision.

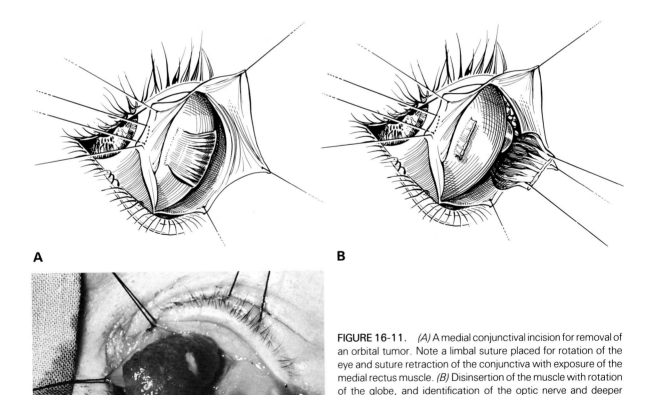

A   **B**

FIGURE 16-11. *(A)* A medial conjunctival incision for removal of an orbital tumor. Note a limbal suture placed for rotation of the eye and suture retraction of the conjunctiva with exposure of the medial rectus muscle. *(B)* Disinsertion of the muscle with rotation of the globe, and identification of the optic nerve and deeper orbital space for surgery. *(C)* Removal of a medially located cavernous hemangioma of the orbit through a conjunctival incision.

C

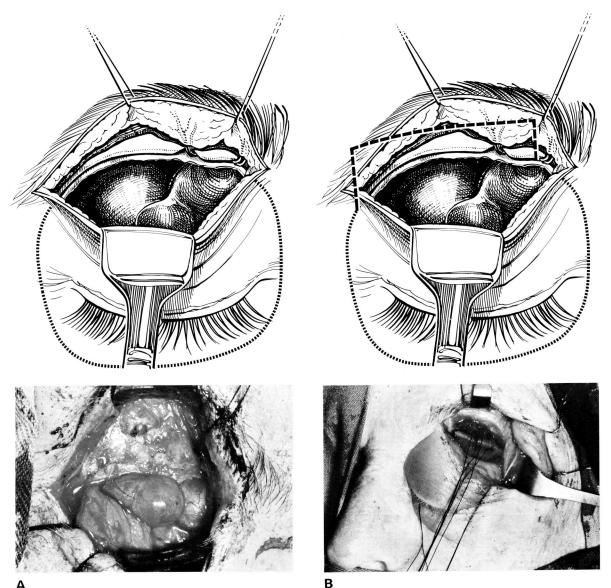

A   **B**

FIGURE 16-12.   *(A, top)* Schematic demonstrates a superior orbital extraperiosteal incision for removal of a tumor. Note distraction of the subcuticular tissues and periorbita with exposure of the supraorbital space and the supraorbital notch. When necessary, it is possible to distract the supraorbital nerve and dissect it free of the orbital contents while removing the tumor, thus avoiding transecting it. *(A, bottom)* A superior orbital schwannoma being removed by such an incision. *(B, top)* Schematic demonstrates the bony incision site to expand the access to the superior orbital space. The supraorbital nerve can be distracted at the time of bony incision. *(B, bottom)* Clinical photograph demonstrates a patient with the bone temporarily excised, allowing greater access to the superior orbital space.

sect the supraorbital nerve when operating on large superior lesions. The nerve can be distracted after unroofing the bony canal or incising the overlying ligament at the time of superior orbital exploration.

Larger explorations through the extraperiosteal space usually require postoperative drainage with a Penrose drain. It should be cautioned that the extraperiosteal approach should not be utilized in biopsy of suspected malignant intraorbital lesions because the periosteum provides a barrier to egress of malignancies.

TRANS-SEPTAL APPROACH

The choice of trans-septal incisions should be based on the natural contours and folds of the lid (see Fig. 16-10), the site of the lesion, and a need to avoid critical structures. Generally speaking, the orbicularis can be easily split by following the contours of the muscle fibers (Fig. 16-13). The levator palpebrae superioris can usually be distracted and structures behind it identified. The surgeon should avoid horizontal incision through the levator or damage to the lateral horn, which will result in ptosis. A surprising degree of exposure can be obtained from an anterior orbital approach, which can easily be enhanced by using traction sutures to distract structures.

Lateral Orbitotomy (Wright Modification)

Patient Preparation

The patient is placed in the reverse Trendelenburg position, and the head is turned to give a clear view of the lateral aspect of the face and orbit (see Fig. 16-1). The face is prepped and a sterile adhesive spray is used to outline the position of the head drape. Adhesive plastic draping can then be placed over the operative field.

Incision

The underlining bony contours are important to establish the incision. The key landmark is the marginal tubercle on the zygomatico-frontal process (Fig. 16-14 A). The incision is outlined with a surgical pen and a saddle suture is placed under the lateral rectus, which later facilitates the identification of the muscle at the beginning of the orbital dissection (Figs. 16-14 B,C,O). The incision begins at the superolateral orbital margin, extending as a lazy S along the zygomatic process to the zygomatic arch, and ending about 35 mm to 40 mm in front of the tragus. It is accomplished with a number 20 blade, and one should attempt to obtain an appropriate depth with one or two sweeps, the assistant placing pressure at the margin of the wound to prevent excessive bleeding. The inci-

sion is deepened until it reaches a level of the fascia overlying the temporalis muscle. Mosquito forceps are then used in clipping and identifying major sources of bleeding, the assistant maintaining a clear field with vacuum suction. Following clipping of the vessels, a unipolar cautery is used to cauterize the vessels through the metallic mosquito forceps, or it may be used directly on some of the bleeding sites.

Fascial Dissection and Exposure

Because the fascial plane is important for later separation of tissue, the level of the incision is carefully established in this plane to minimize sharp dissection in the more critical overlying tissues on later extension of the wound (Figs. 16-14 C, D). Subcuticular dissection is necessary to give adequate mobility to the tissues, and can be aided by blunt dissection with a dry surgical swab. Then, with a fine scissor, the fascia is carefully separated anteriorly over the orbital margin. Therefore, the fully mobilized superficial subcuticular dissection is in the plane of the fascia overlying the temporalis muscle and extends over the superior and inferior orbital margins and posteriorly, taking care to identify and avoid branches of the seventh nerve. The degree of mobilization varies depending on the intrinsic elasticity of the tissue and the size of the bony opening anticipated. The procedure outlined allows for maximum flexibility.

Following full mobilization of the subcuticular tissues, the complete operative site can be exposed. This is facilitated by the use of various retraction methods. The ones we prefer are nonbarbed fish hooks or specially designed skin hooks. The anterior part of the incision, however, is preferably retracted using a 4-0 silk suture as shown (Fig. 16-14 E). This allows for a large and clear field of view of the fully dissected plane in anticipation of the periosteal incision.

Fascial and Periosteal Incision

Figure 16-14 E demonstrates the full extent of the fascial and periosteal incision, which must include a superior relaxing incision at the inferior temporal line and an inferior relaxing incision along the zygomatic arch. These incisions allow for later mobilization of the temporalis muscle in the temporalis fossa. The periosteal incision is accomplished with a number 15 blade, paying close attention to the underlying bony landmarks. It may extend along the zygomatico-frontal process onto the zygomatic arch, thereby accomplishing the relaxing incision described in a single stroke. Alternatively, the inferior relaxing incision could be accomplished with scissors. Another choice could be to expose the entire periosteal and fascial incision site using cutting cautery for accurate and complete hemostasis at the time of incision.

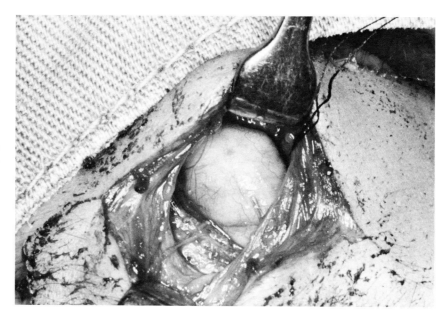

FIGURE 16-13. A direct percutaneous incision for an orbital dermoid.

Bony Exposure

Periosteal elevation is then achieved with a variety of small elevators along with neurosurgical swabs or suction to keep the field clear of oozing that may occur from bone. The anterior part of the periosteal elevation extends around the border of the orbital rim and is carefully dissected until reaching and releasing the loose periorbita on the lateral orbital wall (Fig. 16-14 *F*). During dissection of the lateral periorbita, the zygomaticotemporal and zygomaticofacial nerves and vessels will be encountered and can be clipped and cauterized. The bone superior to the inferior temporal line and that of the anterior portion of the zygomatic arch is then exposed.

Attention should then turn to freeing the temporalis muscle, which cannot be achieved without the previously noted relaxing incisions. The muscles should be elevated to avoid excessive bleeding because the fibers are attached independently to the underlying bone and not as a fascial attachment. Various types of elevators are used; shown are a round elevator (Fig. 16-14 *G*) and a curved type (Fig. 16-14 *H*), which can extend underneath the arch into the temporalis fossa for elevation of muscle. Alternatively, cutting cautery may be used to free the temporalis muscle. The temporalis retractor is then inserted into the fossa allowing a clear view to complete the dissection (Fig. 16-14 *I*).

Bony Incision and Removal

Figure 16-14 *I–J* illustrates the usual site of bony incision, which may be larger and include the superolateral orbit or zygomatic arch (Fig. 16-14 *J*1). In preparation for the bony cut, drill holes may be placed on either side of the anticipated site. Alternatively, drill holes can be made at the time of replacement of bone. The drill is cooled with saline irrigation to avoid heating and bony necrosis. The bone incision can be accomplished either with a radial or a sagittal saw, with irrigation as shown in Figure 16-14 *J*. Vacuum suction is necessary because some diploic bleeding usually occurs at this time.

The fracture is accomplished with a heavy rongeur and occurs along the junction of the zygomatic bone and the greater wing of the sphenoid. The bone is then freed of any remaining attached muscle and removed. Alternatively, the bone can be freed following the incision by the use of a chisel. The posterior bony incision is then extended with a rongeur or drill, which also smoothes and contours the irregular bony margins resulting from the fractures (Fig. 16-14 *K*). Bone wax is usually necessary to stop diploic bleeding after excision of the bone.

Periorbital Incision and Dissection

Figure 16-14 *L* demonstrates the operative site after freeing the temporalis and removing the bone. The periorbital incision can be made either an H or U shape with a large posterior flap. This incision is accomplished by means of scissors and careful dissection of the underlying orbital tissues. As an alternative, the tip of a number 15 scalpel blade can be used as shown (Fig. 16-14 *L*). Following incision, the underlying orbital tissues are carefully freed of the periorbita, and the horizontal incision is performed (Fig. 16-14 *M*) with continued freeing of the at-

(Text continues on p. 596.)

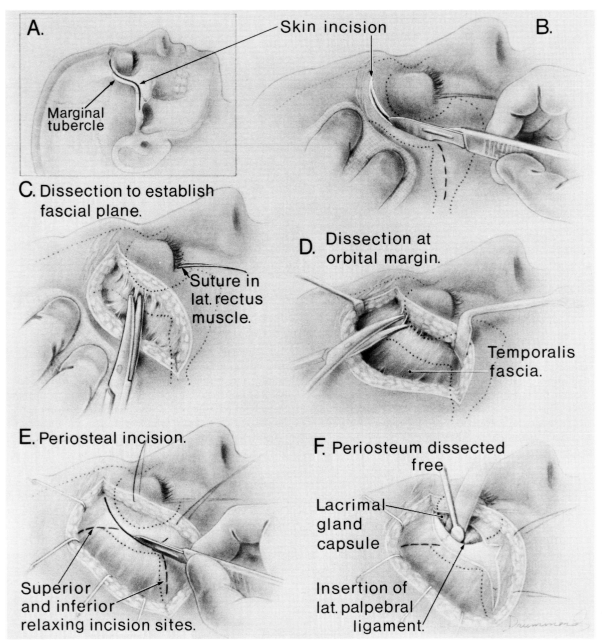

A.

Skin incision

B.

Marginal
tubercle

C. Dissection to establish
fascial plane.

D. Dissection at
orbital margin.

Suture in
lat. rectus
muscle.

Temporalis
fascia.

E. Periosteal incision.

F. Periosteum dissected
free

Lacrimal
gland
capsule

Superior
and inferior
relaxing incision sites.

Insertion of
lat. palpebral
ligament.

FIGURE 16-14.   *(A – Y)* The lateral orbitotomy procedure.

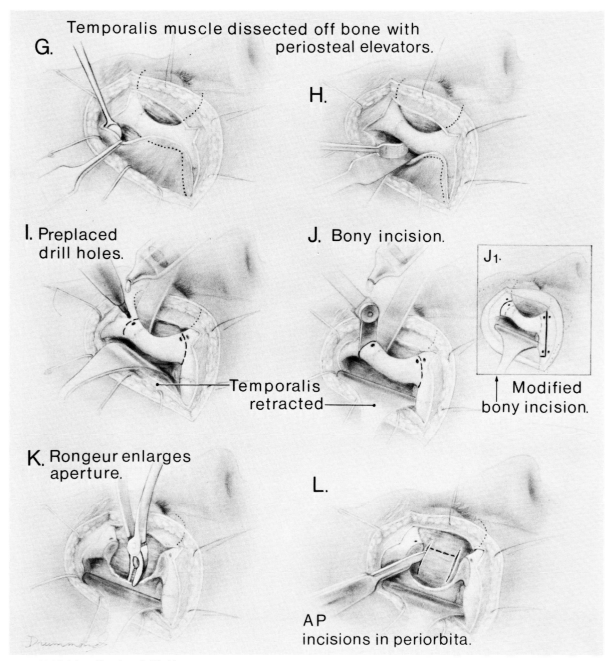

G. Temporalis muscle dissected off bone with periosteal elevators.

H.

I. Preplaced drill holes.

J. Bony incision.

J₁. Modified bony incision.

Temporalis retracted

K. Rongeur enlarges aperture.

L.

AP incisions in periorbita.

FIGURE 16-14. *(Continued) (G–L).*

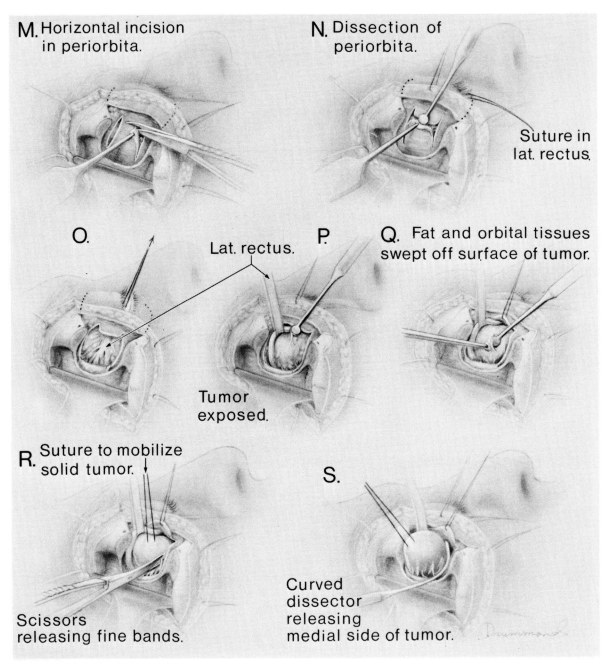

M. Horizontal incision in periorbita.

N. Dissection of periorbita.

Suture in lat. rectus.

O.

Lat. rectus.

Tumor exposed.

P.

Q. Fat and orbital tissues swept off surface of tumor.

R. Suture to mobilize solid tumor.

Scissors releasing fine bands.

S.

Curved dissector releasing medial side of tumor.

FIGURE 16-14. (Continued) (M–S).

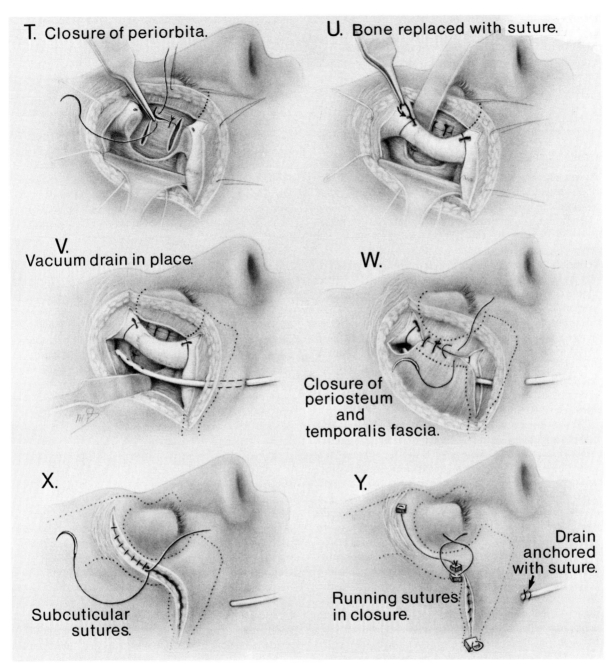

T. Closure of periorbita.

U. Bone replaced with suture.

V.
Vacuum drain in place.

W.
Closure of periosteum and temporalis fascia.

X.
Subcuticular sutures.

Y.
Running sutures in closure.

Drain anchored with suture.

FIGURE 16-14. *(Continued) (T–Y)*.

tached orbital tissues by blunt microdissection (Fig. 16-14 N). Often, small adherent bands within the orbital tissues are noted and can be freed using scissors. The orbital septae and bands are especially dense anteriorly in the regions overlying the lateral rectus muscle and the lacrimal gland. Once incised, the periorbita tends to retract, and orbital fat and tissues billow out through the incision site.

Orbital Dissection

Having retracted the periorbita, the key to orbital dissection is to establish the lateral rectus as a landmark. Your assistant can help to identify the lateral rectus by pulling intermittently on it with the previously placed suture (Fig. 16-14 O). It is most easily defined posteriorly where the septae are more tenuous and the muscle intimate to the periorbita. It can then be dissected free of the surrounding attachments and retracted with umbilical tape as shown (Fig. 16-14 P). Upon entry into the orbit, it is best to establish tissue planes by careful blunt dissection. On occasion one may have to do deeper intraconal dissections to expose a tumor mass or to operate on the optic nerve, in which instance, longer instruments are used. A nasal speculum may be used to retract the orbital fat and find the deeper orbital structures. Another option when operating in the deeper part of the orbit is the use of a fixed retractor for exposure.

When dissecting an orbital tumor there are several principles to keep in mind. Most importantly, you should remain close to the capsule of well-defined masses. In a sense, the surgeon is freeing the mass away from the orbital contents rather than dissecting into the orbital structures themselves. One should start the orbital dissection on the most accessible part of the tumor and gradually free it from the surrounding structures so that you are able to work deeper and deeper into the orbit, thus bringing the tumor out as it is freed. As the dissection progresses, the tumor will deliver itself and become more accessible on the deeper orbital side. The bulk of the dissection can usually be carried out with blunt microdissecting instruments (Figs. 16-14 Q,S). Sometimes, fine bands may have to be freed with scissors as shown (Fig. 16-14 R). Small bands that are more remote can be gently swept forward with the aid of an instrument, identified, and cut with scissors.

The final dissection of a solid benign tumor or a hemangioma may be aided with a suture used to mobilize the mass (Figs. 16-14 R,S). In the case of a cavernous hemangioma, because it is a low-flow lesion the suture has the added benefit of reducing the bulk of the mass by partially exsanguinating it. Another means of traction is the use of a cryoprobe to hold the tumor during mobilization. Excision of cystic lesions of the orbit may also be

facilitated by suction drainage or removal of the contents of the cyst after having delineated the borders of the lesion. As in any other type of ocular surgery, patience is the key to successful orbital technique.

Wound Closure

The periorbita is usually closed using interrupted 5-0 Dexon or catgut suture (Fig. 16-14 T). Following closure of the periorbita, we usually irrigate the wound with antibiotic solution (Bacitracin). The bone is then reinserted into its bed and sutured through drill holes using 3-0 Neurilon (Fig. 16-14 U). Following bone replacement, a vacuum drain is placed in the wound site (temporalis fossa) and extended out through the skin with a fresh trochar incision (Fig. 16-14 V). The drain can either be inserted through the skin inferiorly or superiorly. We find the superior drainage site better for placement in the temporalis fossa. The drain should be anchored to the skin with a suture to avoid pulling it out accidentally during the postoperative period (Fig. 16-14 W). Closure of the periosteum and the fascia overlying the temporalis muscle is accomplished with interrupted 5-0 Dexon suture. Subcutaneous sutures are then placed to approximate the wound, and the skin is closed with interrupted or running subcuticular nylon suture (Fig. 16-14 X). Figure 16-14 Y shows the final wound with the drain in place. The wound is then dressed with locally applied sterile dressings.

Postoperative Care

The site is dressed with care to avoid significant pressure on the wound or orbit. We prefer dressing the wound itself with lateral pressure and avoid direct dressings over the eye postoperatively. The drain is generally left in for 24 hours to 48 hours depending on the amount of postoperative drainage. Dressings are changed within the first 12 hours and ocular function is monitored by assessment of visual acuity, ocular movements, pupillary functions, and degree of orbital edema. When vacuum drains are used the amount of postoperative edema is minimal while the drain is in place, but it tends to increase in the first 24 hours after removal. Swelling can be minimized by the use of cold packs and elevation of the head of the bed. Patients experience very little pain following lateral orbitotomies and usually note some stiffness of the jaw or discomfort on chewing as a result of disinsertion of the temporalis. Following removal of the drain, the region of the lateral incision and the lateral portion of the jaw tend to swell temporarily. The patients are permitted to ambulate as soon as they are able postoperatively.

Complications

Careful preoperative planning, compulsive and meticulous operative technique, and vigilant postoperative care will minimize complications, which are rare in a modern setting. The major complications are tissue damage, inflammation, and hemorrhage.

Operative tissue damage may lead to excessive postoperative edema with compression of orbital structures. Direct injury to the optic nerve from trauma interoperatively may occur or the blood supply can be damaged by excessive manipulation. Although a rare complication, it is a risk when operating on optic nerve lesions or tumors of the apex. Excessive traction or trauma to the ocular muscles may produce a postoperative paresis. Usually this is temporary and avoidable. Most commonly the lateral rectus is involved but superior orbital surgery may lead to damage to the levator. Excessive trauma to, or resection of, the lateral horn of the levator during lacrimal surgery can cause a lateral ptosis. This can be corrected by a lateral plication at a later date. Rarely, the surgeon may encounter a cerebrospinal fluid leak during surgery as a result of a tear in the dura. This is best dealt with by direct closure with the aid of a neurosurgeon. Small leaks can be closed by patching the defect with temporalis fat or cyanoacrylate adhesive. Absolute failure of closure may necessitate a dural patch from above.

Excessive inflammation postoperatively can also seriously compromise ocular function and must be identified and dealt with promptly. Noninfectious causes such as idiopathic inflammatory lesions can be treated with systemic corticosteroids. Infection should be dealt with by use of appropriate antibiotics, drainage, and decompression when necessary. Tissue damage is largely preventable by gentle surgery and the avoidance of excessive or persistent traction on retrobulbar structures.

Postoperative hemorrhage will cause increasing proptosis, ecchymosis, neuropraxia, and pain. The rapidity of onset and development varies depending on the source of bleeding. If the hemorrhage threatens ocular function (as defined by decreasing vision with an afferent pupillary defect) or if it causes severe pain, prompt relief of orbital pressure is necessary. CT scan or ultrasonography may help to locate the blood pool. The decompression can be done through the original incision, and it may be enhanced if necessary by means of alternate routes as for any decompression.

Panoramic Orbitotomy

Panoramic orbitotomy is the preferred route of access to the apical portion of the orbit. The procedure allows for an en bloc excision of the roof and lateral wall of the orbit and a wide view of both the orbit and adjacent

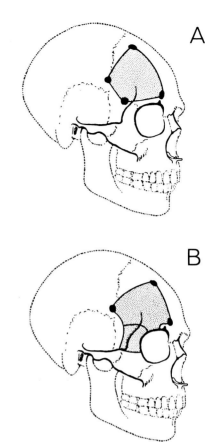

FIGURE 16-15. Schematics for frontal craniotomy *(A)* and panoramic orbitotomy *(B)*. The panoramic orbitotomy allows for excision of the roof and lateral wall of the orbit en bloc, as demonstrated in Figure 16-16.

intracranial structures (Fig. 16-15). Briefly, this approach consists of a coronal incision and removal of the frontal flap in the usual manner followed by dissection of the temporalis fossa and elevation of periorbita from the adjacent bone. An incision is then made along the superomedial wall of the orbit after distracting the frontal lobe from above. The bony incision is extended along the roof of the orbit to the lateral margin near the apex, whence the lateral wall and frontozygomatic process are incised. With removal of the bone a wide view of the roof and lateral orbital structures is obtained (Fig. 16-16). This approach is particularly useful for excision of tumors at the apex of the orbit or for combined intracranial orbital lesions, such as tumors of the optic nerve or sphenoid wing.

When removing the optic nerve the bony canal must be unroofed and the annulus of Zinn incised apically in the orbit. The best site for incision of the annulus is medially between the superior oblique origin and the levator palpebrae-superior rectus origins. The fourth nerve can be seen coursing over these structures to its site of insertion in the posterior third of the superior oblique muscle. It may be necessary to transect the fourth nerve in order to deliver an optic nerve tumor. However, we have been able to avoid this in many circumstances by carefully dissecting the optic nerve within its dural sheath from the annulus, transecting it intracranially, and pulling it forward through the annulus into the orbit, from which it can be removed following transection at the globe and dissection from adjacent structures. It is possible to dissect the posterior ciliary nerves and vessels within the orbit and avoid sectioning them while doing this procedure. This preserves the posterior choroidal blood supply. Intracranially, the neurosurgeon must be careful to identify the origin of the ophthalmic artery from the internal carotid as it courses into the dura of the optic nerve. Frequently, the ophthalmic artery must be transected in order to remove an optic nerve tumor. The rich collateral blood supply of the orbit maintains the circulation. The panoramic orbitotomy is an example of a multidisciplinary operative procedure requiring a neurosurgeon and orbital surgeon.

Combined Procedures

COMBINED MEDIAL AND LATERAL ORBITOTOMY

The combined medial and lateral orbitotomy can be used, particularly in exploration of the nasal apex for optic nerve lesions or tumors (Fig. 16-17). This technique requires an initial lateral orbitotomy and a secondary medial incision either through conjunctiva or skin. Usually, the lesion lies within the muscle cone and the incision medially is through conjunctiva with detachment of the medial rectus muscle. The lateral orbital bone does not necessarily have to be removed, but can be outfractured while it remains attached to the temporalis muscle.

COMBINED LATERAL AND INFERIOR ORBITOTOMY

A lateral orbitotomy can be combined with an inferior fornix-based lid flap. The procedure may be useful in the excision of large, inferiorly located lesions. The technique consists of a standard Berke-Kronlein orbitotomy and the extension of the incision laterally through the fornix to the inferior orbital rim. This transconjunctival incision through the lower fornix is combined with a lateral canthotomy and inferior cantholysis to allow wide exposure of the floor and both medial and lateral wall of

the orbit. Thus, the periosteum can be visualized, elevated, and exposed. Closure requires simple approximation of the conjunctiva and a standard technique for closure of the lateral orbitotomy.

Orbital Decompression

Orbital decompression is done for indications previously discussed. It consists essentially of producing increased space by herniating orbital contents into the adjacent ethmoid, maxillary sinuses, or temporalis fossa. The route and amount of decompression should be individualized based on the indications. In the case of thyroid orbitopathy with optic neuropathy, it is important to achieve adequate decompression at the apex of the orbit. This is best facilitated by ethmoidal and apical maxillary decompression. Additional decompression can be individualized at the time of surgery depending on the degree of proptosis; thus, it can be augmented with inferior or lateral orbitotomy as necessary. I prefer direct percutaneous routes of decompression, because the identification of orbital landmarks is easier by means of these routes. An alternate route for maxillary and ethmoidal decompression is a transantral or Caldwell-Luc approach from below. Generally speaking, I start with medial decompression and augment when necessary with inferior or lateral decompression, respectively. Decompression is also discussed in Chapter 11.

ETHMOIDAL DECOMPRESSION

Patient Preparation

The patient is positioned as previously described (see Fig. 16-1), and a 4% cocaine nasal pack is inserted high in the nasal meatus to reduce vascularity. One percent lidocaine with epinephrine is then injected along the anticipated incision site.

Incision

A Lynch (curved nasal) incision is made medially about 5 mm anterior to the canthus and deepened to the periosteum (Figs. 16-18 A,B). Hemostasis is obtained by means of cautery and the periorbita is exposed. The inferior part of the incision should be carried below the level of the medial canthal ligament.

Periorbital Dissection

The periosteum is then incised with a scalpel and carefully elevated posteriorly (Figs. 16-18 C,D). It is usually tightly adherent to the bone at this site, particularly at the suture lines, the orbital margin, and the anterior and pos-

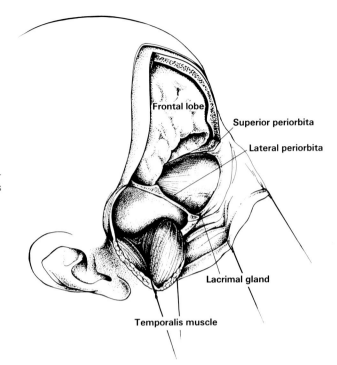

FIGURE 16-16. Schematic shows the exposure of the superior and lateral orbit with retraction of the temporalis. This allows a panoramic access to the orbital contents.

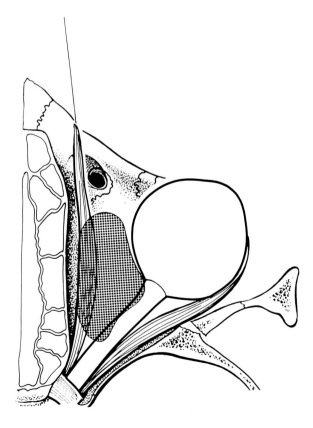

FIGURE 16-17. Combined medial and lateral orbitotomy approach for removal of a medial tumor. The lateral wall may be removed and reinserted later or simply outfractured while attached to the temporalis muscle.

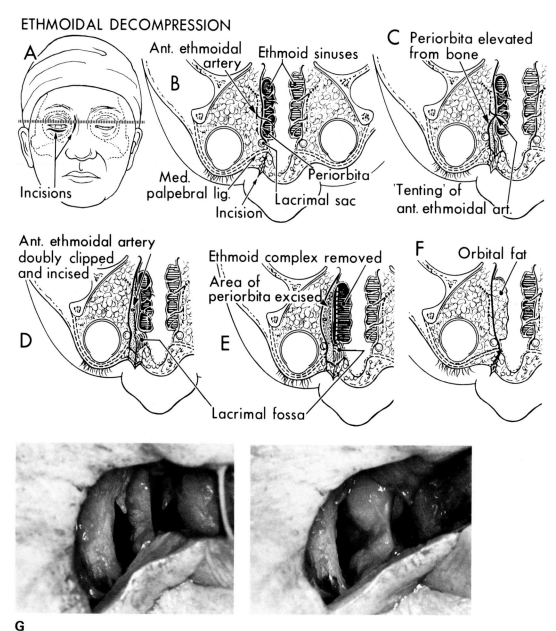

FIGURE 16-18. *(A–F)* Medial and inferior decompression. The posterior portion of the ethmoidal decompression can be extended to allow access to the posteromedial floor for excision. *(G)* Schematic demonstrates a medial decompression before *(left)* and after *(right)* incision of the periorbita, which allows for prolapse of orbital fat.

terior lacrimal crests. The medial canthal ligament is elevated with the periosteum, as is the lacrimal sac within the fossa. Rarely, the trochlea may have to be detached with the periosteum to provide adequate access medially. Posterior to the lacrimal crest the periorbita is much more loosely adherent and is easily dissected free using either an elevator or a fine suction tip. About 1.5 cm to 2.0 cm behind and in line with the superior margin of the lacrimal fossa the periorbita tents, at the site of the anterior ethmoid artery entering the sinus (Fig. 16-18 C). The artery can then be exposed using a vascular retractor (see Fig. 16-6), then doubly clipped with fine vascular clips and incised, freeing the periorbita from the adjacent medial wall. Frequently, there is a small prolapse of orbital fat at this site, which serves as a landmark in later dissection. Following exposure of the entire medial wall, the periorbita can be elevated inferiorly through the same incision, exposing the posterior and medial floor of the orbit. The entire wound site is then retracted using 4-0 silk sutures anteriorly (Fig. 16-18 D).

Ethmoidectomy

The ethmoidectomy is then performed in the following manner (Fig. 16-18 E). A chisel is placed just behind the posterior lacrimal crest and the ethmoid sinuses entered. Using Glasgow, Ostram-Antrum pinch forceps, and Wilde ethmoid forceps and suction, the entire ethmoid complex is then removed taking care to remain below the line of the anterior ethmoid artery, which is the landmark for the level of the cribriform plate, thus avoiding entry into the middle cranial fossa. Rarely, it should be noted that the cribriform plate may bow down into the ethmoid sinuses and can be disrupted at the time of ethmoidectomy. This can be avoided by careful preoperative evaluation of coronal CT scans. In the event of a CSF rhinorrhea, this complication can be handled by patching with orbital fat or a cyanoacrylate adhesive. Failure to occlude the drainage site can also be managed by a strict postoperative rhinorrhea routine until the leakage either stops spontaneously or, in rare circumstances, requires patching from above.

The inferior line of ethmoidectomy incision should be about to the level of the bottom of the lacrimal crest, taking care to avoid entry into the nasal passages because the mucosa of the nose tends to bleed much more vigorously than that of the ethmoid sinuses. The decompression can be augmented by downfracture with or without excision of the medial floor of the orbit into the maxillary sinus. Hemostasis is achieved by removing the lining of the ethmoid sinuses, cauterizing any bleeding sites, and by the use of chemical cautery followed by packing of the sinuses for a short period of time. If the augmenting floor fracture is carefully done, the sinus lining need not be

removed from the maxillary sinus. Once hemostasis is obtained, attention is then turned to decompression of the orbital contents.

Decompression

The periorbita is then incised in an AP direction (Fig. 16-18 F). The line of the superior incision starts just anterior to the previously noted prolapse of fat adjacent to the anterior ethmoid artery. This is carried forward until the periorbita is felt to be adherent to intraorbital structures. The line of the inferior incision is parallel to and at the level of the inferior bony incision. As this incision is accomplished, orbital fat is seen to prolapse into the wound (Fig. 16-18 G). The anterior parts of the incisions are joined, the periorbita dissected free posteriorly to the apex, and the flap removed. The decompression can be enhanced with the use of fine microdissectors above and below the medial rectus muscle. In thyroid orbitopathy there is frequently scarring of the orbital septae; thus, this is an important step to aid decompression. These septae are relatively easily broken down, and if one applies gentle counterpressure on the globe further fat prolapse occurs (see Fig. 16-18 F).

Closure

The anterior periorbita is sutured together and the subcuticular tissues realigned. As long as the anterior periorbita is tightly sutured, it is not necessary to suture the medial canthal ligament because it is firmly adherent to the periorbita. The skin is then closed with either interrupted 6-0 silk sutures or a running nylon suture.

DIRECT INFERIOR DECOMPRESSION

Incision and Periorbital Dissection

The incision for direct inferior decompression can either be subciliary or midway between the lash line and orbital rim through a natural wrinkle line (Figs. 16-18A and 16-19A). Alternatively, an inferior fornix or swinging eyelid incision may be used. It is carried down through the orbicularis, which is elevated from the underlying septum down to the level of the orbital rim. Frequently, prolapsing orbital fat is noted at this point and can be removed as in a blepharoplasty, providing the added advantage of augmenting cosmesis obtained from the procedure. The periorbita is then incised along the rim and freed posteriorly to the apex of the orbit. The periorbita is adherent at the inferior orbital groove where care should be taken to avoid dissection, because the infraorbital nerve is frequently attached along with its vasa nervorum and incision into it may cause vigorous bleeding. This adhesion is an important landmark in helping to

INFERIOR DECOMPRESSION

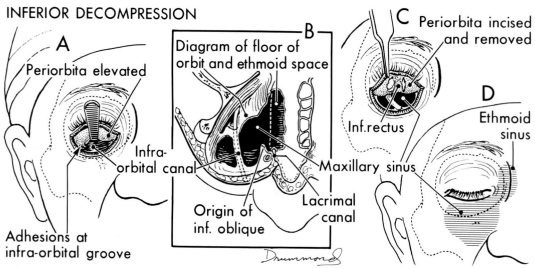

FIGURE 16-19. *(A–C)* A procedure for inferior orbital decompression. *(D)* Outlines the ethmoid and maxillary sinuses as sites for decompression.

identify the infraorbital canal and nerve, which can be seen as a prominent, white opacity in the floor of the orbit (Fig. 16-19 *B*).

Bony Excision

The floor is fractured immediately lateral or medial to the infraorbital canal using a chisel (Fig. 16-19 *B*). Frequently the floor can be elevated from the underlying maxillary sinus lining, and the bone can be easily lifted off the roof of the infraorbital canal. The medial half of the floor of the orbit can then be removed in a similar manner, as can the floor of the infraorbital canal. It is important to avoid the bone just behind the lower part of the lacrimal crest because this is the site of origin of the inferior oblique muscle and removal of this bone may result in motility problems. Having achieved an adequate bony resection, one can then proceed with the periorbital incisions.

Decompression

The periorbita is incised just medial and lateral to the line of the inferior rectus muscle, and blunt intraorbital dissection is carried out and augmented as described for the medial decompression (Fig. 16-19 *C*). The wounds are then closed with subcuticular and skin sutures.

LATERAL DECOMPRESSION

Lateral decompression can be done through the incision and exposure as described in the lateral orbitotomy, or it may be achieved through a Berke-Kronline incision to

avoid visible scarring by using a lid crease. Bony resection can involve the removal of the entire lateral orbital wall or all but the orbital rim itself. Again, it is important to incise the periorbita and dissect the orbital fat above and below the line of the lateral rectus muscle.

COMBINED LATERAL AND MEDIAL DECOMPRESSION

A combined approach by means of a lateral and medial incision can allow access to the floor of the orbit so that all three walls can be removed. Alternatively, a swinging eyelid flap can allow access to all three walls.

Postoperative Care and Complications

Postoperative care and complications are essentially the same as for lateral orbitotomy except that in the case of sinus surgery, postoperative nasal packs may be necessary. For the most part they are infrequently needed if meticulous hemostasis is obtained during surgery. In addition, following sinus surgery the patient should be cautioned to avoid blowing the nose, because air can be forced into the orbit in the early postoperative periods. Antibiotics are used only when specifically indicated on the basis of evidence of infection; they are not used prophylactically. Because many patients requiring orbital decompression have considerable myopathy to begin with, postoperative strabismus with accentuation of the myopathy is frequent following orbital decompression for Graves' disease. In fact, overall about one third of patients with significant preoperative myopathy have in-

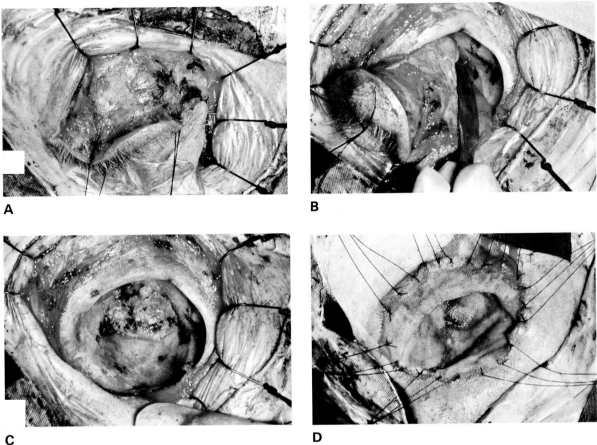

FIGURE 16-20. The stages of orbital exenteration. *(A)* Retraction of the skin and exposure of the subcuticular tissues around the orbit. *(B)* Distraction of the deep superior and medial orbital structures after dissection of the periorbita. *(C)* The deep orbit following excision of the orbital contents. *(D)* Placement of the skin graft within the orbit and attachment to the surrounding skin.

creased deviation following orbital decompression, and they should be warned preoperatively of this risk.

Exenteration

TOTAL EXENTERATION

Total exenteration is accomplished by first mapping the incision site around the orbital rim, which may vary according to the dictates of the primary lesion (Fig. 16-20). Wider margins may be necessary for locally invasive carcinomas or malignancies that come close to the orbital rim. To avoid blood loss, the procedure should be done rapidly and efficiently. The bulk of the blood vessels anteriorly are located in the medial portion of the orbit; therefore, it is useful to perform the incision down to periosteum in the remaining orbit prior to dealing with

the medial portion. The incision is carried down to the level of the periosteum, which is then incised with cutting cautery. The periosteum is elevated to the apex and the lacrimal duct is transected using the cutting cautery. Care should be taken to avoid damage to the very thin medial orbital wall. Once the periorbita has been detached as far back as possible, the orbital contents are excised using large scissors and cautery. When possible, a moderate mass of tissue is left at the apex to act as a bed for graft or granulation tissue. The orbit should be carefully inspected for any evidence of extension of tumor. Because of the thin bone the orbit is a unique site for split-thickness skin grafting, and we usually choose to graft the orbit. Alternatively, the orbit can be left to granulate and epithelialize over the next 8 weeks to 12 weeks. The split-thickness graft can be applied to the orbital bone and sewn to the skin margins, and the orbit can then be packed using antibiotic impregnated gauze. Alternatively, the orbit can be packed, and 3 days to 4 days following exenteration the graft can be applied directly to the granulating bone and pressure dressed without the necessity of suturing the margins. The graft can be harvested at the time of exenteration surgery and applied later as long as it has been refrigerated under sterile conditions. Another slight modification when the primary disease process permits is to dissect out and preserve the supraorbital nerve at the time of surgery to avoid the annoying loss of sensation in the forehead and scalp.

A pressure dressing is applied to the orbit, and is usually removed on the third postoperative day. The orbital packing is removed on the sixth or seventh postoperative day, and any necrotic areas in the graft can be excised. With time an eschar forms, and should be allowed to desquamate spontaneously. The orbit can be gently cleaned every other day with hydrogen peroxide and cotton-tip applicators. Generally between the third and sixth month, the epithelium is stable enough to allow for a fitting of a prosthesis.

SUBTOTAL EXENTERATION

When the lid structures are not involved with the primary neoplasm, they may be preserved by splitting the skin at the lid margins (Fig. 16-21). The incision is carried down through orbicularis and dissected in the plane of the orbital septum to the orbital rim, where the periosteum is incised. The rest of the subtotal exenteration procedure is the same as described for exenteration. The lids can then be used either to line the orbit (which is then packed), or an Allen orbital implant may be placed in the orbit and the lids sewn over it.

SUPEREXENTERATION

Malignant lesions of the lacrimal gland may require en bloc excision, or superexenteration, of the entire orbit within its bony confines, particularly the superior and lateral portions (Fig. 16-22). This is a multidisciplinary procedure involving a neurosurgeon, orbital surgeon, and facial reconstructive surgeon. We proceed by first making the periorbital skin incision. It should be carried out laterally beyond the zygomaticofacial and zygomaticotemporal nerves, because they pass through the lacrimal gland and may be involved by carcinoma (especially adenoid cystic carcinoma). The excision should also include the anterior portion of the temporalis muscle, which relates immediately to the zygomaticotemporal nerve and vessel. A coronal flap is then prepared and a frontal craniotomy carried out. The brain is retracted intradurally. Only the medial portion of the orbit is entered, where the periorbita is elevated to guide the bony excision supero-

medially. The bone is then excised from above and below in the superomedial orbit. The inferomedial orbit is then dissected free of the periorbita, and an en bloc bony excision carried out along the floor of the orbit through the upper portion of the zygomatic arch. The posterior roof of the orbit is incised to the region of the superior orbital fissure and connected to a bony cut deep in the temporalis fossa at the most posterior reaches of the lateral wall of the orbit. This incision is carried out from the roof and temporalis fossa to avoid entering the orbit. The orbit then is completely free for en bloc excision.

There are a number of reconstructive options for repairing the defect. It can either be filled with a delto-pectoral myocutaneous vascularized flap or with an advancement flap from the forehead. We prefer the tubular graft because it produces a better cosmetic result. Additionally, a more recently described procedure utilizes an extended trapezius musculocutaneous flap. We have also used bone from the posterior plate of the frontal craniotomy flap to perform a primary bone reconstruction of the orbit. The reconstruction can also be accomplished by using rib grafts. If the superficial temporal artery has been preserved, a free myocutaneous vascular flap may potentially be obtained and used.

Exenteration and superexenteration are chilling and mutilating procedures necessitated by the gravity of the primary disease process. It is important to spend an adequate amount of time with the patient to ensure that he understands the necessity of the procedure, the nature of the reconstructive options, the length of postoperative care, and the quality of prosthetic devices available. In addition, patients should be carefully monitored in the postoperative period for an expected depression following the loss of a vital organ.

Aspiration Needle Biopsy

Fine-needle aspiration biopsy is an ancillary technique for the orbital surgeon. In particular, this method of biopsy is useful for establishing a diagnosis of malignant secondary orbital neoplasia; thus, it may circumvent the need for further surgery. It should be avoided when the lesion is believed to be locally resectable, encapsulated, dense, or cicatrizing.

The method consists of the insertion a 22-gauge or 23-gauge thin needle into the suspected orbital mass, and aspiration of a core biopsy. The needle is attached to a 20-ml syringe and a pistol-grip holder (Fig. 16-23). As long as the needle is firmly attached to the syringe, a pistol-grip holder is not absolutely necessary. The needle is inserted into the orbital mass, and its position within the lesion is determined by CT scan or ultrasonography when necessary. The surgeon can usually feel the mass on entry. During insertion into the tumor, a firm negative

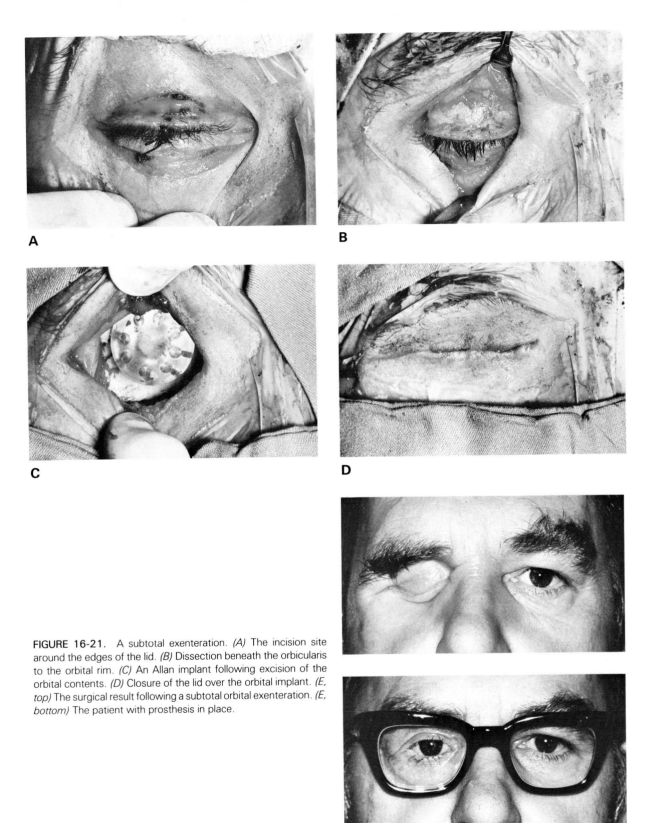

FIGURE 16-21. A subtotal exenteration. (A) The incision site around the edges of the lid. (B) Dissection beneath the orbicularis to the orbital rim. (C) An Allan implant following excision of the orbital contents. (D) Closure of the lid over the orbital implant. (E, top) The surgical result following a subtotal orbital exenteration. (E, bottom) The patient with prosthesis in place.

605

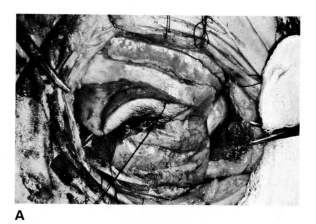

A

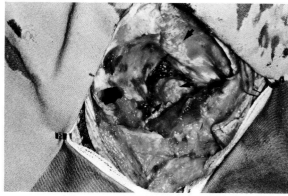

B

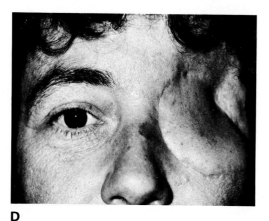

C   D

FIGURE 16-22.   The various stages of superexenteration. *(A)* The exenteration site prepared following a coronal flap excision of frontal bone with exposure of the anterior cranial dura. *(B)* The orbit after orbitectomy. The only bone remaining is in the medial wall. *Arrows* point to frontal and temporal dura. Apex of orbit superior and inferior orbital fissure and contents are shown. *(C)* The patient with a deltopectoral tubular graft. *(D)* The patient after separation of the tubular graft.

pressure is applied and the needle is removed and reinserted into the mass several times without removing it from the orbit. Negative pressure is released before the needle is removed from the orbit to avoid aspirating the core biopsy into the syringe.

A cytology technician should be present at the procedure. The technician can quickly prepare the slides, both air dry and fix them in 95% alcohol, and stain them. The needle is then flushed to obtain any remaining material. The core biopsy is then routinely fixed and embedded in paraffin, or it may even be studied by electron microscopy, histochemistry, and immunohistochemistry.

Endoscopy of the Orbit

Norris has described an endoscope for use in orbital surgery. The instrument has the advantage of being small; thus, it requires a tiny incision. It provides a view through the fiberoptic tip. The instrument requires infusion of saline during the procedure and has numerous attachments for biopsy and removal of foreign bodies. It has been used in cases of trauma, fistula, foreign bodies, and biopsy, and for exploring tumors. It is particularly useful in following the tract of a foreign body. The major limitation of this instrument is the need for infusion, which can lead to swelling of the orbital structures, thus limiting the length of the procedure.

Recent Advances in Treatment of Major Deformities of the Orbit

Donald Fitzpatrick and Jack Rootman

The evolution of the discipline of craniofacial surgery has led to the development of a wide variety of dramatic techniques for the management of congenital (craniofa-

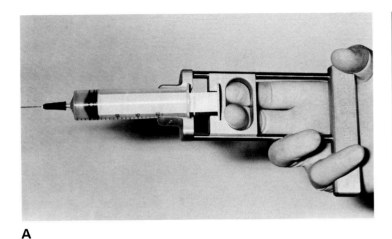

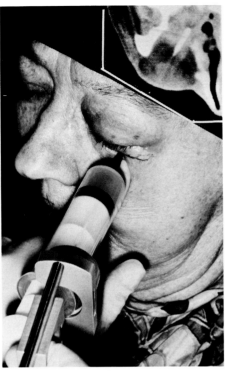

B

FIGURE 16-23. *(A)* Handle used for aspiration needle biopsy of the orbit. *(B)* Placement of the needle in the tumor. *(Inset)* CT scan for guiding aspiration needle biopsy.

cial dysostosis, hypertelorism, and exorbitism), traumatic (dystopia, enophthalmos), or tumor-related (orbitectomy) problems. In particular, it has permitted reconstruction of major craniofacial defects, which often jointly involve the orbit and facial structures. The procedures are properly the domain of a team that may, on occasion, involve the orbital surgeon. One lesson we have learned from these new techniques is that osteotomies of facial bones in childhood reconstruction do not lead to subsequent failure of growth. Thus, although rarely necessitated, bony entry into the orbit in childhood can be safely carried out.

These techniques have also been applied to the repair of major traumatic and postneoplastic defects with autogenous bone or exogenous alloplastic materials. Alloplastic implants can now be designed with the aid of computerized three-dimensional reconstructive technologies that allow for determination and matching of exact bony contours and volume needs. The best results from reconstruction can usually be obtained when missing components are replaced with like components, that is, skin with skin, soft tissue with soft tissue, and bone with bone.

REQUIREMENTS OF RECONSTRUCTION

The basic requirement for reconstruction may include bony support, soft tissue lining of or external cover for the orbit, and plastic repair of lids. Bone reconstruction is necessary to support and protect orbital structures and to provide a normal aesthetic contour. Soft tissue requirements include mucous membrane lining and soft tissue cover for bone grafts or following en bloc excision of orbit. Plastic repair of the eyelids may be necessary following surgical or traumatic malpositioning or damage to lid structures.

TECHNIQUES FOR RECONSTRUCTION

Bone

Bony contours and deficits may be reconstructed using free, nonvascularized bone grafts obtained from rib, iliac crest, and cranial bone. The last has some advantages in that it is handy when a coronal incision has been made and it seems to be less subject to resorption. Nonvascularized bone grafts are not suitable for irradiated beds where cranial bone on a pedicle of temporal fascia is preferable. Alloplastic materials such as Silastic and Proplast may also be used to augment deficient bony contours.

Soft Tissue

Full- and split-thickness skin or mucosal grafts may be used to replace missing eyelid skin or conjunctiva. How-
(Text continues on p. 610.)

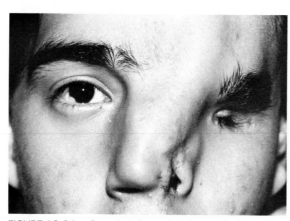
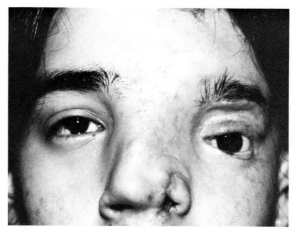

FIGURE 16-24. Case 1: Left anophthalmia and micro-orbit with extreme contraction before *(left)* and after *(right)* reconstructive surgery.

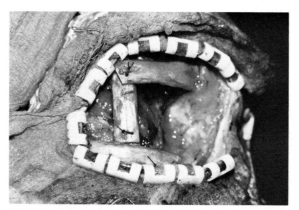
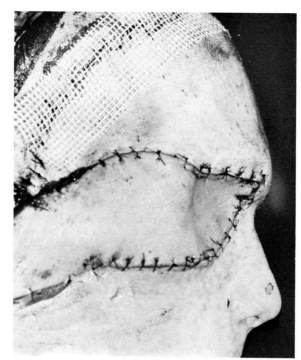

FIGURE 16-25. Case 2. *(Left)* Reconstruction of the bony orbit with split cranial bone and rib grafts following superexenteration. *(Right)* A sternomastoid myocutaneous flap was used as an external cover for the reconstruction.

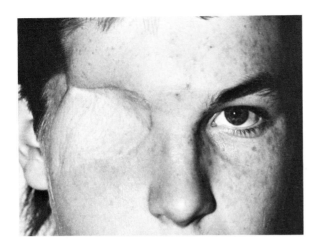

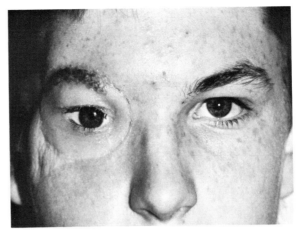

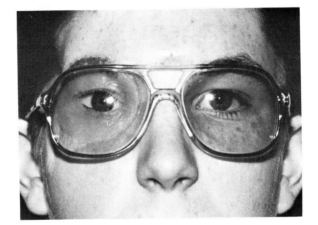

FIGURE 16-26. Case 2, continued. *(Top left)* Photograph of the patient in Figure 16-25 shows the final reconstruction. *(Top and bottom right)* The patient with a prosthesis in place.

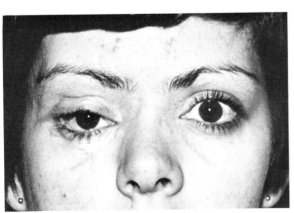

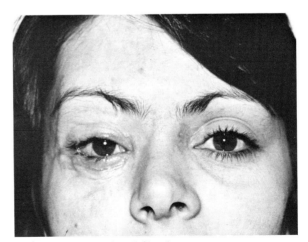

FIGURE 16-27. Case 3: A patient with vertical orbital dystopia and orbital volume loss before *(left)* and after *(right)* augmentation of the orbital floor and elevation of the globe.

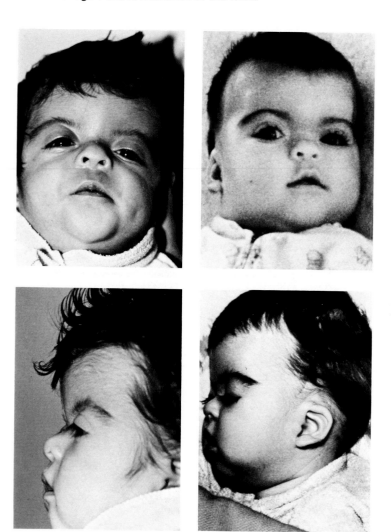

FIGURE 16-28. *(Left)* Case 4: A 3-month-old girl with Crouzon's disease and shallow orbits. *(Right)* The same patient 3 months after osteotomies of the roof and lateral wall of the orbit, with advancement of the anterior portion of the roof, the supraorbital bar, and lateral margin.

ever, such grafts are not suitable in irradiated beds, and tissue with its own blood supply should be used in this situation. Flaps may include skin and subcutaneous tissue, fascia, or muscle and may be of local, regional, or distant origin. Local donor sites in the orbital region may be from the eyelids, the forehead, and the cheeks. Regional flaps include postauricular flaps, flaps of temporalis fascia or muscle, and flaps of pericranium. Distant flaps include sternomastoid myocutaneous and deltopectoral flaps. Free tissue transfer may also be appropriate at times. A dorsalis pedis flap (skin and soft tissue based on the dorsalis pedis artery of the foot), or a radial arm flap (skin and soft tissue based on the radial artery of the forearm) may be transferred to the orbital region by microvascular anastomosis to the superficial temporal artery. Such cover may be useful following en bloc orbitectomy.

CASE REPORTS

The reconstructive techniques mentioned above can best be illustrated by several cases. Case 1 is a 19-year-old man with a congenital left anophthalmia and micro-orbit with extreme contraction (preventing use of an ocular prosthesis) and downward displacement. The deformity was associated with a naso-ocular bony cleft. Expansion of the bony orbit was undertaken by an intracranial approach. At a second stage, the palpebral fissure was widened and orbital mucosal grafts were done. A left brow lift and full-thickness skin graft were done to replace a portion of the upper eyelid, and a medial canthopexy was performed to bring the canthus closer to the nose. The procedure reduced the disfigurement and permitted him to wear an ocular prosthesis (Fig. 16-24).

Case 2 was a 15-year-old boy who had a right en bloc

orbitectomy for adenoid cystic carcinoma of the lacrimal gland. The bony framework was reconstructed by using split cranial bone grafts for the orbital floor and roof and split rib for the superior, lateral, and inferior orbital margins. The temporalis muscle was transposed into the orbital space through the deficient lateral wall, and temporalis fascia was used to cover the lateral bone grafts. A sternomastoid myocutaneous flap was then used as external cover for the entire reconstruction (Fig. 16-25). This "distant" flap was carried out in two stages: the first was done to obtain cover and the second was done 3 weeks later to divide the flap. The donor site was closed primarily without skin grafting. Postoperatively, he was fitted with a prosthesis worn externally and camouflaged by glasses (Fig. 16-26).

Case 3 is that of a 23-year-old woman who had posttraumatic vertical orbital dystopia and orbital volume loss as a result of displacement of the floor and lateral wall. Split rib grafts were used to augment the orbital floor, reduce the orbital volume, and elevate the globe. Medial and lateral canthopexies were done to elevate the ligaments and a dermis-fat graft was used in the upper eyelid to augment deficient soft tissue contour in this region. A full-thickness skin graft in the lower eyelid was used to correct ectropion and lower lid retraction (Fig. 16-27).

Case 4 is a 3-month-old girl with Crouzon's disease and shallow orbits as a result of premature closure of coronal and basal suture lines. The supraorbital region, in particular, is retruded and exorbitism is present bilaterally. The deformity could be expected to become more pronounced with growth. In one bilateral procedure at 3 months of age, the orbits were expanded by performing osteotomies of the roof and lateral wall of the orbit with advancement of the anterior portion of the roof, the supraorbital bar, and the lateral margin. This is done by a combined intracranial and plastic surgical approach pioneered by Paul Tessier. In addition, the coronal sutures were released. When done in infancy, the procedure is usually sufficient to prevent the gross exorbitism seen in untreated Crouzon's disease, but may not prevent subsequent midfacial retrusion (Fig. 16-28).

Bibliography

Berke RN: A modified Kronlein operation. Arch Ophthalmol 51:609,1954

Henderson JW, Farrow GM: Orbital Tumors, p 567. New York, Thieme-Stratton, 1980

Housepian EM, Trokel SL, Jakobiec FO et al: Tumors of the orbit. In Youmans JR (ed): Neurological Surgery, 2nd ed, Vol 5, p 3024. Philadelphia, WB Saunders, 1982

Jones BR: Surgical approaches to the orbit. Trans Ophthalmol Soc UK 90:269, 1970

Jones IS: Deep Orbital Surgery. In Soll DB (ed): Management of Complications in Ophthalmic Plastic Surgery, p. 259. Birmingham, Alabama, Aesculapius, 1976

Kennerdell JS, Maroon JC: Microsurgical approach to intraorbital tumors. Arch Ophthalmol 94:1333, 1976

Kennerdell JS et al: Fine needle aspiration biopsy. Arch Ophthalmol 97:1315, 1979

Kennerdell JS, Maroon JC, Dekker A et al: Microsurgery and fine needle aspiration biopsy of orbital tumors. Trans Pa Acad Ophthalmol Otolaryngol 32, No. 2:147, 1979

Krohel GB, Stewart WB, Chavis RM: Orbital Disease: A Practical Approach. New York, Grune & Stratton, 1981

Leone CR: Surgical approaches to the orbit. Ophthalmology 86:930, 1979

Linberg JV, Orcutt JC, VanDyk HJL: Orbital Surgery. In Duane TD, Jaeger EA (eds): Clinical Ophthalmology, Vol 5. Philadelphia, Harper & Row, 1985

Maroon JC, Kennerdell JS: Surgical approaches to the orbit: Indications and techniques. J Neurosurg 60:1226, 1984

Maroon JC, Kennerdell JS: Microsurgical approach to orbital tumors. Clin Neurosurg 26:479, 1979

McCarthy JG, Grayson B, Bookstein F et al: Le Fort III advancement osteotomy in the growing child. Plast Reconstr Surg 74:343, 1984

McCord CD: Surgical Approaches to Orbital Disease. In McCord CD (ed): Oculoplastic Surgery, p. 285. New York, Raven Press, 1981

McCord CD: A combined lateral and medial orbitotomy for exposure of the optic nerve and orbital apex. Ophthalmic Surg 9:58, 1978

McCord CD, Moses JL: Exposure of the inferior orbit with fornix incision and lateral canthotomy. Ophthalmic Surg 10:53, 1979

Norris JL: Orbital endoscopy. Trans Pac Coast Oto-Ophthalmol Soc 59:145, 1978

Norris JL: Endoscopic orbital surgery: Report of a case. Arch Ophthalmol 99:1400, 1981

Norris JL, Cleasby GW: An endoscope for ophthalmology. Am J Ophthalmol 85:420, 1978

Norris JL, Cleasby GW: Endoscopic orbital surgery. Am J Ophthalmol 91:249, 1981

Norris JL, Stewart WB: Bimanual endoscopic orbital biopsy: An emerging technique. Ophthalmology 92, No. 1:34, 1985

Rosen HM: The extended trapezius musculocutaneous flap for cranio-orbital facial reconstruction. Plast Reconstr Surg 75:318, 1985

Schafer ME: Craniofacial surgery: Its evolution and application. Neurologic Clinics 3, No. 2:331, 1985

Stallard HR: Eye Surgery, 4th ed. Baltimore, Williams & Wilkins, 1965

Stewart WB: Ophthalmic Plastic and Reconstructive Surgery. San Francisco, American Academy of Ophthalmology, 1984

Stewart WB, Krohel GB, Wright JE: Lacrimal gland and fossa lesions, and approach to diagnosis and management. Ophthalmology 86:886, 1979

Tse DT, Panje WR, Anderson RL: Cyanoacrylate adhesive used to stop CSF leaks during orbital surgery. Arch Ophthalmol 102:1337, 1984

Wolfley DE: The lid crease approach to the superomedial orbit. Ophthal Surg 16, No. 10:652, 1985

Wright JE: The role of surgery in the management or orbital tumours. Proceedings 2nd Symposium on Orbital Disorders, Amsterdam, 1973 (Basel, Karger, 1975). Mod Probl Ophthal 14:553

Wright JE: Orbital surgery. In Silver B (ed): Ophthalmic Plastic Surgery, 3rd ed, p 213. American Academy of Ophthalmology Manual, 1977

Wright JE, Steward WB: Orbital surgery. In Tenzel RR (ed): Ocular Plastic Surgery, International Ophthalmology Clinics 18, No. 3:149, Fall, 1978

Wright JE: Surgical exploration of the orbit. Trans Ophthalmol Soc UK 99:238, 1979

Index

Note: Page numbers followed by *t* or *f* indicate tables or figures, respectively.

ISBN 0-397-50651-1

90000